DISEASES
of the
HUMAN BODY

DISEASES
of the
HUMAN BODY

CAROL WARDEN-TAMPARO, B.S., Ph.D., CMA-A
Chair, Business Division
Instructor, Medical Assisting
Highline Community College
Seattle, Washington

MARCIA A. LEWIS, R.N., M.A., Ed.D., CMA-AC
Instructor, Medical Assisting
Olympic College
Bremerton, Washington

 F.A. DAVIS COMPANY • Philadelphia

Printed in the United States of America

Last digit indicates print number: 10 9 8 7 6 5 4 3 2

Library of Congress Cataloging-in-Publication Data

Warden-Tamparo, Carol, 1940–
    Diseases of the human body / Carol Warden-Tamparo, Marcia A. Lewis.
        p.   cm.
    Includes bibliographies and index.
    ISBN 0-8036-5642-4
    1. Pathology—Handbooks, manuals, etc. 2. Internal medicine—Handbooks, manuals, etc. I. Lewis, Marcia A. II. Title.
    [DNLM: 1. Disease—examination questions. 2. Disease—outlines. QZ 18 W265d]
    RB30.W37   1989
    616—dc10
    DNLM/DLC
    for Library of Congress   88-36757
                                                                           CIP

THIS BOOK IS DEDICATED TO

Lyle and Lee Chermak
Married March 27, 1937

and

Keith and Beulah Nelson
Married March 30, 1938

Without them, we wouldn't be.
Thanks, Mom and Dad!

Carol and Marti

▬▬ *Note to Instructors*

*E*very reasonable effort has been made to assure the information in *Diseases of the Human Body* is accurate, up-to-date, and in accord with accepted standards. Not all authorities agree, however, on the etiologies, signs and symptoms, or the diagnostic and treatment procedures for many of the medical conditions presented here. In cases when conflicting information was noted, the authors attempted to present the consensus from among the authorities consulted.

Preface

*T*his text provides clear, succinct, and basic information about common medical conditions. *Diseases of the Human Body* is carefully formulated to meet the unique educational and professional needs of medical assistants and other medical office personnel. The book focuses on human diseases that are frequently first diagnosed or treated in the medical office setting. Each entry considers what the disease is, how the health care provider might diagnose and treat the disease, and the likely consequences of the disease for the person experiencing it.

Following an overview of the causes of diseases, neoplasms, and congenital diseases, the coverage of major conditions is organized by body systems. This pattern of organization is easily integrated with medical terminology or anatomy and physiology courses that medical assisting students often take concurrently with their study of human disease. Within the body system chapters, each disease condition is highlighted following a logical, seven-part format consisting of:

- Description
- Etiology
- Signs and Symptoms
- Diagnostic Procedures
- Treatment
- Prognosis
- Prevention

The balance of information in each of these subsections varies according to the relative frequency and severity of the condition. In every case, however, the information selected is chosen to reflect the medical assistant's need for thorough, yet concise information about the condition in question. Each prevention entry, as well as the concluding chapters on pain management and holistic health, can be usefully combined with units on patient teaching within the students' curriculum.

The organization of the text is thoroughly contemporary and designed to help students retain and understand basic concepts within the context of their profession. These features include clear chapter outlines, study questions, and end-of-chapter glossaries (when glossary terms are first mentioned in the text, they appear in bold-face type). A 24-page color atlas of the human body and carefully chosen illustrations are included to reinforce essential anatomical concepts underlying the discussions of human disease. Moreover, the appendix provides succinct descriptions of the common diagnostic procedures mentioned within the text.

The study of human disease is never easy. But we have attempted in every instance to make it clear and accessible by selecting information that will benefit the student as well as the medical office professional.

Carol Warden-Tamparo
Marcia A. Lewis

Acknowledgments

We are fellow instructors. We are friends. We write "together"—not separately. We live 50 miles across the Puget Sound from each other. So we write—and write. We process words on a KayPro and a Wang. And we drive—and drive. We share homes and meals. We share good times of laughter and play. We write to the accompaniment of great music. We share sad times and tedious times. We agree and we agree to disagree. We are co-authors.

And as co-authors, we have many people to thank for their support, their help, and their belief in us. First, to F. A. Davis Company/Publishers go our thanks for their belief that we did indeed have a good idea and the capability to realize it.

Second, we would like to thank our dedicated, expert reviewers, who helped shape the format and content of this book: Harriet L. Carlin, CMA-AC, Pacific Medical Services; Juanita Bryant, CMA-AC, Cabrillo College; Ann Frazier, R.N., B.S., M.A., Detroit College of Business; Barbara Herlihy, R.N., Ph.D., Incarnate Word College; Thomas R. Klobchar, PA-C, M.S., Gannon University; Phyllis E. Parks, B.S., M.A., CMA-AC, Northwestern Michigan College.

Third, we feel deep appreciation for the continued support of our families, Les and Martiann Lewis, Jayne and Duuana Warden, and Tom Tamparo. There are reflections of a humorous, beautiful, lovable 8-year-old named Martiann saying, "But, Mommie, you see more of Carol than you do of me!" Then there is a never-failing, stubborn, truthful husband, Les, saying, "When are you going to be home?" (in one breath, then gathering his second breath to say) "So what's your next project going to be?" For Duuana, 22, and Jayne, 24, it was a time of transition—a time of becoming mature adults and striking out on their own. A time for saying, "We better go now while Mom has the book to keep her glued together." So the tears flowed as the furniture moved, and the writing continued.

In addition, thanks to our students, who questioned our mentality—teaching, parenting, and being students ourselves. "Were we (or are we?!) nuts?" they wondered. Our students continually gave us their suggestions and their help. They are our inspiration.

Finally, we would like to acknowledge all the authors of the many reference resources we used in preparing this book. The content of our book is not new. We have not blazed a new trail. Rather, we have presented this material in a new manner and style. We hope you like it, too.

Contents

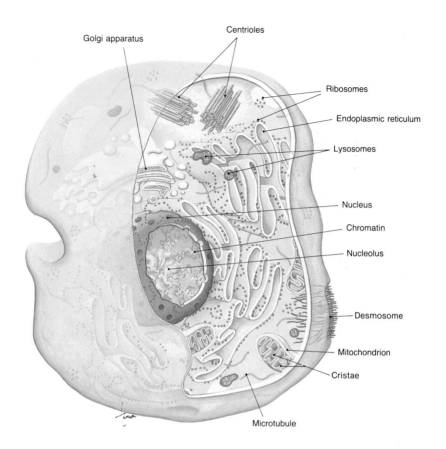

Plate 1.   The Cell.

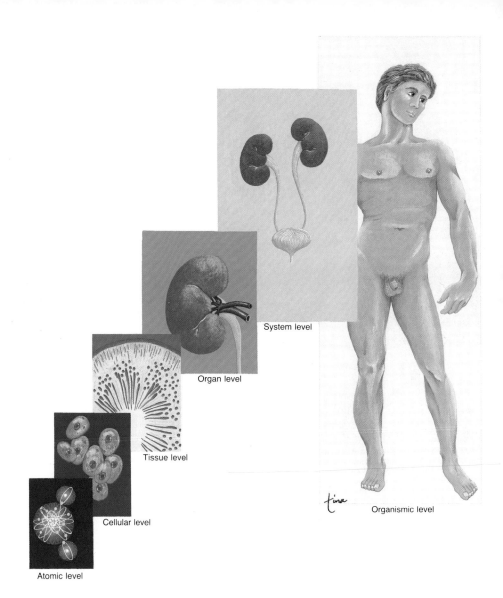

System level

Organ level

Tissue level

Cellular level

Atomic level

Organismic level

Plate 2.   Levels of Organization of the Body.

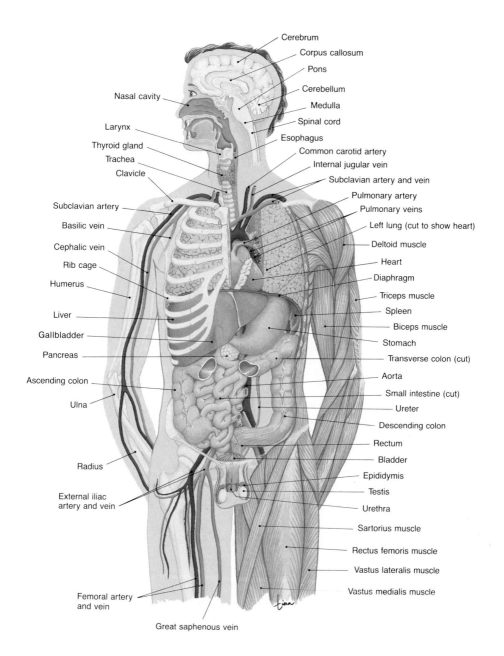

Plate 3.   Overview of Some of the Body's Organs and Structures.

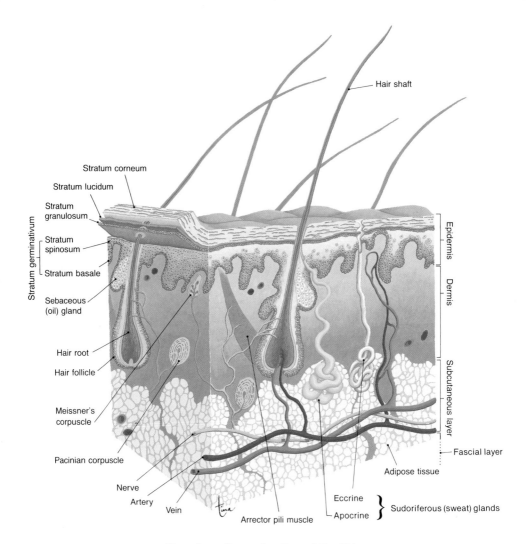

Plate 4.   Cross-Section of the Skin.

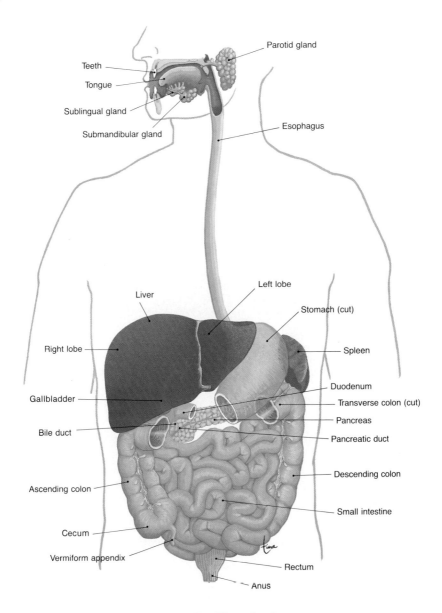

Plate 5. The Digestive System.

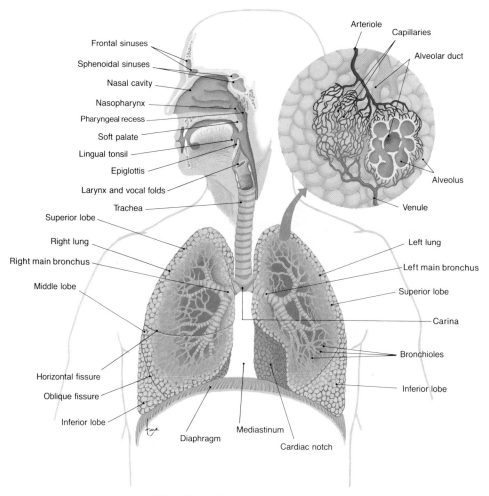

Plate 6.   The Respiratory System.

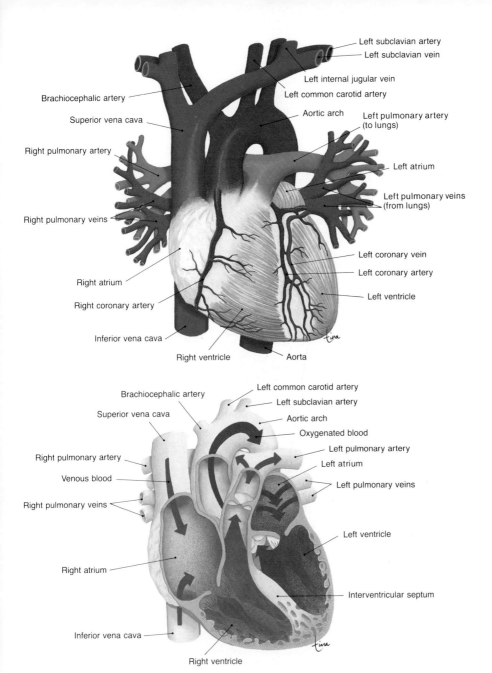

Plate 7. **The Exterior of the Heart, and Blood Flow Through the Heart.**

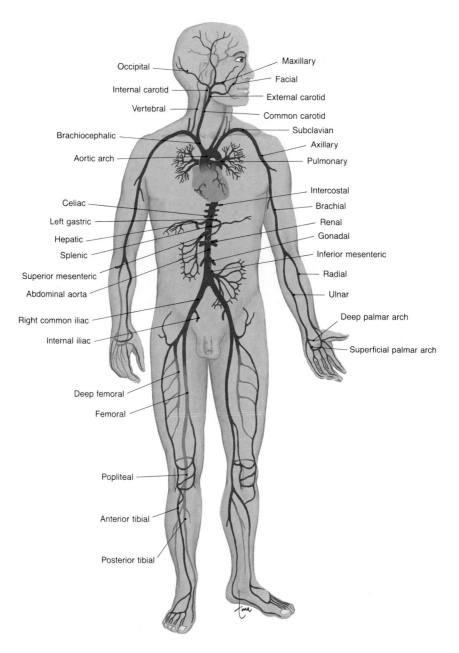

Plate 8.   The Arteries.

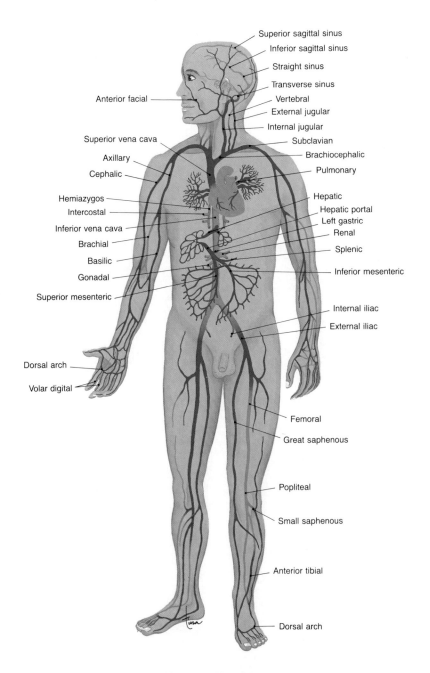

Superior sagittal sinus
Inferior sagittal sinus
Straight sinus
Transverse sinus
Anterior facial
Vertebral
External jugular
Internal jugular
Superior vena cava
Subclavian
Axillary
Brachiocephalic
Cephalic
Pulmonary
Hemiazygos
Hepatic
Intercostal
Hepatic portal
Inferior vena cava
Left gastric
Brachial
Renal
Basilic
Splenic
Gonadal
Inferior mesenteric
Superior mesenteric
Internal iliac
External iliac
Dorsal arch
Volar digital
Femoral
Great saphenous
Popliteal
Small saphenous
Anterior tibial
Dorsal arch

Plate 9.   The Veins.

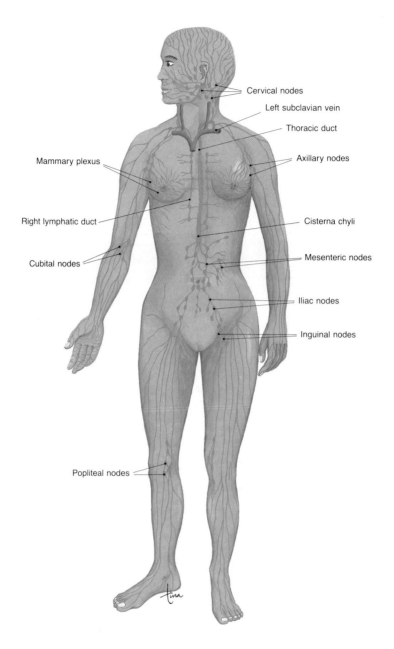

Cervical nodes

Left subclavian vein

Thoracic duct

Mammary plexus

Axillary nodes

Right lymphatic duct

Cisterna chyli

Cubital nodes

Mesenteric nodes

Iliac nodes

Inguinal nodes

Popliteal nodes

Plate 10.   The Lymphatic System.

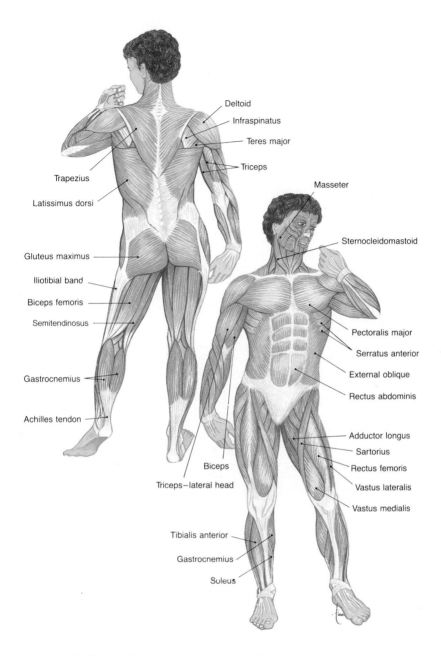

Plate 11.   Posterior and Anterior Views of the Muscles.

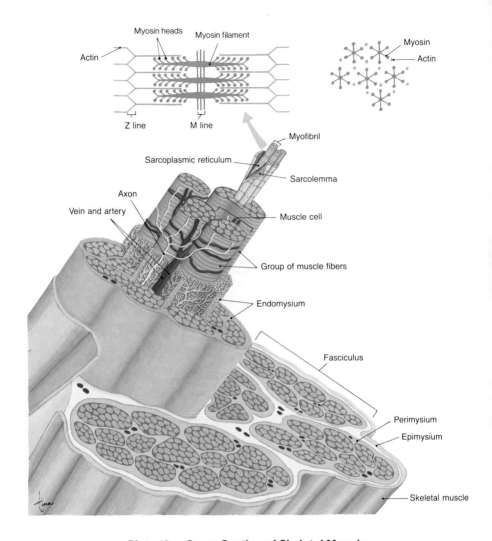

Plate 12.   Cross-Section of Skeletal Muscle.

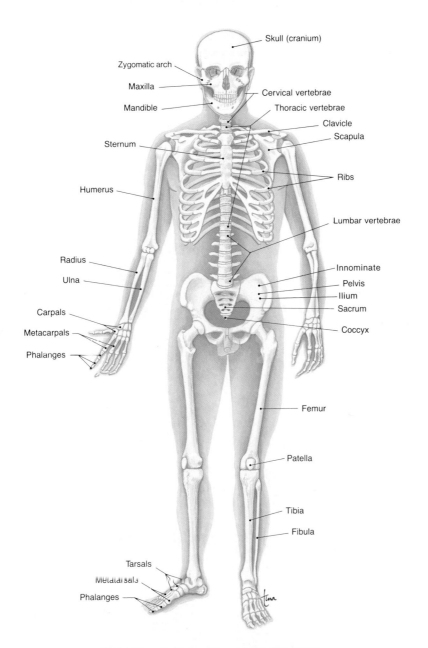

Skull (cranium)

Zygomatic arch

Maxilla

Mandible

Cervical vertebrae

Thoracic vertebrae

Clavicle

Scapula

Sternum

Ribs

Humerus

Lumbar vertebrae

Radius

Ulna

Innominate

Pelvis

Ilium

Sacrum

Carpals

Coccyx

Metacarpals

Phalanges

Femur

Patella

Tibia

Fibula

Tarsals

Metatarsals

Phalanges

Plate 13.   Anterior View of the Skeleton.

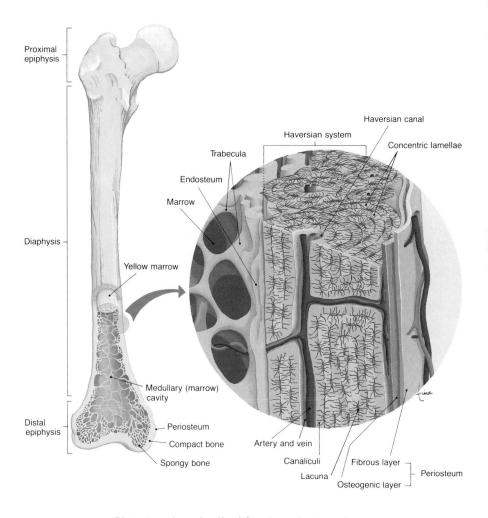

Plate 14.   Longitudinal Section of a Long Bone.

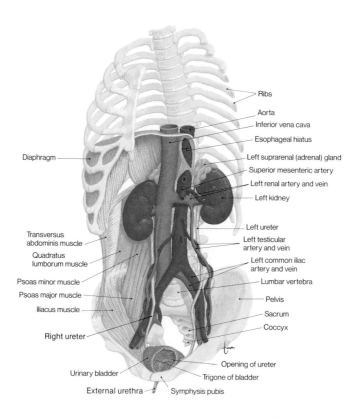

Ribs
Aorta
Inferior vena cava
Esophageal hiatus
Left suprarenal (adrenal) gland
Superior mesenteric artery
Left renal artery and vein
Left kidney
Diaphragm
Left ureter
Left testicular artery and vein
Transversus abdominis muscle
Left common iliac artery and vein
Quadratus lumborum muscle
Lumbar vertebra
Psoas minor muscle
Pelvis
Psoas major muscle
Sacrum
Iliacus muscle
Coccyx
Right ureter
Opening of ureter
Urinary bladder
Trigone of bladder
External urethra
Symphysis pubis

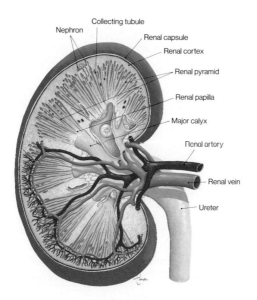

Collecting tubule
Nephron
Renal capsule
Renal cortex
Renal pyramid
Renal papilla
Major calyx
Renal artery
Renal vein
Ureter

Plate 15.   The Urinary System, and the Kidney.

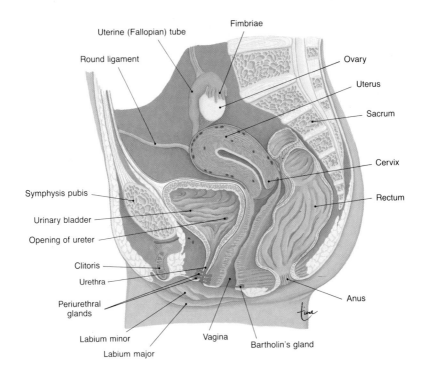

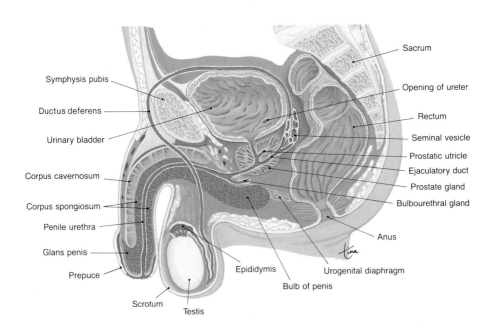

Plate 16. The Female and Male Reproductive Systems.

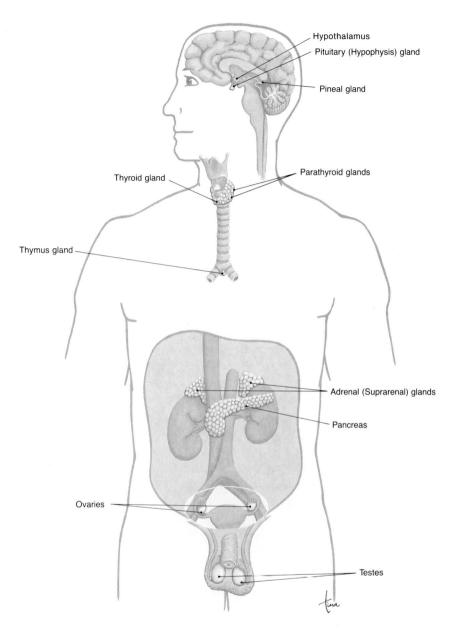

Hypothalamus

Pituitary (Hypophysis) gland

Pineal gland

Parathyroid glands

Thyroid gland

Thymus gland

Adrenal (Suprarenal) glands

Pancreas

Ovaries

Testes

Plate 17.   The Endocrine System.

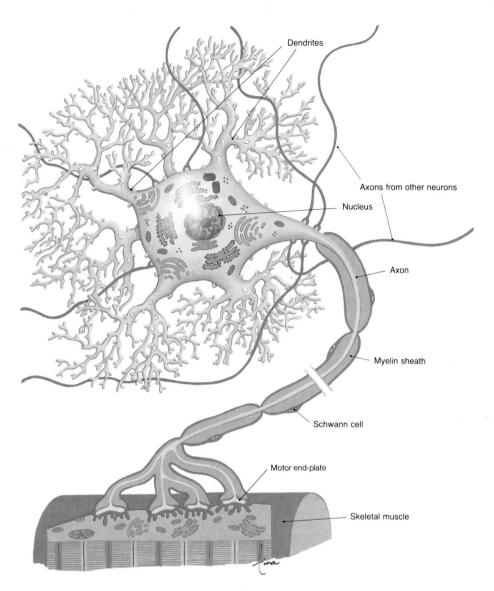

Dendrites

Axons from other neurons

Nucleus

Axon

Myelin sheath

Schwann cell

Motor end-plate

Skeletal muscle

Plate 18.   A Motor Neuron.

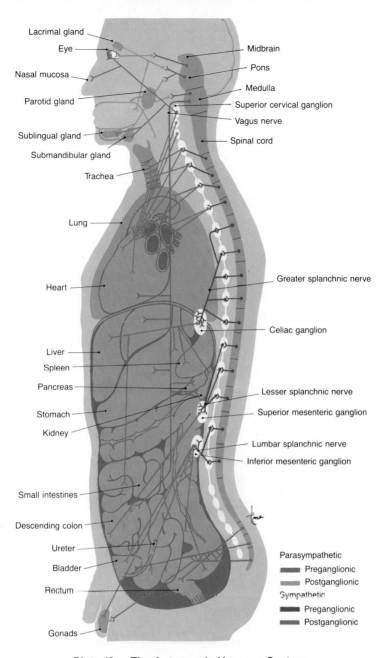

Plate 19.   The Autonomic Nervous System.

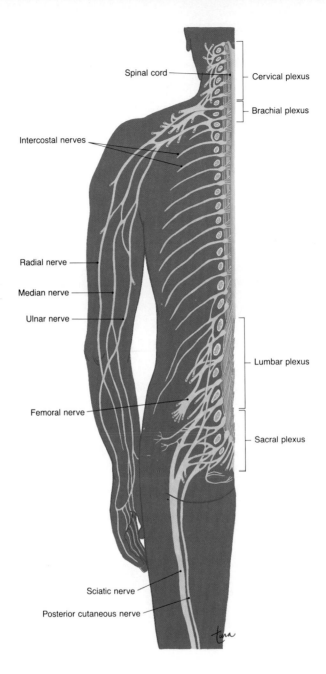

Spinal cord

Cervical plexus

Brachial plexus

Intercostal nerves

Radial nerve

Median nerve

Ulnar nerve

Lumbar plexus

Femoral nerve

Sacral plexus

Sciatic nerve

Posterior cutaneous nerve

Plate 20.   The Nervous System.

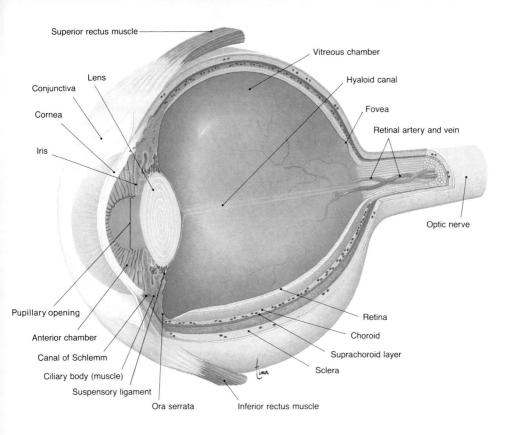

Superior rectus muscle

Vitreous chamber

Conjunctiva

Lens

Hyaloid canal

Cornea

Fovea

Retinal artery and vein

Iris

Optic nerve

Pupillary opening

Anterior chamber

Retina

Canal of Schlemm

Choroid

Ciliary body (muscle)

Suprachoroid layer

Suspensory ligament

Sclera

Ora serrata

Inferior rectus muscle

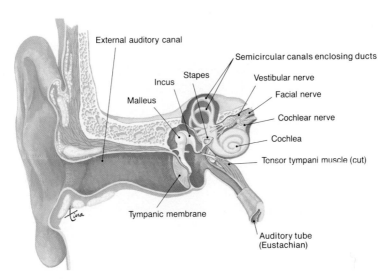

External auditory canal

Semicircular canals enclosing ducts

Stapes

Vestibular nerve

Incus

Facial nerve

Malleus

Cochlear nerve

Cochlea

Tensor tympani muscle (cut)

Tympanic membrane

Auditory tube
(Eustachian)

Plate 21.   The Eye, and the Ear.

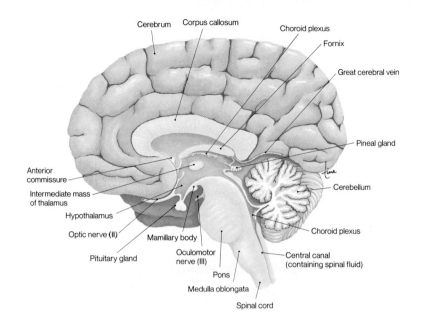

Cerebrum
Corpus callosum
Choroid plexus
Fornix
Great cerebral vein
Pineal gland
Cerebellum
Choroid plexus
Central canal (containing spinal fluid)
Anterior commissure
Intermediate mass of thalamus
Hypothalamus
Optic nerve (II)
Mamillary body
Pituitary gland
Oculomotor nerve (III)
Pons
Medulla oblongata
Spinal cord

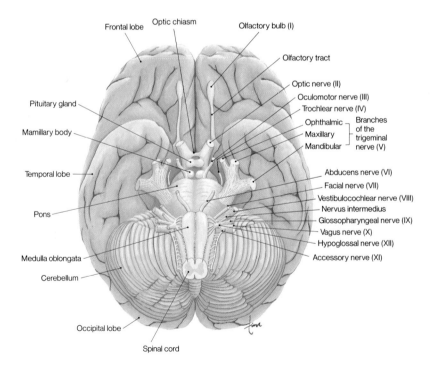

Frontal lobe
Optic chiasm
Olfactory bulb (I)
Olfactory tract
Optic nerve (II)
Oculomotor nerve (III)
Trochlear nerve (IV)
Ophthalmic
Maxillary
Mandibular
Branches of the trigeminal nerve (V)
Pituitary gland
Mamillary body
Temporal lobe
Pons
Medulla oblongata
Cerebellum
Occipital lobe
Spinal cord
Abducens nerve (VI)
Facial nerve (VII)
Vestibulocochlear nerve (VIII)
Nervus intermedius
Glossopharyngeal nerve (IX)
Vagus nerve (X)
Hypoglossal nerve (XII)
Accessory nerve (XI)

Plate 22.   Cross-Sections of the Brain, and the Cranial Nerves.

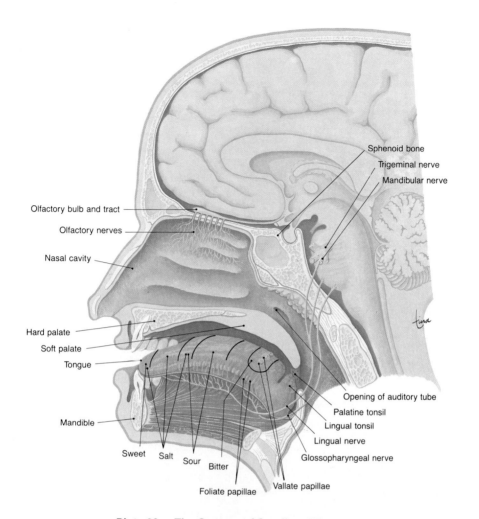

Sphenoid bone
Trigeminal nerve
Mandibular nerve

Olfactory bulb and tract

Olfactory nerves

Nasal cavity

Hard palate

Soft palate

Tongue

Mandible

Opening of auditory tube

Palatine tonsil

Lingual tonsil

Lingual nerve

Glossopharyngeal nerve

Sweet   Salt   Sour   Bitter

Foliate papillae   Vallate papillae

Plate 23.   The Centers of Smell and Taste.

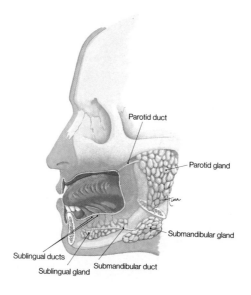

Parotid duct
Parotid gland
Submandibular gland
Sublingual ducts
Sublingual gland
Submandibular duct

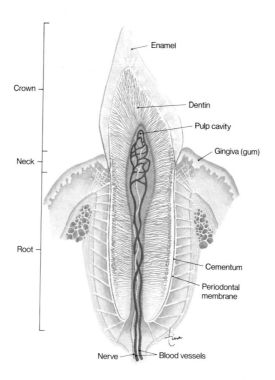

Enamel
Crown
Dentin
Pulp cavity
Neck
Gingiva (gum)
Root
Cementum
Periodontal membrane
Nerve
Blood vessels

Plate 24.   The Salivary Glands, and the Tooth.

Chapter 1

Causes of Disease

LEARNING OBJECTIVES

Upon successful completion of this chapter, you will
- Define disease.
- Contrast illness and disease.
- List and briefly explain at least seven causes of diseases.
- Restate at least three predisposing factors of disease.
- Describe DNA's genetic-related activity.
- Distinguish between genotype and phenotype.
- Identify the three classifications of hereditary diseases.
- Describe how infections are transmitted.
- Name at least four groups of microorganisms.
- Identify the most likely anatomic sites for traumatic injuries.
- Recall at least six chemical agents/irritants that may cause disease.
- Contrast neoplasm and cancer.
- Define benign and malignant tumors.
- Identify three means of protection afforded by the immune system.
- Differentiate between
  - ☐ Natural and acquired immunity.
  - ☐ Humoral and cell-mediated immunity.
  - ☐ B-cell and T-cell immunity.
- Name three classifications of immune-related diseases.

1

■ Identify a disease associated with each type of allergy.
■ Describe how anaphylactic shock can occur in any of the allergic reactions.
■ Name four categories of immunodeficiency-related diseases.
■ Explain mental and emotional factors as a cause of illness.
■ Give three examples of nutritional imbalance.
■ Define idiopathic and iatrogenic causes of disease.

INTRODUCTION

A rapid growth in medical research and a phenomenal development in technology accompanied by society's increased awareness of wellness and health have not been able to eradicate disease from our lives. Disease is a pathologic condition of the body in response to an alteration in the normal body harmony. Causes of disease may be the direct result of trauma, physical agents, and poisons or the indirect result of genetic anomalies and metabolic and nutritional disturbances.

Keep in mind that there is a difference between illness and disease. *Illness* describes the condition of a person who is experiencing a disease. It is more aptly thought of as how individuals perceive themselves as suffering from a disease. A *disease,* on the other hand, is known by its medical classification and distinguishing features. For most health care providers, a disease is easier to treat than an illness. Proper and effective medical management should deal with both the disease and the illness.

Fear, anxiety, embarrassment, or concern about the cost of treatment or about possible disfigurement may be some of the troubling emotions persons feel when faced with an illness. Some will desire to know everything about their particular disease; others will chose complete ignorance. Most expect the medical community to have a "cure"; few fully understand the importance of their participation in the "getting well" process.

This chapter provides a brief synopsis of the causes of disease. When considering the disharmony that occurs in the body in the form of disease, remember the harmony that exists most of the time.

PREDISPOSING FACTORS

A *predisposing factor* is a condition or situation that may make a person more susceptible to disease. Some predisposing factors include age, sex, heredity, and environment. For example, an infant's immune system is not fully developed and functioning at birth. Consequently, any undue exposure to disease-producing agents could cause drastic effects. Newborns do have residual immunity provided by their mothers for a short time, but they need to be protected by immunizations and proper care.

The elderly have unique problems, too, merely from the aging process. Physiologic changes occur in the body systems, and some may cause functional impairment. For example, the elderly experience problems with temperature extremes, have lowered resistance to disease due to decreased immunity, and have less physical activity tolerance. Certain diseases are more common in the elderly. They include cancer, heart disease, stroke, osteoporosis, senile dementia, and diabetes.

One's sex is a predisposing factor in disease as well. Men have gout more frequently than women, but osteoporosis is more common in women.

Hereditary influences will be discussed later in this chapter. However, if hereditary risks are known, individuals can be better prepared to prevent or treat and cope with such problems.

Environment also may have an effect on disease. Medical care, for example, may be more readily available in cities than in rural settings. Exposure to air, noise, and other environmental pollutants may predispose individuals to disease. No environmental setting is disease-free.

HEREDITARY DISEASES

Hereditary diseases are caused by a person's genetic makeup. It is uncertain to what extent environmental factors influence the course of a hereditary disease, but the two do interact. Hereditary diseases do not always appear at birth. Mild hemophilia and muscular dystrophy, for example, may go undetected until adolescence or adulthood.

All genetic information is contained in deoxyribonucleic acid (DNA), a complex molecular structure found in the nucleus of cells. The DNA itself is incorporated into structures called **chromosomes**. The normal number of chromosomes in human beings is 46 (23 pairs). In the formation of the ovum and sperm cells (sex cells, or gametes), this number is reduced by half, with each gamete having 23 chromosomes. When the two sex cells unite at the time of fertilization, the 23 chromosomes from the ovum combine randomly with the 23 chromosomes from the sperm, producing a cell with a full complement of 46 chromosomes. Two of these chromosomes are responsible for our gender (X,Y).

But what is a gene? A **gene** is a basic unit of heredity. Each gene consists of a fixed segment of the DNA on a specific chromosome. Our physical traits are the result of pairs of genes, both dominant and recessive. Gene pairs are **homozygous** when they are both dominant or both recessive in their expression of a trait. Gene pairs are **heterozygous** if one gene is dominant and one recessive. When trying to determine genetic makeup, a family history is taken to determine a person's **genotype**. Genotype includes all the genes you have inherited from your parents. Your **phenotype** is revealed in your appearance: your hair, the shape of your nose, how tall you are, and so on.

A hereditary disease (sex-linked) can occur when one of the parents contributes a defective gene from the sex chromosome. For example, in color blindness, the inability to distinguish reds from greens is the result of a recessive gene located on the X chromosome. The trait shows up when there is no dominant gene for normal color vision to override the recessive gene.

Changes in the structure of genes, called **mutations**, may cause functional disturbances in the body. Mutations occur when the normal sequence of DNA units is disrupted. How such a disruption is manifested depends on whether the affected gene is dominant or recessive and whether it is homozygous or heterozygous. Why mutations occur is largely unknown, but they could be the result of environmental factors, such as exposure to certain chemicals or radiation.

Classification of Hereditary Diseases

The conventional method of classifying hereditary diseases is to group them into chromosomal, mutational, and polygenic categories.[1]

Chromosomal diseases are caused by abnormalities in the number of chromosomes or by changes in chromosomal structure, such as deletions (missing genes) or translocations (genes shifted from one chromosome to another or to a different location on the same chromosome).

Examples of chromosomal diseases include

■ *Klinefelter's syndrome,* a disease that affects men and occurs when there is an additional X chromosome. The body shape is elongated, the testes are small, the mammary glands are abnormally large, and mental retardation is common.

■ *Turner's syndrome,* a disease that affects women and is characterized by rudimentary or absent ovaries, dwarfism, and other physical abnormalities; it is caused by the loss of the Y chromosome.

■ *Trisomy-21 or Down's syndrome,* a condition in which an individual has three number 21 chromosomes instead of the normal two. The condition is more likely to occur in babies born to women over 40 years old. Infants with this condition typically have sloping foreheads, folds of skin over the inner corners of their eyes, and other physical abnormalities. They generally become moderately to severely retarded.

In *mutation diseases,* the problem is due to a defective gene rather than a defective chromosome. The genetic evidence is clear through testing. Examples include

■ *Phenylketonuria (PKU),* an inability to metabolize an essential **amino acid**, phenylalanine. Without a special diet, mental retardation typically occurs. See Chapter 3.

■ *Cystic fibrosis,* a **chronic**, generalized disease of the **exocrine glands**, primarily affecting the pancreas, respiratory system, and sweat glands. See Chapter 3.

■ *Tay-Sachs disease,* a rare **lipid** abnormality distinguished by progressive neurologic deterioration and a cherry-red spot with a gray border on both retinae. It chiefly affects Jewish infants, resulting in deafness, blindness, and paralysis. Recurrent bronchopneumonia usually causes death before the age of 5.

■ *Sickle cell anemia,* a disease affecting mostly blacks; it occurs because the body produces a defective form of hemoglobin, causing red blood cells to roughen and become sickle-shaped. See Chapter 8.

■ *Hemophilia,* a bleeding disorder caused by a deficiency of specific types of serum proteins called *clotting factors.*

All evidence supports a genetic etiology for *polygenic diseases.* The data, however, are not explicable on the basis of a defect in a single gene, hence the term *polygenic,* meaning pertaining to or caused by several genes. A few examples of these diseases include

■ *Rheumatoid arthritis,* a chronic, **systemic**, inflammatory disease affecting the joints. See Chapter 11.

■ *Gout,* a metabolic disturbance causing the excessive accumulation of uric acid in the body. See Chapter 11.

■ *Hypertension,* or high blood pressure, causing the heart to work against increased circulatory pressure. See Chapter 8.

■ *Diabetes mellitus,* a disorder of carbohydrate, fat, and protein metabolism. The disease is due primarily to insufficient insulin production by the pancreas. See Chapter 10.

■ *Congenital heart anomalies,* including six major anatomic defects that cause circulatory problems. See Chapter 3.

INFECTIONS

Infection is the invasion and multiplication of **pathogenic** microorganisms in the body. Most microorganisms in our bodies are nonpathogenic and, in fact, are often necessary to maintain **homeostasis**. It is when one or more of the factors in the infectious process are present that a microorganism can become a possible pathogen. For example, people serve as hosts for organisms, as do animals. A host does not necessarily have to be "diseased" or "sick," but simply serves as a reservoir for the microorganisms. Transmission can be from coughing, sneezing, or touching something contaminated from the infected host as well as direct contact with the microorganism. If the receiving host is not susceptible, then the microorganism has little chance of becoming a pathogen. The susceptible host, however, may have low resistance and provide the microorganism with a means of entry via an open wound, mouth, ears, eyes, or some other orifice.

Whenever a pathogenic microorganism finds a suitable environment for growth in an appropriate host, disease may result. Growth factors for microorganisms vary and can include the presence of oxygen—or the lack of it—a ready source of food, an optimal temperature, moisture, darkness, and a specific **pH**.

Microorganisms, including those that cause disease, can be classified into six general groups.

Fungi. This group includes yeasts and molds that may be present in the soil, air, and water, but only a few species cause disease. Fungal diseases, called *mycoses,* usually develop slowly, are resistant to treatment, and are rarely fatal. The more common mycoses include histoplasmosis, coccidioidomycosis (see Chapter 7), ringworm, athlete's foot, and thrush.

Rickettsiae. This group of bacteria-like organisms live parasitically inside living cells. They are transmitted by bites from infected lice, fleas, ticks, and mites. Rickettsial diseases include Rocky Mountain spotted fever, typhus, and trench fever. These diseases are more likely to occur where unsanitary conditions prevail.

Protozoa. These are single-celled organisms from the animal kingdom. Malaria, amebic dysentery, and African sleeping sickness are examples of protozoal diseases. *Trichomonas vaginalis* is a protozoon that causes trichomoniasis or vaginitis, a disease fairly common among women.

Viruses. These are the smallest microorganisms, visible only through electron microscopy. They are parasitic, difficult to isolate, and few are susceptible to antibiotics. Viruses may remain dormant in a host for long periods before becoming active. Viral infections include the common cold, yellow fever, measles, mumps, rabies, chickenpox, herpes, poliomyelitis, hepatitis, influenza, and certain types of pneumonia and encephalitis.

Bacteria. These are single-celled organisms of many varieties. Most are nonpathogenic and useful. Bacteria, including those that cause disease, are classified according to their shape:

- *Bacilli* are rod-shaped bacteria. Diseases caused by bacilli include tuberculosis, whooping cough, tetanus, typhoid fever, and diphtheria.
- *Spirilla* are spiral-shaped bacteria. Diseases caused by spirilla include syphilis and cholera.
- *Cocci* are dot-shaped bacteria. Diseases caused by cocci include gonorrhea, meningitis, tonsillitis, bacterial pneumonia, boils, scarlet fever, sore throats, and certain skin and urinary infections.

Helminths. These are a large division of wormlike animals, some of which may live as parasites in humans. They are typically transmitted from person to person via fecal contamination of food, water, or soil. Three classes of helminths may infect humans:

- *Roundworms* resemble earthworms in appearance. Those most frequently affecting humans include pinworms.
- *Tapeworms* are long and narrow, as their name indicates, and they depend on two hosts, one human and one animal from the development of the egg to the larva to the adult. The easiest way to remember their names is by the name of the animal that acts as the second host, i.e., beef tapeworm, pork tapeworm, fish tapeworm, and dog tapeworm.
- *Flukes* are small, leaf-shaped, flat, unsegmented worms. They are not common

in the United States, but they may become a problem for individuals traveling in Asian countries.

With the threat of invasion from any of the microorganisms listed here, be particularly sensitive to prevention of this invasion. Keep in mind the growth factors necessary for microorganisms mentioned earlier in this chapter. It is important to practice cleanliness. Keep your body and work area as clean and free from infection as possible.

Communicable diseases demand an extra measure of caution. It is helpful to know what the infectious period is for the disease so that anyone who has been exposed can be alerted. Isolate the patient to prevent further exposure. **Table 1–1** outlines the incubation period, the onset and duration, and the suggested isolation period for several contagious infections.

Medical office personnel and hospital staff members are required to notify county and state health departments of confirmed cases of certain communicable diseases. This helps monitor epidemics and alerts the medical community to special problems.

Immunizations are important for protection against certain communicable diseases. Medical office personnel keep accurate records of immunizations, but in such a mobile society, parents should keep a separate and complete record of their children's and their own immunizations. Additional health immunizations are required for travel to some foreign countries. County health departments have specific information on recommended or required immunizations for world travel.

TRAUMA

The leading cause of death in the United States for persons under 40 is *physical trauma,* an injury or wound caused by external force or violence. It is the third leading cause of death for individuals over 40, following cardiovascular disease and cancer.[2]

Head Trauma

Injuries to the head include concussion; cerebral contusion; skull, nose, and jaw fractures; and perforated eardrum.

Cerebral contusions and concussions cause the brain to be jostled inside the skull. Cerebral contusions are more serious than concussions because contusions bruise the brain tissue and disrupt normal nerve function. Contusions may cause loss of consciousness, hemorrhage, and even death. Concussions cause temporary neural dysfunction but are not severe enough to cause a contusion. This kind of trauma normally is the result of falls, severe blows to the head area, and automobile

TABLE 1–1. Contagious Infections

Name	Period of Incubation	Time of Eruption	Duration of Eruption	Period of Quarantine or Isolation
Scarlet fever	1–3 days	12–24 h after onset	7–10 days	7 days isolation
Smallpox	8–17 days	3d or 4th day of fever	14–21 days	21 days or until all scabs disappear
Measles (rubeola)	8–13 days	4th day of fever	4–6 days	Isolation from diagnosis until 7 days after appearance of rash; strict isolation from children under 3 years
Rubella	14–21 days	2d day of fever	1–3 days	None, but avoid contact with nonimmune pregnant women
Mumps	12–26 days			Until all swellings have subsided
Whooping cough	About a week			Isolation for 3 weeks after onset of spasmodic cough
Chickenpox	14–21 days	2d day of fever	7–21 days	7 days after onset
Diphtheria	2–5 days			7 days and until two successive nose and throat cultures, 24 h apart, are negative; to be taken after cessation of antibiotic therapy
Typhus fever	7–14 days	3d to 8th day of fever	14 days	None

Typhoid fever	7–21 days	4th day of fever	3–5 days for each crop of spots	Release after three successive negative cultures of urine and feces not less than 24 h apart and not earlier than 1 month after onset

*From Thomas, C. L. (ed.), *Taber's Cyclopedic Medical Dictionary,* ed. 15. F. A. Davis, Philadelphia, 1985, p. 841, with permission.

accidents. If unconsciousness, convulsions, forceful and persistent vomiting, blurred vision, staggering walk, or hemorrhage occur, the person should be taken to a hospital immediately. Allow a physician to determine the seriousness of the event and the proper treatment needed.

Skull fractures often are accompanied by skin wounds. A skull fracture may be accompanied by scalp wounds and profuse bleeding. For example, individuals with nose fractures usually exhibit a nosebleed. Fractures generally are accompanied by pain, tenderness, and swelling of the affected areas. **Reduction** and/or surgery may be required. The patient should be closely monitored in a hospital.

Perforated eardrums normally result from the insertion of sharp objects into the ear canal or from a severe blow to the side of the head. Sudden and excessive changes in air pressure can cause perforation, too. Children suffering from acute otitis media (earache) may suffer a perforated eardrum as a complication of this disease.

Trauma to the Chest

Thoracic injuries usually result from automobile accidents when the driver is thrown against the steering wheel. Penetrating chest injuries often are caused by knife and gunshot wounds. Penetrating chest wounds typically cause a sucking sound as air enters the chest cavity through the chest wall opening. The patient may be in severe pain. **Tachycardia** is apt to occur. There may be a weak pulse, blood loss, and possible **hypovolemic shock**. It is important to control blood loss in penetration wounds.

Nonpenetrating chest injuries such as rib fractures are characterized by a sensation of tenderness and pain that worsens with deep breathing or exertion. A potential complication of rib fractures is the penetration of a rib into the **pleura**, lung tissue, or **myocardium**.

X-ray is necessary to determine the extent and location of damage. An electrocardiogram (ECG) will assess cardiac damage, and blood studies may be performed. Immediate assessment and attendance by a physician are paramount. Surgical repair is often necessary.

Abdominopelvic Trauma

Injuries to the abdominopelvic region may cause hemorrhages within the liver, spleen, pancreas, and kidneys and/or rupture of the stomach, intestine, gallbladder, and urinary bladder. Rupture of the organs results in the spilling of the organs' contents (including bacteria) into the abdominopelvic cavity. This is a major cause of infection. Blood loss and hypovolemic shock are also a concern. Emergency attention is necessary to determine the extent of damage and the necessary treatment. Most abdominal injuries require surgical repair. Prognosis depends on the extent of injury, but prompt attention generally improves the outcome.

Trauma to Extremities

Because sprains, strains, and fractures to the arms and legs are so common to musculoskeletal diseases, they are explained in Chapter 11.

IRRITANTS AND CHEMICAL AGENTS

Irritants and chemical agents can adversely affect the body. The degree to which this occurs depends on many factors. For example, if the person is debilitated, diseased, very young or elderly, has lowered resistance, or is on some medication, chemical agents or irritants may affect the body much more than in the case of a person who is well and healthy.

If the exposure to the irritant is short in duration and frequency and is fairly localized, the damage may be unnoticed or reversible. However, the irritant may cause irreversible systemic damage.

Some of the more common irritants and chemical agents include extreme heat and cold, radiation, extremes in atmospheric pressure, electric shock, poisonings, near-drowning, bites from insects and snakes, asphyxiation, and burns.

Extreme Heat and Cold. Extreme heat may occasion **syncope**, heat cramps, heat exhaustion, and heatstroke. Causes of these heat disorders include overexertion in heat, prolonged heat exposure, salt depletion, dehydration, failure of the body's heat-regulating mechanisms, or a combination of these. Although heat syncope depends on severity of exposure, it generally responds promptly to rest, cooling, and liquids administered orally. The remaining heat disorders may require hospitalization with intravenous (IV) therapy, cooling therapy, increased fluid intake, temperature monitoring, and muscle massaging. Hypersensitivity to heat may remain for some time. Any of these heat disorders can be fatal.

Extreme cold may occasion disorders such as chilblain, frostbite, and hypothermia. Causes include overexposure to cold air, wind, or water. *Chilblain,* a mild frostbite, produces red, itching skin lesions, usually on the extremities, whereas *frostbite,* the freezing of exposed areas, causes tingling and redness followed by paleness and numbness of the affected areas. Untreated, either condition can lead to gangrene and may necessitate amputation. *Hypothermia* is a systemic reaction, and it can be fatal. Treatment of any of the cold disorders includes gradually warming the person, monitoring temperature, protecting the affected part, preventing infection, and administering **analgesics** as necessary.

Radiation. The effects of radiation range from mild to fatal depending on the duration and intensity of exposure and the form of radiating agent. The radiation may be ingested, inhaled, or through direct contact. Causes may include occupational or accidental exposure or the misuse of radiation for diagnostic or treatment purposes. The harmful effects of radiation may be immediate or delayed, **acute** or chronic. Treatment is symptomatic and supportive and may include **antiemetics**, simple and palatable foods, blood transfusions, and emotional support.

Extremes of Atmospheric Pressure. Extremes of atmospheric pressure result from changing too rapidly from a high- to low-pressure or low- to high-pressure environment. Decompression sickness is an occupational hazard for deep-sea divers and airplane pilots who ascend too quickly or for hospital personnel who work with hyperbaric chambers. Systemic damage occurs following rapid decompression when gases dissolved in the blood and other tissues escape faster than can be diffused through respiration. Gas bubbles form in the blood and tissue causing respiratory problems and pain. Treatment consists of emergency oxygen until the person can be transported to a hyperbaric chamber. Recompression, followed by slow decompression, will be done and other supportive measures given.

Electric Shock. Electric shock can occur anywhere there is electricity—home, work, school, or the medical office. The causes of electric shock can be natural (as from lightning) or contrived (due to carelessness or ignorance or from faulty equipment). The victim must be freed from the source of electric current without the rescuer contacting the current, and treatment must begin immediately. Cardiopulmonary resuscitation (CPR) may be necessary. If the damage is severe, hospitalization may be required to observe the patient, treat any burns, and prevent infection.

Poisoning. Poisoning is a common occurrence, especially among curious children. Recently, our society has become increasingly aware of poisonous chemicals that have been dumped or buried and are causing problems. If the soil and water remain contaminated, the ecologic and/or personal damage that can result is frightening.

Poisons may be ingested, inhaled, injected, or absorbed through the skin. The cause is generally accidental, but it can result from occupational hazards of working with toxic chemicals, from improper cooking and canning of food, and from drug overdoses or drug abuse. Treatment consists of first aid measures, identifying and providing the correct antidote if one exists, and supportive measures. The local poison control center offers valuable help. Prompt, correct treatment can save a life.

Near-Drowning. Near-drowning is a common occurrence during the warm summer months and could be prevented in many cases by following water safety precautions. In near-drowning, the person generally aspirates fluid, but the person may have an obstructed airway caused by spasm of the larynx as he or she gasps under water, resulting in **hypoxemia**. Later, within minutes or possibly days of near-drowning, the person may experience respiratory distress. Emergency treatment is critical. Hospitalization may be required for oxygenation, airway maintenance, observation of the cardiovascular status of the patient, and prevention of further complications.

Bites of Insects and Snakes. Insect and snake bites occur more often during the warm summer months. Bee, yellowjacket, wasp, and hornet stings may cause localized pain, but usually they require little more than symptomatic treatment. Allergic reactions and multiple stings, however, are a more serious matter and should be treated as a medical emergency. Snake bites require quick emergency measures to prevent venom absorption and life-threatening symptoms from occurring. Transporting the victim to a hospital is essential to administer the specific antidote. Close observation of the victim is essential whether the insect or snake bite is considered serious or mild.

Asphyxiation. *Asphyxiation,* or lack of oxygen and accumulating carbon dioxide in the blood, may result from near-drowning, **hypoventilation**, airway obstruction, or inhalation of toxic substances. Emergency treatment is generally required, and it may involve removal of any obstruction, CPR, oxygenation, and intubation. Hospitalization may be necessary to stabilize the victim's vital signs. Obviously, any breathing difficulty is frightening to the victim, so reassurance and encouragement are needed.

Burns. Burns are a leading cause of death among children. Tragically, burns usually are preventable by following fire safety guidelines. Burns are classified by extent, depth, patient age, and associated illness and injury. The "rules of nines" is useful for assessing the extent of burns. Figure 1–1 illustrates the "rule of nines" and burn classification criteria. Emergency measures may be necessary to maintain the burn victim's airway, cool the wound, and prevent serious loss of body fluids. Once the victim has been transported to a hospital, frequently a special burn center, the focus is on maintaining fluid balance, prevention of infection, and patient support. Severe burns can be extremely painful and require a lengthy rehabilitation period, including possible skin grafting and plastic surgery. Emotional support is essential.

NEOPLASIA AND CANCER

Neoplasia means new formation or new growth. *Tumor* and *neoplasm* are commonly used synonymously and will be here. Specific neoplastic diseases will be dealt with in Chapter 2. Here we will discuss etiologic factors and their results.

The actual cause of neoplasms is not known; however, alteration in genes does

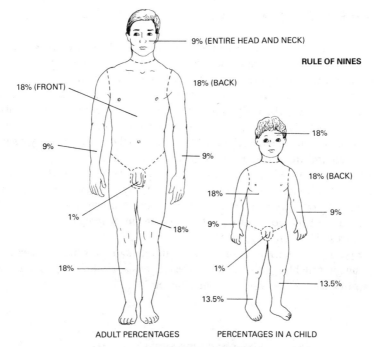

9% (ENTIRE HEAD AND NECK)

RULE OF NINES

18% (FRONT)

18% (BACK)

9%

9%

1%

18%

18%

18%

18%

18% (BACK)

9%

9%

1%

13.5%

13.5%

ADULT PERCENTAGES

PERCENTAGES IN A CHILD

CLASSIFICATION OF BURNS

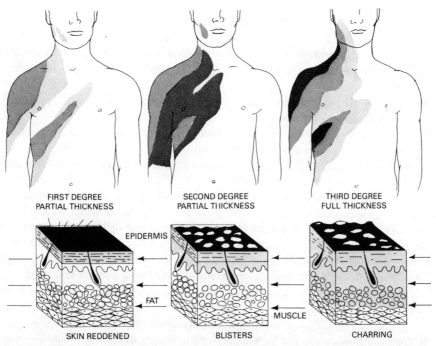

FIRST DEGREE
PARTIAL THICKNESS

SECOND DEGREE
PARTIAL THICKNESS

THIRD DEGREE
FULL THICKNESS

EPIDERMIS

FAT

MUSCLE

SKIN REDDENED

BLISTERS

CHARRING

FIGURE 1–1. The ''Rule of Nines'' and Burn Classification Criteria. (From Thomas, C. L. [ed.], *Taber's Cyclopedic Medical Dictionary,* ed. 15. F. A. Davis, Philadelphia, 1985, p. 243, with permission.)

occur, allowing independent and uncontrollable growth. As was discussed earlier under Hereditary Diseases, an alteration in a gene on a chromosome is a *mutation*. The mutant cell differs from the normal cell in that the abnormal cell is no longer subject to normal control mechanisms. Apparently, mutations such as this occur relatively frequently, but the body is able to destroy the resulting mutant cells as soon as they appear. Therefore, a tumor may represent a failure on the part of the body's immune system. The harmful effects of the neoplastic growth may be from the growth itself and from destruction of surrounding tissue.

The neoplasm may be benign or malignant, depending on its growth pattern. A *benign* tumor is one that remains circumscribed, although it may vary in size from small to large. A *malignant* tumor, or cancer, is one that spreads to other cells, tissues, and parts of the body through the bloodstream or lymphatic system. The spreading process is called **metastasis**.

Cancer is a general term for more than 100 diseases, all of which are characterized by the uncontrollable growth of cells. The diagnosis, treatment, prognosis, and prevention of cancer will be discussed in Chapter 2.

IMMUNE-RELATED FACTORS

The Immune Response

An ideal design for the body would be one that is disease-free. Indeed, a careful study of body chemistry and cells reveals such a blueprint. The body is protected in three ways:

- Normal body structure and function, such as tears, mucous membranes, bones, muscles, and healthy body cells.
- Inflammatory response, in which **leukocytes** rush to a site of infection and engulf invading organisms in a process called **phagocytosis**.
- A specific immune response that causes a protective reaction to a foreign antigen.

The body's immune system is both natural and acquired. Natural immunity is specific to a species. Humans, for example, do not suffer from canine distemper or hoof and mouth disease. Acquired immunity indicates that the body has developed the ability to defend itself against a specific agent. This can occur from having actually had a disease or having received immunizations against a disease. Although the human body does not begin developing **antibodies** until 3 to 6 weeks of age, an infant receives temporary immunity, in utero, because of antibodies produced by its mother's immune system.

There are two different types of acquired immunity.[3]

- *Humoral immunity* is the body's major defense against bacteria. Here the body produces antibodies or **immunoglobulins** that combine with and eliminate the foreign substance or **antigen**. These antibodies are formed by white blood cells called *B-cell lymphocytes*. The humoral response is rapid, beginning immediately or within 48 hours of antigen contact.

Humoral immunity, in the presence of an antigen, causes an antibody to be released, which, in turn, reacts exclusively with that antigen. This binding of antibody to antigen encourages phagocytosis of the antigen and activates the complement system. The complement system is responsible for enzyme development that helps remove the antigen from the body.

■ *Cell-mediated immunity* is action by another group of white cells, called *T-cell lymphocytes*. These are the main protection against viruses, fungi, parasites, some bacteria, and tumors. The T-cells mature in the thymus and are stored in the lymphatic system and spleen.

Cell-mediated immunity is initiated when a T-lymphocyte becomes sensitized by contact with a specific antigen. In response to additional contacts with the antigen, the T-lymphocyte releases sensitized lymphocytes which migrate to the inflammation site. These lymphocytes help to transform local **macrophages** into "killer" T-lymphocytes that are highly phagocytic. The migration of antigens also is prohibited. Some normal tissue can be destroyed during this process, which is very intense.

The ability to generate an immune response is controlled by genetics. Immune response genes regulate B-cell and T-cell proliferation. Therefore, they influence resistance to infection and tumors. The immune response normally recognizes its own body cells, thereby preventing damage to tissue.

While this complex system to protect the body is an example of the disease-free design of the body, the immune response can malfunction. Three main classifications of immunity gone wrong are (1) allergy, when the immune response is inappropriate; (2) autoimmunity, when the immune response is misdirected; and (3) immunodeficiency, when the immune response is inadequate.

Allergy

Allergies that reflect malfunctioning immunity include **urticaria**, or hives. The symptoms include **wheals** surrounded by a reddened area that may cover a small area or the entire body. Causation factors may include foods (especially milk, fish, and strawberries), the presence of pets, insect bites, certain fabrics, inhalants, and cosmetics. Familial history, stress, and general physical condition may predispose to allergies.

Another allergic reaction results from the transfusion of the wrong type of blood or blood components, which become toxic to the body's cells. Transfusion reactions may be mild or severe, depending on the amount of transfused fluid and the person's condition. Symptoms of transfusion reaction range from chills and fever, pain, nausea, and vomiting, to **anaphylaxis** and congestive heart failure. Blood and laboratory tests have to be performed to confirm the type and severity of reaction. The attention of a physician is necessary to prevent complications.

Allergy is also seen in hypersensitivity reactions to drugs. Certain drugs in some people may act as antigens, stimulating the formation of sensitizing antibodies. Although any drug can be the offender, common ones include penicillin, sulfa drugs, and aspirin. The degree of hypersensitivity depends on the extent and duration of exposure to the drug, the person's **atopic** history, age, sex, and underlying disease. Symptoms range from a local rash, **pruritus**, and **erythema** to more severe conditions such as asthma, anemia, or anaphylaxis.

Anaphylactic shock is considered by some authorities as an allergic reaction. This reaction is acute and potentially life-threatening. It may be caused by drug hypersensitivity, foods (the most likely offenders are nuts, legumes, berries, and seafoods), and insect stings (honeybees, wasps, yellowjackets, mosquitoes, ants, and certain spiders). Anaphylaxis may occur after a single exposure to an antigen or following repeated exposures. For this reason, it is important to be alert for an allergic reaction in *any* person at *any* time. In some cases, the reaction may occur within seconds, but usually no later than 40 to 50 minutes following contact with the **allergen**. Cardiovascular symptoms may include hypotension, shock, and cardiac irregularities. Respiratory symptoms may include nasal congestion, profuse watery rhinorrhea, itching, and sudden sneezing. **Edema** of the nose or throat can cause **stridor, dyspnea,** or acute respiratory failure. Gastrointestinal and genitourinary symptoms include stomach cramping, nausea, diarrhea, and urinary urgency and **incontinence**.

Anaphylactic shock is an emergency. It requires immediate countermeasures, which may include injection of epinephrine. It is important to maintain the individual's airway and administer CPR, if necessary, in the event of cardiac arrest.

Autoimmunodeficiency

In autoimmune disease, self-antigens or abnormal immune cells develop that incite the immune response into abnormal or excessive activity of T-cells or B-cells.

Most of the autoimmune diseases are discussed in their respective systems in this book; however, a brief summary of four types follows:

- *Gastrointestinal:* Primary biliary cirrhosis, chronic active hepatitis, ulcerative colitis, and atrophic gastritis. See Chapter 6.
- *Cardiovascular:* Rheumatic fever, pernicious anemia, hemolytic anemia, idiopathic thrombocytopenia, and leukopenia. See Chapter 8.
- *Endocrine:* Juvenile autoimmune diabetes, thyrotoxicosis, and Hashimoto's thyroiditis. See Chapter 10.
- *Musculoskeletal:* Mixed connective-tissue diseases, systemic lupus erythematosus (SLE), and myasthenia gravis. See Chapter 11.
- *Dermatologic:* Dermatomyositis and scleroderma. See Chapter 12.

Immunodeficiency

The immunodeficiency diseases are a result of (1) B-cell deficiency, (2) T-cell deficiency, (3) a B-cell and/or T-cell deficit, and (4) some unknown immunodeficient factor. The majority of immunodeficient diseases are diagnosed by immuno-logic analyses, since many persons are asymptomatic except for recurrent infec-tions. Most immunodeficient patients have impaired resistance to infections, and it is these infectious conditions which may cause death.

One of the most common immunodeficiency diseases is *Hodgkin's disease,* a neoplastic malignancy of the lymph system. It is thought to be an immunode-ficiency due to impaired T-cell function, leaving the person more susceptible to infections. Once a fatal disease, now, with treatment, it is potentially curable even in advanced stages. Hodgkin's will be discussed in detail in Chapter 8, under the lymphatic system.

Acquired Immunodeficiency Syndrome (AIDS) is a disorder first diagnosed in the United States in 1980. AIDS is caused by the human immunodeficiency virus (HIV). HIV is a member of the class of retroviruses. These very simple viruses carry their genetic material in the form of ribonucleic acid (RNA) rather than DNA. HIV predominantly infects cells critical to the operation of the body's immune system called helper T-4 cell lymphocytes. An HIV virus replicates itself by taking over the genetic machinery of the T-cell it invades. The replication process con-tinues until the host cell is destroyed. The newly produced HIV viruses can then infect other T-5 lymphocytes. This progressive and inevitable destruction of T-4 cells leaves the body open to opportunistic infections. In fact, the presence of one or more opportunistic infections, such as *Pneumocystis carinii* pneumonia, is one of the diagnostic criteria of AIDS. A complete presentation of AIDS is given in Chap-ter 5.

Hodgkin's lymphomas, and sometimes lymphosarcomas, are malignant neo-plasms of the lymphoreticular system. Persons with genetic, or acquired, immune deficiency disorders clearly are predisposed to these malignant neoplasms. Signs and symptoms include swelling of lymph glands and those symptoms specific to the affected area. Diagnosis is chiefly by lymph node **biopsy** to differentiate lymphoma from Hodgkin's disease and other causes of **lymphadenopathy**. Identifying the disease involvement is necessary for proper treatment. Chemotherapy and radiation are used with some success. Lymphomas cause more deaths than Hodgkin's dis-ease, with death resulting from complications such as anemia and infections.

MENTAL AND EMOTIONAL FACTORS

To this point, disease etiologies have been traditional and readily identifiable. Such is not the case when discussing the *emotional* or *mental causes of disease,* also termed *psychosomatic illnesses.* The definition is the same no matter which term is used—the expression of an emotional conflict through physical symptoms, both real and imagined.

There appear to be two viewpoints on psychosomatic illnesses:
■ Such illnesses do not exist; what exists in the "head" has little or nothing to do with the rest of the body.
■ The body is a whole, of which the mind is a part. The two cannot be separated.
  Proponents of the first philosophy tend to have a difficult time accepting a need

for personal counseling or psychological and/or psychiatric care. It seems to be easier to accept an illness where the heart wears out and can no longer effectively pump blood through the body than it is to accept a mental breakdown.

Proponents of the second philosophy believe that the body must be treated as a whole; if mental health is not good, physical health suffers. Poor mental health may lead to illness or disease, and vice versa. Proponents of this philosophy believe that emotional, mental, and physical health are equal in value and should be protected, cared for, and treated as such.

From the moment of birth, each of us begins a process of developing a sense of self and self-esteem. Adaptations and adjustments are necessary. When the stimuli are stressful, adaptation occurs to keep the body in a state of well-being. How adaptation occurs is the key to mental health:

> A continuing inability to cope with life and reality induces some degree of mental illness.[4]

Laurence J. Peter and Bill Dana, in their book, *The Laughter Prescription,* say:

> Emotional stress can cause physical deterioration by setting off a complex process that starts in the cerebrum, the thinking part of the brain. Thoughts in the cerebrum can affect the hypothalamus, the part of the brain that regulates body temperature, certain metabolic processes, the autonomic nervous system and chemical balance. Your feelings literally can make you sick or well. Emotional stress is just as real as any kind of physical stress. When you experience sustained anxiety, anger or fear, your physical processes are out of balance and your body cells actually are deteriorating. If degenerative trends are not corrected, you will become susceptible to colds, coronaries and a host of diseases. It is, therefore, important that downward spirals be reversed immediately.[5]

It becomes important, therefore, in considering the etiology of disease, to consider the emotional and mental state of the patient as the direct or indirect cause of a particular ailment.

NUTRITIONAL IMBALANCE

Nutritional imbalance can cause growth problems, specific diseases, and even death. Nutritional imbalances, deficiencies, and excesses are becoming more apparent as causes of health problems. Nutritional deficiencies can cause grave intellectual and physical impairments as well as affect an individual's overall well-being. Causes of nutritional imbalances include starvation, malnourishment, obesity, vitamin and mineral deficiencies and excesses.

Starvation. Starvation does exist in this country, but how much and where are disputable issues. Causes include not enough to eat or an imbalanced diet over a long period of time, causing metabolic and physiologic body changes. A starved person generally is one who does not have adequate food, whereas someone who is malnourished generally has adequate food available but of inadequate nutritive value. Starvation is seen at any age; however, infants and children from 1 to 3 years of age suffer more severely than adults.

Malnourishment. Malnourishment may be due to

- Improper intake of foodstuffs in both quality and quantity, as seen in people suffering from alcoholism, anorexia nervosa, and bulimia or in those who engage in diet faddism.
- Improper intake of foodstuffs because of gastrointestinal problems, as exhibited in the person who has no taste or smell, the postoperative anorexic, or the person who has a lesion in the throat.
- Malabsorption or poor utilization of foodstuffs, as seen when an individual is unable to properly absorb nutrients.
- Increased need for food, as seen in a marathon runner, a person in a febrile state, and a cancer patient with increased needs of certain nutrients.
- Impaired metabolism of foodstuffs, as when both hereditary and acquired biochemical disorders are seen.
- Food and drug interactions, as seen in those taking corticosteroid medications, which are known to deplete muscle protein, lower glucose tolerance, and induce osteoporosis.[6]

Obesity. Obesity has been defined as being 10 to 20 percent above the ideal body weight. Of course, "ideal" is difficult to determine, and factors such as family history and body build need to be considered. The cause of obesity may be too many calories, too little activity, or, less frequently, an endocrine and metabolic problem. Fluid retention may cause an increase in weight, too. Treatment may include lowering caloric intake, increasing physical activity, or in the case of metabolic disorders, correcting the error. If fluid retention is a problem, diuretics may be prescribed, and any underlying cause of the retention should be detected and treated. The prognosis for obesity is not good. While a small percentage of obese individuals are able to lose weight, an even smaller percentage are able to maintain permanent weight reduction.

Vitamin Deficiencies and Excesses. Early signs of *vitamin deficiency* are generally vague and nonspecific. Vitamin-deficiency diseases include *scurvy,* a lack of vitamin C, causing abnormal bone formation and hemorrhages of mucous membranes; *rickets,* a lack of vitamin D (see Chapter 11), and *beriberi,* a lack of vitamin B_1, causing neurologic damage. Treatment typically consists of a diet high in protein and the lacking vitamin. *Vitamin excess* may occur when people take vitamins in an attempt to cover missed or inadequate meals, when they hope to prevent some disease (e.g., the common cold), or when they self-treat a condition. Large doses of some vitamins are toxic and may cause illness, especially when taken over a long period of time.

Mineral Deficiencies and Excesses. Minerals are a vital component of a balanced diet. *Mineral deficiencies* of chloride, potassium, sodium, calcium, and magnesium are the more common ones. Causes include dietary deficiencies and metabolic disorders. Treatment may involve increasing the intake of a deficient mineral through foodstuffs or by medication or treating any underlying metabolic disorder. *Mineral excess* may be caused by diet, medication, or a metabolic error, too. Treatment consists of locating the cause and correcting it. Hospitalization may be required to monitor these minerals and treat the cause.

IDIOPATHIC AND IATROGENIC CAUSES OF DISEASE

Some diseases having no known cause are described as *idiopathic.* Of course, when the cause is unknown, the disease can only be treated symptomatically.

Some diseases are *iatrogenic;* that is, caused by treatment and its effects in patients. This can be seen in the treatment of some cancers, where the chemotherapy drugs used may cause severe anemia, or when hepatitis develops as a result of a blood transfusion.

SUMMARY

The causes of disease are varied, complex, sometimes multiple, and sometimes unknown. When the body is out of harmony, there is a need for care and treatment. Only when the causes of diseases are understood is that care and treatment possible.

REFERENCES

1. Boyd, W., and H. Sheldon, *Introduction to the Study of Disease,* 8th Ed., Lea & Febiger, Philadelphia, 1980, p. 278.
2. *Diseases,* Nursing 83 Books, Intermed Communications, Inc., Springhouse, Pa., p. 116.
3. Crowley, L. V., *Introduction to Human Disease,* Wadsworth Health Sciences Division, Monterey, Calif., 1983.
4. *Diseases,* Nursing 83 Books, Intermed Communications, Inc., Springhouse, Pa., 1983, and Porth, C., *Pathophysiology,* J. B. Lippincott Company, Philadelphia, 1982, p. 74.
5. Peter, L. J., and Bill Dana, *The Laughter Prescription,* Ballantine Books, New York, 1982, p. 22.
6. Chatton, M. J., and P. M. Ullman, "Nutrition: Nutritional and Metabolic Disorders," *Current Medical Diagnosis and Treatment, 1984,* Lange Medical Publications, Los Altos, Calif., 1985, p. 794.

REVIEW QUESTIONS

Matching

_____	1. Genetic constitution of organism
_____	2. Describes condition of a sick person
_____	3. DNA sequence is disrupted
_____	4. Smallest parasitic organism
_____	5. Not in harmony
_____	6. Contains all hereditary information
_____	7. Worms
_____	8. Leukocytes rush to site and phagocytize invading organism
_____	9. Caused by treatment
_____	10. Helps assess extent of burns

a. Disease
b. Illness
c. Genotype
d. DNA
e. Mutation
f. Virus
g. Helminths
h. "Rule of nines"
i. Inflammatory response
j. Iatrogenic
k. Homeostasis
l. Phenotype

Short Answer

1. List nine causes of diseases/disorders:
   a.
   b.
   c.
   d.
   e.
   f.
   g.
   h.
   i.

2. The leading cause of death in the United States for those under 40 is

   _____.

3. Predisposing factors of disease are
   a.
   b.
   c.
   d.

True/False

T F 1. Extremes in cold are chilblain, frostbite, and hypothermia
T F 2. Burns are a leading cause of death in children.
T F 3. Neoplasia is defined as cancer.
T F 4. Humoral immunity is the body's major defense against bacteria.
T F 5. Allergy is an example of an inappropriate immune response.

Multiple Choice

Place a checkmark by *all* the *correct* answers.

1. Phagocytosis
   a. is a process of devouring foreign substances.
   b. is accomplished by neutrophils and macrophages.
   c. depends on the lymphatic system.
   d. activates the complement system.

2. B-cell lymphocytes
   a. provide cell-mediated immunity.
   b. are responsible for acquired humoral immunity.
   c. are the first and most rapid response of antigen contact.
   d. are processed in the thymus.

3. Cell-mediated immunity
   a. is responsible for rejection of transplanted organs.
   b. may be referred to as T-cell immunity.
   c. is initiated when a T-lymphocyte is sensitized by contact with a specific antigen.
   d. is highly effective against fungal and viral invasion and cancer.

4. Three main classifications of immunity gone wrong are
   a. allergy
   b. pneumoconioses
   c. autoimmunity
   d. immunodeficiency

Discussion/Further Study

Contact your county health department to determine the number of diagnosed AIDS cases in your geographic location. How does this number compare with the previous 2 years? What percent of increase/decrease is indicated? What might be the cause of this increase/decrease?

ANSWERS

Matching

1. c
2. b
3. e
4. f
5. a

6. d
7. g
8. i
9. j
10. h

Short Answer

1. a. genetic factors
   b. infections
   c. trauma
   d. chemical agents and irritants
   e. neoplasia/cancer
   f. immune-related factors
   g. mental & emotional factors
   h. nutritional imbalance
   i. idiopathic/iatrogenic

2. Trauma

3. a. age
   b. sex
   c. heredity
   d. environment

True/False

1. True
2. True
3. False
4. True
5. True

Multiple Choice

1. a, b, and d
2. b and c
3. a, b, c, and d
4. a, c, and d

GLOSSARY

ACUTE: Designating a disease having rapid onset, severe symptoms, and a short course. (Compare with *Chronic*.)

ALLERGEN: Any substance that, when introduced into the body, is capable of inducing an allergic reaction.

AMINO ACID: Any one of a large group of organic compounds constituting the primary building blocks of proteins.

ANALGESIC: A drug or other agent used to relieve pain.

ANAPHYLAXIS: An allergic reaction of the body to a foreign protein or other substance. Sometimes used to refer exclusively to a sudden, unusually severe, and possibly life-threatening allergic reaction.

ANTIBODY: A protein substance produced by the body's immune system in response to and interacting with a specific antigen.

ANTIEMETIC: A drug or other agent used to prevent or stop vomiting.

ANTIGEN: Any substance that, when introduced into the body, causes the production of a specific antibody by the immune system.

ATOPIC: Pertaining to the hereditary predisposition to develop a certain type of allergy.

BIOPSY: Excision of a small piece of living tissue for microscopic examination. Usually performed to establish a diagnosis.

CHROMOSOME: In human cells, a linear structure in the nucleus composed of DNA and proteins, bearing part of the genetic information of the cell. Each human cell (except for egg or sperm cells) has 46 chromosomes, occurring in 23 pairs.

CHRONIC: Designating a disease showing little change or of slow progression. (Compare with *Acute*.)

DYSPNEA: Labored or difficult breathing, generally indicating an insufficient amount of oxygen in the blood.

EDEMA: A local or generalized condition in which body tissues accumulate an excessive amount of fluid.

ERYTHEMA: Diffused redness of the skin.

EXOCRINE GLANDS: Glands that release their secretions into the digestive tract or to the outer surface of the body.

GENE: One of the units of heredity, located at a definite position on a particular chromosome.

GENOTYPE: A description of the combination of genes of an individual, either with respect to a single trait or with respect to a larger set of traits. (Contrast with *Phenotype*.)

HETEROZYGOUS: Possessing different genes from each parent for a particular trait.

HOMEOSTASIS: The tendency of the body systems to maintain stability even though they are exposed to continually changing outside forces.

HOMOZYGOUS: Possessing identical genes from each parent for a particular trait.

HYPOVENTILATION: Reduced rate and depth of breathing.

HYPOVOLEMIC SHOCK: A condition of severe physiologic distress caused by a decrease in the circulating blood volume so large that the body's metabolic needs cannot be met.

HYPOXEMIA: Insufficient oxygenation of the blood.

IMMUNOGLOBULIN: One of a family of closely related though not identical proteins that are capable of acting as antibodies.

INCONTINENCE: Inability to control the passage of urine, semen, or feces due to one or more physiologic or psychologic conditions.

LEUKOCYTE: Any of the white cellular components of blood or lymph.

LIPID: Any one of a group of fats or fatlike substances.

LYMPHADENOPATHY: Disease of the lymph nodes.

MACROPHAGE: Any of the class of cells within the body tissues having the ability to engulf particulate substances and microorganisms.

METASTASIS: Movement of bacteria or body cells, especially cancer cells, from one part of the body to another. Typically by way of the circulatory system.

MUTATION: A permanent change in a gene potentially capable of being transmitted to offspring.

MYOCARDIUM: The middle layer of the walls of the heart, composed of cardiac muscle.

PATHOGENIC: Capable of causing disease.

pH: The degree of acidity or alkalinity of a solution, expressed in numbers from 0 to 14. Increasing acidity is expressed as a number less than 7 and increasing alkalinity as a number greater than 7. Maximum acidity is pH 0, and maximum alkalinity is pH 14. A pH of 7 is neutral.

PHAGOCYTOSIS: Ingestion and digestion of bacteria, other cells, and particles by a class of cells called phagocytes.

PHENOTYPE: The observable physical characteristics of an individual, determined by the combined influences of the individual's genetic makeup and the effects of environmental factors. (Contrast with *Genotype*.)

PLEURA: The saclike membrane enveloping each lung and lining the adjacent portion of the thoracic cavity, the two layers forming a potential space, the pleural cavity.

REDUCTION: The restoration or rejoining of fractured bones to their normal position.

PRURITUS: Severe itching.

STRIDOR: Harsh sound during respiration; high-pitched and resembling the blowing of wind.

SYNCOPE: Temporary loss of consciousness due to inadequate blood flow to the brain; fainting.

SYSTEMIC: Pertaining to or affecting the body as a whole.

TACHYCARDIA: Abnormally rapid heart beat; generally defined as exceeding 100 beats per minute.

URTICARIA: A vascular reaction of the skin characterized by the temporary eruption of wheals. Hives.

WHEAL: Local area of edema on the skin often attended by severe itching.

Chapter 2
Neoplasms

LEARNING OBJECTIVES

Upon successful completion of this chapter, you will
- Define neoplasm.
- Compare benign and malignant tumors.
- Recall death statistics on cancer.
- Identify at least eight suggestions for cancer prevention.
- List the seven warning signals of cancer.
- Describe the three main classifications for cancer.
- Identify the grading and staging of neoplasms and their use.
- List at least four possible causes of cancer.
- Discuss three major forms of cancer treatment and their advantages and disadvantages.
- Describe circumstances in which a physician and patient may choose a combination of the three major cancer treatments.

INTRODUCTION

Some new growth in our bodies is necessary and advantageous. Bone and skin repair is an example. Other new growth (neoplasm) could be frightening, perplexing, and life-threatening. *Neoplasm* is a new formation or new growth that serves no useful purpose. In fact, the growth is uncontrollable and progressive, and it may be detrimental to other parts of the body. The term *tumor*, a swelling or enlargement, may be used interchangeably with neoplasm.

A tumor may be benign or malignant depending on its growth pattern, cell characteristics, potential for **metastasis**, tendency to recur, and capacity to cause death. A *benign* tumor is one that grows slowly, and the cells resemble normal cells of the tissue from which the tumor originated. The tumor usually is **encapsulated** and does not infiltrate surrounding tissue; it does not tend to recur when removed. A favorable recovery is usual.

A *malignant* tumor, by comparison, is one that is invasive, grows rather rapidly, is sometimes **anaplastic**, and has the capability of metastasizing through the blood or lymph. These tumor cells are not normal. If untreated, a malignancy generally will progress and death frequently results. We commonly refer to malignant tumors as *cancer*. Henceforth in this chapter, the two terms will be used interchangeably.

Cancer is such a focus of attention in American society because of its toll in lives, the suffering it causes, and the economic losses it produces. Cancer strikes people of all ages, both men and women, and is the second leading cause of death in the United States, preceded only by heart disease. According to the American Cancer Society, the disease strikes approximately 1 in 3 Americans. Figure 2–1 *(top)* illustrates the estimated incidence of cancer by site and sex.

> Twenty percent of Americans die from cancer; this amounted to 450,000 deaths in 1984. Half of the deaths were due to the three most common types of cancer: lung, breast, and colon-rectum. Lung cancer is more prevalent in males, while breast cancer is the commonest form of malignancy in females. Cancer of the colon and rectum is equally common in males and females.[1]

Medical researchers have continued to develop improved treatment procedures for various forms of cancer. Five-year survival rates, for example, are improving for uterine, breast, cervical, prostate, bladder, colon, and rectal cancers. The overall death rate from cancers that typically occur before age 45 has declined. Figure 2–1 *(bottom)* illustrates the estimated deaths from cancer by site and sex. Figure 2–2 illustrates the 5-year cancer survival rates for selected sites by race.

CANCER RISK FACTORS
AND PREVENTIVE MEASURES

The use of tobacco is a significant factor in the cause of respiratory cancers. A high incidence of colon cancer may be linked to a highly refined, low-fiber diet, which is very popular in American households. And although not reported statistically, the incidence of skin cancers has a direct relationship to society's high regard for a sun tan.

The American Cancer Society recommends the following preventive measures:

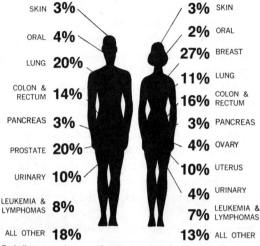

SKIN **3%**	**3%** SKIN
ORAL **4%**	**2%** ORAL
	27% BREAST
LUNG **20%**	**11%** LUNG
COLON & RECTUM **14%**	**16%** COLON & RECTUM
PANCREAS **3%**	**3%** PANCREAS
	4% OVARY
PROSTATE **20%**	**10%** UTERUS
URINARY **10%**	**4%** URINARY
LEUKEMIA & LYMPHOMAS **8%**	**7%** LEUKEMIA & LYMPHOMAS
ALL OTHER **18%**	**13%** ALL OTHER

Excluding non-melanoma skin cancer and carcinoma in situ of uterine cervix.

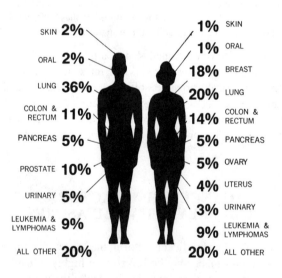

SKIN **2%**	**1%** SKIN
ORAL **2%**	**1%** ORAL
	18% BREAST
LUNG **36%**	**20%** LUNG
COLON & RECTUM **11%**	**14%** COLON & RECTUM
PANCREAS **5%**	**5%** PANCREAS
	5% OVARY
PROSTATE **10%**	**4%** UTERUS
URINARY **5%**	**3%** URINARY
LEUKEMIA & LYMPHOMAS **9%**	**9%** LEUKEMIA & LYMPHOMAS
ALL OTHER **20%**	**20%** ALL OTHER

FIGURE 2–1. *Top,* Estimated 1987 cancer incidence by site and sex. *Bottom,* Estimated 1987 cancer deaths by site and sex. Cancer Statistics, 1987, American Cancer Society, New York, NY. (Adapted from Thomas, C. L. [ed.], *Taber's Cyclopedic Medical Dictionary,* ed. 15. F. A. Davis, 1985, p. 259.)

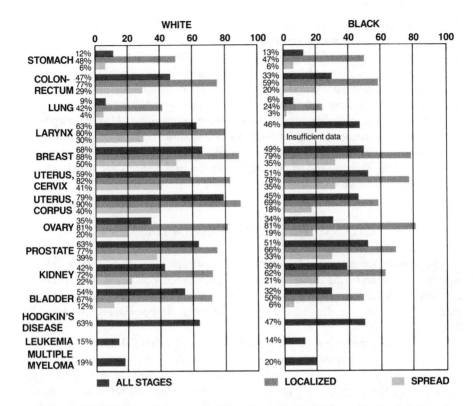

FIGURE 2–2. Five-year cancer survival rates (adjusted for normal life expectancy) for selected sites by race. (From Cancer Facts and Figures, American Cancer Society, 1984, p. 12, with permission.)

- Do not smoke. The risk of developing lung cancer increases 15 times for the smoker.
- Limit alcoholic intake. Heavy drinking increases the risk of cancer of the esophagus, mouth, throat, larynx, and liver.
- Protect skin from excessive sun exposure.
- Refuse needless x-rays. Special precautions must be taken to protect the unborn child if x-rays are necessary.
- Limit exposure to chemicals such as asbestos, aniline dyes, arsenic, chromium, nickel compounds, vinyl chloride, benzene, and certain products of coal, lignite, oil shale, and petroleum.
- Take hormone therapy to relieve menopausal symptoms only as long as necessary.
- Avoid heavily polluted air and long exposure to household solvent cleaners, paint thinners, etc.

■ Follow label instructions carefully when using pesticides, fungicides, and other home garden and lawn chemicals.

■ Monitor caloric intake, and exercise properly. Eat less fatty foods and more high-fiber foods such as bran, whole grains, and fibrous vegetables and fruits.

■ Women should regularly perform breast self-examination.

■ Have regular checkups by physicians. For women over 50, the doctor may recommend a **mammogram** as part of the routine examination. Also, the **Pap test** should be performed at regular intervals. Men should be regularly checked for prostate cancer. A rectal examination should be part of every medical checkup for men and women, and stool samples should be examined for blood, which may be an indication of colon cancer.

CLASSIFICATION OF NEOPLASMS

Neoplasms are classified for diagnostic, treatment, and research purposes as well as to aid in reporting cancer statistics. One commonly accepted system classifies neoplasms according to the type of body tissue in which they appear. Using this method, neoplasms are divided into three categories: carcinomas, sarcomas, and leukemias.

Carcinomas, the largest group, are solid tumors of **epithelial** tissue of external and internal body surfaces. Benign tumors of epithelial origin usually are named using the suffix *-oma* added to the type of tissue involved. For example, an *adenoma* is a benign tumor of a gland. Malignant tumors of epithelial origin, however, are named using the term *-carcinoma* added to the type of tissue involved. An *adenocarcinoma* is a malignant tumor of a gland. Such terminology often is confusing for the layperson, who may believe that *all* tumors are cancerous.

Sarcomas, less common than carcinomas, arise from supportive and connective tissue such as bone, fat, muscle, and cartilage. Again, benign tumors of connective tissue are named by appending the suffix *-oma* to the type of tissue involved, and malignant tumors of connective tissue are named by adding the term *-sarcoma* to the type of tissue involved. Thus, *osteoma* is a benign tumor of bone; *osteosarcoma* is a malignant tumor of bone.

Leukemias, the third classification of neoplasms, are sometimes considered to be sarcomas. But the fact that leukemias do not form solid tumors suggests the need for a separate category. Leukemias arise from the body's blood-forming tissues within the bone marrow. The abnormal tissue proliferates, crowding out normal blood-forming cells, and releases large quantities of abnormal leukocytes into the circulating blood.

Leukemias are further subdivided into chronic and acute forms. The chronic leukemias include chronic myelocytic leukemia and chronic lymphocytic leukemia. The acute leukemias include acute myeloblastic leukemia and acute lymphoblastic leukemia. The pathologic course of leukemia is characterized by the infiltration of leukemic cells into numerous organs, which subsequently become enlarged, soft, and pale. The lymph nodes, spleen, and bone marrow are particularly susceptible. No organ is exempt from this infiltration, however.

GRADING AND STAGING OF NEOPLASMS

Pathologists grade neoplasms by studying the microscopic appearance of suspected tumor cells to determine their degree of anaplasia. The grading helps in the diagnosis and in the treatment planning. Usually four grades are used as follows:

- Grade I: Tumor cells are well **differentiated**, closely resembling normal parent tissue.
- Grades II and III: Tumor cells are intermediate in appearance, moderately or poorly differentiated.
- Grade IV: Tumor cells are so anaplastic that recognition of the tumor's tissue origin is difficult.

Persons with Grade I tumors typically have a high survival rate, whereas persons with Grade IV tumors have a much poorer likelihood of survival. Grading also is used when evaluating cells from body fluids in preventive screening tests, such as **Pap smears** of the uterine cervix.

Staging neoplasms involves estimating the extent to which a tumor has spread. As with grading, staging is important in determining a proper course of treatment. The *TNM system* was developed by the International Union Against Cancer and the American Joint Committee on Cancer Staging and End-Stage Reporting. In this system, tumors are staged according to three basic criteria: **T** refers to the size and extent of the primary tumor, **N** indicates the number of area lymph nodes involved, and **M** refers to any metastasis of the primary tumor.

ETIOLOGY OF NEOPLASMS

As discussed in Chapter 1, the actual cause of neoplasms is not known, but some alteration in the cell chromosomes does occur, allowing independent and uncontrollable cell growth. Such a mutated cell is abnormal in that it is not subject to normal control mechanisms. It is suspected that mutations occur fairly frequently, but that the body's immune response is able to destroy the abnormal cells as soon as they occur. Therefore, a malignancy may represent a failure of the body's immune system.

There is some evidence that viruses may cause some kinds of cancers, and this is an area of active research. It has been shown that viruses can cause tumors in animals. The same proof is not so clear in humans, however. A herpes-like virus, the Epstein-Barr virus, often associated with infectious mononucleosis, is thought to be a causative factor in Burkitt's lymphoma.* The herpes simplex virus appears to be more common in individuals with cervical cancer.

It is a debatable issue whether heredity has any importance in the cause of cancer. There are, however, a few examples deserving discussion. Cancer of the breast generally is more common in female relatives of affected women than in the general population. The uncommon cancer polyposis coli[†] is inherited through an autosomal dominant trait which eventually leads to carcinoma of the colon. Another rare cancer, retinoblastoma,[‡] is inherited as a Mendelian dominant trait and usually is present at birth.

Carcinogens were mentioned briefly earlier in this chapter. Hundreds of carcinogenic compounds that act directly on the cells to cause cancer have been identified. The process may take many years to occur in humans; the process may stop at any point and occasionally may be reversible. Generally, there will be a progressive evolution of cancer cells through different states—**hyperplasia**, **dysplasia**, carcinoma **in situ**, to carcinomas that metastasize.

Chronic irritation probably is not considered an etiology of cancer, but a precursor in some instances. A chronic irritation that is not eliminated can cause abnormal cell changes that may become cancerous. For example, chronic skin ulcers sometimes are complicated by the development of squamous cell carcinomas.

DIAGNOSIS OF NEOPLASMS

Early recognition of the cancer warning signals is essential. The American Cancer Society lists several signs of cancer, the initial letters of which form the acronym **CAUTION**:

- **C**hange in bowel or bladder habits.
- **A** sore that does not heal
- **U**nusual bleeding or discharge
- **T**hickening or lump in breast or elsewhere
- **I**ndigestion or difficulty in swallowing
- **O**bvious change in a wart or mole
- **N**agging cough or hoarseness

Responsibility for early detection lies with the individual. Because any delay in the diagnosis and treatment of cancer can significantly alter the disease course, the American Cancer Society recommends that females regularly do breast self-examination and undergo the Pap test and that males perform a testicular self-examination and undergo a rectal examination at regular intervals.

---

*A malignant neoplasm composed of undifferentiated lymphoreticular cells that form a large osteolytic lesion in the jaw or an abdominal mass. It is seen chiefly in Africa.

[†]A highly malignant condition marked by multiple adenomatous polyps lining the intestinal muscosa, beginning about puberty.

[‡]A tumor arising from retinal germ cells, a common malignancy of the eye in childhood.

To help in the diagnosis of the disease, a Pap test and a biopsy may be performed. The Pap test was developed by Dr. George N. Papanicolaou (1883–1962) to detect cancer, commonly of the uterus and cervix. It is a simple test using an **exfoliative cytology** staining procedure, and it can be performed on any body **excretion**, such as urine and feces; secretion, such as sputum, prostatic fluid, and vaginal fluid; or tissue scrapings, such as from the uterus or the stomach. The specimen sample is placed on a slide, stained, and studied under the microscope for abnormal cells. For a person at average risk who has had two negative Pap tests 1 year apart, the American Cancer Society recommends subsequent Pap tests every 3 years. The Pap test is highly effective in detecting early cancer of the cervix or the uterus.

In a **biopsy**, a live tissue sample is taken for microscopic examination. The tissue may be obtained by needle aspiration, endoscopy, or surgical incision. In *needle aspiration,* the tissue is obtained by application of suction through a needle attached to a syringe. In *endoscopy,* the tissue is removed by the appropriate instrument, such as a bronchoscope or cystoscope. In *surgical excision,* the tissue is removed from the body by surgical cutting, sometimes allowing the removal of the entire tumor at the same time.

TREATMENT OF NEOPLASMS

Treatment of cancer is continually changing as new technology develops. The treatment may offer symptomatic relief to the patient, be used in conjunction with some primary course of treatment, and, perhaps, cure the cancer. The three major types of treatment against cancer include surgery, radiation therapy, and chemotherapy. The physician may recommend one or any combination of these three treatment procedures in order to combat a particular form of cancer.

Surgery

Surgery now is more precise because of improved diagnostic equipment and operating procedures and advancements in pre- and postoperative care. Surgery for cancer may be specific, **palliative**, or preventive.

Specific surgery is done to remove all the cancerous tissue and cure the patient. The types of cancers that respond well to this type of surgery are those of the lung, skin, stomach, large intestine, breast, and endometrium.

Palliative surgery is done to sustain the cancer patient or to alleviate the pain that directly or indirectly results from the cancer. Examples include treating complications of cancer such as abscesses, intestinal perforation and bleeding, or intestinal obstructions. In advanced cancers, palliative surgery may be done to sever nerves to alleviate pain.

Preventive surgery may be done to prevent the development of cancer. For example, polyps of the colon may be removed because they are thought to be pre-cancerous.

Types of surgery include excisional, or *en bloc*, which is done during a radical mastectomy, colectomy, or gastrectomy. *Cryosurgery* involves freezing the malignancy with a liquid nitrogen probe. This method is especially favored in cancers of the brain or bladder tissue. *Electrosurgery* is the burning of cancer tissue. This is the preferred method of treating cancers of the rectum.

Radiation Therapy

Radiation may be used alone or in combination with other forms of cancer treatment. About half of all cancer victims receive some type of radiation therapy. The radiation may be externally or internally applied. In the external mode, an x-ray machine or **radioisotope** elements may be used. In the internal mode, a radio-isotope is placed into catheters, beads, seeds, ribbons, or needles and implanted inside the body.

The goal of radiation therapy is to destroy as much of the tumor as possible without affecting surrounding healthy tissue. Unfortunately, some cancers are situated where radiation would cause serious harm to surrounding tissues. Moreover, some cancers are *radioresistant,* meaning they are not affected by the safe dosage range of radiation.

The effects of radiation on the body include cell death as radioactive energy disrupts DNA and interferes with cell replication and growth. Recovery from radiation damage to normal tissue does occur between doses, but the degree varies depending on the radiosensitivity of the normal tissue. The radiation dose is determined by the size, type, and location of the tumor.

The adverse effects of radiation generally occur in the skin, mucous membranes, and bone marrow. Hair may begin to fall out, erythema may develop, and eating may be difficult because of the nausea, vomiting, and mucosal damage to the mouth and stomach. These distressing side effects generally reverse, either between radiation treatments or after the therapy is complete.

New developments in cancer radiology are continually appearing for both curative and palliative purposes. For example, the *cyclotron,* which produces an intense beam of fast neutrons, is under investigation to treat cancer. The neutrons deposit 50 to 100 times more energy in cells than do x-rays in conventional radiotherapy treatments; thus they are better able to kill many tumors, especially deep-seated tumors.

Chemotherapy

Chemotherapy may be used alone or in combination with other cancer treatments. It is especially effective against cancers that spread, such as leukemias and some solid cancers, including choriocarcinoma and Hodgkin's disease. As with radiation, chemotherapeutic drugs affect normal cellular growth and replication, especially of rapidly proliferating cells. Many of the chemotherapeutic drugs are experimental and can only be used by oncologists. Chemotherapeutic drugs of similar action generally are grouped together.

Most of these drugs are toxic and have adverse effects on the gastrointestinal tract, skin, and bone marrow. The most common side effects of chemotherapeutic drugs include nausea, vomiting, **anorexia**, anemia, **leukopenia**, and loss of hair. The person receiving chemotherapy will be monitored closely with laboratory testing and physical examination in order to evaluate the efficacy of the treatment and to detect potentially serious side effects.

SUMMARY

Cancer is a life-threatening disease that can strike any person at any age. It can strike with or without warning. Early detection and prompt treatment are the best course of action. If the spread is not controlled or checked, cancer can result in death. However, many cancers can be cured if detected and treated promptly.

REFERENCE

1. Petersdorf, R. G., et al., *Harrison's Principles of Internal Medicine,* McGraw-Hill Book Company, New York, 1987, p. 422.

REVIEW QUESTIONS

Short Answer

1. _____ is a new formation that serves no useful purpose; it is uncontrollable and progressive.
2. _____ is a new formation that grows slowly; cells resemble cells of tissue from which the tumor originates.
3. _____ is a new formation that is invasive, grows rather rapidly, is anaplastic and is capable of metastasis.
4. _____ are the major site of cancer in males.
5. _____ , _____ , and _____ are the three most common cancer sites for females.

6. List the seven warning signs of cancer which make the acronym CAUTION:

C

A

U

T

I

O

N

7. Name at least three recommendations for prevention of cancer:

a.

b.

c.

Matching

Match the following definitions with their correct cancer classification.

_____ 1. Largest group of cancers, solid tumors of epithelial tissue

     a. Carcinomas

     b. Sarcomas

     c. Leukemias

_____ 2. Neoplasms of blood-forming tissues

_____ 3. Cancers made up of supportive and connective tissue

4. Define TNM:

   T:

   N:

   M:

Multiple Choice

Place a checkmark by *all* the *correct* answers.

1. Which of the following are diagnostic tools of neoplasms:

     a. Early recognition of cancer warning signals

     b. Breast self-examination

     c. Testicular self-examination

     d. Pap test

     e. Biopsy by needle aspiration, endoscopy, or surgical incision

2. Which of the following are treatments for cancer.

     a. Surgery

     b. Radiation

     c. Chemotherapy

     d. Biopsy

     e. Immunotherapy

ANSWERS

Short Answer

1. Neoplasm
2. Benign neoplasm
3. Malignant neoplasm

4. Lungs
5. Breast, colon, and rectum
6. Change in bowel or bladder habits.
   A sore that does not heal
   Unusual bleeding or discharge.
   Thickening or lump in breast or elsewhere.
   Indigestion or difficulty in swallowing.
   Obvious change in a wart or mole.
   Nagging cough or hoarseness.
7. a. Don't smoke.
   b. Limit alcohol intake.
   c. Protect your skin from excessive sun exposure.
   d. Refuse needless x-rays.
   e. Limit exposure to chemicals.
   f. Avoid heavily polluted air.
   g. Follow label instructions carefully on all containers.
   h. Monitor caloric intake and exercise properly.

Matching

1. A
2. C
3. B
4. TNM system relates to staging of neoplasms for more accurate diagnosis and treatment of the cancer. *T* refers to size and extent of the primary tumor. *N* refers to the number of area lymph nodes involved. *M* refers to any metastasis of the primary tumor.

Multiple Choice

1. All are correct.
2. a, b, c, and e.

GLOSSARY

ANAPLASIA: An irreversible change in the structure of mature cells, resulting in the loss of their characteristic appearance and specialized function.

ANOREXIA: Loss of appetite for food.

BIOPSY: Removal of a small piece of living tissue for microscopic examination.

CARCINOGEN: Any substance or agent that can produce or incite cancer.

DIFFERENTIATION: The process whereby cells take on functions and forms different from those of the cells from which they originated.

DYSPLASIA: Alteration in size, shape, and organization of mature cells.

EN BLOC: In surgery, to remove as one piece.

ENCAPSULATION: Enclosure in a layer of tissue not normal to the part.

EPITHELIAL: Pertaining to the layer of cells forming the outer surface of the body, the lining of the body cavities, and principal tubes and passageways.

EXCRETION: The process of eliminating or getting rid of waste products of the body.

EXFOLIATIVE CYTOLOGY: The microscopic examination of cells that have shed or scaled off the surface epithelium. Performed for diagnostic purposes.

HYPERPLASIA: Excessive proliferation of normal cells.

IN SITU: In position, localized.

LEUKOPENIA: An abnormal decrease in the number of circulating white blood cells.

MAMMOGRAM: A low-dosage diagnostic x-ray of the breast.

METASTASIS: Movement of bacteria or body cells, especially cancer cells, from one part of the body to the other, typically by way of the circulatory system.

PALLIATIVE: Treatment provided to relieve the symptoms of a disease rather than curing the disease.

PAPANICOLAOU TEST (SMEAR): A diagnostic test for the early detection of cancer cells. Abbreviation: Pap test, Pap smear.

RADIOISOTOPE: Radioactive form of an element. Some are commonly used for diagnostic or therapeutic purpose.

Chapter 3
Congenital Diseases

LEARNING OBJECTIVES

Upon successful completion of this chapter, you will
- Describe the three types of cerebral palsy.
- Identify the signs and symptoms of spina bifida, meningocele, and myelomeningocele.
- Recall the diagnostic procedures used for hydrocephalus.
- Identify the etiology of pyloric stenosis.
- Discuss Hirschsprung's disease.
- Review the prevention of erythroblastosis fetalis.
- Compare and contrast the congenital defects of the heart.
- Define cryptorchidism.
- Explain why Wilm's tumor is a congenital problem.
- Compare and contrast the congenital defects of the ureter, bladder, and urethra.
- List the four common forms of clubfoot.
- Recall the etiology of congenital hip dysplasia.
- Describe the signs and symptoms of cystic fibrosis.
- Restate the diagnostic procedures for PKU.

INTRODUCTION

In Chapter 1, a basic description of genetic factors relating to the body's disease processes was given. Here, *congenital diseases* refer to those problems which are present at birth, brought about by genetic causes, nongenetic causes, or a combination of the two. Their clinical manifestations may be minor and inconsequential, or they may be life-threatening. Some may be detected at birth; others are not apparent until later in infancy or childhood. However, all congenital diseases require the attention of physicians and the involvement of the entire family.

NERVOUS SYSTEM DISEASES

Cerebral Palsy

Description: Cerebral palsy is bilateral, symmetrical, nonprogressive paralysis resulting from developmental defects of the brain or trauma at birth.

Etiology: Cerebral palsy is caused by central nervous system damage prior to or following birth. The occurrence of cerebral palsy is highest in premature infants, and it is the most common cause of crippling in children. There are three types: spastic, athetoid, and ataxic.

Signs and Symptoms: *Spastic cerebral palsy* affects the majority of victims and is characterized by hyperactive reflexes, rapid muscle contraction, muscle weakness, and underdevelopment of limbs. Children with this form of cerebral palsy typically walk on their toes, crossing one foot in front of the other.

Athetoid cerebral palsy affects far fewer children and is characterized by involuntary muscle movements and **dystonia**. The arms are more often affected than the legs, and speech may be difficult. The body movements in athetoid cerebral palsy are increased during times of stress and not apparent during sleep.

Even fewer persons show signs of *ataxic cerebral palsy.* They have difficulty with balance and coordination and show signs of **nystagmus**, muscle weakness, and tremor. Sudden movements almost always are impossible.

A few children will exhibit signs of all three types of cerebral palsy. Mental retardation, seizure disorders, and impaired speech often are present.

Diagnostic Procedures: Careful neurologic assessment, including examination and history, is necessary. Spontaneous movement and behavior of the child are observed for characteristic signs, such as (1) inability to suck or keep food in the mouth, (2) difficulty in voluntary movements, (3) difficulty separating legs during diaper changes, and (4) use of only one hand or both hands, but not the legs. A diagnostic test often performed on infants at 6 months of age involves placing a diaper or light blanket over their face. A child with cerebral palsy will have difficulty removing the blanket or will use only one hand to do so.

Treatment: Cerebral palsy has no cure, and treatment is directed toward helping children overcome any functional or intellectual disability. The treatment process typically involves the entire family. Treatment may include the use of braces and special appliances, range-of-motion exercises, orthopedic surgery, and medications to decrease seizures and spasticity.

Prognosis: The prognosis varies. If impairment is mild, a near normal life may be possible.

Prevention: Early prenatal care and good maternal health are preventive measures.

Neural Tube Defects: Spina Bifida, Meningocele, Myelomeningocele

Description: Spina bifida, meningocele, and myelomeningocele are developmental defects of the first trimester of pregnancy that are characterized by incomplete closure of the bones encasing the spinal cord. *Spina bifida occulta* is the most common but least severe of these defects. It is marked by an incomplete closure of one or more vertebrae, with no protrusion of the spinal cord or **meninges**. In *meningocele,* the incomplete closure of the vertebrae is accompanied by a protrusion of the spinal fluid and meninges into an external sac. *Myelomeningocele* results when the external sac contains meninges, cerebrospinal fluid, and a portion of the spinal cord or its nerve roots.

Etiology: The cause is essentially unknown. Risk factors associated with these conditions include exposure to radiation, viruses, and genetic factors.

Signs and Symptoms: Spina bifida occulta may show no visible signs or may be manifested by a dimple in the skin, hair tuft, or port-wine nevi along the posterior surface of the body in the midline above the buttocks. In meningocele and myelomeningocele, a saclike structure protrudes from the spinal area. Spina bifida and meningocele may cause little or no neurologic deficit, but myelomeningocele frequently results in permanent neurologic difficulties.

Diagnostic Procedures: Prenatal detection of some open neural tube defects is possible through ultrasound examination between the fourteenth and sixteenth weeks of gestation. Following birth, meningocele and myelomeningocele are obvious upon examination. Spina bifida occulta may not be evident upon visual inspection. Accordingly, x-rays, pinprick examination of the legs and trunk, and myelography are other procedures used to diagnose the condition.

Treatment: Spina bifida occulta usually requires no treatment. Meningocele and myelomeningocele require surgical repair of the sac and supportive measures to promote independence and to decrease the possibility of complications.

Prognosis: The prognosis is dependent on the extent of neurologic deficit that accompanies the condition. The prognosis is worse for individuals with open spinal lesions and much better for those with only spina bifida occulta. In the latter, many affected individuals may be able to live a normal life. In the most severe cases, waist supports, leg braces, and management of fecal incontinence and neurogenic bladder are necessary.

Prevention: Since spinal cord defects occur more often in offspring of women who have previously had a child with a similar defect, genetic counseling may be helpful.

Hydrocephalus

Description: Hydrocephalus is a condition marked by too much cerebrospinal fluid in the ventricles of the brain. The condition is called *noncommunicating hydrocephalus* when there is an obstruction in cerebrospinal fluid flow. If the problem is faulty absorption of cerebrospinal fluid, the condition is called *communicating hydrocephalus.*

Etiology: Nomcommunicating hydrocephalus may result from problems in fetal development, infection, tumor, or a blood clot. In communicating hydrocephalus, faulty absorption of the cerebral spinal fluid may be a consequence of surgery to repair myelomeningocele or a meningeal hemorrhage.

Signs and Symptoms: The classic symptom of noncommunicating hydrocephalus is the enlarged head; communicating hydrocephalus produces bulging **fontanelles** as the only visible sign. The scalp skin may be thin and fragile looking with the veins clearly visible. Hydrocephalic infants often have high-pitched cries and abnormal muscle tone in their legs.

Diagnostic Procedures: The abnormally large head suggests the diagnosis. Skull x-rays, ventriculography, angiography, and pneumocephalography also may be used.

Treatment: Surgical correction is the treatment of choice for hydrocephalus. A shunt is usually placed from the affected ventricles of the brain into the peritoneal cavity or into the right atrium of the heart, where the excess fluid makes its way into venous circulation.

Prognosis: The prognosis is guarded even with early detection and surgical correction. Mental retardation, vision loss, and impaired motor function often occur. Without surgery, the mortality rate is high.

Prevention: There is no known prevention.

DIGESTIVE SYSTEM DISEASES

Pyloric Stenosis

Description: Pyloric stenosis is narrowing of the **pyloric sphincter.** This condition causes obstruction of the flow of **chyme** into the small intestine and is much more common in males than in females.

Etiology: The cause is unknown, but it may be hereditary in nature.

Signs and Symptoms: The classic symptom is **projectile vomiting**, beginning about the second to fourth week after birth. The infant may eject vomitus a distance of 3 to 4 feet. Signs of dehydration and starvation may be evident if the pyloric sphincter closes completely. There may be decreased elasticity of the skin, abdominal distension, and a palpable tumor in the **epigastrium**.

Diagnostic Procedures: The patient history and physical examination may suggest the condition. Other studies may include upper gastrointestinal x-rays and laboratory tests, with the latter being used to detect dehydration and electrolyte imbalances. Pyloric stenosis must be distinguished from feeding difficulties associated with colic or disturbed mother–child relationships.

Treatment: The standard treatment is incision and suture of the pyloric sphincter. The procedure, called *pyloromyotomy,* is relatively simple, safe, and effective.

Prognosis: The prognosis is excellent with proper care and surgical correction.

Prevention: There is no known prevention.

Hirschsprung's Disease
(Congenital Aganglionic Megacolon)

Description: Hirschsprung's disease is the obstruction and dilation of the colon with feces as a result of inadequate intestinal motility. The condition is due to an absence of autonomic **parasympathetic ganglion** cells in the colorectal walls, resulting in the absence of **peristalsis** in the affected portion. Consequently, feces is not moved past the aganglionic segment of the colon. Pressure from accumulating feces then distends the preceding portion of the colon. The amount of intestinal wall affected varies from only the internal sphincter to the entire colon. The disease more frequently affects whites and females. Often, the disease occurs with other congenital anomalies.

Etiology: The cause of the disease is unknown, but it appears to be hereditary.

Signs and Symptoms: Clinical manifestations typically appear during infancy, but they may not appear until adolescence. In infancy, signs and symptoms include severe abdominal distension, feeding difficulties, fever, failure to thrive, and explosive watery diarrhea. In adolescence, symptoms may include chronic constipation, abdominal distension, and palpable fecal masses. The child also may be anemic and appear poorly nourished.

Diagnostic Procedures: Diagnosis is confirmed by a rectal biopsy revealing the absence of ganglion cells in the colorectal wall. A barium enema, upright x-rays of the abdomen, or rectal manometry may be ordered.

Treatment: Medical or surgical treatment may be tried. Medical treatment includes enemas, stool softeners, and a low-residue diet. Surgery may be performed to remove the aganglionic portion of the bowel and to improve functioning of the internal sphincter. A temporary **colostomy** or **ileostomy** may be necessary.

Prognosis: With prompt treatment, the prognosis is good. If untreated, death is likely from enterocolitis, severe diarrhea, and shock.

Prevention: There is no known prevention.

CARDIOVASCULAR DISEASES

Erythroblastosis Fetalis
(Hemolytic Disease of the Newborn)

Description: *Erythroblastosis fetalis* is a disease of the newborn characterized by excessive rates of red blood cell destruction **(hemolysis).** The condition is caused by an incompatibility between maternal and fetal blood, especially an Rh factor or ABO incompatibility. During a first pregnancy, an Rh⁻ female becomes sensitized to Rh⁺ blood antigens that the fetus has inherited from the father. The maternal blood develops antibodies against the fetal red cell antigens. Usually this process, called **isoimmunization**, does not affect the fetus of a first pregnancy, because the initial sensitization generally does not occur until the onset of labor. During subsequent pregnancies with an Rh incompatible fetus, the maternal antibody crosses the placenta and reacts with the Rh antigen on the fetal red cells. The resulting antigen/antibody reaction causes hemolysis of fetal red cells. A transfusion with Rh⁺ blood prior to pregnancy also may sensitize the mother.

ABO incompatibility occurs when the major blood group antigens of the fetus are different from those of the mother. (The major blood groups are A, B, AB, and O.) An example of this incompatibility is a mother with O blood and an infant with A blood. Although ABO incompatibilities are more likely to occur than Rh incompatibilities, the effects of ABO incompatibilities are far less severe, often remaining subclinical.

Signs and Symptoms: Jaundice may appear within 3 to 24 hours after birth. The spleen and liver may be enlarged. In severely affected infants, **pallor**, anemia, edema, **petechiae**, lethargy, and convulsions may result.

Diagnostic Procedures: A maternal history and blood typing of both mother and father are essential. A history of blood transfusions may be indicative, too. A direct Coomb's test, bilirubin test, and hematocrit of the infant's blood may be done for diagnosis.

Treatment: The goal of treatment is to stop the hemolytic process. An **exchange transfusion** is frequently the treatment of choice. Albumin infusions, to aid in the binding of **bilirubin**, and **phototherapy** may be used, too. If severe hemolysis is detected in utero, the delivery may be advanced 2 to 4 weeks, or an intrauterine peritoneal transfusion may be tried and repeated until the fetus can be safely delivered.

Prognosis: The prognosis for an infant with ABO incompatibility is generally good. The prognosis for an infant with an Rh incompatibility is always guarded, with the outcome depending on the exact nature of the Rh incompatibility and the degree of damage done to other body tissues.

Prevention: Prevention includes early prenatal care with blood typing. In the event of Rh incompatibility, Rh immune globulin (RhoGAM) may be given to the mother after delivery to prevent isoimmunization to Rh^+ antigens.

Congenital Heart Defects

Description: Congenital heart defects can be broadly classified according to whether or not poorly oxygenated blood entering from the veins mixes in the heart with the freshly oxygenated blood reentering the systemic circulation. *Acyanotic* defects are those in which there is no mixing of poorly oxygenated blood with the blood reentering the systemic circulation. *Cyanotic* defects are those in which poorly oxygenated blood does mix with the blood reentering the systemic circulation.

Acyanotic defects include

- *Ventricular septal defect (VSD),* a congenital heart defect in which there is an abnormal opening between the right and left ventricle. The extent of the opening may vary from pin size to complete absence of the ventricular septum, creating one common ventricle. This defect typically accompanies other congenital anomalies, especially Down's syndrome, or renal and other cardiac defects. VSD is the most commonly occurring congenital heart defect.
- *Atrial septal defect (ASD),* an abnormal opening between the right and left atria. The size and location of the opening determines the severity of the defect.
- *Coarctation of the aorta,* a malformation in a portion of the wall of the aorta that causes narrowing of the aortal **lumen** at the point of the defect. Consequently, blood pressure is increased proximal to the defect and decreased distal to it.
- *Patent ductus arteriosus (PDA),* a defect resulting from the failure of the ductus arteriosus to close after birth. During the prenatal period, much of the fetal circulation bypasses the lungs through this blood vessel that connects the pulmonary artery to the aorta. When this fetal structure fails to close after birth, blood from the aorta flows back into the pulmonary artery.

Cyanotic defects include

- *Tetralogy of Fallot,* a combination of four congenital heart defects, including (1) pulmonary stenosis, a narrowing of the opening into the pulmonary artery from the right ventricle; (2) ventricular septal defect, an abnormal opening in the septum between the left and right ventricles; (3) dextroposition of the aorta, in which the opening of the aorta bridges the ventricular septum, receiving blood from both the left and right ventricles; and (4) right ventricular **hypertrophy**. Tetralogy of Fallot is the most common cyanotic heart defect.
- *Transposition of the great vessels,* a condition in which the two major arteries of the heart are reversed, with the aorta arising from the right ventricle and the

pulmonary artery from the left ventricle. The result is two noncommunicating circulatory systems—one circulating blood in a closed loop between the heart and lungs and the other, between the heart and systemic circulation.

Etiology: The etiology of congenital heart defects is unknown, but genetic anomalies are strongly suspected. Predisposing factors may include maternal **rubella**, diabetes, alcoholism, poor maternal nutrition, or pregnancy in women over 40 years old.

Signs and Symptoms of Acyanotic Defects:

■ *VSD:* The classic clinical feature is a loud, harsh systolic murmur heard during **auscultation**.

■ *ASD:* The classic clinical feature is a crescendo-decrescendo type of systolic ejection murmur.

■ *Coarctation of the aorta:* The clinical features vary with age. A murmur may or may not be present. An infant may exhibit dyspnea, pulmonary edema, **tachypnea**, and failure to thrive. Symptoms appearing after adolescence may include dyspnea, **claudication**, headache, **epistaxis**, and hypertension.

■ *PDA:* The clinical feature is a "machinery" murmur usually associated with a **thrill**, and often accompanied by a widened pulse pressure.

Signs and Symptoms of Cyanotic Defects:

■ *Tetralogy of Fallot:* **Cyanosis** is often evident at birth or within several months of birth and is considered the hallmark of the disorder. The child may exhibit clubbing of the fingers and delayed physical growth and development.

■ *Transposition of the great vessels:* The infant is typically severely cyanotic at birth. Signs of congestive heart failure and **cardiomegaly** follow.

Diagnostic Procedures: A patient history and physical examination are essential and may be all that is necessary to diagnose tetralogy of Fallot. Other diagnostic procedures may include x-rays, heart catheterization, electrocardiogram (ECG), phonocardiogram, and echocardiogram. Laboratory studies may be ordered for determining the degree of cyanosis and for detecting possible acidosis.

Treatment: Surgery is usually the treatment of choice for a congenital heart defect. Surgery may be performed soon after birth, or it may be delayed until the child is old enough to withstand corrective surgery.

Prognosis: The prognosis is dependent on the type of defect, its location, and its severity. If the defect is small, the prognosis is often good; otherwise, the prognosis is guarded.

Prevention: There is no known prevention other than proper prenatal care and minimizing suspected risk factors.

GENITOURINARY DISEASES

Undescended Testes (Cryptorchidism)

Description: This congenital condition is the failure of one or both testes to descend into the scrotal sac from the abdominal cavity. The condition may be unilateral or bilateral.

Etiology: The cause is essentially unknown, but it may be linked to inadequate or improper hormone levels in the fetus. The testes normally descend into the scrotal sac during the eighth month of gestation, so the condition is most often seen in premature births.

Signs and Symptoms: When the condition is unilateral, the testis on the affected side is not palpable in the scrotum. In bilateral cryptorchidism, the scrotum will appear underdeveloped.

Diagnostic Procedures: Physical examination reveals cryptorchidism. A serum gonadotropin test will confirm the presence of testes, since it assesses the level of circulating hormone produced by the testes.

Treatment: In many cases, the testes will descend during the infant's first year. Otherwise, the treatment of choice is human chorionic gonadotropin hormone therapy. If the testis(es) does not eventually descend as a result of hormonal treatment, surgical correction before age 5 may be attempted.

Prognosis: The prognosis is good with proper attention. Corrected cryptorchidism does not cause sexual dysfunction later. Testes that have not descended by the time of adolescence will atrophy, causing sterility.

Prevention: Since the cause is essentially unknown, prevention also is unknown.

Wilm's Tumor

Description: Wilm's tumor is a malignant neoplasm of the kidneys occurring primarily in children. Wilm's tumor is considered a congenital anomaly because it forms during embryonic life. The neoplasm then lies dormant until later in childhood. It is more common in children with other congenital anomalies.

Etiology: The cause is unknown.

Signs and Symptoms: The classic sign is a firm, smooth, palpable mass in the abdomen. Hypertension and vomiting may be present, too. There may be pain and **hematuria**.

Diagnostic Procedures: The palpable mass is suggestive of the diagnosis, but intravenous pyelography and a 24-hour urine specimen may be required. The latter is to rule out **neuroblastoma**.

Treatment: The treatment of choice is surgical removal of the tumor, the affected kidney if necessary, and any accessible metastatic sites, such as the adrenal glands. Radiation therapy and chemotherapy usually follow surgery.

Prognosis: With treatment, prognosis is good. Wilm's tumor has a high survival rate. When the tumor is localized, the 5-year survival rate is 90 percent; with other metastasis, it is 50 percent.

Prevention: There is no known prevention.

Congenital Defects of the Ureter, Bladder, and Urethra

The causes of congenital defects of the ureter, bladder, and urethra are unknown. Some of the problems are obvious at birth; others are not apparent until later when they produce symptoms. The following is a brief discussion of the most common congenital urinary tract anomalies, together with their symptoms and possible treatments.

Duplicated ureter means that each kidney has two ureters rather than one. Sometimes the two ureters join before they enter the urinary bladder. The common symptoms may include frequent urinary infections, urinary frequency and urgency, diminished urine output, and flank pain. Surgery is the treatment of choice.

Retrocaval ureter occurs when the right ureter passes behind the inferior vena cava before entering the urinary bladder. The symptoms may include **hydroureter**, right flank pain, urinary tract infection, **renal calculi**, and hematuria. Surgical resection and **anastomosis** of the ureter constitute the treatment of choice.

Ectopic orifice of the ureter occurs when the ureteral opening inserts into the vagina in females or in the prostate or vas deferens in males. The symptoms may include urinary obstruction, reflux, incontinence, flank pain, and urinary urgency. Resection and ureteral reimplantation into the bladder are necessary for correction.

Stricture or stenosis of the ureter means that one of the ureters is tightened or partially closed. The affected ureter may become enlarged, and **hydronephrosis** may result. Surgical repair is necessary. A nephrectomy may be required if severe renal damage has occurred as a result of hydronephrosis.

Ureterocele is the bulging of the ureter into the urinary bladder, sometimes almost filling the bladder. There will be urinary obstruction difficulties and recurrent urinary tract infections. Surgical repair or resection of the ureterocele is necessary.

Exstrophy of the bladder is a congenital malformation in which the lower portion of the abdominal wall and the anterior wall of the bladder are missing. Consequently, the inner surface of the posterior wall of the bladder is everted through the opening in the abdominal wall. In effect, the bladder appears turned inside out. The skin covering the hole in the abdominal wall is easily **excoriated** by accumulating urine, and infection typically results. Surgical closure of the defect is necessary. Reconstruction of the bladder and abdominal wall is required, and urinary diversion may be necessary.

Congenital bladder diverticulum is caused by a pouching out (diverticulum) of the bladder wall. Fever, urinary frequency, and pain on urination are common. Surgery is the treatment of choice to correct the herniation.

Hypospadias is an abnormal opening of the male urethra onto the undersurface of the penis or of the female urethra into the vagina. *Epispadias* is an abnormal opening of the male urethra onto the upper surface of the penis or of the female urethra through a fissure in the labia minor and clitoris. In all these instances, normal urination is difficult or impossible. Surgical repair is almost always necessary.

MUSCULOSKELETAL DISEASES

Clubfoot (Talipes)

Description: *Clubfoot* is a nontraumatic, frequently occurring congenital deformity in which the foot is permanently bent forward. The four basic forms are (1) *talipes varus,* an inversion or inward bending of the foot, (2) *talipes valgus,* an eversion or outward bending of the foot, (3) *talipes equinus,* or plantar flexion, in which the toes are lower than the heel, and (4) *talipes calcaneus,* or dorsiflexion, in which the toes are higher than the heel.[1] An individual also may have a combination of these basic forms, e.g., talipes equinovarus, in which the toes point downward and the body of the foot bends inward.

Etiology: The exact cause is unknown, but a combination of genetic and environmental factors in utero have been implicated.

Diagnostic Procedures: The deformity is commonly obvious at birth.

Treatment: Treatment is aimed at correcting the deformity and maintaining the corrected position. Simple manipulation and casting may be done and repeated several times. Corrective surgery may be required. Maintenance treatment includes special exercises, night splints, and orthopedic shoes. Close follow-up observation is essential.

Prognosis: The prognosis is good with prompt treatment.

Prevention: There is no known prevention.

Congenital Hip Dysplasia

Description: Hip dysplasia is an abnormality of the hip joint that may take three forms: (1) unstable hip dysplasia, in which the hip can be dislocated manually; (2) incomplete dislocation, in which the **femoral head** is on the edge of the **acetabulum**; and (3) complete dislocation, in which the femoral head is outside the acetabulum.

Etiology: The cause is not known; however, two possible etiologies have been proposed. First, hormones which relax the maternal ligaments during labor also may relax the hip ligaments of the infant. Second, hip dislocation may result if the fetus is not positioned correctly within the uterus prior to and during birth.

Signs and Symptoms: The signs are typically quite obvious when children attempt to walk if the condition has not been discovered prior to that time.

Diagnostic Procedures: Observations during physical examination may suggest the diagnosis, but a positive Ortolani's or Barlow's sign will confirm the diagnosis.

Treatment: It is important for treatment to begin as soon as possible. Prior to 3 months of age, treatment requires closed reduction of the dislocation followed by the use of a splint-brace for 2 to 3 months. If the child is much older, open reduction followed by casting may be necessary.

Prognosis: When the condition occurs prior to age 5, the prognosis is excellent. If not treated promptly, abnormal development of the hip and permanent disability may result.

Prevention: There is no known prevention.

METABOLIC ERRORS

Cystic Fibrosis

Description: *Cystic fibrosis* is a congenital disorder of the **exocrine** glands characterized by the production of copious amounts of abnormally thick secretions of mucus, especially in the lungs and pancreas.

Etiology: The disease is caused by an underlying biochemical defect transmitted as an **autosomal recessive trait**.

Signs and Symptoms: The signs of cystic fibrosis may appear soon after birth or take some time in developing, but since all exocrine glands can be affected, the symptoms can be quite numerous. The sweat glands and respiratory and gastrointestinal functions most commonly are affected. The sweat glands typically exhibit increased concentrations of salt in sweat. Respiratory symptoms may include wheezy respirations, a dry cough, dyspnea, and tachypnea stemming from accumulations of thick secretions in the **bronchioles** and **alveoli** of the lungs. Gastrointestinal symptoms may include intestinal obstruction, vomiting, constipation, electrolyte imbalance, and the inability to absorb fats. Fibrous tissue and fat slowly replace the normal saclike swellings found in the pancreas, resulting in pancreatic insufficiency characterized by insufficient insulin production.

Diagnostic Procedures: The presence of abnormal quantities of salt concentrated in sweat in a child, accompanied by pulmonary and pancreatic insufficiencies, confirms the diagnosis. Family history may show siblings or other relatives with cystic fibrosis.

Treatment: The treatment for cystic fibrosis is largely supportive. Patient management includes generous salting of food to replace salt lost in sweat, physical therapy to combat pulmonary dysfunction, loosening and removal of mucopurulent secretions, and oxygen therapy. Vitamin and oral pancreatic supplements may be given. Both the family and the patient require emotional support.

Prognosis: The prognosis is poor. There is no cure for cystic fibrosis, and about half of all children with this disease die by age 16. Cystic fibrosis is the most common fatal genetic disease. Death is usually due to such complications as shock and arrhythmias that may occur during hot weather due to profuse sweating. Serious, often fatal respiratory complications include pneumonia, emphysema, and atelectasis. Gastrointestinal complications include rectal prolapse and malnutrition.

Prevention: There is no known prevention. Genetic counseling may be advisable in families known to be at risk.

Phenylketonuria (PKU)

Description: *Phenylketonuria* is an autosomal recessive defect resulting in an error in phenylalanine metabolism.

Etiology: During normal metabolic processes, the enzyme phenylalanine hydroxylase converts the amino acid phenylalanine to tyrosine, another amino acid. In PKU, this enzyme is not produced by the body, causing phenylalanine to accumulate in the blood and urine. Mental retardation will result if the condition is not quickly corrected. The full extent of cerebral damage is complete by 2 or 3 years of age and is irreversible.

Signs and Symptoms: The infant is typically asymptomatic until about 4 months of age, when signs and symptoms of mental retardation, such as hyperactivity, personality disorders, macrocephaly, and irritability, begin to appear. There is often a characteristic musty odor to the child's perspiration and urine due to the presence of phenylacetic acid, a metabolite of phenylalanine.

Diagnostic Procedures: An elevated blood phenylalanine level and urine phenylpyruvic acid level present at birth will confirm the diagnosis. Repeated testing may need to be done.

Treatment: Treatment consists of following a protein-restrictive diet for 3 to 6 years and, some authorities maintain, for life. Most natural proteins need to be restricted, since phenylalanine is a component of most proteins. Serum phenylalanine levels need to be monitored to determine the efficacy of the diet.

Prognosis: The sooner the protein-restrictive diet is started, the better is the prognosis. If the disease is detected and treated before 2 years of age, the chances of the child achieving normal intelligence are good. The protein-restrictive diet will not reverse any existing mental retardation, but it will prevent further progression.

Prevention: Prevention includes genetic counseling and PKU testing at birth.

REFERENCE

1. Whaley, L.F. and D.L. Wong, *Nursing Care of Infants and Children,* CV Mosby, St Louis, 1979, p. 392.

REVIEW QUESTIONS

Multiple Choice

1. Select all the correct statements concerning cerebral palsy:
   a. Caused by central nervous system damage prior to birth.
   b. May be spastic, athetoid, and ataxic.
   c. A neurologic assessment is the most common diagnostic tool.
   d. Is curable.
   e. No known prevention.

2. Select all the correct signs and symptoms of cystic fibrosis:
   a. Intestinal obstruction
   b. Vomiting
   c. Constipation
   d. Wheezy respirations
   e. A dry cough
   f. Dyspnea
   g. Tachypnea
   h. Electrolyte imbalance
   i. Inability to absorb fats
   j. Deficient insulin

3. Select all the correct answers from the following statements concerning erythro-blastosis fetalis:
   a. It is a hemolytic disease of the newborn.
   b. The fetal blood cells build antibodies against maternal cells.
   c. It affects the fetus in the first pregnancy.
   d. ABO incompatibility is more common than an Rh type.
   e. Jaundice is a common symptom.
   f. Phototherapy is the treatment of choice.

Matching

1. Select the correct definition for these spinal cord defects.

   _____ Incomplete closure of one or more vertebrae   a. Meningomyelocele

   _____ Incomplete closure of vertebrae with   b. Meningocele
   protrusion of spinal fluid and meninges into   c. Spina bifida occulta
   sac

   _____ External sac contains meninges, cerebral
   spinal fluid, and portion of cord and nerve
   roots

2. Match the following congenital defects of the heart with their definitions.

   _____ Abnormal opening between the two atria   a. ventricular septal defect

   _____ Fetal ductus arteriosus fails to completely   b. atrial septal defect
   close   c. coarctation of the aorta

   _____ Abnormal opening between the right and   d. patent ductus
   left ventricles   arteriosus

   _____ Localized narrowing of aorta   e. tetralogy of Fallot

Short Answer

1. The two different types of hydrocephalus are _____ and _____ .
2. The characteristic symptom in pyloric stenosis is _____ .
3. Another name for undescended testes is _____ .
4. What does PKU stand for? Describe it.
5. Name at least three congenital defects of the ureter, bladder, and urethra.
   a.
   b.
   c.
6. List the four most common forms of clubfoot or talipes.
   a.
   b.

   c.

   d.

7. List the three forms of congenital hip dysplasia.

   a.

   b.

   c.

ANSWERS

Multiple Choice

1. a, b, c, and e
2. All the symptoms are possible in cystic fibrosis.
3. a and e

Matching

1, c, b, and a
2. b, d, a, and c

Short Answer

1. Noncommunicating (where there is an obstruction in cerebral spinal fluid flow) Communicating (where there is faulty absorption of cerebral spinal fluid)
2. Projectile vomiting (due to increased size of the pyloric muscle)
3. Cryptorchidism
4. Phenylketonuria. It is an inherited genetic defect due to an error in phenylalanine metabolism. Phenylalanine hydroxylase, an enzyme, is needed to convert phenylalanine to tyrosine. In PKU, this enzyme is absent, causing phenylalanine to accumulate in the blood and urine.
5. Duplicated ureter, retrocaval ureter, ectopic orifice of ureter, stricture or stenosis of ureter, ureterocele, exstrophy of the bladder, congenital bladder diverticulum, hypospadias, and epispadias.
6. a. Talipes varus
   b. Talipes valgus
   c. Talipes equinus
   d. Talipes calcaneus or dorsiflexion
7. a. Unstable hip dysplasia (where the hip can be dislocated manually)
   b. Incomplete dislocation (where the femoral head is on the edge of the acetabulum)
   c. Complete dislocation (where the femoral head is outside the acetabulum)

GLOSSARY

ACETABULUM: The rounded cavity on the outer surface of the hip bone that receives the head of the femur.

ALVEOLI (PULMONARY): The microscopic air sacs in the lungs, through whose walls the exchange of carbon dioxide and oxygen occurs.

ANASTOMOSIS: Surgical, traumatic, or pathologic formation of a connection between two normally separate tubular structures or organs in the body.

AUSCULTATION: Listening to sounds produced by the internal organs or other body parts for diagnostic purposes.

AUTOSOMAL RECESSIVE TRAIT: A trait, carried in a chromosome other than the sex (x and y) chromosome, that expresses itself only when a dominant gene is not present.

BILIRUBIN: An orange to yellow compound in the blood plasma produced by the breakdown of hemoglobin following the normal or pathologic destruction of red blood cells. It is collected by the liver to produce bile.

BRONCHIOLE: One of the many smaller passages conveying air within the lung.

CARDIOMEGALY: Increased volume or size of the heart muscle tissue.

CHYME: The nearly liquid mixture of partially digested food and gastric secretions found in the stomach and duodenum during the digestion of a meal.

CLAUDICATION: Lameness; limping

COLOSTOMY: A surgically created opening in a portion of the large intestine (colon), brought to the abdominal surface for the purpose of evacuating feces. May be temporary or permanent. (Compare with *Ileostomy.*)

CYANOSIS: A bluish discoloration of the skin and mucous membranes due to an increased proportion of unoxygenated hemoglobin in the blood.

DYSTONIA: Impaired or disordered muscle tone.

EPIGASTRIUM: Region of the abdomen over the pit of the stomach.

EPISTAXIS: Hemorrhage from the nose; a nosebleed.

EXCHANGE TRANSFUSION: The repeated removal of small amounts of blood from an individual and its replacement with like amounts of donor blood. Usually performed until a one or two blood volume exchange is achieved.

EXCORIATION: Abrasion of the skin or of the surface of any organ by trauma, chemical agents, burns, or other causes.

EXOCRINE: Pertaining to glands that release their secretions into the digestive tract or to the outer surface of the body.

FEMORAL HEAD: The top or head of the femur, commonly called the thigh or leg bone.

FONTANELLES: Incompletely ossified spaces or soft spots between the cranial bones of the skull of a fetus or infant.

GANGLION: A mass of nerve-cell bodies lying outside the brain and spinal cord.

HEMATURIA: Blood in the urine.

HEMOLYSIS: The rupturing of red blood cells with the resulting release of hemoglobin into the plasma.

HYDRONEPHROSIS: Swelling of the renal pelvis of the kidney with urine due to obstructed outflow.

HYDROURETER: The swelling of the ureter with urine due to obstructed outflow.

HYPERTROPHY: An increase in size or volume of an organ or other body structure produced entirely by an increase in the size of existing cells, not by an increase in the number of cells.

ILEOSTOMY: A surgically created opening in the lower small intestine (ileum), brought to the abdominal surface for the purpose of evacuating feces. May be temporary or permanent. (Compare with *Colostomy.*)

ISOIMMUNIZATION: Immunization of an individual against the blood group antigens (e.g., Rh antigens) of another individual.

LUMEN: The space within an artery, vein, intestine, or other tubular structure.

MENINGES: The three membranes covering the brain and spinal cord.

NEUROBLASTOMA: A malignant, highly invasive tumor composed of embryonic cells of the central nervous system, primarily affecting infants and children.

NYSTAGMUS: Rhythmic, involuntary movement of the eyeball.

PALLOR: Lack of color; paleness, as of the skin.

PARASYMPATHETIC: Referring to a portion of the autonomic (involuntary) nervous system. Activity of the parasympathetic nerves produces affects such as constriction of the pupil of the eye and slowed heart rate.

PERISTALSIS: The involuntary wavelike contractions occurring along the walls of the hollow tubes of the body, especially the esophagus, stomach, and intestines.

PETECHIAE: Small, round, purplish hemorrhagic spots on the skin.

PHOTOTHERAPY: Treatment of disease by exposure of the skin to natural or artificial light.

PROJECTILE VOMITING: Vomiting in which the stomach contents are ejected with great force.

PYLORUS (PYLORIC SPHINCTER): The lower opening of the stomach leading into the duodenum. The pylorus is closed most of the time by the pyloric sphincter, a ring of muscles that opens at intervals to allow the flow of chyme into the duodenum.

RENAL CALCULI: Small crystalline masses formed by the pathologic accumulation of mineral salts in the kidney; kidney stones.

RUBELLA: German measles.

TACHYPNEA: Abnormal, very rapid breathing.

THRILL: An abnormal tremor accompanying a vascular or cardiac murmur felt on palpation.

Chapter 4

Urinary System Diseases

LEARNING OBJECTIVES

Upon successful completion of this chapter, you will
■ Identify the major diseases of the kidney.
■ Name the most common diagnostic procedures to detect kidney and kidney-related diseases.
■ List at least three characteristics common to polycystic kidney disease.
■ Identify complications of kidney-related diseases.
■ Compare and contrast pyelonephritis and glomerulonephritis.
■ Recall infectious precursors to kidney-related diseases.
■ Explain why women are more prone to urinary tract infections.
■ List the characteristics unique to nephrotic syndrome.
■ Name at least three causes of uremia.
■ Describe how acute tubular necrosis occurs.
■ Discuss the complications of renal calculi.
■ Identify possible treatments for renal calculi.
■ Repeat the common signs and symptoms of urinary tract diseases.
■ Describe the prognosis of lower urinary tract infections.
■ Define neurogenic bladder.
■ Compare and contrast the malignant tumors of the bladder and of the kidney.

56

■ Distinguish between the two types of kidney dialysis.
■ List at least four common complaints of the urinary system.

INTRODUCTION

The urinary system is responsible for the production and elimination of urine. The organs of this system include two kidneys, two ureters, the urinary bladder, and the urethra. Figure 4–1 illustrates the interior and exterior features of the urinary system organs.

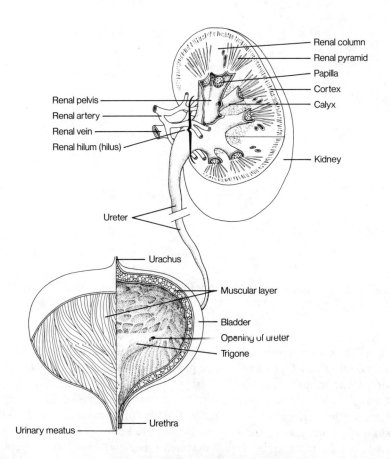

FIGURE 4–1. Urinary system structures. (Modified from Gylys, B. A., and Wedding, M., *Medical Terminology: A Systems Approach,* ed. 2. F. A. Davis, Philadelphia, 1988, p. 241.)

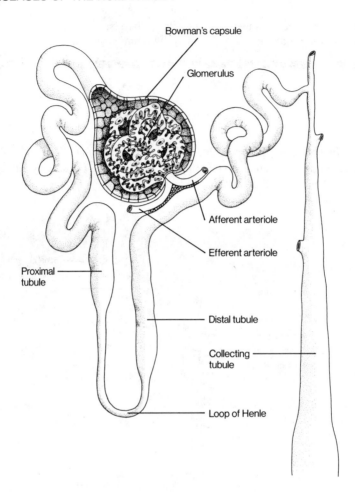

Bowman's capsule

Glomerulus

Afferent arteriole

Efferent arteriole

Proximal tubule

Distal tubule

Collecting tubule

Loop of Henle

FIGURE 4–2. A Nephron. (Modified from Gylys, B. A., and Wedding, M., *Medical Terminology: A Systems Approach,* ed. 2. F. A. Davis, Philadelphia, 1988, p. 242.)

The kidneys help to regulate the water, **electrolyte**, and acid-base content of the blood and selectively filter out the waste products of metabolism. They also play an important role in regulating blood pressure. Each kidney contains over 1 million nephrons (Figure 4–2), which are the principal functional units of the kidney. It is here that the three-part process of selective filtration of wastes, reabsorption of vital minerals and fluid, and secretion of urine takes place.

It is worth emphasizing the reabsorption process of the kidneys' nephrons. Were it not for this process, the body would rapidly be depleted of its fluid. Typically, only 1 percent of the fluid passing through a nephron is excreted as urine.

KIDNEY DISEASES

Polycystic Kidney Disease

Description: *Polycystic kidney disease* is a developmental defect of the collecting tubules in the cortex of the kidneys. Groups of tubules that fail to empty properly into the renal pelvis slowly swell into multiple, grapelike, fluid-filled sacs or cysts. The pressure from the expanding cysts slowly destroys adjacent normal tissue, progressively impairing kidney function. Both kidneys are usually affected.

Etiology: There are two forms of the disease, each due to a genetic defect. The more common adult form, usually manifested during midlife, is an **autosomal dominant** defect. The much less common infant and childhood forms, manifested at birth or during childhood, are **autosomal recessive defects**. The following discussion pertains to the more frequently occurring adult form.

Signs and Symptoms: The disease is usually asymptomatic until midlife. Then the patient may complain of colicky abdominal and **lumbar** pain or mention seeing blood in the urine or passing renal calculi.

Diagnostic Procedures: The patient history may reveal a family tendency for renal disease. The physical examination may reveal palpably enlarged kidneys and **hypertension.** The physician may order an intravenous pyelogram, ultrasound examination, or CT scan to detect enlarged kidneys and the presence of cysts. Urinalysis may be ordered to evaluate renal function and to detect hematuria.

Treatment: No treatment will stop the course of the disease. Treatment goals involve guarding against or managing urinary tract infections and controlling secondary hypertension. Urine cultures should be performed at regular intervals. In the event of renal failure, renal dialysis or kidney transplantation may be attempted to prolong life.

Prognosis: The prognosis is poor. Kidney function is progressively impaired, leading to renal failure, **uremia**, and eventual death.

Prevention: No prevention is known. Genetic counseling may be indicated for families at risk.

Pyelonephritis (Acute)

Description: *Pyelonephritis* is inflammation of the kidney and renal pelvis due to infection. One or both kidneys may be affected. The infection can result in the destruction or scarring of renal tissue, impairing kidney function. It is the most common type of kidney disease and is far more common in women than in men.

Etiology: Pyelonephritis is most commonly due to infection by the bacteria *Escherichia coli*. Staphylococcal and streptococcal bacteria are less frequent agents of infection. The bacteria typically ascend to the kidneys from the lower urinary tract, but they also may enter the kidneys through the blood or lymph.

Women are most at risk, particularly those who are pregnant or practice poor genital hygiene. In men, pyelonephritis may arise as a complication of prostate enlargement. Any catheterization of the urinary tract also increases the likelihood of infection.

Signs and Symptoms: The individual experiencing acute pyelonephritis may complain of nausea, vomiting, diarrhea, chills, fever, and lumbar pain. These symptoms may be accompanied by **pyuria, dysuria**, and **nocturia**.

Diagnostic Procedures: The physical examination may reveal tenderness during palpation of abdominal or lumbar areas. Culture and sensitivity tests are performed on a clean-catch urine specimen. Urinalysis also may reveal **casts** and **hematuria**. X-ray studies may be necessary.

Treatment: Antibiotic therapy is usually the treatment of choice.

Prognosis: The prognosis is variable. Acute pyelonephritis frequently subsides in a few days, even without treatment with antibiotics. Reinfection is likely, however. Repeated infection may lead to a chronic form of the disease, causing enough destruction of kidney tissue to produce renal failure.

Prevention: Individuals should practice proper genital hygiene to avoid introducing bacteria into the urinary tract.

Glomerulonephritis (Acute)

Description: *Glomerulonephritis* is the allergic inflammation of the glomeruli in the kidney's nephrons. The rate of filtration of the blood is reduced, causing retention of water and salts. Resulting injury to the glomeruli may allow red blood cells and serum protein to pass into the urine. Both kidneys are affected.

Etiology: The disease is caused by circulating antigen-antibody complexes that become trapped within the network of the capillaries of a glomerulus. The complexes are produced as a consequence of an infection elsewhere in the body, most frequently following an infection of the upper respiratory tract by streptococcal bacteria. Other bacteria, however, as well as certain viruses and parasites also may induce glomerulonephritis. The disease also may arise as a consequence of various multisystem diseases such as lupus erythematosus. (see Chapter 11.)

Signs and Symptoms: There may be headaches from secondary hypertension, puffy eyes due to **edema** from leaky, inflamed capillaries; pain in the lumbar region from swollen kidneys, and **oliguria** due to the nephron damage. There also may be malaise, **anorexia**, and a low-grade fever.

Diagnostic Procedures: A detailed patient history is important and may reveal a recent streptococcal infection of the upper respiratory tract. Blood tests may show elevated blood urea nitrogen, creatinine, and a rapid sedimentation rate. Urine may be described as "bloody," "coffee-colored," or "smoky." KUB x-rays may reveal bilateral kidney enlargement. A renal biopsy may be necessary to confirm the diagnosis. New methods of fluorescent and electron microscopy have been helpful in distinguishing between different forms of glomerulonephritis.

Treatment: Treatment goals are generally supportive. The physician may prescribe diuretics to control edema and hypertension. Bed rest is usually indicated. Dietary restrictions on salt, protein, and fluid intake may be advised. If an underlying streptococcal infection can be confirmed, antibiotics may be prescribed.

Prognosis: The prognosis is generally good. Most patients with acute glomerulonephritis experience a resolution of symptoms within a few weeks of onset. Children generally recover more rapidly than adults. A few cases, though, may progress into a chronic form of the disease. Repeated acute attacks also may induce the onset of chronic glomerulonephritis.

Prevention: Prompt treatment of any streptococcal pharyngitis or other upper respiratory tract infection is important.

Nephrotic Syndrome

Description: *Nephrotic syndrome* is a disease of the basement membrane of the glomerulus. (The basement membrane surrounds each of the many fine capillaries comprising a glomerulus.) The disease is characterized by severe **proteinuria**, often to the extent that the body cannot keep up with the protein loss (**hypoalbuminemia**). The disease is further characterized by **hyperlipemia**, lipiduria, and generalized edema.

Etiology: Nephrotic syndrome may result from a variety of disease processes having the capacity to damage the basement membrane of the glomerulus. Between 70 and 75 percent of the cases of nephrotic syndrome result from some form of glomerulonephritis. The syndrome also may arise as a consequence of diabetes mellitus, systemic lupus erythematosus, neoplasms, or reactions to drugs or toxins. The disease is occasionally idiopathic in origin.

Signs and Symptoms: Edema is the most common symptom, and it may be either slow in onset or sudden. As body fluid accumulates, the patient may experience shortness of breath and anorexia. **Ascites**, hypertension, **pallor**, and fatigue may result.

Diagnostic Procedures: Nephrotic syndrome may be difficult to diagnose. Urinalysis may reveal proteinuria and increased casts. Blood serum tests may show decreased albumin levels and increased cholesterol. Renal biopsy is important in reaching a definitive diagnosis.

Treatment: Treatment is symptomatic and supportive. The physician will attempt to manage the edema and hyperlipemia. High-protein diets, vitamin supplementation, and salt restriction may be prescribed. Any underlying disease or condition determined to be responsible for the nephrotic syndrome must be treated as well.

Prognosis: The prognosis varies according to the underlying cause and the age of the patient. The prognosis is good for children. With adults, nephrotic syndrome is frequently a manifestation of a serious, progressive kidney disorder or a disorder elsewhere in the body leading to renal failure. Renal vein thrombosis is a complication that significantly worsens the prognosis.

Prevention: Nephrotic syndrome may possibly be avoided through prompt diagnosis and treatment of underlying disorders having the capacity to produce this syndrome.

Chronic Renal Failure (Uremia)

Description: *Chronic renal failure* (CRF) is the gradual, progressive deterioration of kidney function. Nitrogenous end products of metabolism such as **urea** and **creatinine** accumulate in the blood, eventually reaching toxic levels (thus the alternate name *uremia*). As kidney function diminishes, every organ in the body is affected, accounting for the host of symptoms presented by an individual with CRF.

Etiology: Chronic renal failure is most frequently initiated by chronic glomerulonephritis. Other causes include diabetes mellitus, polycystic kidney disease, **nephrosclerosis**, hypertension, and chronic pyelonephritis.

Signs and Symptoms: The patient may complain of progressive weakness and lethargy, weight loss, anorexia, diarrhea, hiccups, pruritus, and **polyuria**. The individual with CRF also may appear mentally confused and have skin that is pallid and scaly.

Diagnostic Procedures: The patient history may reveal a previous renal disease or other predisposing disorder. The physical examination may reveal one or more of the presenting signs and symptoms, along with hypertension. Blood testing typically reveals elevated serum creatinine, blood urea nitrogen, and potassium levels, along with decreased hemoglobin and hematocrit. Urinalysis may reveal proteinuria and urine that is highly diluted. X-rays such as KUB, intravenous pyelogram (IVP), and renal scintiscans may be done to determine the extent of renal damage.

Treatment: Treatment is generally directed at relieving symptoms and guarding against complications. Dietary restrictions of protein, sodium, and potassium intake may be attempted. **Antiemetics** may be prescribed for nausea. Hypertension must be controlled. Dialysis or kidney transplantation may be attempted to prolong life.

Prognosis: The prognosis is poor. A variety of complications often cause death before complete kidney failure occurs. Chief among these are infections, while others include a spectrum of cardiovascular, blood, and gastrointestinal abnormalities.

Prevention: No prevention is known, other than prompt treatment of underlying disorders that may eventually lead to chronic renal failure.

Acute Tubular Necrosis

Description: *Acute tubular necrosis* (ATN) is the rapid destruction or degeneration of the tubular segments of nephrons in the kidneys. ATN is characterized by a sudden deterioration in renal function resulting in the accumulation of nitrogenous wastes in the body. Impaired or interrupted renal function from ATN is considered reversible.

Etiology: The majority of cases of ATN are due to renal **ischemia**, the interruption or impairment of blood flow in and out of the kidneys. While there can be numerous causes for such impairment, renal ischemia leading to ATN is most frequently produced by severe bodily trauma or as a complication following surgery. The renal tubules also can be damaged in other ways. ATN may be toxin-induced (exposure to solvents, heavy metals, certain antibiotics). It also may be caused by transfusion reactions or arise as a complication of pregnancy.

Signs and Symptoms: Since renal failure affects the function of nearly every organ in the body, the individual with ATN may present with a host of widely distributed symptoms. Principal symptoms include oliguria and **anuria**. Other generalized symptoms include weakness, mental confusion, and edema.

Diagnostic Procedures: The patient history may indicate the individual as being at risk for ATN, e.g., after trauma, after surgery, after transfusion, or during pregnancy. The clinician also may seek to determine if the individual could have been exposed to any toxins or was taking certain antibiotics. The clinician also will attempt to eliminate any underlying kidney diseases or urinary tract obstructions as possible causes for the renal failure. Diagnostic tests ordered may include urinalysis, revealing dilute urine with red blood cells and casts. Blood tests will often indicate increased blood urea nitrogen and creatinine or reveal disturbances in the electrolyte balance of the blood.

Treatment: The clinician will generally attempt to promote proper renal circulation if the ATN is due to ischemia. If the ATN is toxin induced, dialysis may be attempted to cleanse the blood. Otherwise, treatment is largely supportive until kidney funciton increases. Supportive treatment may include dietary modifications and carefully controlling fluid intake.

Prognosis: The prognosis is guarded. Before adequate renal function resumes (highly variable period), many individuals with ATN die from complications. These may include cardiovascular complications, gastrointestinal disorders, blood abnormalities, and infections.

Prevention: Prevention includes avoiding exposure to toxins and careful monitoring of individuals known to be at risk.

Renal Calculi (Uroliths or Kidney Stones)

Description: A *renal calculus* is a concentration of various mineral salts in the kidney or elsewhere in the urinary tract.

Etiology: Renal calculi form as a result of a disturbance in the kidneys' delicate balancing act of preventing water loss while at the same time eliminating water-soluble mineral wastes. Many factors, such as prolonged dehydration or immobilization, can upset this balance. The balance also may be upset by underlying diseases such as gout, **hyperparathyroidism,** Cushing's syndrome, or urinary tract infections and neoplasms. The condition appears to be hereditary for certain types of stones, with men much more commonly afflicted than women. In many instances, though, no specific cause can be pinpointed.

Signs and Symptoms: A person having renal calculi may remain asymptomatic for long periods. If a stone or calculus fragment lodges in a ureter, however, the individual may complain of intense flank pain and urinary urgency. Less common presenting symptoms include nausea, vomiting, chills and fever, hematuria, and abdominal distension.

Diagnostic Procedures: The patient history may reveal a familial tendency toward the formation of kidney stones. A urinalysis may be ordered to detect elevated levels of red or white blood cells in the urine or to check for the presence of protein, pus, and bacteria. A KUB x-ray or IVP may be ordered to determine the locations of calculus formation. Blood testing may be helpful in confirming imbalances of minerals in the blood or the existence of other metabolic disorders.

Treatment: Treatment is directed at clearing obstructive stones and preventing the formation of new ones. Increased fluid intake may enhance elimination of stones in some case, but large stones may require surgical intervention, especially if renal function is threatened. New techniques, such as ultrasonic percutaneous lithotripsy, pulverize stones in place, allowing them to be passed in the urine. Antibiotics may be prescribed if it is determined that the calculus buildup is due to bacterial infection. Analgesics may be necessary for relief of intense pain.

Prognosis: The prognosis is good if urinary tract obstruction is prevented and underlying disorders are promptly treated.

Prevention: An adequate daily fluid intake is the best way to minimize the chance of stone formation, especially among individuals at risk.

Hydronephrosis

Description: *Hydronephrosis* is the distension of the renal pelvis and calyces of a kidney due to pressure from accumulating urine. The pressure impairs, and may eventually interrupt, kidney function. One or both kidneys may be affected.

Etiology: Hydronephrosis is caused by a urinary tract obstruction. In children, the obstruction is usually the result of some congenital defect in urinary tract structure. In adults, the obstruction is more often acquired, resulting from blockage by **uroliths** or neoplasms. Urinary tract obstruction in men may be produced by benign or malignant enlargement of the prostate, whereas women may experience urinary tract obstruction as a complication of pregnancy. Underlying disorders such as neurogenic bladder also may allow urine to accumulate to the extent that it produces hydronephrosis.

Signs and Symptoms: If the obstruction is above the opening of the bladder, only one kidney may be affected and the person may be asymptomatic for a prolonged period ("silent" hydronephrosis). Symptoms may be severe, however, especially if both kidneys are affected. The person may complain of intense flank pain, nausea, vomiting, oliguria or anuria, and hematuria.

Diagnostic Procedures: A thorough physical examination of all urogenital structures will be performed. An intravenous or retrograde pyelogram may be ordered to visualize obstructions. Urinalysis may reveal hematuria, pus, and bacteria, as well as assist in determining the extent of any impairment of renal function.

Treatment: Treatment goals include removing the obstruction, preventing complications, and treating underlying disorders. Catheterization may be attempted for the immediate relief of urinary pressure. Analgesics may be prescribed. Surgery is sometimes required. Treatment procedures for renal stones were discussed earlier.

Prognosis: The prognosis is variable, depending on whether one or both kidneys are affected, whether the obstruction can be removed, and whether permanent renal damage has occurred.

Prevention: There are no specific preventative measures.

LOWER URINARY TRACT INFECTIONS (CYSTITIS AND URETHRITIS)

Description: *Cystitis,* inflammation of the bladder, and *urethritis,* inflammation of the urethra, are common lower urinary tract infections (UTI). Together these diseases account for the majority of office visits by individuals experiencing urinary tract problems.

Etiology: Infection by the bacteria *Escherichia coli* accounts for the majority of cases of cystitis and urethritis. Other causative organisms may include *Proteus, Klebsiella, Enterobacter,* and *Pseudomonas* bacteria. These organisms typically ascend the urinary tract from the opening of the urethra, but they also may be introduced as a result of urinary tract catheterization. Urethritis also may be caused by sexually transmitted organisms such as *Chlamydia trachomatis* and *Neisseria gonorrhoeae* (the agents of chlamydia and gonorrhea, respectively).

Women are far more susceptible to ascending urinary tract infections than men. This is due in part to a shorter urethra and the comparative ease with which fecal contaminants can be spread from the anus to the opening of the vagina. Finally, both women and men are more at risk of contracting a lower urinary tract infection as a complication of any disorder that obstructs normal urinary flow.

Signs and Symptoms: The person presenting with cystitis may complain of dysuria, urinary frequency and urgency, and pain above the pubic region. Cloudy, bloody, or foul-smelling urine also may be noted. The individual with urethritis will typically present similar symptoms, with the exception that the quality of the urine is often not affected. Any other symptoms, such as fever, nausea, vomiting, and low back pain, may indicate a simultaneous upper UTI such as pyelonephritis.

Diagnostic Procedures: The patient history may reveal past urinary tract infections, recent catheterization, or a change in sexual partners. A urinalysis is necessary to identify the organism responsible for the infection, as well as the presence of red and white blood cells. Sensitivity tests are necessary to prescribe the appropriate antimicrobial agent.

Treatment: Antibiotics or sulfa drugs appropriate to combat the particular causative organisms may be prescribed. Fluid intake may be increased to promote urinary outflow. Any underlying disorders that are detected must be treated as well. Analgesics may be prescribed for short-term pain relief.

Prognosis: If no complications arise, the prognosis for complete recovery from cystitis and urethritis is quite good. Reinfection in susceptible individuals is likely, however.

Prevention: Preventive measures include maintaining adequate fluid intake, complete emptying of the bladder, and avoiding "holding urine." Proper feminine hygiene, including wiping the perineum from front to back and cleansing well after a bowel movement, will lessen the chance of introducing disease-causing microorganisms into the vagina. Women with a history of lower urinary tract infection also may be placed on a long-term course of antibiotics.

NEUROGENIC BLADDER

Description: *Neurogenic bladder* is any loss or impairment of bladder function caused by central nervous system injury or damage to nerves supplying the bladder. Impaired bladder function may be manifested as either loss of voluntary control of **micturition** or loss of the autonomic reflex, producing the sensation that the bladder is full.

Etiology: Physical trauma to the spinal cord is a frequent cause of neurogenic bladder. Other causes may include nerve damage as a consequence of chronic alcoholism or heavy metal poisoning. Metabolic disorders, such as diabetes mellitus or hypothyroidism, and collagen diseases, such as systemic lupus erythematosus, also may cause this disorder. Neurogenic bladder also may arise as a consequence of multiple sclerosis, **dementia**, and Parkinson's disease.

Signs and Symptoms: An individual with neurogenic bladder may complain of mild to severe urinary **incontinence**, inability to empty the bladder completely, difficulty in starting or stopping voiding, and bladder spasms.

Diagnostic Procedures: Neurogenic bladder often is difficult to diagnose. A detailed patient history and a physical examination that includes a neurologic evaluation are essential. Special tests that may be ordered include a CT scan of the brain, a spinal tap, or cystometry.

Treatment: Treatment goals include preventing complications from urinary tract infection and controlling incontinence through learning special bladder evacuation techniques. Any underlying diseases that are detected will be treated. Various forms of drug therapy or surgery may be attempted to restore bladder function.

Prognosis: The prognosis depends on whether the damage to the nerves supplying the bladder is reversible. Such complications as urinary tract infections and the formation of renal calculi worsen the prognosis. If the disorder is of the form in which sensation of a full bladder is lost, urine may back up, causing hydronephrosis and possible renal failure.

Prevention: There is no specific prevention other than prompt treatment of diseases that may produce nerve damage leading to neurogenic bladder.

TUMORS OF THE URINARY SYSTEM

Tumors of the urinary tract may be benign or malignant; however, the small benign adenomas or fibromas are not clinically significant. The most common malignant tumor of the kidney is adenocarcinoma, followed by Wilm's tumor (discussed in Chapter 3). Tumors of the lower urinary tract are more common than those of the kidney and will be discussed after adenocarcinoma.

Adenocarcinoma of the Kidney (Hypernephroma)

Description: *Adenocarcinoma of the kidney,* or *hypernephroma,* is a malignant neoplasm of the epithelium of a nephron's proximal convoluted tubule. The disease frequently metastasizes to the lungs, liver, brain, and bone marrow.

Etiology: The cause of hypernephroma is not known, but there appears to be a genetic predisposition to the disease. Other risk factors may include exposure to smoke or heavy metals. Adenocarcinoma tends to occur more frequently in men than in women, especially in later midlife.

Signs and Symptoms: An affected individual typically remains asymptomatic until later stages of the disease. Then gross, painless hematuria is the most common presenting symptom. Later on, the individual may report intermittent fever and flank pain.

Diagnostic Procedures: Physical examination may reveal a palpably enlarged kidney in later stages of the disease; x-ray may confirm this. IVP and CT scan of the kidney may be employed to confirm the presence of a renal tumor.

Treatment: Nephrectomy is a common treatment procedure, whether or not the tumor has metastasized. If it is determined that metastasis has occurrred, radiation therapy may be attempted and various palliative measures will be undertaken.

Prognosis: The prognosis varies depending on the staging of the tumor. The 5-year survival rate is about 60 percent if the tumor is confirmed within the affected kidney, dropping to less than 5 percent if extensive metastasis has occurred.[1]

Prevention: No prevention is known.

Tumors of the Bladder

Description: *Tumors of the bladder* arise from the epithelial cell membrane lining the bladder interior. These neoplasms are almost always malignant, and they metastasize readily. Bladder tumors are staged according to their depth of penetration.

Etiology: The cause of bladder tumors is unknown. Predisposing factors may include exposure to certain types of industrial chemicals, and there is an association with cigarette smoking. Individuals with chronic cystitis also seem prone to develop bladder tumors. The disease affects men three times more frequently than women and generally appears after the age of 40.

Signs and Symptoms: Many persons are asymptomatic until advanced stages of the disease. For those presenting with symptoms, however, painless, gross hematuria is the most common indicator. Less frequently, the individual may complain of dysuria, urinary frequency and urgency, or nocturia.

Diagnostic Procedures: The patient history may reveal occupational exposure to certain industrial chemicals. A complete physical examination and a urinalysis to detect hematuria will be performed. Cystoscopy and biopsy of the suspected lesion are usually required to reach a definite diagnosis.

Treatment: The tumor may be surgically removed by **transurethral resection** or fulguration (electrical destruction). For advanced cases, radical **cystectomy** may be required, followed by radiation or chemotherapy treatment.

Prognosis: The prognosis varies, depending on the depth of penetration of the tumor. While the immediate prognosis for an individual with a superficial bladder tumor may be good, there is still a great likelihood of recurrence within 3 years. When the tumor penetrates the bladder more deeply or has metastasized, the prognosis is poor, with a low 5-year survival rate.

Prevention: The best prevention is to minimize risk factors by protecting oneself from exposure to industrial chemicals and by not smoking.

SPECIAL FOCUS:
TREATMENT OF RENAL FAILURE

Dialysis

The blood of an individual experiencing acute or chronic renal failure typically contains high concentrations of metabolic waste products. Dialysis may be attempted to remove these wastes. In its broadest sense, *dialysis* is a process in which water-soluble substances diffuse across a semipermeable membrane. Renal dialysis involves diffusing dissolved substances in the blood across such a semipermeable membrane to remove toxic materials and to maintain proper fluid, electrolyte, and acid-base balances. Two methods are currently used to dialyze the blood: *peritoneal dialysis* and *hemodialysis*.

Peritoneal Dialysis

This process uses a person's own peritoneum as the dialyzing membrane. A plastic tube is inserted through the patient's abdomen into the peritoneal cavity and sutured in place. A dialyzing fluid is passed through the tube into the person's peritoneal cavity and left there for a prescribed period. During this time, wastes diffuse across the peritoneal membrane into the fluid. The contaminated fluid is then drained and replaced with fresh solution. This process can be performed manually or automatically by machine; generally, it is repeated three times a week or as often as required.

A newer form of peritoneal dialysis is *continuous ambulatory dialysis.* After the infusion of the fluid, the dialysis bag can be rolled up and put around the individual's waist, allowing freedom of movement.

Hemodialysis (Extracorporeal Hemodialysis)

In this process, blood is drawn outside the person's body for dialysis in an artificial kidney, or *dialyzer,* and then returned to the individual by means of tubes connected to the person's circulatory system. This form of dialysis treatment takes from 3 to 5 hours, about half the time of peritoneal dialysis. It is the preferred dialysis method in cases of acute renal failure.

Kidney Transplantation

When treating serious kidney disease with a combination of dialysis and transplantation, the results, in many instances, have been promising. Kidney transplantation is being used increasingly despite the technical and immunologic risks associated with the procedure.

The donor of a kidney can be either a close relative of the person receiving the kidney or a recently deceased person (cadaver donor). If the donor and recipient are related, the graft has a better chance of survival. "One study of renal transplants illustrated this fact by showing that 60 percent of kidneys donated by siblings, 50 percent of those donated by parents, and 30 percent of cadaver kidneys remained functional after 5 years."[2]

Any kidney will contain antigens foreign to the recipient, however, unless it is donated by an identical twin. Once the donor antigens are in the recipient, a rejection process begins in which the recipient's immune system produces antibodies that lead to the destruction of the tissue of the transplanted kidney. Immunosuppressive drugs may be administered to combat this process. Still, some recipients may reject the kidney. Once rejection occurs, the donated kidney is removed, and the patient must resume dialysis.

For those persons who do not reject the donor kidney, life can seem relatively normal. But immunosuppressive drugs must be continued indefinitely, making the person more susceptible to infections and other diseases. Sometimes, too, the underlying disease process that destroyed the original kidney may destroy the donor kidney as well.

COMMON SYMPTOMS OF URINARY SYSTEM DISEASES

Individuals may present with the following common complaints, which deserve attention from health professionals:

■ Any change in normal urinary patterns, such as nocturia, hematuria, dysuria, or urgency and frequency
■ Pain in the lumbar region varying from slight tenderness to intense pain
■ Fever
■ Nausea and vomiting or anorexia
■ Malaise, fatigue, and lethargy

Serious urinary system diseases also may produce circulatory system and respiratory system symptoms. These symptoms might include hypertension, edema, ascites, and shortness of breath.

REFERENCES

1. Petersdorf, R.G., et. al., *Harrison's Principles of Internal Medicine,* McGraw-Hill Book Company, New York, 1987, p. 1220.
2. Boyd, H. Sheldon, *Introduction to the Study of Disease,* 9th Ed., Lea & Febiger, Philadelphia, 1984, p. 180.

REVIEW QUESTIONS

Multiple Choice
Select the best answer:
1. The kidney is responsible for
   a. regulation of body fluids.
   b. filtration of wastes from blood.
   c. regulation of blood pressure.
   d. all of the above.
   e. only a and b of the above.

2. Of the fluid that passes through the nephron, _____ percent becomes urine.
   a. 1
   b. 5
   c. 10
   d. 50
   e. 98

3. Urinary tract infections
   a. are more common in males.
   b. usually exhibit dysuria, urgency, and frequency.
   c. commonly are caused by a virus.
   d. do not respond to antibiotic therapy.
   e. have a poor prognosis.

4. The two forms of dialysis are
   a. peritoneal and hemodialysis.
   b. perineal and hemodialysis.
   c. peritoneal and extracorpeal.
   d. perineal and extracorpeal.
   e. a and c of the above.

5. The inability to control urine excretion is called
   a. incontinence
   b. micturition
   c. ischemia
   d. anuria
   e. nocturia

Matching

_____ 1. Nocturia
_____ 2. Anuria
_____ 3. KUB
_____ 4. Ascites
_____ 5. Uremia
_____ 6. Micturition
_____ 7. Pruritus
_____ 8. Pyuria
_____ 9. Oliguria
_____ 10. Hematuria

a. No urinary output
b. Accumulation of serous fluid in abdominal cavity
c. Blood in urine
d. Urination
e. Excessive urination at night
f. Kidneys, ureters, and bladder
g. Scanty urine
h. Urine in blood
i. Pus in urine
j. Itching

Fill in the Blanks

Select from the following:

nephrotic syndrome
pyelonephritis
renal calculi
polycystic kidney
uremia

acute tubular necrosis (ATN)
intravenous pyelogram (IVP)
neurogenic bladder
glomerulonephritis
urinary tract infection (UTI)

1. A disease which exhibits multiple, grapelike, fluid-filled sacs or cysts in the kidney cortex is _____ .
2. When the body cannot keep up with the loss of protein in the urine, _____ is the result.
3. Chronic renal failure often is referred to as _____ .
4. The most common cause of acute renal failure is _____ .
5. Intense pain with urinary frequency, nausea, vomiting, fever, hematuria, and flank pain may indicate _____ .
6. A disorder often difficult to diagnose which is related to any nerve dysfunction of the bladder is _____ .
7. Contrast medium injected intravenously and x-rays taken as the medium clears from the blood is _____ .
8. The most common type of kidney disease is _____ .
9. Headaches from secondary hypertension and puffy eyes due to edema from leaky capillaries may indicate _____ .
10. UTI refers to _____ .

Answers
Multiple Choice
1. d
2. a
3. b
4. e
5. a

Matching
1. e
2. a
3. f
4. b
5. h
6. d
7. j
8. i
9. g
10. c

Fill in the Blanks
1. polycystic kidney
2. nephrotic syndrome
3. uremia
4. acute tubular necrosis (ATN)
5. renal calculi
6. neurogenic bladder
7. intravenous pyelogram (IVP)
8. pyelonephritis
9. glomerulonephritis
10. urinary tract infection

GLOSSARY

ANOREXIA: Loss of appetite for food.

ANTIEMETIC: A drug or other agent used to prevent or stop vomiting.

ANURIA: Cessation of urine production by the kidney.

ASCITES: Abnormal accumulation of fluid in the peritoneal cavity.

AUTOSOMAL DOMINANT DEFECT: A defect that will be expressed in the offspring even though it is carried on only one of the homologous chromosomes.

AUTOSOMAL RECESSIVE DEFECT: A defect carried in a chromosome other than a sex (x and y) chromosome that sometimes expresses itself only when a dominant gene is not present.

CASTS (URINARY): An abnormal component of urine formed from proteins that have precipitated in the renal tubules.

CREATININE: A nitrogen-based compound formed in muscle tissue, passed to the bloodstream, and excreted in the urine. Elevated levels of creatinine in the blood may indicate a kidney disorder.

CYSTECTOMY: As used here, excision of the urinary bladder or a part of it.

DEMENTIA: An irreversibly deteriorating mental state characterized by impaired memory, judgment, and ability to think, caused by cerebral damage due to an organic brain disease.

DYSURIA: Painful or difficult urination, symptomatic of numerous conditions.

EDEMA: Excessive accumulation of fluid in bodily tissues. May be localized or general.

ELECTROLYTES: As used here, the ionized salts present in blood, tissue fluids, and within cells. They are involved in all metabolic processes and are essential to the normal functioning of all cells.

HEMATURIA: Blood in the urine.

HYPERLIPEMIA: Excess levels of fatlike substances called lipids in the blood.

HYPERPARATHYROIDISM: As used here, oversecretion of parathyroid hormone by the parathyroid glands as a consequence of chronic renal disease. Hyperparathyroidism results in a rise in blood calcium and a drop in blood phosphorus levels. Calcium is removed from bones, resulting in increased fragility.

HYPERTENSION: Persistently high arterial blood pressure.

HYPOALBUMINEMIA: Abnormally low levels of a protein called albumin in the blood plasma.

INCONTINENCE: Inability to control the passage of urine, semen, or feces due to one or more physiologic or psychologic conditions.

ISCHEMIA: A temporary deficiency of blood in a body part due to a constriction or obstruction of a blood vessel.

LUMBAR: Pertaining to the part of the back between the thorax and pelvis.

MICTURITION: Urination.

NEPHROSCLEROSIS: Hardening of structures within the kidney, generally associated with hypertension and disease of the renal arterioles.

NOCTURIA: Excessive urination at night.

OLIGURIA: Reduced urine secretion.

PALLOR: Lack of color; paleness, as of the skin.

POLYURIA: Excessive formation and discharge of urine.

PROTEINURIA: Excessive levels of serum protein in the urine.

PYURIA: Pus in the urine.

TRANSURETHRAL RESECTION: Surgical procedure in which a portion of the prostate is removed using an instrument passed up through the urethra.

UREA: The chief nitrogenous constituent of urine.

UREMIA: Toxic condition associated with chronic renal failure and produced by excess levels of urea, creatinine, and other nitrogen-based compounds in the blood.

UROLITH: A concretion, or stone, within the urinary tract.

Chapter 5

Reproductive System Diseases

LEARNING OBJECTIVES

Upon successive completion of this chapter, you will
- Describe the twofold function of human sexuality.
- List the three components of sexual health identified by the World Health Organization.
- Discuss the three factors which cause dyspareunia.
- Compare impotence in males to frigidity in females.
- Identify the possible causes for premature ejaculation.
- List the factors which contribute to both female and male fertility.
- Identify the classic symptoms of infertility.
- Discuss diagnostic procedures used to identify infertility in the male and female.
- Describe the necessity for a complete sexual history when obtaining a patient's medical history.
- List the seven sexually transmitted diseases (STDs).
- Contrast the causes of STDs.
- Identify the diseases related to the prostate gland.
- Discuss the complications of prostate-related disorders.
- Restate the common causes of epididymitis and orchitis.
- Compare the diseases related to a female's menses.
- List the characteristic signs and symptoms of ovarian cysts or tumors.
- Define endometriosis.
- Identify a primary complication of endometriosis.
- Describe the most common tumor in females.
- List the causes of pelvic inflammatory disease.
- Discuss the signs and symptoms of menopause.
- Identify the diagnostic procedures used for diagnosing breast-related diseases.
- List the three reasons for breast reconstruction.
- Recall the possible causes of spontaneous abortion.
- Define ectopic pregnancy.
- Compare preeclampsia to eclampsia.
- Compare placenta previa and abruptio placentae.
- Define PROM.
- List the most common reasons for cesarean birth.
- Recall at least six common complaints of the reproductive system.

INTRODUCTION

The only mammals known to express caring and loving in the sexual act are human beings. For males and females, the function of sexuality is twofold—reproductive and the enhancement of caring and pleasure.

The World Health Organization identifies the following as components of sexual health:[1]

■ The enjoyment and control of sexual and reproductive behavior according to personal and social ethics.

■ Freedom from fear, shame, guilt, misconceptions, and other psychologic factors which inhibit sexual response and can impair sexual relationships.

■ Freedom from organic disorders, diseases, and deficiencies that may interfere with either sexual or reproductive functions.

Experiences of arousal, plateau, orgasm, and resolution characterize the stages of the human sexual response cycle. *Arousal,* or excitement, is psychologically determined, whereas the remaining stages have both psychologic and physiologic components. The major physiologic processes of the sexual response cycle include **vasoconstriction** and **myotonia.** Sexual dysfunction may result if some physical or mental condition arises that interferes with any of these stages.

SEXUAL DYSFUNCTION

An important consideration in the treatment of any sexual dysfunction is a sensitivity to open communication of the problem. Both the patient and the physician may have difficulty in raising questions regarding sexual functions. If this occurs, dysfunctions may go undetected and untreated.

All health care professionals need to be alert to patients' signals and questions that may indicate a sexual concern. Patients often feel more comfortable raising a question to someone other than the physician. Therefore, it is important that the physician include a detailed sexual history in a patient's medical history. All health professionals need to feel comfortable initiating questions about sexual function. Health care that treats the total person cannot ignore the human sexual response and its function or dysfunction.

Dyspareunia (Painful Intercourse)

Description: *Dyspareunia* is the occurrence of pain in women during sexual intercourse.

Etiology: Painful intercourse may result from any of the following causes.

■ *Anatomic:* Congenital deformities of the vagina, an intact hymen

■ *Pathologic:* Scar tissue, genitourinary tract infections, pelvic inflammatory disease, abnormal growths

■ *Psychosomatic:* Fear of pain or injury, feelings of guilt or shame, lack of arousal resulting in insufficient lubrication, ignorance of sexual anatomy and physiology, fear of pregnancy

Signs and Symptoms: The individual may experience mild to severe discomfort during or after intercourse. Vaginal itching or burning also may occur.

Diagnostic Procedures: A physical examination will be performed and diagnostic tests ordered to detect any underlying anatomic or pathologic causes of the dyspareunia. A detailed sexual history is important to help reveal any psychologic factors that may be causing the disorder.

Treatment: Individuals may be instructed to use creams or water-soluble jellies for lubrication prior to intercourse. Medications may be prescribed if any infections are detected. Excision of any scars and gentle stretching of the vaginal orifice may be needed. Education about the sexual response and counseling or psychotherapy may be indicated.

Prognosis: The prognosis is good with adequate treatment, proper education, and sensitivity on the part of the woman's sexual partner.

Prevention: Preventive measures include prompt treatment of any infections or inflammatory diseases of the genitourinary tract.

Impotence

Description: *Impotence* is the inability of a male to achieve or sustain an erection.

Etiology: Impotence may be psychologic or physiologic in cause. Psychologic causes include anxiety or depression. Physiologic causes include certain pharmacologic agents, drug abuse, diabetes mellitus, surgical complications, spinal cord and disk injuries, and neurologic, endocrine, or urologic disorders.

Signs and Symptoms: The individual may express a loss of sexual desire or the inability to achieve or maintain an erection even though aroused.

Diagnostic Procedures: The diagnostic procedures will help to differentiate between physiologic and psychologic causes of the impotence. They will typically include a physical examination, medical history, and detailed sexual history.

Treatment: Treatment of impotence may include therapy to correct any underlying physiologic disorders and counseling or psychotherapy to alleviate psychologic problems. The surgical implantation of a penile prosthesis is a treatment option for individuals when impotence is due to untreatable neurologic or vascular disorders.

Prognosis: The prognosis is variable, depending on how long the patient has suffered from the dysfunction and how severe it is.

Prevention: Prompt treatment of any physiologic cause is important.

Frigidity

Description: *Frigidity* is partial or complete failure to attain or maintain the vaginal lubrication-swelling response of sexual excitement until completion of the sex act.

Etiology: *Frigidity* may be caused by physiologic factors, especially diseases that produce nerve damage, such as diabetes mellitus or multiple sclerosis. Drug reactions, pelvic infections, and vascular disease also may produce frigidity. More commonly, however, frigidity is due to psychologic factors such as anxiety, depression, sexual misinformation, poor sexual techniques, and early traumatic sexual experiences.

Signs and Symptoms: A female may express a loss of sexual desire or report slow sexual arousal. She may lack the vaginal lubrication and vasocongestive response of sexual arousal.

Diagnostic Procedures: A physical examination, medical history, and a detailed sexual history are needed to differentiate physiologic causes from psychologic causes.

Treatment: The treatment of frigidity is directed toward correcting underlying physiologic disorders or alleviating any psychologic problems. The latter may involve therapy for both partners.

Prognosis: In the absence of nerve damage, the prognosis is good if the female has had some sexual arousal previously. Psychologic causes may require lengthy treatment.

Prevention: Early treatment of any physiologic or psychologic problem is the best prevention.

Premature Ejaculation

Description: *Premature ejaculation* is the expulsion of seminal fluid prior to complete erection of the penis or immediately following the beginning of sexual intercourse.

Etiology: Psychologic factors of premature ejaculation include anxiety or guilt feelings about sex. Negative sexual relationships, such as may exist when a male unconsciously dislikes females or seeks to deny his partner's need for sexual gratification, also may induce premature ejaculation. Pathologic factors are rare, but they may be linked to degenerative neurologic disorders, urethritis, or prostatitis.

Signs and Symptoms: Ejaculation during foreplay, prior to complete erection of the penis, or as soon as **intromission** occurs are the classic symptoms.

Diagnostic Procedures: Physical examination and laboratory tests may be ordered to rule out any pathologic causes. A detailed sexual history is important to adequately assess this dysfunction.

Treatment: An intensive program of psychotherapy may be necessary. It is important that both partners be involved in the treatment and that they understand that the condition is reversible.

Prognosis: The prognosis is excellent with proper treatment and understanding on the part of both partners. A positive self-image should be encouraged by explaining that premature ejaculation is a disorder that does not reflect on one's masculinity.

Prevention: No prevention is known.

Male and Female Infertility

Description: *Infertility* is diagnosed as the failure to become pregnant after 1 year of regular, unprotected intercourse. About 10 percent of couples are infertile. Female fertility normally peaks at 24 years of age and diminishes after 30, with pregnancy occurring rarely after the age of 50. Hormonal balances, the ovulation cycle, and vaginal secretions determine female fertility. A female is most fertile within 24 hours of ovulation.

Male fertility peaks usually at age 25 and declines after age 40. Sperm count, semen composition, and bodily hormonal changes affect male fertility. Greatest fertility for a male occurs when he has sexual intercourse four times a week.

Etiology: Causes of infertility in females include hormonal problems, nutritional deficiencies, infections, tumors, and anomalies of the reproductive organs. In males, persistent infertility may be caused by sperm deficiencies, congenital abnormalities, endocrine imbalances, and chronic inflammation of the testes, epididymis, or vas deferens.

Signs and Symptoms: There is typically no obvious sexual dysfunction on the part of either the male or female other than the female's inability to conceive.

Diagnostic Procedures: In a female, a complete medical, surgical, and gynecologic history and examination are essential. Laboratory studies ordered may include urinalysis, complete blood count, and the serology test for syphilis. Hysterosalpingography may be necessary to detect uterine abnormalities. An analysis of cervical mucus just prior to ovulation and within 6 hours after **coitus** may be done. Vaginal smears or an endometrial biopsy may be required. Tests may be performed to determine if the fallopian tubes are patent or obstructed, or a laparoscopy may be ordered to detect endometriosis.

In a male, a complete ejaculate following sexual abstinence of 4 days should be examined within 1 to 2 hours of collection. A complete physical examination including rectal and genital palpation is essential. Laboratory studies may include urinalysis, complete blood count, and the serology test for syphilis. A testicular biopsy may be performed if **azoospermia** or **oligospermia** is determined. Cystoscopy and catheterization of ejaculatory ducts may be ordered to detect any occlusion or stenosis of the tubes.

Treatment: The treatment of infertility is dependent on the cause. In a female, treatment may include any of the following:

■ Salpingostomy
■ Lysis of adhesions
■ Removal of ovarian abnormalities
■ Correction of endocrine imbalance
■ Alleviation of **cervicitis**
■ Microsurgical excision of tubal obstructions

  In a male, treatment may include any of the following:
■ Surgical correction of any abnormality

- Correction of testicular hypofunction secondary to **hypothyroidism**
- Surgical correction of **varicocele** or **hydrocele**
- Prompt treatment of mumps orchitis[2]

Prognosis: About 50 percent of those couples who are treated for infertility achieve pregnancy. The remainder of the cases are untreatable and complicated.

Prevention: Prevention of infertility in females and males generally involves avoiding the causative factors leading to acquired infertility, such as infections, drugs and alcohol, trauma, and environmental agents.

SEXUALLY TRANSMITTED DISEASES (STDs)

Gonorrhea

Description: *Gonorrhea* is a contagious bacterial infection of the epithelial surfaces of the genitourinary tract in males and females. It is currently the most prevalent sexually transmitted (venereal) disease in the United States.

Etiology: Gonorrhea is caused by the bacterium *Neisseria gonorrhoeae*. The disease is transmitted during sexual intercourse with an infected partner or by other forms of intimate sexual contact. Infants born of infected mothers can contract gonorrhea during vaginal delivery, with the bacteria infecting the conjunctivae, respiratory tract, or anal canal.

Signs and Symptoms: The signs and symptoms of gonorrhea will vary according to the site and duration of the infection, the particular characteristics of the infecting strain, and whether the infection remains localized or becomes systemic. It is worth emphasizing, however, that many cases of gonorrhea, especially in females, are asymptomatic or produce symptoms that are so slight that they are ignored by the infected individual.

The presenting symptoms of an infected male are typically those of acute urethritis: **purulent** urethral discharge, **dysuria**, and urinary frequency. A purulent discharge from the pharynx or rectum with accompanying pain may be the presenting symptoms among infected homosexual men.

The symptoms of an infected female are typically those of acute cervicitis: purulent vaginal discharge, dysuria, urinary frequency, or abnormal menstrual bleeding. Other symptoms may include pelvic pain with muscular ridigity or abdominal tenderness and distension.

In the newborn, **gonorrheal ophthalmia neonatorum** may produce a purulent discharge from the eyes 2 to 3 days after birth. Eyelid edema may be evident as well.

Diagnostic Procedures: Bacterial cultures from the site of infection will generally establish the diagnosis.

Treatment: Antibiotics will be given, with various penicillins or tetracycline being the drugs of choice. Patients are advised to have a second culture 1 to 2 weeks after the first and then again in about 6 months to ensure that they no longer have the disease.

Prognosis: The prognosis is good with prompt diagnosis and treatment of localized gonorrheal infections. Systemic gonorrheal infections may produce joint destruction or potentially life-threatening complications such as meningitis or endocarditis. Pelvic inflammatory disease is a serious complication of gonorrheal infection among women, producing fever, nausea, vomiting, and tachycardia.

Prevention: The use of condoms and the tracing of the sexual contacts of an infected individual aid in preventing the spread of gonorrhea. Instillation of a 1% silver nitrate solution in the eyes of the newborn has reduced the incidence of gonococcal ophthalmia neonatorum.

Genital Herpes

Description: *Genital,* or *venereal, herpes* is a highly contagious viral infection of the male and female genitalia. Unlike other sexually transmitted diseases, genital herpes tends to spontaneously recur. The disease has two stages. During the active stage, characteristic skin lesions and other accompanying symptoms may occur. During the latent stage, the individual is asymptomatic. The incidence of genital herpes is steadily increasing in the United States.

Etiology: Genital herpes is caused by the herpes simplex virus (HSV). Although two strains of the virus—designated HSV-1 and HSV-2—may produce the disease, most cases of genital herpes are attributable to HSV-2. The disease is transmitted by direct contact with infected bodily secretions. Infection typically occurs during sexual intercourse, but it may possibly occur from contact with infected personal care items or clothing. A particularly life-threatening form of the disease can occur in infants infected by the virus during vaginal birth.

Signs and Symptoms: During the active phase of the disease, males and females may present with characteristic skin **lesions** on their genitals. These appear as multiple, shallow ulcerations, **pustules,** or erythematous **vesicles**. The vesicles tend to rupture upon urination, causing acute pain and consequent itching. Other generalized symptoms may include fever, headache, malaise, muscle pain, anorexia, and dysuria. **Leukorrhea** may be a further symptom in women.

Diagnostic Procedures: Physical examination for evidence of the characteristic lesions is usually sufficient for diagnosis. Scraping and biopsy of the ulceration may be required to confirm the diagnosis.

Treatment: Treatment of genital herpes is generally symptomatic. Topical medications may be ordered to reduce edema and pain. The individual should be encouraged to keep any lesions clean and dry. Treatment with new classes of antiviral drugs has shown promise in reducing the active phase of the disease, although these will not eradicate the virus. Secondary infections need to be prevented or speedily managed.

Prognosis: Genital herpes cannot be cured. The prognosis varies according to the individual's age, the severity of the infection, and the individual's immunologic response. It is estimated that as many as 80 percent of individuals with primary genital herpes infections will experience a recurrence within 12 months. Very serious complications can result if the virus spreads systemically. The virus is also associated with cervical cancer.

Prevention: No proven method of prevention among adults has been established other than avoiding sexual intercourse with infected individuals. Transmission of the disease to infants can be minimized through cesarean delivery when it is known that the mother is infective.

Genital Warts

Description: *Genital warts* are circumscribed, elevated skin lesions, usually seen on the external genitalia or near the anus. Their incidence is increasing in the United States.

Etiology: Genital warts are caused by several types of human **papillomaviruses** (HPV). They are typically spread from person to person during sexual intercourse. These warts have a prolonged incubation period of 1 to 6 months.

Signs and Symptoms: The patient may be asymptomatic or experience tenderness in the area of the wart. Genital warts appear as solitary or clustered lesions. In males, the warts typically occur at the end of the penis, but they may appear anywhere along the penis as well. They also may appear in the perianal area, especially among homosexual males. In women, the warts typically appear near the opening of the vagina, and they commonly spread to the perianal area. The warts may vary in size from tiny to 3 or 4 inches in diameter.

Diagnostic Procedures: The characteristic appearance and location of the lesions are usually sufficient for diagnosis. Scrapings from wart cells may help in confirming the diagnosis.

Treatment: No form of treatment is especially effective. Topical medication may be applied or surgery, **cryosurgery, electrocautery,** or **debridement** may be attempted. Small warts may require no treatment.

Prognosis: The prognosis is variable. Spontaneous "cures" occur in about half of the cases, but the remainder may be unresponsive to any form of treatment.

Prevention: There is no known prevention other than avoiding sexual intercourse with infected individuals.

Syphilis

Description: *Syphilis* is a highly infectious, chronic, sexually transmitted disease characterized by lesions that may involve any organ or tissue.

Etiology: Syphilis is caused by the bacterium *Treponema pallidum.* The bacteria are transmitted by direct contact with infected lesions, typically through sexual intercourse or through contact with infected bodily fluids. Syphilis also may be contracted as a consequence of transfusion with infected blood (a rare occurrence). In pregnant women, *Treponema pallidum* can cross the placenta and infect the fetus, causing serious fetal damage.

The bacteria rapidly penetrate skin or mucous membrane. From the point of infection, they spread into the lymphatic system and the blood, producing a systemic infection. Typically, the bacteria will have been carried throughout the body long before the first clinical symptoms appear.

Signs and Symptoms: When untreated, syphilis typically progresses through three clinical stages, each with characteristic signs and symptoms. Note, however, that some infected individuals will be asymptomatic or present with symptoms that are not readily evident upon casual inspection.

Primary syphilis is characterized by the appearance of a distinctive, painless lesion, called a **chancre,** at the point of infection. In males, the chancre typically appears on the penis. The chancre also may appear on the anus or within the rectum of homosexual males. Among females, the lesion typically appears on the labia of the vagina or within the vagina or cervix. Among both men and women, chancres also may appear on the lips, tongue, fingers, or nipples. The appearance of the chancre also may be accompanied by regional **lymphadenopathy.** It must be emphasized that the chancres are *highly contagious.*

Secondary syphilis can produce a host of symptoms, many of which may be mistaken for other diseases. Most frequently, though, individuals at this stage of the disease will present with a skin rash characterized by uniform **macular, papular, pustular,** or nodular lesions. These typically, but not exclusively, appear on the palms or soles. In moist areas of the body, these lesions may erode and become contagious. Various general or systemic manifestations may accompany the rash, including headache, malaise, gastrointestinal upset, sore throat, fever, **alopecia,** and brittle nails.

After the manifestations of secondary syphilis subside, a *latent* stage of the disease begins in which the infected individual is generally asymptomatic. The bacteria may remain latent indefinitely. But in roughly half of untreated individuals with latent syphilis, manifestations of the final, or *tertiary,* stage of the disease begin to appear 2 to 7 years after the initial infection. In tertiary syphilis, the *Treponema* bacteria may cause life-threatening damage to the aorta of the heart, the central nervous system, or the musculoskeletal system. No organ system is immune from damage, however. Consequently, the symptoms of tertiary syphilis mimic the symptoms of other organ system diseases, making diagnosis difficult.

Diagnostic Procedures: The most sensitive test available for detecting syphilis is the *fluorescent treponemal antibody-absorption (FTA–ABS) test.* A Venereal Disease Research Laboratories (VDRL) and cerebrospinal fluid (CSF) examination also may be performed.

Treatment: Penicillin G is the antibiotic of choice for treatment of all stages of syphilis. Tetracycline or erythromycin may be used in the event of allergic reaction to penicillin. Any lesions should be kept as dry and clean as possible. Regular

VDRL testing typically accompanies the drug therapy in order to be certain that the *Treponema* bacteria have been eradicated.

Prognosis: The prognosis varies with the age of the affected individual and with the stage at which the disease is detected and treated. The prognosis for complete recovery is very good for adults treated for primary and secondary syphilis. While tertiary disease also can be successfully treated, any organ system damage that may have occurred to that point is generally irreversible. Untreated, the disease may lead to life-threatening heart, central nervous system, or musculoskeletal disorders. The prognosis is poor for a fetus infected with syphilis, with spontaneous abortion or stillbirth occurring in nearly 20 percent of cases.

Prevention: The use of condoms during sexual intercourse can reduce the possibility of transmitting or acquiring syphilis. Contact tracing of intimate partners and serologic screening, though, remain the most important methods in limiting the spread of this disease.

Trichomoniasis

Description: *Trichomoniasis* is a protozoal infestation of the vagina, urethra, or prostate.

Etiology: *Trichomonas vaginalis,* a motile protozoan, is the cause of trichomoniasis. The disease usually is transmitted by sexual intercourse and affects 10 to 15 percent of sexually active persons. Women may increase their susceptibility to *Trichomonas* infection by using vaginal sprays and over-the-counter douches. These preparations may change the natural flora of the vagina sufficiently enough to create a more hospitable enviornment for the parasite.

Signs and Symptoms: Nearly half of females with trichomoniasis are asymptomatic for the first 6 months. When symptoms occur, they are usually those of acute vaginitis: a strong-smelling, greenish yellow, frothy vaginal discharge, possibly accompanied by itching, swelling, dyspareunia, and dysuria. Symptoms may persist for several months if untreated.

In most males, the disease may be asymptomatic. When symptoms are present, they are typically those of urethritis, such as dysuria and urinary frequency.

Diagnostic Procedures. Diagnosis of trichomoniasis is facilitated by microscopic examination of vaginal or urethral discharges. The disease also may be detected through urinalysis.

Treatment: Treatment of both partners with antiparasitic drugs usually cures trichomoniasis. After treatment, both sexual partners should have a follow-up examination.

Prognosis: The prognosis is good with proper treatment. Reinfection may occur, however.

Prevention: Persons can reduce the risk of infection by wearing cotton and loose-fitting underwear that allows ventilation, since bacteria grow in warm, dark, and moist places. Cleanliness is also important.

Chlamydial Infections

Description: *Chlamydial infection* is a sexually transmitted infection causing inflammation of the urethra and epididymis in men and inflammation of the cervix in women. Chlamydial infections are now highly prevalent and among the most potentially damaging of all the STDs in the United States.

Etiology: Chlamydial infection is caused by the bacterium *Chlamydia trachomatis.*

Signs and Symptoms: An individual may be asymptomatic or present with very mild symptoms. Thus this disease is sometimes called the "silent" STD. Clinical manifestations in many women may resemble those of gonorrhea. These include itching and burning in the genital area, mucopurulent vaginal discharge, and cervicitis. In men, urethritis and epididymitis may result.

Diagnostic Procedures: Diagnosis can be confirmed by cytologic and serologic studies.

Treatment: The recommended treatment is an antibiotic such as tetracycline or erythromycin. Both partners should be treated simultaneously.

Prognosis: The prognosis is good if treatment is instituted early. If left untreated, complications include disease of the fallopian tubes, pelvic inflammatory disease, and infertility in women. Men may become sterile.

Prevention: The use of condoms during sexual intercourse can reduce the possibility of transmitting or acquiring chlamydial infection. Contact tracing of intimate partners and serologic screening, though, remain the most important methods of limiting the spread of this disease.

Acquired Immune Deficiency Syndrome (AIDS)

Description: *Acquired immune deficiency syndrome* (AIDS) is a severe illness associated with a human immune-deficiency virus (HIV) infection. The Surgeon General of the United States estimates that by the end of 1991, 270,000 cases of AIDS will have occurred in the United States and 5 to 10 million Americans will have been infected with HIV. An estimated 179,000 deaths from AIDS will have occurred by 1991, only 10 years after AIDS was first recognized.

The majority of individuals suffering from AIDS are male homosexuals and bisexuals, followed by intravenous drug users. Other individuals at risk are sexual partners of those infected with HIV, persons who have received blood products and transfusions infected with HIV (before screening of blood and blood products was possible), and children born to mothers infected with HIV.

Etiology: HIV belongs to the group of retroviruses. These viruses carry their genetic material in the form of RNA rather than DNA. HIV infects a class of cells called helper T-4 lymphocytes, taking over the genetic machinery of the infected cells. The result is that copies of the virus are replicated within the cell. The cell is killed, and the newly produced viruses then infect other T-4 lymphocytes.

AIDS is deadly because T-4 lymphocytes are an important component of the body's immune response. They recognize foreign antigens, activate antibody-producing B-cell lymphocytes, and defend against parasitic infections. When T-4 lymphocyte function is impaired, the means is provided for **opportunistic infections** to invade and cause serious illness.

Signs and Symptoms: AIDS usually produces a spectrum of clinical manifestations. The pulmonary, gastrointestinal, and neurologic systems may be involved, and several forms of malignancy and chronic illnesses may result:

- *Pulmonary symptoms* include shortness of breath, dyspnea, coughing, chest pain, and fever caused by a variety of opportunistic infections. The most common pulmonary infection is *Pneumocystis carinii* pneumonia, which has a mortality rate of 60 percent.
- *Gastrointestinal symptoms* of AIDS may include loss of appetite, nausea, vomiting, oral candidiasis, and chronic diarrhea. Diarrhea occurs in over half of all AIDS patients.
- *Neurologic symptoms* may include memory loss, headache, depression, fever, confusion, and visual disturbances.
- *Malignancies* commonly associated with AIDS include Kaposi's sarcoma, a neoplasm evidenced by multiple vascular nodules in the skin and other organs. This malignant neoplasm is especially prevalent in the lymph nodes, the gastrointestinal tract, and the lungs. The purple lesions characterizing Kaposi's sarcoma may appear on the skin and grow rapidly until wounds are produced that increase the patient's susceptibility to infections.
- *Chronic illness.* Because AIDS patients are often severely immunocompromised, nearly all eventually develop one or more chronic opportunistic infections during the course of the disease. Such illnesses may complicate treatment and produce debilitating symptoms.

Diagnostic Procedures: It is necessary to obtain a complete patient history (including risk factors) and perform a physical examination. Laboratory studies are essential to determine the extent of immune system impairment, the presence of any opportunistic infections, and the presence of HIV antibodies.

Treatment: Currently there is no effective treatment to stop the HIV infection and the immunodeficiency it causes. It is important to manage the opportunistic infections and malignancies as aggressively as possible, using antimicrobial agents for infections and radiation therapy or chemotherapy for the malignancies. Chronic illnesses may require symptomatic treatment for malnutrition, weakness, immobility, diarrhea, skin lesions, and altered mental state.

Prognosis: To date there have been no reports of spontaneous reversal of the immune deficiency that characterizes AIDS. Recurrent bouts of opportunistic infections, with or without malignancies, ultimately cause the death of the patient.

Researchers are looking for ways to halt the immunodeficiency virus. A promising recent development is the antiviral drug azidothymidine (AZT), which appears to be effective in preventing the virus from replicating in some individuals. Experiments have been attempted with interferon in an attempt to reconstitute and enhance the operation of the immune system. Other experimental treatments have included bone marrow transplantation and infusions of lymphocytes.

Prevention: The use of condoms for any form of sexual intercourse is essential. Body fluids and items such as used hypodermic needles should be considered potentially infective. Blood products from blood donors are now screened by the enzyme-linked immunosorbent assay (ELISA) test to detect the presence of HIV antibodies.

Common Symptoms of STDs

Individuals with STDs may present with the following common symptoms, which deserve attention from health professionals:
■ Dysuria, **hematuria**, urinary frequency or incontinence, purulent discharge, or burning and itching upon urination
■ Pelvic or genital pain
■ Any skin ulcerations in the genital area
■ Fever and malaise
■ Dyspareunia

MALE REPRODUCTIVE DISEASES

Prostatitis

Description: *Prostatitis* is inflammation of the prostate gland (Figure 5–1). The condition may be acute or chronic, the latter being more common in men over 50 years old.

Etiology: Prostatitis may be either bacterial or nonbacterial in origin. Bacterial causes of the disease include *E. coli, Proteus, Staphylococcus, Streptococcus,* or *Pseudomonas.* Routes of infection can be either via the urethra or bloodstream. In nonbacterial prostatitis, no infectious agent is detectable.

Signs and Symptoms: Low back pain, **myalgia**, perineal fullness or pain, fever, dysuria, urethral discharge, and urinary frequency are common symptoms of acute prostatitis. The prostate, when palpated, may be enlarged, tender, and boggy. An individual with chronic protatitis may be asymptomatic or experience sporadic, mild forms of acute symptoms.

Diagnostic Procedures: Urinalysis, urine culture, and a rectal examination help in diagnosing prostatitis. Abnormally high urine leukocyte counts in the absence of detectable bacteria are indicative of nonbacterial prostatitis.

Treatment: Antimicrobial therapy is initiated, and the patient is usually advised to rest and increase fluid intake. **Analgesics, antipyretics** and stool softeners also may be ordered. Sitz baths may be recommended.

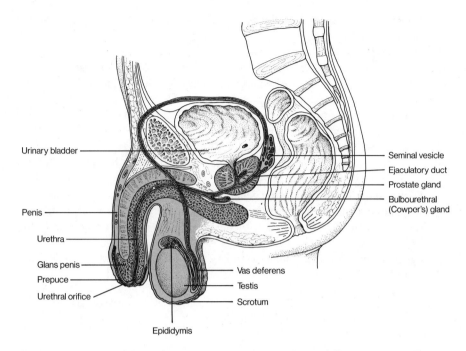

Urinary bladder

Penis

Urethra

Glans penis

Prepuce

Urethral orifice

Seminal vesicle

Ejaculatory duct

Prostate gland

Bulbourethral
(Cowper's) gland

Vas deferens

Testis

Scrotum

Epididymis

FIGURE 5–1. The male reproductive system. (Modified from Gylys, B. A. and Wedding, M. E., *Medical Terminology: A Systems Approach,* ed. 2. F. A. Davis, Philadelphia, 1988, p. 244.)

Prognosis: Acute prostatitis responds well to treatment; however, chronic prostatitis does not. Complications may include epididymitis, cystitis, and urethritis. Chronic prostatitis predisposes to recurrent urinary tract infections, urethral obstruction, and acute urinary retention.

Prevention: Early treatment of urinary tract infections is the best prevention.

Epididymitis

Description: *Epididymitis* is inflammation of the epididymis due to infection. The condition is typically unilateral.

Etiology: *Chlamydia trachomatis* and *Neisseria gonorrhoeae* are the most common infectious agents causing epididymitis among sexually active males. Other bacterial causes of this condition include *E. coli, Staphylococcus,* and *Streptococcus.* Epididymitis can occur as a result of prostatitis, a urinary tract infection, mumps, tuberculosis, or sexually transmitted diseases such as gonorrhea and syphilis. Trauma, prostatectomy, or the prolonged use of an indwelling catheter may predispose to epididymitis.

Signs and Symptoms: The epididymis may become enlarged, hard, and tender, causing pain. Scrotal and groin tenderness, fever, and malaise also may occur. Groin tenderness is the result of enlarged lymph nodes in the groin. Patients may "waddle" as they walk, trying to protect the scrotal area.

Diagnostic Procedures: Urinalysis and urine cultures help in the diagnosis. An increased leukocyte count is common.

Treatment: Antimicrobial therapy appropriate for the particular causative agent will be initiated. A scrotal support and analgesics may be helpful. Bed rest may be necessary in the acute phase.

Prognosis: The inflammation generally responds well to therapy, but portions of the epididymis may be scarred. Consequently, sterility may result if treatment is delayed, especially if the disease is bilateral. Orchitis may develop as a further complication.

Prevention: Early treatment of urinary tract infection is the best prevention. The use of a condom during sexual intercourse is recommended.

Orchitis

Description: *Orchitis* is inflammation of the testes due to infection. The condition may be either bilateral or unilateral.

Etiology: Orchitis typically arises as a consequence of infection from mumps virus. Other viruses and bacteria also can produce this condition. Orchitis also may accompany a case of epididymitis. Scrotal trauma may predispose an individual to orchitis.

Signs and Symptoms: Unilateral or bilateral testicular swelling or tenderness with acute pain are the common presenting symptoms of orchitis. These symptoms are typically accompanied by chills, fever, malaise, nausea, and vomiting.

Diagnostic Procedures: The individual's clinical history may reveal a recent or ongoing case of mumps or other related disease. Testicular examination will suggest the diagnosis. Serology, urinalysis, or throat cultures may be used to isolate mumps virus or identify other causative agents.

Treatment: No specific treatment is effective against mumps virus–induced orchitis. Treatment is typically supportive. Analgesics and antipyretics may be prescribed. Certain adrenal steroid drugs may be used to reduce swelling and fever in severe cases. Bed rest is generally indicated, and the wearing of a scrotal support may be helpful. If the orchitis is bacterial in origin, the appropriate antibiotic therapy should be instituted.

Prognosis: .The prognosis is good. Atrophy of the affected testicle occurs in half the cases, but complete sterility is unusual.

Prevention: To prevent mumps orchitis, the mumps vaccine is recommended for prepubertal males and all adult males who have not had clinical mumps.

Benign Prostatic Hyperplasia (BPH)

Description: *Benign prostatic hyperplasia* is the overproliferation of cells within the inner portion of the prostate. The condition is normal in males over 60 years of age. It is only clinically significant if the enlarging, hyperplastic portion of the prostate obstructs urinary outflow.

Etiology: The etiology of BPH is not well understood, but it seems to be due to metabolic and hormonal changes associated with aging. In clinically significant BPH, the gland compresses the urethra or the neck of the bladder, obstructing urinary flow. Less frequently, the enlarged portion of the prostate may press against the rectum, causing constipation.

Signs and Symptoms: The individual may report symptoms of urinary obstruction, such as difficulty in initiating urination or in completely emptying the bladder. Other symptoms may include dysuria, urinary frequency, or urinary or fecal incontinence. In severe cases of BPH-caused urinary obstruction, the individual may present with symptoms of hydronephrosis or pyelonephritis.

Diagnostic Procedures: Symptomatology of the patient and a rectal examination may be sufficient for diagnosis. However, urinalysis, urine culture, intravenous pyelogram (IVP), and cystoscopy may be ordered to confirm the diagnosis. Prostatic biopsy may be required to ensure that prostatic carcinoma is not causing enlargement.

Treatment: Symptomatic treatment may include prostatic massage, catheterization, and sitz baths. Various surgical procedures such as transurethral resection may be done to remove urinary tract obstruction. Regular sexual intercourse may help to relieve prostatic congestion.

Prognosis: Prognosis is good with surgical intervention, and the mortality rate is low. If untreated, infections may ascend to the kidney, or various urinary obstructive disorders may result. Complications include cystitis, dilation of the ureters, hydronephrosis, pyelonephritis, and uremia.

Prevention: No specific prevention is known, but older men should be encouraged to have a regular prostate examination in order to detect any enlargement.

Prostatic Cancer

Description: *Prostatic cancer* is a malignant neoplasm of the prostate tissue. The majority of these neoplasms are classified as adenocarcinomas. Prostatic cancer is the third leading cause of cancer deaths in males (after lung and colon cancers). Prostate cancer tends to metastasize, often spreading to the bones of the spine or pelvis before it is detected. The disease is rare before the age of 50.

Etiology: The cause of prostatic cancer is not known. No specific risk factors, other than the increasing incidence with age, have been identified.

Signs and Symptoms: Most individuals with prostatic cancer are asymptomatic on diagnosis. When symptoms are present, they are typically those of urinary obstruction, such as dysuria, difficulty in voiding, urinary frequency, or urinary retention. Hip or back pain may be present in advanced stages of the disease.

Diagnostic Procedures: A rectal examination will help in diagnosing the tumor. A biopsy is essential for confirmation of the diagnosis. A CT scan or ultrasonography may be useful in localizing and gauging the extent of the tumor.

Treatment: The course of treatment selected will depend on the stage of the disease and the patient's physical condition and age. Surgery may be performed to remove the prostate and adjacent affected tissues. Various hormonal therapies also may be attempted to limit prostatic cell growth, including orchidectomy and estrogen therapy. Radiation therapy may be tried in some cases, and this further helps to relieve bone pain. Chemotherapy may be used in treating advanced stages of the disease.

Prognosis: The earlier the cancer is detected, the better is the prognosis. But generally, the prognosis is poor, with most affected individuals dying within 3 to 4 years.

Prevention: There is no known prevention other than early detection through routine physical examination. A prostate examination should be a regular part of the physical examination for every man over 40.

Testicular Cancer

Description: *Testicular cancer* is a malignant neoplasm of a testis. There are various forms of the disease, classified according to the type of testicular tissue from which the malignancy originates. The disease primarily affects young to middle-age men and is rare over the age of 40.

Etiology: The cause of cancer of the testes is essentially unknown. Predisposing factors include **cryptorchidism**, even after this condition has been surgically corrected. Other risk factors include a prior history of mumps or an inguinal hernia during childhood.

Signs and Symptoms: The first sign often is a smooth, firm, painless mass in the testicles. Later symptoms may include breast enlargement and nipple tenderness.

Diagnostic Procedures: Diagnosis generally is through palpation of the testes. Further tests may be necessary to differentiate the cell type of the mass.

Treatment: Treatment may include any combination of surgery, radiation, and chemotherapy as determined by the tumor cell type and staging.

Prognosis: The prognosis varies according to the cancer's type and staging. Cure rates of roughly 90 percent can be expected following the successful treatment of early-stage testicular cancers.

Prevention: While no specific prevention is known, early detection is crucial to successful treatment. Men should be encouraged to perform a testicular self-examination on a regular basis.

Common Symptoms of Male Reproductive Diseases

Males may present with the following common complaints, which deserve attention from health professionals:
- Any urinary complaints such as frequency, urgency, incontinence, dysuria, etc.
- Pain in any of the reproductive organs
- Swelling or enlargement of any of the reproductive organs
- Any sexual dysfunction such as impotence

FEMALE REPRODUCTIVE DISEASES

Premenstrual Syndrome (PMS)

Description: *Premenstrual syndrome* is a cluster of symptoms that regularly recur several days prior to the onset of menstruation. PMS appears more frequently in females during their thirties and forties. (Refer to Figures 5–2 and 5–3 to review the structure of the female reproductive system.)

Etiology: The cause of PMS is not clearly understood. Some theories suggest that the condition may be attributable to water retention, estrogen-progesterone imbalance, psychologic factors, or dietary deficiencies.

Signs and Symptoms: The particular assortment of symptoms and their severity vary from woman to woman. Symptoms associated with PMS include
- Irritability
- Sleeplessness
- Fatigue
- Depression
- Headaches
- Vertigo
- Syncope
- Lowered resistance to infections
- Abdominal bloating and weight gain
- Heart palpitations
- Acne
- Swollen and tender breasts
- Easily bruised skin
- Alterations in appetite (e.g., cravings for sweet or salty foods)

Diagnostic Procedures: Diagnosis depends on the timing of the symptoms rather than on the appearance of any specific set of symptoms. Consequently, the affected individual should be encouraged to keep a journal recording the onset, duration, and intensity of all symptoms. Evaluation of estrogen and progesterone levels in the blood to check for imbalances should be performed.

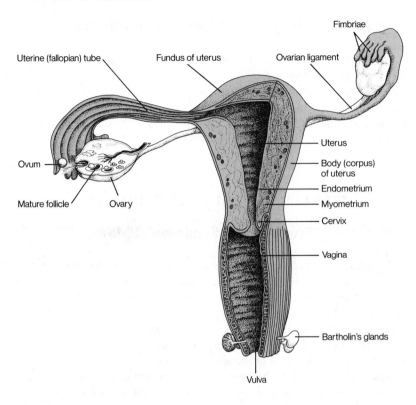

FIGURE 5–2. The female reproductive system (front view). (Modified from Gylys, B. A. and Wedding, M. E., *Medical Terminology: A Systems Approach,* ed. 2. F. A. Davis, Philadelphia, 1988, p. 270.)

Treatment: There is no one effective treatment for PMS. A reduction of salt intake for 2 weeks prior to menses will minimize water retention. Avoidance of stimulants (coffee, nicotine, and alcohol) is beneficial for some. Proper diet, exercise, and sufficient amounts of rest are important.

Prognosis: The prognosis is variable. The disorder is considered chronic but will cease at menopause and does not have long-term effects.

Prevention: There is no known prevention.

Amenorrhea

Description: *Amenorrhea* is the absence of **menarche** beyond age 18 (*primary* amenorrhea) or the absence of menstruation for 6 months in a woman who has previously had regular, periodic menses (*secondary* amenorrhea).

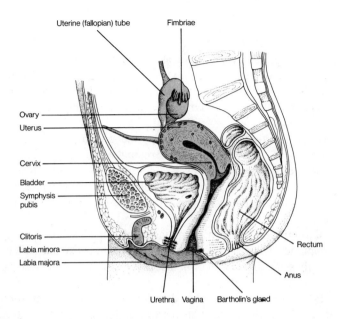

FIGURE 5–3. The female reproductive system (side view). (Modified from Gylys, B. A. and Wedding, M. E., *Medical Terminology: A Systems Approach,* ed. 3. F. A. Davis, Philadelphia, 1988, p. 269.)

Etiology: Medically significant primary or secondary amenorrhea may be caused by a variety of hormonal imbalances capable of preventing ovulation. Several forms of congenital anatomic defects, such as the absence of a uterus, also may cause amenorrhea. The condition is also associated with endometrial problems, ovarian or pituitary tumors, malnutrition, psychologic stress, or too much physical exercise.

Signs and Symptoms: A young woman reporting delayed menarche or a woman reporting skipped periods should be carefully assessed for amenorrhea.

Diagnostic Procedures: A thorough pelvic examination will rule out pregnancy and anatomic abnormalities. Analysis of blood and urine samples may reveal hormonal difficulties. X-rays and laparoscopy with a biopsy may be necessary to detect tumors.

Treatment: Hormone therapy usually starts the menstrual cycle, but some causes of this disorder may require more aggressive treatment, such as surgery.

Prognosis: Prognosis is good when the underlying cause can be determined and corrected. It is important that an accurate record of the menstrual cycle be kept to aid in the detection of amenorrhea.

Prevention: Preventive measures include adequate diet, reduction of psychologic stress, and a balanced physical exercise program.

Dysmenorrhea

Description: *Dysmenorrhea* is pain associated with menstruation. It is one of the most frequent gynecologic disorders. Dysmenorrhea is divided into primary and secondary categories. *Primary* dysmenorrhea is not associated with any identifiable pathologic disorder, whereas *secondary* dysmenorrhea accompanies some underlying disease condition.

Etiology: A specific cause of primary dysmenorrhea is difficult to pinpoint. Hormonal imbalances such as increased **prostaglandin** secretions may be the cause. Secondary dysmenorrhea arises as a consequence of some other problem, such as endometriosis, cervical **stenosis**, or pelvic inflammatory disease. Secondary dysmenorrhea is occasionally associated with the presence of uterine polyps or benign tumors.

Signs and Symptoms: Sharp, cramping pains in the lower abdominal area are the classic symptoms. The pain may radiate to the thighs, back, and genitalia. These symptoms usually start just prior to or immediately after menses and subside within 18 to 24 hours.

Diagnostic Procedures: A detailed history and pelvic examination will be performed to determine the cause. Laparoscopy and dilation and curettage (D&C) may be attempted.

Treatment: Analgesics usually are sufficient for relieving the pain of this disorder. Aspirin, moreover, when taken prior to menses, is an inhibitor of prostaglandins. Heat applied to the abdomen may provide comfort. Sometimes sex steroid therapy (oral contraceptives) may be prescribed to relieve pain by suppressing ovulation. Uterine **leiomyomas** may require surgery.

Prognosis: The prognosis is good. Primary dysmenorrhea may disappear after a female becomes sexually active or gives birth to a child.

Prevention: Correction of any hormonal imbalance may be helpful in prevention.

Ovarian Cysts and Tumors

Description: Benign *cysts* of the ovary are derived from ovarian follicles and the **corpus luteum**. These cysts may occur anytime from puberty to menopause. Nonneoplastic cysts (*tumors*) usually are small and produce few symptoms. True ovarian neoplasms may be benign, malignant, cystic, or solid. Dermoid or benign cystic **teratomas** also are common in the ovary.

Etiology: The etiology of ovarian cysts and tumors is not known.

Signs and Symptoms: Large cysts may produce pelvic pain, low back pain, and dyspareunia. Cysts that are mobile and can twist may produce a colicky, acute abdominal pain.

Diagnostic Procedures: Visualization of the ovaries through laparoscopy or sonography may indicate ovarian cysts.

Treatment: Cysts may disappear spontaneously or may require drug-induced ovulation therapy or surgical resection. If any question exists regarding malignancy, surgery may be necessary for diagnosis as well as treatment.

Prognosis: Prognosis varies according to whether the diagnosis indicates nonneoplastic cysts or a true ovarian neoplasm, either benign or malignant.

Prevention: There is no known prevention.

Endometriosis

Description: *Endometriosis* is the appearance and growth of endometrial tissue in areas outside the **endometrium**, the uterine cavity's lining. The misplaced endometrial tissue generally is found within the pelvic area, but it can appear anywhere in the body. Despite its location at an **ectopic** site, the tissue still responds to the hormonal signals of the female's menstrual cycle, but the "menstruating" tissue cannot be sluffed off through the vagina. This situation gives rise to a variety of symptoms and may lead to scarring of the ectopic site. Endometriosis is a disease of females during their active reproductive years.

Etiology: The cause of endometriosis is still not known, although various theories have been proposed.

Signs and Symptoms: Dysmenorrhea will occur, producing constant pain in the lower back and the vagina. There will be pain at the ectopic site during menses.

Diagnostic Procedures: Diagnosis usually occurs by visualizing the ectopic deposits within the pelvis through laparoscopy. Palpation may detect tender nodules or areas of the pelvis. These nodules become more tender during menses.

Treatment: Hormone therapy that will completely suppress the menstrual cycle may be recommended. Birth-control pills will suppress endometriosis as well. Surgery, which may involve a **panhysterosalpingo-oophorectomy,** may be indicated.

Prognosis: The prognosis varies according to the location of the ectopic sites and the intensity of symptoms experienced by each affected individual. A primary complication of endometriosis is infertility. Females who have not had a child may be advised not to postpone pregnancy.

Prevention: It may be best for adolescents to use sanitary napkins rather than tampons to prevent displacement of the endometrial lining.

Uterine Leiomyomas

Description: *Uterine leiomyomas* are often mislabeled as fibroids or fibroid tumors. They are not composed of fibrous tissue, however. Rather, they are composed of smooth muscle tissue. These benign tumors may vary in size, number, and location within the uterine muscle. They are the most common tumor in females, but they tend to calcify after menopause.

Etiology: The etiology of leiomyomas is not known.

Signs and Symptoms: Frequently, leiomyomas are asymptomatic. If symptoms do occur, they may include pelvic pressure, urinary frequency, constipation, and **menorrhagia**. A palpable mass may be detected.

Diagnostic Procedures: The patient's symptoms and a thorough history and physical examination, including palpation of the tumor, are essential for diagnosis. Additional tests may include a dilation and curettage (D&C) to detect submucosal leiomyomas in the endometrial cavity or laparoscopy to visualize leiomyomas on the surface of the uterus.

Treatment: Treatment is dependent on the female's age, **parity**, desire to have children, tumor status, and the severity of symptoms. If the tumors are small, no treatment may be necessary. A pelvic examination every 6 to 12 months may then be advised. Surgical removal of the tumors may be done or a hysterectomy performed.

Prognosis: The prognosis is good. Only a very small percentage of leiomyomas develop into a malignancy.

Prevention: No prevention is known.

Pelvic Inflammatory Disease (PID)

Description: *Pelvic inflammatory disease* is an acute or subacute, recurrent or chronic infection of the fallopian tubes, ovaries, and adjacent tissues.

Etiology: The causes of PID include (1) infections following **parturition**, (2) infections from *Neisseria gonorrhoeae, Chlamydia trachomatis, Pseudomonas,* and *E. coli,* and (3) iatrogenic causes, such as following **conization** or cervical cauterization or insertion of an IUD or biopsy curet.

Signs and Symptoms: This disease may exhibit both acute and chronic symptoms. Acute symptoms include sudden pelvic pain, a purulent and foul-smelling vaginal discharge, fever, sexual dysfunction, **metrorrhagia**, and rebound pain. Chronic symptoms such as cervical **dysplasia** and laceration may go undetected for an indefinite period of time.

Diagnostic Procedures: Diagnosis includes taking a smear of uterine secretions for culture. Ultrasonography may be used to identify any uterine mass. PID may occur along with conditions such as salpingo-oophoritis, cervicitis, and endometritis.

Treatment: Appropriate antibiotics are the best treatment for PID. Supplemental therapy may include analgesics and bed rest. Surgery may be necessary to prevent **septicemia.**

Prognosis: The prognosis of PID is good when treatment is instituted early and few complications occur.

Prevention: There is no known prevention.

Menopause

Description: *Menopause* is the cessation of menses and ovarian function, with a resultant increased loss of estrogen.

Etiology: Menopause occurs naturally in females between the ages of 40 and 50. It also can be surgically induced by oophorectomy or can result from malnutrition, severe stress, or a disease that has an adverse affect on hormone balance.

Signs and Symptoms: Menstruation irregularities, a decrease in the amount of menstrual flow, and finally, cessation of menses are the common series of symptoms. These occur over a period of months or years. Other changes can occur in the body systems as well, producing hot flashes, syncope, **tachycardia**, loss of elasticity in the skin, reduction of size and firmness of breast tissue, some atrophy of the genitalia, and a decrease in secretion from the Bartholin's gland.

Diagnostic Procedures: A careful patient history usually will suggest menopause. Blood serum levels will be checked for increase production of **follicle-stimulating hormone** (FSH) and **luteinizing hormone** (LH).

Treatment: Some individuals need no treatment; others may require hormone replacement therapy or counseling. A female requiring hormone replacement therapy should be informed of the possible increased risks of endometrial cancer and should be monitored carefully.

Prognosis: The prognosis is generally good.

Prevention: Menopause cannot be prevented, but it is important to recognize that emotional mood swings may occur.

Abnormal Premenopausal and Postmenopausal Bleeding

Premenopausal or *postmenopausal bleeding* is bleeding occurring at times other than during the normal menstrual flow. Either condition may be troublesome or cause few problems. However, these conditions should be investigated to determine the underlying cause. **Oligomenorrhea**, menorrhagia, metrorrhagia, or a brownish spotting from the vagina are the most common signs. To help assess the problem, it is important to monitor the dates of abnormal bleeding and the number of tampons or pads used a day. A dilation and curettage (D&C) may be necessary to relieve bleeding.

Common Symptoms of Female Reproductive System Diseases

Females may present with the following common symptoms, which deserve attention from health professionals:

- Pre- and postmenstrual complaints such as amenorrhea, dysmenorrhea, oligomonorrhea, and metrorrhagia; skin changes; and psychologic reactions to hormonal changes
- Lower abdominal or pelvic pain
- Any abnormal vaginal discharge or itching
- Fever
- Dyspareunia or any sexual dysfunction
- Breast changes, such as unusual swelling, lumpiness, mass formation, pain, or nipple abnormalities

DISEASES OF THE BREASTS

Mammary Dysplasia or Fibrocystic Disease

Description: *Fibrocystic disease of the breast* is a generalized diagnosis for a condition in which there are palpable cysts in the breasts that fluctuate in size with the menstrual cycle. Other benign changes in the breast epithelium include **papillomatosis**, fibrosis, and **hyperplasia**. The condition is sometimes known as "chronic cystic mastitis." The disease is seen more frequently in females 30 to 50 years old and rarely after menopause. (Refer to Figure 5–4 for a review of the structure of the breast.)

Etiology: The causes of fibrocystic diseases are not well understood, but they are linked to the hormonal changes associated with ovarian activity.

Signs and Symptoms: The upper, outer quadrant of the breast is the most frequent segment involved. There may be widespread lumpiness or a localized mass. Pain, tenderness, and a nipple discharge may be present. The mass tends to grow in size and becomes tender just before the menstrual period.

Diagnostic Procedures: Mammography may be used to help in the diagnosis, but biopsy is essential to confirm the diagnosis. The clinical picture of pain, fluctuation in size, and lumpiness help to differentiate mammary dysplasia from breast cancer.

Treatment: Breast aspiration may be attempted to remove the watery fluid typically contained in most lesions. Breast pain may be alleviated with a good supportive bra worn both day and night. Caffeine intake may be restricted, since some studies indicate that its elimination aids in reduction of dysplasia.

Prognosis: The prognosis is good, although exacerbations may continue until menopause, after which they subside. Cancer of the breast is more common in females who also have mammary dysplasia.

Prevention: There is no known prevention. Monthly self-examination of the breast is advised.

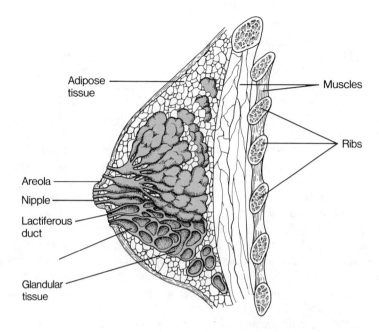

FIGURE 5–4. The breast. (Modified from Gylys, B. A. and Wedding, M. E., *Medical Terminology: A Systems Approach,* ed. 2. F. A. Davis, Philadelphia, 1988, p. 68.)

Benign Fibroadenoma

Description: A *fibroadenoma* is a benign, well-circumscribed tumor of fibrous and glandular breast tissue. It is a common tumor occurring in females 20 years after puberty.

Etiology: The cause is unknown.

Signs and Symptoms: The breast mass is typically round, firm, discrete, and relatively movable. It is nontender and usually discovered by accident.

Diagnostic Procedures: Due to its distinctive characteristics, the tumor is not difficult to diagnose, but it must be differentiated from a cyst or carcinoma through biopsy.

Treatment: The mass is excised under local anesthesia.

Prognosis: The prognosis is good following excision of the tumor.

Prevention: There is no known prevention.

Carcinoma of the Breast

Description: *Breast cancer* encompasses a variety of malignant neoplasms of the breast. It is the most common site of cancer in females and was the leading cause of cancerous deaths among females in the United States, having been surpassed recently by lung cancer.

Etiology: The exact causes of breast cancer are unknown, although hereditary patterns to the disease are quite obvious. Those at greatest risk of developing breast cancer include women over the age of 50 who have not had children or women who have not had children until after age 30. Other risk factors include a history of chronic breast disease, exposure to high doses of radiation, especially during adolescence, and obesity. The risk of breast cancer increases with age.

Signs and Symptoms: Breast changes such as a lump, thickening, dimpling, swelling, skin irritation, distortion, retraction or scaliness of the nipple, nipple discharge, pain, or tenderness are the most common signs and symptoms. Advanced symptoms include edema, redness, nodularity, or ulceration of the skin and enlargement or shrinkage of the breast.

Diagnostic Procedures: The best method of early detection continues to be the monthly breast self-examination. Mammography, ultrasonography, or thermography are also frequently used screening methods. Diagnosis, however, must be made without delay because of the possibility of metastasis. Biopsy is essential for definitive diagnosis. Diagnosed breast cancer will be staged and typed according to its pattern of growth.

Treatment: Treatment may be curative or palliative. If the cancer is advanced, palliative treatment is indicated. Curative treatment nearly always involves surgical management of the cancer, but no single procedure is now recognized as ideal for all affected individuals. Surgical options range from removing the affected breast, underlying chest muscles, and associated lymphatics (called a *total radical mastectomy*) to removing only the tumor and immediately adjacent breast tissue (called a *lumpectomy*). In most cases, surgery will be followed by a course of radiation therapy or chemotherapy).

The tumor tissue will be tested for the presence of hormone receptors in order to determine if the tumor is estrogen- or progesterone-dependent. If this is the case, hormonal manipulation such as removal of the ovaries or adrenal glands and administration of testosterone may be attempted to halt tumor regrowth or to prevent its spread.

Prognosis: The most reliable indicator of the prognosis is the stage of the breast cancer. In the early stages, the prognosis is good, especially if no metastasis has occurred. According to the American Cancer society, the 5-year survival rate for localized breast cancer has risen to 87 percent. If the cancer has spread, however, the rate is reduced to 47 percent.

Prevention: There is no known prevention of breast cancer.

SPECIAL FOCUS: BREAST RECONSTRUCTION

Breast reconstruction may be performed to augment, reduce, or repair the breast. New developments in plastic surgery have greatly reduced the risks of the procedure and provide a female with a choice about her body's appearance. Whatever the reason for the reconstruction, females need to be emotionally prepared for the surgery and especially well informed of its potential results.

DISORDERS OF PREGNANCY AND DELIVERY

Spontaneous Abortion

Description: *Spontaneous abortion,* or *miscarriage,* is the expulsion of the **conceptus** before viability. As many as 10 to 30 percent of pregnancies may end in spontaneous abortion. The incidence is higher in first pregnancies.

Etiology: Spontaneous abortion may be a result of (1) defective development of the embryo (chromosomal abnormalities), (2) faulty implantation of the fertilized ovum, (3) placental problems, (4) maternal infections, (5) hormonal imbalances, and (6) trauma.

Signs and Symptoms: A pink or brown discharge may precede the onset of cramping and increased vaginal bleeding. The cervix will dilate, and the uterine contents will be expelled. The discharge may appear as a clotty menstrual flow.

Diagnostic Procedures: Evidence of the expelled uterine contents, pelvic examination, and laboratory studies will confirm the occurrence of a spontaneous abortion.

Treatment: Bed rest may be required for as long as spotting continues. Hospitalization may be necessary to control hemorrhage. If remnants of the conceptus persist in the uterus, dilation and curettage should be performed.

Prognosis: The prognosis for full recovery is good, barring any complications.

Prevention: The progression of a spontaneous abortion usually cannot be prevented.

Abortions are performed on a voluntary basis also. It is not the purpose of this book to discuss the methods or legality of voluntary abortion.[3]

A female who has had an abortion, whether spontaneous or voluntary, will typically benefit from emotional support and counseling. Most females grieve the loss of their unborn and need to recognize the psychologic and physiologic aspects of their grief.

Ectopic Pregnancy

Description: *Ectopic pregnancy* occurs when the fertilized ovum implants somewhere other than the uterine cavity. The most common ectopic site is within one of the fallopian tubes. Less frequently, ectopic implantation may occur in an ovary or the abdominal cavity.

Etiology: Ectopic pregnancy is often due to scarring or inflammation of the fallopian tubes as a result of infection, or it may be due to congenital malformations of the tubes. In general, any factor that impedes the migration of the fertilized ovum into the uterus before attachment takes place increases the likelihood of an ectopic pregnancy.

Signs and Symptoms: Signs of early pregnancy may be present. There also may be abdominal pain and tenderness, as well as slight vaginal bleeding. A rupture of a fallopian tube due to the developing conceptus is life-threatening and will cause severe abdominal pain and intraabdominal bleeding.

Diagnostic Procedures: A pelvic examination and a careful patient history may suggest ectopic pregnancy. A serum pregnancy test and an ultrasound likely will be used in this determination. Laparoscopy and exploratory laparotomy also may help in the diagnosis of this condition.

Treatment: Laparotomy is frequently necessary. A ruptured fallopian tube may need to be removed. All attempts will be made to save the ovary. Transfusion of whole blood may be necessary in the event of severe intraabdominal bleeding or hypovolemic shock.

Prognosis: The prognosis is good when emergency treatment is sought quickly and without delay.

Prevention: Prompt treatment of any genitourinary infection may help reduce the likelihood of ectopic pregnancy.

Toxemia of Pregnancy (Preeclampsia and Eclampsia)

Description: *Toxemia of pregnancy* is a hypertensive disorder that may develop during the third trimester. Most health care professionals prefer to use the more precise terms of *preeclampsia* and *eclampsia* to designate the condition. *Preeclampsia* is the initial cluster of symptoms, characterized by hypertension, edema, and proteinuria. *Eclampsia* is the subsequent group of symptoms, characterized by convulsions and coma. Eclampsia is a medical emergency. The condition is more likely to occur in **primagravidae** or in women over 30 who have had multiple pregnancies.

Etiology: The cause of preeclampsia and eclampsia is not known, but it may be related to malnutrition, especially a lack of protein in the diet. Predisposing factors include preexisting vascular and renal disease.

Signs and Symptoms: Hypertension, generalized edema, proteinuria, and sudden weight gain are the classic symptoms of preeclampsia. Headache, vertigo, malaise, irritability, epigastric pain, and nausea also may occur. Eclampsia symptoms may include tonoclonic convulsions, coma, rhonchi, **nystagmus**, and **oliguria** or **anuria**.

Diagnostic Procedures: Elevated—especially steadily rising—blood pressure, proteinuria, and oliguria are suggestive of preeclampsia. The clinical picture of convulsions confirms a diagnosis of eclampsia.

Treatment: In preeclampsia, the goal of treatment is to prevent eclampsia and to deliver a normal baby. Bed rest is advised, with sedatives prescribed. Antihypertensives may be necessary. The fetus will be delivered as soon as it is judged viable. With the onset of eclampsia, the patient will be hospitalized and intensive treatment instituted. Immediate termination of the pregnancy is indicated, whether or not the fetus is judged viable.

Prognosis: The prognosis is good for preeclampsia. In eclampsia, the maternal mortality rate is about 15 percent.

Prevention: Adequate nutrition, good prenatal care, and control of high blood pressure during pregnancy are important. Early treatment of preeclampsia can prevent eclampsia.

Placenta Previa

Description: In *placenta previa,* the placenta is implanted abnormally low in the uterus so that it covers all or part of the internal cervical os, or opening. This condition is dangerous because the placenta may prematurely separate from the uterus, causing maternal hemorrhaging and interrupting oxygen to the fetus.

Etiology: The cause is unknown, but predisposing factors include multiparity, advanced maternal age, previous uterine surgery, and early or late fertilization.

Signs and Symptoms: A typical symptom is slight, painless bleeding, generally occurring in the third trimester, that may become more severe. The fetus may present in a variety of positions, but the situation is not critical as long as fetal heart tones remain strong.

Diagnostic Procedures: Ultrasonography will help in the diagnosis, as will careful pelvic examination.

Treatment: Hospital treatment is aimed at controlling and treating any blood loss, delivering a healthy infant, and preventing complications. A cesarean section may be necessary.

Prognosis: The maternal prognosis depends on the amount of bleeding; the fetal prognosis depends on gestational age, blood loss, and consequences of possible anoxia. Complications include shock and maternal or fetal death. With prompt and effective treatment, however, both mother and child usually survive.

Prevention: There is no known prevention.

Abruptio Placentae

Description: *Abruptio placentae* is the premature separation of a normally implanted placenta from the uterine wall about the twentieth week of gestation. The condition is most common in primagravidae.

Etiology: The cause is unknown, but predisposing factors include trauma, chronic hypertension, and preeclampsia or eclampsia.

Signs and Symptoms: Abruptio placentae is characterized by abdominal pain, tenderness of the uterus, hemorrhage, and the onset of shock.

Diagnostic Procedures: Ultrasonography, pelvic examination, and patient history will help confirm the diagnosis.

Treatment: The goals of treatment are to control the bleeding, deliver a healthy infant, and to prevent complications. Hospitalization is required, and a cesarean section is typically performed.

Prognosis: The maternal prognosis is good if the bleeding can be controlled. The fetal prognosis depends on its gestational age and the amount of blood loss. Complications include **disseminated intravascular coagulation** (DIC) and renal failure.

Prevention: There is no known prevention.

Premature Labor/Premature Rupture of Membranes (PROM)

Description: *Premature rupture of membranes* is early rupture of the placenta. *Premature labor* is the early onset of rhythmic uterine contractions after fetal viability but before fetal maturity.

Etiology: These conditions may be caused by "incompetent cervix," preeclampsia, multiple pregnancy, abruptio placentae, anatomic malformations, infections, or fetal death.

Signs and Symptoms: There may be a blood-tinged flow from the vagina with uterine contractions and cervical dilation and **effacement**. Premature rupture of the membranes is marked by the flow of amniotic fluid from the vagina.

Diagnostic Procedures: Diagnosis is confirmed by prenatal history and physical examination. Ultrasonography also may be used.

Treatment: Attempts will be made to suppress premature labor by requiring bed rest and appropriate drug therapy. PROM typically requires induction of labor or cesarean delivery.

Prognosis: The maternal prognosis is good with proper attention and care. The fetal prognosis depends on gestational age.

Prevention: The best prevention is good prenatal care.

Common Symptoms of Disorders of Pregnancy and Delivery

Pregnant females may present with the folloiwng common complaints, which deserve attention from health professionals:
- Abdominal pain, tenderness, or cramping
- Unusual discharge, pink or brown in color, or clotted
- Hypertension, rapid weight gain, edema, and malaise to indicate possible toxemia

SPECIAL FOCUS: CESAREAN BIRTH

In a *cesarean birth,* an incision is made through the abdomen and uterus to remove the fetus and placenta. The most common situations requiring cesarean birth include malpresentation of the fetus, fetal distress, a maternal pelvis too small to accommodate the fetal head, the presence of sexually transmitted disease organisms in the birth canal, preeclampsia or eclampsia, and previous cesarean births. Prolonged labor, abnormal fetal heart actions, and maternal distress are also indicators for a possible cesarean birth.

Ultrasound and x-ray may be helpful in making a decision about cesarean delivery. Amniocentesis also may be used. Maternal complications of the procedure may include cardiovascular and pulmonary difficulties and urinary tract infections.

REFERENCES

1. World Health Organization, *Education and Treatment in Human Sexuality: The Training of Health Professionals* (Report of a WHO Meeting, Technical Report Series No. 572), Geneva, WHO, 1975.
2. Krupp, M. A., and M. J. Chatton, *Current Medical Diagnosis and Treatment,* Lange Medical Publications, Los Altos, Calif., 1984, pp. 468–469.
3. A suggested source of information on the subject is Lewis, M. A. and C. D. Warden, *Law and Ethics in the Medical Office: Including Bioethical Issues,* 2d Ed., F. A. Davis Company, Philadelphia, 1988.

REVIEW QUESTIONS

Short Answer

1. List the two functions of sexuality in humans.
   a.
   b.
2. Name three inflammatory diseases of the male reproductive system. Distinguish them.
   a.
   b.
   c.
3. List two common diagnostic procedures for prostatic cancer.
   a.
   b.
4. What is the difference between amenorrhea and dysmenorrhea?
5. Spell out the following abbreviations:
   a. BPH:
   b. PMS:
   c. PID:

Matching

Match the definitions with the correct sexual dysfunction:

_____ 1. Erectile dysfunction in males
_____ 2. Sexual dysfunction in females
_____ 3. Ejaculation immediately or prior to intromission

a. Dyspareunia
b. Impotence
c. Premature ejaculation
d. Alopecia
e. Coitus
f. Frigidity

Match the causes with the corresponding sexually transmitted diseases:

_____ 4. Disease caused by various types of papillomaviruses
_____ 5. Disease caused by a motile protozoan
_____ 6. Disease caused by bacteria
_____ 7. Disease caused by simplex virus
_____ 8. Autoimmune disease caused by virus

a. Herpes, type II
b. Genital warts
c. Gonorrhea
d. Chlamydial Infection
e. Syphilis
f. Trichomoniasis
g. AIDS

Match the three disorders of the breast with the correct signs and symptoms:

_____ 9. Breast is round, firm, discrete, and relatively movable; nontender
_____ 10. Widespread lumpiness in the upper, outer quadrant of the breast
_____ 11. Breast dimpling, swelling, skin irritation, nipple discharge

a. Mammary dysplasia
b. Benign fibroadenoma
c. Carcinoma of the breast

Match the following diseases/conditions with their common diagnostic procedures:

_____ 12. Ultrasound and x-ray
_____ 13. Pelvic exam, lab studies, and evidence of expelled uterine contents
_____ 14. Prenatal history, physical examinations, and ultrasound
_____ 15. Pelvic exam, patient history, serum PG test, and ultrasound
_____ 16. Proteinuria, oliguria, and high blood pressure readings

a. Abortion
b. Toxemias
c. Cesarean birth
d. PROM
e. Ectopic pregnancy

True/False

T F 1. Benign cysts of the ovary are derived from ovarian follicles and the corpus luteum.

T F 2. Large ovarian cysts may produce pelvic pain and dyspareunia.

T F 3. The cause of endometriosis is bacterial in nature.

T F 4. Endometriosis most frequently occurs postmenopausally.

T F 5. Uterine leiomyomas are composed of fibrous tissue.

T F 6. Frequently leiomyomas are asymptomatic.
T F 7. Menopause is the cessation of ovarian function with an increase in estrogen.

ANSWERS

Short Answer
1. Reproduction and enhancement of caring and pleasure.
2. Prostatis, epididymitis, and orchitis. Prostatitis is inflammation of the prostate that may result from urethritis or directly from the bloodstream. Epididymitis is inflammation of the epididymis resulting from prostatitis, UTI, trauma, or secondary to an infection elsewhere in the body. Orchitis is inflammation of the testes caused by injury or mumps.
3. Rectal examination and rectal biopsy.
4. Amenorrhea, the absence of menstruation, is an abnormal condition which occurs at any time other than before puberty, after menopause, or during pregnancy. Dysmenorrhea is painful menstruation or cramps.
5. a. Benign prostatic hyperplasia
   b. Premenstrual syndrome
   c. Pelvic inflammatory disease

Matching
1. b
2. f
3. c
4. b
5. f
6. c, d, and e
7. a
8. g
9. b
10. a
11. c
12. c
13. a
14. d
15. e
16. b

True/False
1. T
2. T
3. F
4. F
5. F
6. T
7. F

GLOSSARY

ALOPECIA: Absence or loss of hair, especially on the head.

ANALGESIC: A drug or agent that relieves pain.

ANTIPYRETIC: A drug or other agent that reduces fever.

ANURIA: Cessation of urine production by the kidney.

AZOOSPERMIA: Absence of spermatozoa in the semen.

CERVICITIS: Inflammation of the cervix.

CHANCRE: A firm, red, ulcerated sore. A chancre is the primary indication of syphilis, occurring at the point of entry of the infection.

COITUS: Sexual intercourse.

CONCEPTUS: The products of conception from fertilization to birth.

CONIZATION: The surgical removal of a cone of tissue, such as excision of cervical tissue.

CORPUS LUTEUM: A small yellow structure on the ovary formed from the mass of follicle cells left behind after an ovum is released. It secretes hormones necessary for the maintenance of pregnancy.

CRYOSURGERY: A technique used to destroy tissue by application of extreme cold. The cold is typically produced by use of a probe through which liquid nitrogen circulates.

CRYPTORCHIDISM: Failure of one or both testicles to descend into the scrotum.

DEBRIDEMENT: The removal of dead or damaged tissue or other matter, especially from a wound.

DISSEMINATED INTRAVASCULAR COAGULATION (DIC): A pathologic form of coagulation of the blood that is diffuse rather than localized. The process damages rather than protects the area involved, and several clotting factors are consumed to such an extent that generalized bleeding may occur.

DYSURIA: Difficult or painful urination, symptomatic of numerous conditions.

ECTOPIC: Arising or occurring at an unusual location or in a tissue structure where it is not normally found.

EFFACEMENT: The dilation of the cervix.

ELECTROCAUTERY: A technique used to destroy tissue by means of an instrument containing an electrode heated to red hot temperatures by an electric current.

ENDOMETRIUM: The mucous membrane lining the inner surface of the uterus.

FOLLICLE-STIMULATING HORMONE (FSH): A secretion of the pituitary gland that stimulates the growth and maturation of the graafian follicles in the ovary or stimulates the production of sperm in the testes.

GONORRHEAL OPHTHALMIA NEONATORUM: In the newborn, the severe, hyperacute inflammation of the membrane lining the inner surface of the eyelids and covering the white of the eye. Caused by infection with gonococci, and usually contracted during vaginal birth from an infected mother.

HEMATURIA: Blood in the urine.

HYDROCELE: As used here, the painless swelling of the scrotum caused by the accumulation of fluid in the membrane surrounding a testicle.

HYPERPLASIA: The overproliferation of normal cells within a normal tissue structure.

HYPOTHYROIDISM: Underactivity of the thyroid gland, marked by underproduction of the hormone thyroxine.

INTROMISSION: As used here, the insertion of the penis into the vagina.

LEIOMYOMA: Tumor of the smooth-muscle tissue.

LESION: Any discontinuity or disruption of tissue caused by disease or trauma.

LEUKORRHEA: Whitish or yellowish mucous discharge from the vagina. While generally considered a normal secretion of the vagina, leukorrhea may indicate an underlying disorder if the flow markedly increases or changes color, thickness, or odor or is accompanied by a burning sensation or the presence of blood.

LUTEINIZING HORMONE (LH): A secretion of the hypothalamus that stimulates development of the corpus luteum. (See *Corpus luteum.*)

LYMPHADENOPATHY: Disease of the lymph nodes, usually manifested as swelling of the nodes.

MACULA: A small-colored spot or thickening.

MENARCHE: The initial menstrual cycle, marking the onset of fertility.

MENORRHAGIA: Excessive menstrual flow, either in duration or quantity, or both.

METRORRHAGIA: Uterine bleeding, especially at a time other than the menstrual period.

MYALGIA: Muscular pain or tenderness.

MYOTONIA: Any disorder involving sustained involuntary contractions of muscle.

NYSTAGMUS: Rhythmic, involuntary movement of the eyeball.

OLIGOMENORRHEA: Abnormally infrequent menstrual flow.

OLIGOSPERMIA: Deficient quantity of spermatozoa in the seminal fluid.

OLIGURIA: Reduced urine secretion.

OPPORTUNISTIC INFECTIONS: Infections with any organism, but especially fungi and bacteria, that occur due to the opportunity afforded by the altered physiologic state of the host.

ORCHIDECTOMY: Surgical removal of a testicle.

PANHYSTEROSALPINGO-OOPHORECTOMY: Surgical removal of the entire uterus, including the cervix, ovaries, and fallopian tubes.

PAPILLOMATOSIS: The widespread formation of warts.

PAPILLOMAVIRUSES: A family of viruses that cause warts or benign epithelial tumors in humans and animals.

PAPULE: A red, raised area of the skin, generally small and solid.

PARITY: The condition of having borne viable offspring.

PARTURITION: Act of giving birth.

PRIMAGRAVIDA: A woman during her first pregnancy.

PROSTAGLANDINS: A class of chemically related fatty acids present in many body tissues, having the ability to stimulate smooth-muscle contractions, lower blood pressure, and regulate or influence many other body functions.

PURULENT (DISCHARGE): Containing pus.

PUSTULE: Small, raised area of the skin filled with pus or lymph.

SEPTICEMIA: A condition associated with the presence or proliferation of disease-causing microorganisms or the accumulation of their toxins in the blood. Commonly called "blood poisoning."

STENOSIS: An abnormal constriction or narrowing in an opening or passageway of the body.

TACHYCARDIA: Abnormally rapid heart beat; generally defined as exceeding 100 beats per minute.

TERATOMA: A tumor composed of a number of different tissue types, none of which is normally found in the area of occurrence. Teratomas usually occur in the testes or ovaries.

VARICOCELE: Dilation of the complex network of veins that comprise part of the spermatic cord, forming a palpable swelling within the scrotum.

VASOCONSTRICTION: Decrease in the diameter of blood vessels.

VESICLE: A small, fluid-filled blister.

Chapter 6

Digestive System Diseases

LEARNING OBJECTIVES

Upon successful completion of this chapter, you will
- Define periodontitis.
- List the three types of hiatal hernias.
- Identify at least four causes of gastritis.
- Discuss the signs and symptoms of gastroenteritis.
- Describe the destructive process which causes gastric ulcers.
- Describe the symptoms for appendicitis.
- Discuss the inflammatory pattern of Crohn's disease.
- List at least three predisposing factors of ulcerative colitis.
- Restate the cause and treatment for abdominal hernias.
- Identify populations at high risk for colorectal cancer.
- Describe the condition of hemorrhoids.

113

■ Compare and contrast anorexia nervosa and bulimia.
■ Explain the symptoms of malabsorption syndrome.
■ Define duodenal ulcer.
■ Discuss the treatment of duodenal ulcers.
■ Review causes of irritable bowel syndrome.
■ Define diverticulitis.
■ Describe diarrhea as a symptom.
■ Restate the seriousness of pancreatitis.
■ Recall the incidence of pancreatic cancer.
■ Discuss the relationship between cholecystitis and cholelithiasis.
■ Describe cirrhosis and its treatment.
■ Name two complications of cirrhosis.
■ Define the different types of hepatitis.
■ List at least three common complaints of the digestive system.

INTRODUCTION

The digestive system consists of the set of organs and glands associated with the ingestion and digestion of food and the absorption of nutrients (Figure 6–1). This system also eliminates solid wastes from the body. It may be the system most abused. Whether eating foods of little value or a well-balanced diet, the task of the digestive system is the same—to nourish the cells of the body.

UPPER GASTROINTESTINAL TRACT

Periodontitis

Description: *Periodontitis* is a disease of the mouth characterized by the inflammation and subsequent degeneration of the peridental membrane, alveolar bone, cementum, and adjacent gingivae (gingivitis). Figure 6–2 illustrates the location of these structures. As the disease progresses, pus typically forms in pockets that open between the gingivae and the tooth sockets. The supporting bone is reabsorbed and the teeth become loose, eventually falling out.

Etiology: Periodontitis is a consequence of poor oral hygiene, calculus, food impaction, malocclusion, poor fillings, and inadequate diet. The destruction of the gingivae and alveolar bone is caused by masses of bacteria adhering at the gumline of the teeth (plaque) and calculus (calcified plaque). Individuals with Down's syndrome seem particularly susceptible to periodontal disease, as are those with certain systemic diseases such as diabetes mellitus.

Signs and Symptoms: The disease causes red, swollen gingivae that easily bleed with any pressure. In advanced cases, the gingivae may appear ulcerated, and

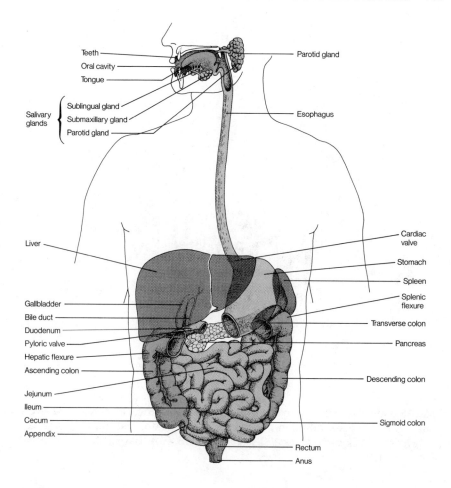

Teeth
Oral cavity
Tongue

Salivary glands
Sublingual gland
Submaxillary gland
Parotid gland

Parotid gland

Esophagus

Liver

Cardiac valve
Stomach
Spleen
Splenic flexure

Gallbladder
Bile duct
Duodenum
Pyloric valve
Hepatic flexure
Ascending colon
Jejunum
Ileum
Cecum
Appendix

Transverse colon
Pancreas

Descending colon

Sigmoid colon

Rectum
Anus

FIGURE 6–1. The digestive system. (Modified from Gylys, B. A. and Wedding, M. E., *Medical Terminology: A Systems Approach,* ed. 2. F. A. Davis, Philadelphia, 1988, p. 92.)

individual teeth may be loose. Strong **halitosis** also may occur with these symptoms. Fever may accompany end-stage periodontitis.

Treatment: Treatment is aimed at reestablishing a healthy oral environment. This includes removing plaque and calculus, scaling, curettage for control of infection, and root planing.

Prognosis: The prognosis is good with early treatment. However, tooth loss in end-stage periodontal disease is almost inevitable. Systemic bacterial infection (bacteremia) is a possibly serious complication of end-stage periodontitis.

Prevention: The disease is easily preventable by following proper oral hygiene procedures such as regular brushing and flossing, accompanied by regular

STRUCTURE OF TOOTH

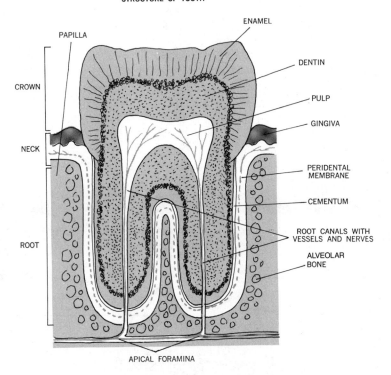

FIGURE 6–2. The tooth. The gingiva, peridental membrane, cementum, and alveolar bone are structures involved in periodontal disease. (Modified from Thomas, C. L. [ed.], *Taber's Cyclopedic Medical Dictionary,* ed. 15. F. A. Davis, 1985, p. 1749, with permission.)

dental care to remove plaque and calculus. Poor occlusion should be corrected, crooked teeth straightened, and missing teeth replaced with bridgework. A well-balanced diet should be encouraged.

Gastritis

Description: *Gastritis* is the inflammation and erosion of the gastric mucosa.

Etiology: The etiology of gastritis is varied and complex. Irritating foods, alcoholic beverages, aspirin, and ingested poisons can cause gastritis. It can be secondary to elevated blood pressure in the portal vein, sprue, and influenza. In many cases, though, gastritis is idiopathic.

Signs and Symptoms: The acute form of gastritis may feature gastrointestinal bleeding, belching, **epigastric** pain, and **hematemesis** or vomiting. The chronic form of gastritis may exhibit no symptoms. When symptoms do develop, they may be hard to pinpoint. A person may experience a loss of appetite, a ''full'' feeling in the stomach, or have vague epigastric pain.

Diagnostic Procedures: The patient history may suggest this disorder. Gastroscopy will help confirm the diagnosis, and x-ray will rule out other diseases with similar symptoms.

Treatment: Symptoms will be relieved by eliminating the irritant or cause. In the event of ingestion of toxic substances, an antidote or **antiemetic** may be prescribed. **Anticholinergics** and antacids may relieve distress, too.

Prognosis: The prognosis is good with proper treatment.

Prevention: Prevention includes avoiding gastric irritants. Taking prescribed steroid medications with milk or food and avoiding aspirin-containing substances will be helpful.

Gastroenteritis

Description: *Gastroenteritis* is inflammation of the stomach and small intestine.

Etiology: Causes of gastroenteritis include infection from bacteria, amebae, parasites, and viruses. The ingestion of toxins, allergic reactions to certain foods, and drug reactions also may produce this disease. Certain cases may be largely due to psychologic factors.

Signs and Symptoms: The etiology of the particular case will determine, in part, the signs and symptoms, which may include diarrhea, cramping, nausea, vomiting, malaise, fever, and rumbling stomach sounds.

Diagnostic Procedures: The patient history may suggest gastroenteritis. A stool and/or blood culture will identify any bacteria or parasite. An endoscopy may be performed.

Treatment: Treatment is symptomatic. Fluid and nutritional support is important to minimize electrolyte and fluid imbalances. **Antidiarrheals** and antiemetics may be prescribed.

Prognosis: The prognosis varies with the etiology but is generally good once the cause has been isolated and treatment has begun.

Prevention: People traveling in underdeveloped countries should be especially careful of contaminated water or food. All perishable food should be properly refrigerated, and hands should be washed thoroughly before handling food.

Gastric Ulcer (Peptic Ulcer of the Stomach)

Description: A *gastric ulcer* is a lesion in the mucosal lining of the stomach. In this disease, a patch of mucosal tissue becomes necrotic and is subsequently eroded by the acids and pepsins released within the stomach. Put simply, the stomach begins digesting itself.

Etiology: Gastric ulcers represent a breakdown in the balance between acid-pepsin secretion and mucosal defense in the stomach. The causes of this breakdown are not clear, but they seem related to chronic oversecretion of gastric juices, stress, and hereditary factors. Reactions to drugs such as **salicylates** and smoking and alcohol may be contributing factors.

Signs and Symptoms: Persistent "heartburn" and indigestion are the classic symptoms. There may be nagging stomach pain as well. Gastrointestinal bleeding, nausea, vomiting, and weight loss may be additional symptoms. The onset of symptoms is more common about 2 hours after meals and after the consumption of orange juice, coffee, aspirin, or alcohol.

Diagnostic Procedures: A barium x-ray and an upper gastrointestinal endoscopy are the most frequent methods used to diagnose a gastric ulcer. Biopsy will rule out malignancy.

Treatment: Treatment of gastric ulcers is aimed at reduction of acid secretions, healing of the mucosal lining, and relief of symptoms. Treatment may consist of the use of antacids or the prescription of a class of drugs known as H2 receptor antagonists that inhibit the release of stomach acid. Mucosal defense may be improved by the ingestion of coating agents such as carafates. The prescription of anticholinergic drugs or tranquilizers may be effective but is controversial due to possible side effects. Bland diets may have some limited benefit, but affected individuals should be advised to avoid alcohol, caffeine, and smoking. Surgical management of a gastric ulcer is generally avoided unless it proves malignant or if perforation occurs.

Prognosis: The prognosis varies. Gastric ulcers are frequently chronic, tending to heal and then reform in the same location. Complications of gastric ulcers include hemorrhage and perforation, both potentially life-threatening situations. Gastric ulcers must be carefully monitored for signs of malignancy.

Prevention: There is no known prevention, although a change to a less stressful lifestyle may be helpful.

Hiatal Hernia

Description: A *hiatal hernia* is the protrusion of some portion of the stomach into the thoracic cavity through the opening in the diaphragm through which the esophagus passes (the esophageal hiatus). There are three varieties of hiatal hernia: (1) in *sliding hernias* (most common), the gastroesophageal junction and the upper portion of the stomach slide upward through the esophageal hiatus; (2) in *paraesophageal*, or "*rolling*," *hernias*, the gastroesophageal junction remains fixed, but some portion of the stomach passes through the esophageal hiatus; and (3) in *mixed hernias*, the characteristics of sliding and paraesophageal hernias are combined. Figure 6–3 illustrates the configuration of hiatal hernias. The incidence of hiatal hernias increases with age.

Etiology: The cause of hiatal hernias is unclear. They may be due to intraab-

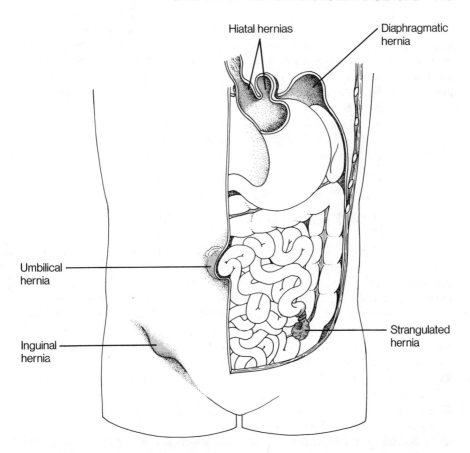

FIGURE 6–3. Hernias and their locations. (From Gylys, B. A. and Wedding, M. E., *Medical Terminology: A Systems Approach,* ed. 2. F. A. Davis, Philadelphia, 1988, p. 99, with permission.)

dominal pressure or weakening of the gastroesophageal junction caused by trauma or the loss of muscle tone.

Signs and Symptoms: Over half of those having hiatal hernias may remain asymptomatic. If symptoms are present, they commonly include heartburn—aggravated by reclining—chest pain, **dysphagia**, esophageal **reflux**, or severe pain if a large portion of the stomach is caught above the diaphragm.

Diagnostic Procedures: Diagnosis of hiatal hernias will be made by chest x-ray, barium x-ray, esophagoscopy, and pH studies of any reflux (to eliminate the possibility of gastric ulcer).

Treatment: The important goal in treatment is to alleviate symptoms. Surgery is not the first choice for treatment unless strangulation of the hernia is evident or symptoms cannot be controlled. An attempt is made to reduce episodes of reflux through dietary modification or by strengthening the lower esophageal sphincter with medication. Activity restrictions may be indicated, and the person may be advised to avoid tight or restrictive clothing. Stool softeners, laxatives, and antacids may be prescribed. Avoiding food intake before sleep and elevating the head of the bed may be advised.

Prognosis: The prognosis is good with proper treatment. Strangulation of the hernia is a serious, possibly life-threatening complication.

Prevention: No prevention is known.

LOWER GASTROINTESTINAL TRACT

Malabsorption Syndrome

Malabsorption syndrome encompasses a host of diseases of the small intestine, characterized by the impaired passage of nutrients, minerals, or fluids through intestinal tissue into the blood or lymph. Possible causes of malabsorption syndrome include

- Inadequate digestion caused by gastrectomy or pancreatic deficiencies.
- Inadequate absorptive surface as a result of intestinal resection or bypass.
- Mucosal absorptive defects caused by various inflammatory disorders or biochemical or genetic defects.
- Reduced concentrations of **bile** as a result of liver disease, bile duct obstruction, bacterial reduction of bile salts, or drug reactions.
- Endocrine or metabolic disorders such as diabetes mellitus or hyperparathyroidism.
- Lymphatic disorders.
- Cardiovascular disorders.

The signs and symptoms of malabsorption syndrome are legion and vary with the specific pathophysiology of the case, but typically they include chronic diarrhea and abnormal bowel movements. The treatment and prognosis of malabsorption syndrome also vary with etiology. A common malabsorption disorder, celiac sprue, is discussed in the following section.

Celiac Sprue (Gluten-Induced Enteropathy)

Description: *Celiac sprue* is a disease of the small intestine marked by malabsorption, gluten intolerance (a protein found in wheat and wheat products), and damage to, and characteristic changes in, the mucosal lining of the intestine. Because of the gluten intolerance characterizing celiac sprue, the disease is sometimes referred to as *gluten-induced* **enteropathy**.

Etiology: The cause of celiac sprue is not clearly understood. The gluten-induced damage to the intestine's mucosal lining may result from either a toxic or immunologic reaction to this protein. The disease may be inherited, since the incidence is high among siblings. Females are affected twice as frequently as males.

Signs and Symptoms: Symptoms of celiac sprue may include weight loss, **anorexia**, abdominal distension, flatulence, intestinal bleeding, peripheral neuritis, dermatitis, and muscle wasting. The condition is also marked by the passage of diarrheal, abnormally large stools that are characteristically light yellow to gray, greasy, and foul-smelling. The resultant chronic malnutrition may cause mineral depletion that may be revealed as bone pain, tenderness, compression deformities, and **tetany**.

Diagnostic Procedures: The disease often is difficult to diagnose and differentiate from other intestinal disorders. If malabsorption is indicated, two criteria must be met for a definitive diagnosis of celiac sprue: (1) biopsy of the small intestine indicating destruction of **villi**, and (2) remission of symptoms and improvement in the condition of the villi after institution of a gluten-free diet.

Laboratory tests may show a decrease in minerals and a deficiency of vitamins B, D, and K. A D-xylose test may indicate a decrease in intestinal absorption. X-rays may reveal demineralization of bone, collapsed vertebrae, and osteoid seams.

Treatment: Treatment consists of strict adherence to a gluten-free diet. A few persons who do not experience improved small bowel function after instituting a gluten-free diet may be treated with corticosteroid drugs.

Prognosis: With proper treatment, the prognosis is good. Symptomatic relief often occurs within a few weeks, but improvement in tests of absorption function and small bowel tissue characteristics may not occur for months, sometimes years. If persons go on and off the diet, tissue regeneration may no longer be possible. Persons with celiac sprue have an increased incidence of abdominal lymphoma and carcinomas later in life. Individuals who develop gastrointestinal symptoms while in remission on a gluten-free diet should be carefully evaluated for malignancy.

Prevention: There is no known prevention of the disease.

Duodenal Ulcer (Peptic Ulcer of the Duodenum)

Description: A *duodenal ulcer* is a circumscribed, crater-like lesion in the mucous membrane of the short, wide segment of the small intestine called the *duodenum.* Duodenal ulcers tend to be chronic and recurrent. They are a major health problem in the United States, but have been declining in frequency. More common in males, they can occur anytime from infancy to later life. The majority of these ulcers appear in the first few inches of the duodenum.

Etiology: The cause is obscure, but it may be due to hypersecretion of stomach acids, damage to duodenal tissue, or critical illness. Genetic factors and smoking are associated with the likelihood of developing the disease. Precipitating factors include trauma, infections, and physical or emotional stress.

Signs and Symptoms: Symptoms produced by duodenal ulcers may be vague, absent, typical, or atypical. Typical symptoms include chronic, periodic heartburn pain that may radiate into the back region. Nausea, vomiting, and epigastric tenderness and guarding also may occur. Usually the symptoms appear 45 minutes to 1 hour after eating and may be relieved by milk, antacids, and vomiting.

Diagnostic Procedures: Diagnosis is difficult, since duodenal ulcers may be confused with gastric ulcers, gastritis, or irritable bowel syndrome, especially if the symptoms are atypical. Laboratory findings may reveal anemia, **occult blood** in stools, and hypersecretion of stomach acids. X-rays are essential to differentiate the disease from other disorders, but they may not always show an ulcer. Endoscopy will be used if x-rays do not confirm the diagnosis.

Treatment: General rest is advised, with alleviation of as much anxiety as possible. Restriction of alcohol, smoking, and some medications such as salicylates and **rauwolfia** is recommended. Dietary measures include a well-balance diet and restriction of coffee, tea, colas, or other foods known to aggravate symptoms. Prescribed medications may include antacids, coating agents such as carafate, antihistamine drugs, especially H2 blocking agents that reduce stomach acid secretions, prostaglandins, and anticholinergic drugs. **Gastrectomy** may be performed in a small percentage of cases, usually if perforation of the duodenal wall occurs.

Prognosis: Duodenal ulcers generally have a chronic course. Many can be controlled, however, by medical treatment. Complications that may worsen the prognosis include hemorrhage, perforation, and bowel obstruction.

Prevention: There is no specific prevention. A change to a less stressful lifestyle, however, may be helpful if the cause is psychologic.

Acute Appendicitis

Description: *Acute appendicitis* is an inflammation of the vermiform appendix.

Etiology: Appendicitis may be initiated by obstruction of the interior of the appendix by a **fecalith**, neoplasm, foreign body, or worms. In many cases, though, ulceration of the mucosal lining of the appendix appears to be the causative factor. Regardless of the etiology, the course of the disease is the same. Bacteria multiply and invade the appendix wall, compromising circulation to the organ. Necrosis of appendiceal tissue, gangrene, and eventual perforation occur. Perforation of the appendix is life-threatening because the infection is then able to spread into the peritoneal cavity.

Signs and Symptoms: The classic symptoms are right upper quadrant abdominal pain and pain localized in the lower right quadrant. Nausea, vomiting, and anorexia will likely occur. Fever, **malaise**, diarrhea, or constipation are less frequent symptoms.

Diagnostic Procedures: Physical examination and the characteristic symptomatology generally indicate appendicitis. Tenderness upon pressure on **McBur-**

ney's point, and the patient's ability to pinpoint the area of maximum tenderness are the strongest diagnostic indicators of appendicitis. Laboratory findings may reveal **leukocytosis** and **pyuria**. Hospitalization and observation may be necessary to differentiate appendicitis from other abdominal disorders. Abdominal and rectal examinations and complete blood counts may need to be repeated.

Treatment: Appendectomy is the choice treatment.

Prognosis: With early diagnosis and treatment, the prognosis is good. If the appendix ruptures, however, peritonitis may ensue, greatly increasing the likelihood of death.

Prevention: No prevention is known.

Irritable Bowel Syndrome

Decription: *Irritable bowel syndrome* (IBS) is a symptom complex marked by abdominal pain and altered bowel function—typically constipation, diarrhea, or alternating constipation and diarrhea—for which no organic cause can be determined. The disease is chronic, with the onset of symptoms usually occurring in early adulthood and lasting intermittently for years. IBS is the most frequently occurring gastrointestinal disorder in the United States. Its management often proves frustrating to patient and physician alike.

Etiology: The cause of IBS is unknown, but it is suspected that the disease may arise from a number of underlying disorders. What is known is that IBS is associated with a change in colonic motility, either decreased motility or increased motility. The disease also has a strong psychologic component, with certain personality types more frequently affected than others. But whether psychologic factors actually cause the disease or merely aggravate its manifestations has not been resolved.

Signs and Symptoms: The hallmark of IBS is abdominal pain with constipation or constipation alternating with diarrhea. The totally diarrheal form of IBS is often painless. Heartburn, abdominal distension, back pain, weakness, faintness, and **tachycardia** also may accompany the primary symptoms. Stool may be reported as mucous-covered. Symptoms usually are experienced as acute attacks that subside within 1 day, but recurrent exacerbations are likely.

Diagnostic Procedures: The chronic, intermittent nature of the symptoms without obvious cause suggests the diagnosis. However, irritable bowel syndrome must be differentiated from other gastrointestinal diseases. A careful patient history, especially of psychologic factors, is essential. A complete blood count and stool examination for occult blood, ova, parasites, and pathogenic bacteria will help rule out closely related conditions. Sigmoidoscopy, colonoscopy, barium enema, and rectal biopsy may provide similarly useful information.

Treatment: There is no one successful treatment for controlling IBS. Dietary modification may be attempted, such as avoiding irritating foods or adding fiber if constipation is a symptom. The patient is advised to get adequate sleep and exercise and alleviate any stress. A sedative or antispasmodic drug may be ordered. Educating the patient about the chronic but benign nature of the disease is an essential part of the treatment process.

Prognosis: Because IBS cannot be cured, the prognosis varies according to how successfully the symptoms can be controlled. There is a higher incidence of diverticulitis and colon cancer in patients with irritable bowel syndrome. Accordingly, regular checkups including sigmoidoscopy and rectal examination are important.

Prevention: There is no known prevention.

Crohn's Disease (Regional Enteritis, Granulomatous Colitis)

Description: *Crohn's disease* is a chronic inflammation of the ileum, but it may affect any portion of the intestinal tract. Crohn's disease is distinguished from closely related bowel disorders by its inflammatory pattern. This includes inflammation extending through all layers of the intestinal wall, resulting in a characteristic thickening or toughening of the wall and narrowing of the intestinal lumen. The inflammation tends to be patchy or segmented (compare with Ulcerative Colitis).

Etiology: The cause of Crohn's disease is not known, but genetic, immunologic, infectious, and psychologic factors have been proposed.

Signs and Symptoms: Signs and symptoms include anorexia, flatulence, malaise, weight loss, and colicky or steady abdominal pain in the right lower quadrant. The pain may be mild or severe. Diarrhea may occur, followed by intervening periods of normal bowel function or constipation.

Diagnostic Procedures: Crohn's disease is diagnosed by differentiating its characteristic pattern of inflammation from those of other bowel disorders. Barium enema, sigmoidoscopy, and colonoscopy may be necessary. Only a biopsy provides a definitive diagnosis.

Treatment: Treatment of Crohn's disease is symptomatic and supportive. Dietary management may include a low-residue diet or total **parenteral** hyperalimentation to let the intestine "rest." Corticosteroids and antimicrobial agents also may be used when the disease is acute. Changes in lifestyle may be encouraged. Surgical treatment of the disease is usually reserved to manage complications, but **colectomy** or **ileostomy** may be necessary in persons with extensive disease.

Prognosis: The prognosis is dependent on the severity of the initial onset of the disease and its clinical history. The prognosis worsens over time. Complications may include intestinal obstruction and **fistula** formation, resulting in peritonitis and sepsis.

Prevention: There is no known prevention.

Ulcerative Colitis

Description: *Ulcerative colitis* is a chronic inflammation and ulceration of the colon, often beginning in the rectum or sigmoid colon and extending upward into the entire colon. Ulcerative colitis is distinguished from closely related bowel disorders by its characteristic inflammatory pattern. The inflammation only involves the mucosal lining of the colon, which exhibits erythema and numerous hemorrhagic ulcerations. In addition, the affected portion of the colon is uniformly involved, with no patches of healthy mucosal tissue evident (compare with Crohn's Disease).

Etiology: The etiology of ulcerative colitis is unknown, but predisposing factors may include a family history of the disease, bacterial infection, allergic reactions to certain foods, emotional stress, and autoimmune factors.

Signs and symptoms: The classic symptom is recurrent bloody diarrhea, often containing pus and mucus, accompanied by abdominal pain. Other symptoms may include fever, weight loss, and signs of dehydration. There is a tendency toward periodic exacerbation and remission of symptoms.

Diagnostic Procedures: The disease is diagnosed by the characteristics of the inflammatory process. Sigmoidoscopy may reveal the mucosal lining to be friable (easily broken or pulverized). Colonoscopy may be necessary to determine the extent of the disease. A biopsy may be done at the same time to rule out carcinoma.

Treatment: The treatment program generally includes measures to counteract nutritional losses, restore blood volume, and control the inflammation. This typically includes parenteral hyperalimentation, blood transfusions, and the use of various anti-inflammatory drugs. Hospitalization may be necessary during a severe attack. Surgical excision and resection of the colon are reserved for management of complications.

Prognosis: The prognosis for an individual with ulcerative colitis depends on the severity of the acute episodes of the disease. Complications may be life-threatening and include anemia and perforated colon with resulting **toxemia**. Persons with ulcerative colitis run a greater than normal risk of developing colorectal cancer. An annual colonoscopy is advised.

Prevention: There is no known prevention.

Diverticulitis

Description: *Diverticulitis* is the acute inflammation of small, pouchlike herniations in the intestinal wall called *diverticula* (Figure 6–4). The diverticula may form anywhere along the intestinal tract but most commonly develop in the colon. The presence of diverticula (diverticulosis) usually does not produce symptoms; rather, it is the infection of the diverticula that produces the clinically significant condition.

Etiology: The cause of diverticulitis is not clearly understood, but it probably involves intestinal matter accumulating within a diverticulum to form a small fecalith. Bacteria multiply around the fecalith, attacking the inner surface of the diverticulum, resulting in inflammation that may lead to perforation. The formation of diverticula and, hence, the incidence of diverticulitis may be due in part to a diet of highly refined, low-residue foods.

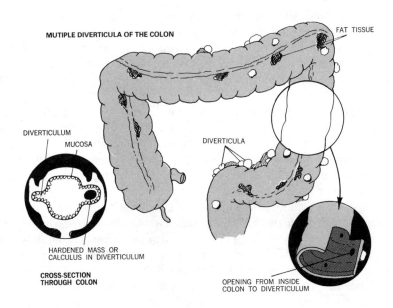

MUTIPLE DIVERTICULA OF THE COLON

FAT TISSUE

DIVERTICULUM

MUCOSA

DIVERTICULA

HARDENED MASS OR
CALCULUS IN DIVERTICULUM

CROSS-SECTION
THROUGH COLON

OPENING FROM INSIDE
COLON TO DIVERTICULUM

FIGURE 6–4. Diverticula of the colon. (From Thomas, C. L. [ed.], *Taber's Cyclopedic Medical Dictionary,* ed. 15. F. A. Davis, Philadelphia, 1985, p. 484, with permission.)

Signs and Symptoms: The symptoms of diverticulitis vary from case to case in both intensity and duration. Typically, though, an acute attack is characterized by fever, pain in the lower abdomen that worsens following a bowel movement, and abdominal muscle spasms, guarding, and tenderness. The person usually experiences constipation, but diarrhea may sometimes occur instead.

Diagnostic Procedures: Sigmoidoscopy and colonoscopy are useful in the diagnosis of diverticulitis. A barium enema or a biopsy of the diverticula may be attempted, but not if the disease is in the active phase because of the possibility of perforation and hemorrhage. Blood testing may reveal an elevated erythrocyte sedimentation rate (ESR), leukocytosis, and the presence of occult blood.

Treatment: Treatment of uncomplicated diverticular disease consists of a high-residue diet that includes bran, bulk additives, and stool softeners. Anticholinergic drugs or antibiotics may be ordered. If perforation or hemorrhage occur, hospitalization, surgery, and blood transfusions may be necessary.

Prognosis: The prognosis becomes less favorable with advancing age. Proper dietary measures and antibiotics can generally forestall acute episodes of the disease. Perforation of the intestinal wall in diverticulitis can lead to acute peritonitis, sepsis, and shock.

Prevention: There is no known prevention.

Hemorrhoids

Description: *Hemorrhoids are dilated, tortuous veins in the mucous membrane of the anus or rectum. There are two kinds: external hemorrhoids,* those involving veins below the anorectal line; and *internal hemorrhoids,* those involving veins above or along the anorectal line.

Etiology: Straining at stool, constipation, prolonged sitting, and anorectal infections are contributing factors of hemorrhoids. Loss of muscle tone due to old age, pregnancy, and anal intercourse are other considerations.

Signs and Symptoms: There may be rectal bleeding and vague discomfort. In some cases, the hemorrhoids may protrude from the anus. There may be a discharge of mucus from the rectum, too.

Diagnostic Procedures: Physical examination will reveal external hemorrhoids. Proctoscopy will reveal internal hemorrhoids.

Treatment: Treatment generally includes measures to ease pain and discomfort, such as taking warm sitz baths. A high-roughage diet and using stool softeners also may be recommended. Protruding hemorrhoids may be reduced manually with a lubricated gloved finger, by reduction and taping the buttocks together, by rubber band ligation, or by cryosurgery. In the event of severe complications or chronic discomfort, complete internal or external hemorrhoidectomy may be advised.

Prognosis: With proper treatment, the prognosis is good. Complications may include **pruritus**, fecal incontinence, anorectal infections, prolapse and strangulation of the hemorrhoidal vein, and secondary anemia due to chronic blood loss.

Prevention: Prevention includes avoiding straining at stool and adherence to a proper diet and exercise regimen.

Abdominal Hernias

Description: An *abdominal hernia* is the protrusion of an internal organ, typically a portion of the intestine, through an abnormal opening in the musculature of the abdominal wall. Abdominal hernias are categorized according to the location of the herniation and include umbilical, inguinal, and femoral hernias (Figure 6–3). Inguinal hernias are the most common.

Etiology: Hernias may result from a congenital weakness in the abdominal wall or muscle. Heavy lifting, pregnancy, obesity, and straining at stool are predisposing factors.

Signs and Symptoms: Inguinal and umbilical hernias are evidenced by a lump appearing over the herniated area which tends to disappear when the person is supine. Sharp, steady, accompanying pain may be present in the groin. Strangulation of a herniated portion of the intestine will cause severe pain and can cause bowel obstruction (Figure 6–3).

Diagnostic Procedures: Physical examination will reveal the herniated area. A patient history of a sharp abdominal pain when lifting or straining also may help confirm the diagnosis. An x-ray will be ordered if bowel obstruction is suspected.

Treatment: Umbilical hernias may require only taping or binding the affected area until the hernia closes. Femoral and inguinal hernias require reduction of the hernia and trussing the weakened portion of the abdominal wall. Herniorrhaphy is the corrective surgery indicated.

Prognosis: The prognosis is excellent with proper treatment and care.

Prevention: Preventive measures include following recommended guidelines for lifting heavy objects, maintaining a soft stool consistency, and practicing moderate exercise.

Colorectal Cancer

Description: *Colorectal cancer* is the collective designation for a variety of malignant neoplasms that may arise in either the colon or rectum.

Etiology: The cause of colorectal cancer is unknown, but there is a higher incidence in societies that have a diet high in red meat and low in fiber. Other predisposing factors include diseases of the digestive tract, a history of irritable bowel syndrome, and familial **polyposis**. The incidence of colorectal cancer increases after the age of 40.

Signs and Symptoms: Symptoms are vague in the early stages. Later symptoms may include **pallor, ascites, cachexia, lymphadenopathy**, and **hepatomegaly**. Any significant change in bowel habits should be regarded as suspicious. This may include alternating states of diarrhea and constipation and the presence of blood in the stool.

Diagnostic Procedures: Digital examination of the rectum may be sufficient to detect many tumors. Testing for occult blood in the stool is the most effective diagnostic indicator of colorectal cancer. Sigmoidoscopy and colonoscopy are also helpful in detection. Barium x-ray can locate lesions that are manually or otherwise visually undetectable.

Treatment: Surgery to remove the tumor and adjacent tissues is the treatment of choice. Chemotherapy and radiation therapy also may be used.

Prognosis: The prognosis varies. This cancer tends to progress slowly and remains localized for a fair length of time. If diagnosed early, colorectal cancer is potentially curable in about 85 percent of cases.

Prevention: A high-fiber, low-fat diet may reduce the risk of colorectal cancer for some individuals.

Diarrhea

Description: *Diarrhea* is the frequent passage of feces, with an accompanying increase in fluidity and volume. Diarrhea is not a disease. It is, rather, a symptom of another underlying condition. "Normal" bowel habits vary widely; consequently, what is considered diarrhea in some individuals may be normal in others.

Etiology: Diarrhea is the result of an abrupt increase in intestinal motility. The highly liquid content of the small intestine is rushed through the colon without sufficient time for fluid reabsorption, resulting in the watery stools characteristic of diarrhea. Numerous diseases and conditions can cause the necessary increase in intestinal motility. These include malabsorption syndrome, gastritis, lactose intolerance, irritable bowel syndrome, gastrointestinal tumors, diverticular disease, viral and bacterial infections of the intestine, parasitic infections, psychogenic disorders, food allergies, and a variety of medications.

Signs and Symptoms: The diarrhea may vary in fluidity and volume. It may be accompanied by flatulence, abdominal distension, fever, headache, anorexia, vomiting, malaise, and **myalgia**.

Diagnostic Procedures: The clinical history of the diarrhea involves determining whether its onset was abrupt or gradual, acute or chronic. The characteristics of the diarrheal stools also will be evaluated. To help determine underlying causes, bacterial cultures and microscopic examination of the stools may be performed. Additional tests include proctoscopy, radiologic studies, and tests for occult blood.

Treatment: Treatment goals in diarrhea include relief of symptoms and correction of underlying disorders.

Prognosis: The prognosis is dependent on the cause. Possible complications include dehydration and **electrolyte** imbalances.

Prevention: Cases of diarrhea due to infectious agents can often be prevented by following proper hygiene and sanitation procedures. Cases due to allergic reactions can be prevented by avoiding known allergens.

ACCESSORY ORGANS OF DIGESTION: PANCREAS, GALLBLADDER, AND LIVER

Acute Pancreatitis

Description: *Acute pancreatitis* is a severe, often life-threatening inflammation of the pancreas (Figure 6–5). In this disease, pancreatic enzymes that normally remain inactive until reaching the duodenum begin digesting pancreatic tissue, causing varying degrees of edema, swelling, tissue necrosis, and hemorrhaging.

Etiology: The causes of this autodigestive process in acute pancreatitis are not well understood. A number of conditions, though, are known to lead to the disease. The chief among these is alcoholism. Other conditions include **gallstones**, trauma to the abdomen, viral infections, drug reactions, systemic immunologic disorders, pancreatic cancer, or complications from a duodenal ulcer. Acute pancreatitis is on occasion idiopathic.

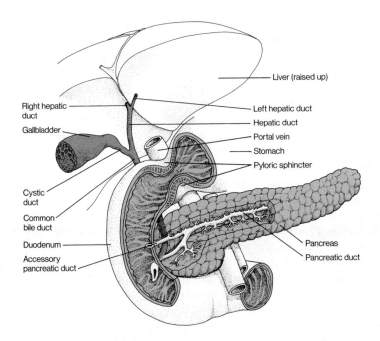

Liver (raised up)

Right hepatic duct

Gallbladder

Left hepatic duct

Hepatic duct

Portal vein

Stomach

Pyloric sphincter

Cystic duct

Common bile duct

Duodenum

Accessory pancreatic duct

Pancreas

Pancreatic duct

FIGURE 6–5. The accessory organs of digestion: the pancreas, liver, and gallbladder. (Modified from Gylys, B. A. and Wedding, M. E., *Medical Terminology: A Systems Approach,* ed. 2. F. A. Davis, Philadelphia, 1988, p. 94.)

Signs and Symptoms: The most important symptom of acute pancreatitis is the sudden onset of severe, persistent abdominal pain that is centered over the epigastric region and that may radiate toward the back. Severe attacks of acute pancreatitis also may cause abdominal distension, nausea, vomiting, fever, tachycardia, and shock.

Diagnostic Procedures: A clinical history of acute onset of the characteristic abdominal pain may suggest the diagnosis. A blood test revealing an elevated level of the enzyme amylase in the serum generally confirms the diagnosis. Ultrasonography and abdominal CT scans may reveal pancreatic enlargement. Leukocytosis may be an additional finding.

Treatment: Treatment is largely symptomatic and supportive or may be directed at controlling any complications. Analgesic drugs, intravenous administration of fluids, and fasting with parenteral hyperalimentation may be tried.

Prognosis: The prognosis is guarded. Acute pancreatitis is usually self-limiting, and pancreatic function is eventually restored. A host of possible complications, however, may worsen the prognosis, and about 10 percent of individuals with acute pancreatitis die, usually from respiratory distress or shock.

Prevention: There is no known prevention.

Chronic Pancreatitis

Description: *Chronic pancreatitis* is the slow, progressive destruction of pancreatic tissue, accompanied by variable amounts of inflammation, fibrosis, and dilation of the pancreatic ducts. As with acute pancreatitis, the damage to the pancreas is thought to result from autodigestion by pancreatic enzymes (see Acute Pancreatitis).

Etiology: While the exact cause is unclear, the leading etiologic factors in chronic pancreatitis appear to be alcoholism in adults and cystic fibrosis in children. The etiologic factors implicated in acute pancreatitis also may play a limited role. In contrast to the acute form of the disease, however, many cases of chronic pancreatitis are idiopathic.

Signs and Symptoms: Severe, persistent abdominal pain, often worsening following a meal, is the primary symptom of chronic pancreatitis, although this pain may be less specifically focused than in acute pancreatitis. Other symptoms may include weight loss, anorexia, and abnormal bowel movements. Advanced pancreatic destruction may be manifested by **jaundice**.

Diagnostic Procedures: Treatment is generally directed at pain management and correcting any nutritional disorders resulting from malabsorption. Pain relief may be accomplished either through drug therapy or various surgical procedures. Pancreatic enzyme replacement therapy helps to correct malabsorption problems and also may provide additional pain relief.

Prognosis: The prognosis is poor for individuals with chronic pancreatitis caused by alcoholism, with a mortality rate approaching 50 percent. Others may do well, although therapy must be maintained indefinitely. Diabetes mellitus is a possible complication of chronic pancreatitis (see Diabetes Mellitus in Chapter 10).

Prevention: There is no known prevention other than alcohol avoidance.

Pancreatic Cancer

Description: *Pancreatic cancer* is a neoplasm, usually an adenocarcinoma, occurring most frequently in the head of the pancreas. Pancreatic cancer is the fourth leading cause of cancer deaths in the United States. The highest incidence is among people 60 to 70 years of age.

Etiology: The etiology is not known, but cigarette smoking, exposure to occupational chemicals, a diet high in fats, and heavy coffee intake are associated with an increased incidence of pancreatic cancer.

Signs and Symptoms: The classic symptoms are abdominal pain, anorexia, jaundice, and weight loss. Other symptoms include weakness, fatigue, diarrhea, nausea and vomiting, and boring pain in the midback. If the disease affects the islets of Langerhans, symptoms of insulin deficiency appear. These symptoms include glucosuria, **hyperglycemia**, and glucose intolerance.

Diagnostic Procedures: A gastrointestinal x-ray series may be ordered. Ultrasonography, CT scanning, and endoscopic retrograde cholangeopancreotography (ERCP) are useful in establishing a diagnosis. Percutaneous needle aspiration biopsy of the affected portion of the pancreas is used to confirm the diagnosis.

Treatment: Treatment usually is palliative, since most pancreatic cancers are diagnosed after they have metastasized to the lungs, liver, and bones. If surgical resection is possible, localized tumors will be removed. Radiation therapy and multidrug chemotherapy may be given. It is important to manage the patient's pain and to correct any nutritional deficits.

Prognosis: The prognosis is poor, since 80 to 85 percent of patients have advanced disease when first diagnosed.

Prevention: There is no known prevention.

Cholelithiasis

Description: *Cholelithiasis* is the formation or presence of stonelike masses called gallstones within the gallbladder or bile ducts. These stones may be formed of either cholesterol or calcium-based (pigmented) compounds and range from a few millimeters to a few centimeters in size. Cholelithiasis is a common condition in the United States, with women affected more than twice as frequently as men. Most individuals with gallstones remain asymptomatic. Clinically significant symptoms result when a gallstone obstructs a biliary duct.

Etiology: The cause of cholelithiasis is not well understood. Any factors that cause the bile to become overladen with cholesterol may increase the likelihood of the formation of cholesterol-based gallstones. Such factors include obesity, high-calorie diets, certain drugs, oral contraceptives, multiple pregnancies, and increasing age. The production of calcium-based (pigmented) gallstones is even less well understood, but it may be related to genetic factors, hemolytic disease, alcoholic cirrhosis, or persistent biliary tract infections.

Signs and Symptoms: As mentioned previously, many individuals with gallstones remain asymptomatic. If bile ducts are obstructed, though, a classic "gallbladder attack," more properly referred to as biliary colic, may result. The telltale symptom is the acute onset of upper right quadrant abdominal pain radiating to the shoulder and back. Nausea and vomiting may accompany the attack. Flatulence, belching, and heartburn also may occur at intervals. Gallbladder attacks typically tend to follow ingestion of large meals or fatty foods. The pain and other symptoms of an attack gradually subside on their own over a period of several hours.

Diagnostic Procedures: A clinical history of the characteristic pain of biliary colic suggests a diagnosis of gallstones. Various methods of visualizing the stones are employed for a definitive diagnosis. These typically include a gallbladder ultrasound, oral cholecystogram, radioisotope scintiscans, or a plain abdominal x-ray.

Treatment: Cholecystectomy is the treatment of choice for symptomatic cholelithiasis. Surgical treatment for asymptomatic individuals remains controversial.

An alternative approach in such cases involves dissolving cholesterol-based stones through bile acid therapy. This therapy inhibits the synthesis and secretion of cholesterol within the liver, altering the composition of the bile. Existing stones may be decreased in size or dissolved entirely.

Prognosis: The prognosis is generally good with prompt treatment. Complications may include cholecystitis (see Acute Cholecystitis) and pancreatitis.

Prevention: No prevention is known.

Acute Cholecystitis

Description: *Acute cholecystitis* is a severe inflammation of the interior wall of the gallbladder.

Etiology: The majority of cases of acute cholecystitis are a consequence of the obstruction of bile ducts by gallstones. The resulting inflammation may result from the increased pressure of accumulating bile within the gallbladder, chemical changes in the bile that erode the gallbladder tissue, or secondary infection from multiplying bacteria. Some forms of the disease are not caused by obstructing gallstones. These cases may be due to obstruction of bile ducts by neoplasms or to vascular disease, diabetes mellitus, parasitic infections, and various systemic diseases. The risk of nonobstructive, acalculous forms of acute cholecystitis is increased in burn patients and following trauma or surgery.

Signs and Symptoms: A characteristic symptom of acute cholecystitis is the gradual onset of upper right quadrant pain that usually remains localized over the area of the gallbladder. Unlike the pain of biliary colic, it does not tend to subside after a few hours (see Biliary Colic). Anorexia, nausea, vomiting, and a low-grade fever and chills also may accompany the pain.

Diagnostic Procedures: Diagnosis of acute cholecystitis is usually suggested on the basis of the characteristic pain. In most cases, gallbladder enlargement is palpable. Laboratory findings typically reveal leukocytosis and elevated serum **bilirubin** and serum aminotransferase levels. Visualization of obstructing gallstones in suspected cases of acute cholecystitis is typically performed through radioisotope scintiscans, gallbladder ultrasound, or abdominal x-ray.

Treatment: Cholecystectomy is the treatment of choice.

Prognosis: The prognosis is generally good with prompt treatment. Complications from perforation of the gallbladder include possibility of peritonitis.

Prevention: There is no known prevention.

Cirrhosis

Description: *Cirrhosis* is a chronic, irreversible, degenerative disease of the liver characterized by the replacement of normal liver cells with fibrous scar tissue and other alterations in liver structure. Cirrhosis is the consequence of the repeated traumatizing of hepatic tissue by toxins, infectious agents, metabolic diseases, and circulatory disorders.

Etiology: Cirrhosis has a diverse set of etiologies. The most common cause of cirrhosis is chronic alcoholism. Other forms of cirrhosis, classified by their pathogenesis, include biliary cirrhosis, which is manifested by **cholestasis**; postnecrotic cirrhosis, resulting from hepatitis; pigment cirrhosis (hemochromatosis), which is due to a genetic disorder of iron metabolism; or cardiac cirrhosis, caused by congestive heart failure. Cirrhosis also may be idiopathic in origin.

Signs and Symptoms: The person may be asymptomatic for a prolonged period, or symptoms may be vague or unspecific. Symptoms may include nausea, vomiting, anorexia, dull abdominal ache, weakness, fatigability, weight loss, pruritus, peripheral neuritis, bleeding tendencies, jaundice, and edema of the legs.

Diagnostic Procedures: Palpation will reveal the liver as enlarged and firm—if not hard—with a blunt edge. Plain abdominal x-rays also may show an enlarged liver. A liver scan and biopsy are essential for diagnosis. Laboratory findings may reveal anemia, folate deficiency, **hemolysis**, and blood loss. Elevated serum glutamic-oxaloacetic transaminase (SGOT), **alkaline phosphatase**, and bilirubin levels may be present.

Treatment: Treatment is aimed at the cause of the cirrhosis in an attempt to prevent further liver damage. Adequate rest and diet are essential, as is restriction of alcohol. Vitamin and mineral supplements may be prescribed. In the event of gastric upset or internal bleeding, antacids may be given.

Prognosis: The prognosis is poor in advanced cirrhosis, especially for alcoholic cirrhosis should the person continue drinking. Hematemesis, jaundice, and ascites are unfavorable signs. Elevated blood pressure in the portal vein, called *portal hypertension*, is a common complication of cirrhosis. As a consequence, blood pressure increases within the spleen, causing **splenomegaly**, and blood bypasses the liver, producing ascites or esophageal **varices**. Hemorrhage of esophageal varices often requires emergency treatment.

Prevention: There is no known prevention unless alcohol is a contributing factor.

Acute Viral Hepatitis

Description: *Acute viral hepatitis* is an infection and subsequent inflammation of the liver by one of several viruses. Viral hepatitis is designated hepatitis A, hepatitis B, or non-A, non-B hepatitis according to the viral pathogen responsible for the case.

Etiology: *Hepatitis A virus* (HAV) is an RNA virus passed from the body in the feces. Therefore, it is most frequently spread through the fecal-oral route, following ingestion of contaminated water, milk, or food. HAV is highly contagious and is responsible for epidemic outbreaks of the disease.

Hepatitis B virus (HBV) is a DNA virus that is present in all bodily fluids of an infected individual. Its mode of transmission, therefore, is largely parenteral, spread through contact with contaminated blood or blood products, contaminated hypodermic needles or intimate personal contact—especially between sexual partners. Those most at risk of contracting type B hepatitis include health care workers, IV drug users, male homosexuals, infants of infected mothers, and dialysis patients. Type B hepatitis may progress to a chronic disease, and certain individuals may become asymptomatic carriers of the virus.

Non-A, non-B hepatitis is a diagnosis of exclusion, that is, a case of hepatitis in which neither the HAV or HBV viruses can be detected. It appears to be transmitted parenterally, almost exclusively as a result of transfusion with infected blood and blood products. Indeed, non-A, non-B hepatitis accounts for the greatest percentage of post transfusion cases of the disease in the United States.

Signs and Symptoms: Symptoms occur suddenly in type A hepatitis and more slowly for type B. Non-A, non-B hepatitis has clinical symptoms similar to type B, but it is milder. Initial symptoms are flulike, vague, and include malaise, fatigue, anorexia, myalgia, **lassitude**, fever, dark-colored urine, clay-colored stools, and jaundice. An aversion to smoking and certain foods is common.

Diagnostic Procedures: A clinical history of exposure to jaundiced persons, recent blood transfusions, or IV drug use may suggest a diagnosis of hepatitis. The liver may be enlarged and tender. Splenomegaly may occur. Laboratory findings in most forms of hepatitis will include **proteinuria** and **bilirubinuria**. Increased levels of SGOT, serum glutamic-pyruvic transaminase (SGPT), alkaline phosphatase, and **gamma globulin** also may be evident. Liver biopsy and liver scintiscan help to confirm the diagnosis.

Treatment: There is no specific treatment for hepatitis. Rather, the disease is treated by general measures. Bed rest, adequate diet, and fluid intake are advised. Antiemetics may be ordered. Corticosteroids may be used in more serious cases, but they are controversial. The disease needs to be reported to the public health department for proper follow-up because of the possibility of contagion.

Prognosis: Because type A hepatitis tends to be mild and self-limiting, the prognosis is generally good. Type B hepatitis may produce more serious symptoms and ensuing complications; hence, the prognosis for this form of the disease is more guarded, especially among the aged and those with previously existing medical conditions.

Prevention: Prevention for all forms of hepatitis includes proper hygienic practices, especially when using needles for injections and when handling human secretions. When individuals are exposed to type A hepatitis, immune serum globulin (ISG) may be administered as a preventive measure. Hepatitis B immune globulin (HBIG) provides similar protection following accidental exposure to HBV. The best protection against HBV, however, is provided by a new type B vaccine. Its use is recommended for those in high-risk groups, such as health care professionals. No preventive measures exist for the non-A, non-B form of hepatitis other than following proper hygienic procedures and avoiding transfusion with commercially acquired blood.

SPECIAL FOCUS: EATING DISORDERS

Anorexia Nervosa

Description: *Anorexia nervosa* is a complex psychogenic eating disorder characterized by an all-consuming desire to remain thin. It is also marked by weight loss, clinical evidence of semistarvation, amenorrhea, and an alteration in body image. Anorexia nervosa should not be confused with simple **anorexia**, a loss of appetite symptomatic of one of many possible underlying physical diseases. On the contrary, most individuals with anorexia nervosa never suffer a loss of appetite. The disorder primarily affects young women around the age of puberty. Men are rarely afflicted with the condition.

Etiology: The cause of anorexia nervosa is not known, although most health professionals believe it is essentially a psychiatric disorder. A female's socioeconomic status, family background, and cultural conditioning may be predisposing factors in development of the conditon.

Signs and Symptoms: A loss of at least 25 percent of original body weight, in the absence of any detectable underlying medical disorder, may suggest a diagnosis of anorexia nervosa. Evidence of food avoidance, vomiting, and excessive exercise also suggest the diagnosis. In severe cases, a host of secondary symptoms may be evident as a result of metabolic and hormonal disturbances resulting from malnutrition. The affected individual also may tend to deny feelings of hunger and will typically claim to be overweight despite physical evidence to the contrary.

Diagnostic Procedures: No specific diagnostic tests exist for anorexia nervosa, but blood testing may reveal associated nutritional anemia and vitamin or mineral deficiencies.

Treatment: Medical treatment of anorexia nervosa generally involves reversing the effects of malnutrition. Noncooperation on the part of the affected individual, however, typically makes treatment of this disorder a difficult, uncertain matter. Intensive individual or family psychotherapy may be recommended. Hospitalization may be required in the event of severe weight loss and malnutrition. Providing the individual with nutritional guidelines and information about proper eating habits also may be useful in the recovery process.

Prognosis: The prognosis varies. Relapses are frequent. Death may occur from malnutrition and complications such as hypothermia and cardiac disturbances in as many as one-quarter of diagnosed cases.

Prevention: No specific prevention is known, but it seems helpful that an individual develop a sense of self-esteem that is not attached to a thin, "model-like" body image.

Bulimia

Description: *Bulimia* is a psychogenic eating disorder characterized by repetitive gorging of food, followed by self-induced vomiting. The condition also may involve laxative abuse. Whereas the individual with anorexia nervosa seems obsessed with becoming even thinner, the person with bulimia has a morbid fear of becoming fat. Other behavioral abnormalities include obsessive secrecy about the condition and also may involve food stealing. The disorder principally affects young women.

Etiology: The cause of bulimia is not known. As is the case with anorexia nervosa, most health professionals believe bulimia is essentially a psychiatric disorder.

Signs and Symptoms: Most persons with bulimia hide the behavioral evidence of their condition, and they are often of normal weight or even slightly overweight upon diagnosis. They may still exhibit signs of malnutrition, however, since the "binge" diet of a bulimic individual is often wildly unbalanced, usually consisting of "junk" foods such as donuts, ice cream, and candy. Owing to the high sugar content of the binge diet and the subsequent reflux of gastric juices during vomiting, the bulimic person typically has a high incidence of dental caries. Reflux of gastric secretions also may produce a chronic sore throat. Menstrual irregulariries are much less common in bulimia than in anorexia nervosa.

Diagnostic Procedures: Blood testing may reveal **hypokalemia** and **alkalosis** as a consequence of vomiting and laxative abuse. Other tests may reveal cardiac arrhythmias or evidence of renal dysfunction.

Treatment: Long-term psychotherapy is usually indicated. As with the anorexic person, noncooperation on the part of the bulimic patient generally makes treatment difficult and frustrating.

Prognosis: The prognosis is guarded. Persons with bulimia may die suddenly from cardiac arrhythmias brought about by hypolakemia. They also have twice as great an incidence of suicide as compared with anorexics. Other complications may include pneumonia, rupturing of the esophagus or stomach, and pancreatitis.

Prevention: There is no specific prevention for bulimia.

COMMON SYMPTOMS
OF DIGESTIVE SYSTEM DISEASES

Individuals may present with the following common symptoms, which deserve attention from health professionals:
■ Loss of appetite and weight loss
■ Nausea and vomiting
■ Any change in bowel habits, such as diarrhea, constipation, and flatulence
■ Blood or mucus in the stool
■ Fever
■ Pain in the area of the gastrointestinal tract
■ Heartburn, indigestion, dysphagia, and any discomfort after eating certain foods
■ Malaise, loss of strength, and fatigability
■ **Diaphoresis**

REVIEW QUESTIONS

Short Answer

1. Identify three functions of the gastrointestinal tract:

   a.

   b.

   c.

2. Name an upper gastrointestinal tract disease related to the teeth: _____ .

3. Common diagnostic procedures used to diagnose disease of the upper gastrointestinal tract include:

   a.

   b.

   c.

4. Common symptoms of gastric and duodenal ulcers include:

   a.

   b.

Matching

_____ 1. Most common malabsorption disorder

_____ 2. Examination of colon using fiberoptic endoscope

_____ 3. Exhibits classic symptom of right upper abdominal pain

_____ 4. Chronic hepatic disease

_____ 5. Person with abnormal fear of becoming fat

_____ 6. Inflammation of gallbladder

_____ 7. Acute infection and inflammation of the liver

_____ 8. Inflammation of stomach and bowel

_____ 9. Associated with a change in colonic motility

a. Gastroenteritis

b. Celiac sprue

c. Appendicitis

d. Irritable bowel syndrome

e. Colonoscopy

f. Cholecystitis

g. Cirrhosis

h. Viral hepatitis

i. Bulimia

j. Duodenal ulcer

k. Hemorrhoids

Discussion/Further Study

Compare and contrast irritable bowel syndrome, Crohn's disease, and ulcerative colitis.

ANSWERS

Short Answer

1. a. Digestion

   b. Absorption

   c. Elimination of solid wastes

2. Periodontitis

3. a. X-ray
   b. Endoscopy
   c. pH studies or analysis

4. a. Indigestion
   b. Heartburn

Matching

1. b	6. f
2. e	7. h
3. c	8. a
4. g	9. d
5. i	

Discussion/Further Study

Irritable bowel syndrome: Chronic bowel disease; unknown etiology; abdominal pain; diarrhea; biopsy may be done; stool may contain mucus. *Crohn's disease:* Chronic bowel disease; inflammation; unknown etiology; abdominal pain; diarrhea; biopsy necessary for diagnosis. *Ulcerative colitis:* Chronic bowel disease; inflammation; unknown etiology; abdominal pain; diarrhea; biopsy may be done; bloody stool; rectum and sigmoid colon is primary.

GLOSSARY

ALKALINE PHOSPHATASE: An enzyme essential in the calcification of bone and in other metabolic processes. Excessive blood serum levels of alkaline phosphatase may indicate liver or pancreatic disease.

ALKALOSIS: Excessive alkalinity of body fluids due to accumulation of alkalines or reduction of acids.

ANOREXIA: Loss of appetite for food.

ANTICHOLINERGIC: Drug that reduces smooth-muscle spasms in the intestine and reduces salivary secretions.

ANTIDIARRHEAL: Drug or other agent used to prevent or treat diarrhea.

ANTIEMETIC: Drug or other agent used to prevent or relieve nausea and vomiting.

ASCITES: Abnormal accumulation of fluid in the peritoneal cavity.

BILE: A thick, brownish yellow to greenish yellow alkaline fluid produced by the liver, stored and concentrated in the gallbladder, and discharged into the duodenum. It is important as a digestive juice, facilitating the digestion of fats by the intestine.

BILIRUBIN: An orange to yellow-colored compound in the blood plasma, produced by the breakdown of hemoglobin following the normal or pathologic destruction of red blood cells. It is collected by the liver to produce bile.

BILIRUBINURIA: The presence of bilirubin in the urine. May be indicative of a liver or blood disorder.

CACHEXIA: A marked wasting away of the body, usually as a consequence of chronic disease.

CHOLESTASIS: A halt in production and secretion of bile by the liver.

COLECTOMY: Surgical removal of all or a portion of the colon.

DIAPHORESIS: Sweating, especially when profuse or medically induced.

DYSPHAGIA: Difficulty in swallowing or inability to swallow.

ELECTROLYTE: As used here, the ionized salts present in blood, tissue fluids, and within cells. Electrolytes are involved in all metabolic processes and are essential to the normal functioning of all cells.

ENTEROPATHY: Any disease of the intestine.

EPIGASTRIC: Pertaining to the epigastrium, the region of the abdomen over the pit of the stomach.

FECALITH: A hard, solid intestinal mass formed around a core of fecal material.

FISTULA: An abnormal tubelike passage from a normal cavity or tube to a free surface or to another cavity.

GALLSTONES: A stonelike mass that forms in the gallbladder.

GAMMA GLOBULIN: A class of proteins formed in the blood that function as antibodies. Ability to resist infection is related to the concentration of these proteins.

GASTRECTOMY: Surgical removal of all or a portion of the stomach.

HALITOSIS: Foul-smelling breath.

HEMATEMESIS: Vomiting blood.

HEMOLYSIS: The rupturing of red blood cells with the resulting release of hemoglobin into the plasma.

HEPATOMEGALY: Enlargement of the liver.

HYPERGLYCEMIA: Abnormally high levels of sugar in the blood. (See *Diabetes mellitus*.)

HYPOKALEMIA: Extreme potassium depletion in the circulating blood, commonly manifested by episodes of muscular weakness or paralysis and tetany.

ILEOSTOMY: A surgically created opening in the lower small intestine (ileum), brought to the abdominal surface for the purpose of evacuating feces. May be temporary or permanent.

JAUNDICE: A condition characterized by the yellowish discolorization of the skin, whites of the eyes, and bodily fluids resulting from the accumulation of bilirubin in the blood. Caused by any of several disease processes in which the normal production and secretion of bile are disrupted.

LASSITUDE: A state of exhaustion or profound listlessness.

LEUKOCYTOSIS: A temporary increase in the number of white cells in the blood typically, but not exclusively, caused by the presence of infection.

LYMPHADENOPATHY: Disease of the lymph nodes, usually manifested by swelling of the nodes.

MALAISE: A generalized feeling of illness, discomfort, or depression indicative of some underlying disease or disorder.

McBURNEY'S POINT: A point of special abdominal tenderness indicating acute appendicitis. It lies over and corresponds with the normal position of the appendix.

MYALGIA: Muscle pain or tenderness.

OCCULT BLOOD: Minute quantities of blood in feces, urine, and gastric fluid, detectable only by microscopic examination or chemical test.

PALLOR: Lack of color; paleness, as of the skin.

PARENTERAL: Taken into the body or administered by some route other than the digestive system, e.g., intravenous, subcutaneous, intramuscular, or mucosal.

POLYPOSIS: The formation of numerous small growths or masses on a mucous membrane surface.

PROTEINURIA: Excessive levels of serum protein in the urine.

PRURITUS: Severe itching.

PYURIA: Pus in the urine.

RAUWOLFIA (SERPENTINA): A plant whose roots are used to derive a number of hypotensive agents.

REFLUX: A flowing back or return flow of fluid or other matter.

SALICYLATES: A class of compounds used for their pain relieving, fever reducing, and anti-inflammatory properties, e.g., aspirin.

SPLENOMEGALY: Enlargement of the spleen.

TACHYCARDIA: Abnormally rapid hearbeat, generally defined as exceeding 100 beats per minute.

TETANY: A nervous condition characterized by sharp, painful, periodic muscle contractions, particularly those of the extremities.

TOXEMIA: A condition in which poisonous products of body cells at a local source of infection or derived from the growth of microorganisms are spread throughout the body in the blood. Commonly called *blood poisoning.*

VARICES: Abnormally dilated and twisted veins, arteries, or lymph vessels.

VILLI (INTESTINAL): The tiny finger-like projections lining the interior of the small intestine that absorb fluid and nutrients.

Chapter 7

Respiratory System Diseases

LEARNING OBJECTIVES

Upon successful completion of this chapter, you will
■ Define epistaxis.
■ List the causes of sinusitis.
■ Describe the treatment for laryngitis.
■ Identify the confirming diagnosis of mononucleosis.
■ Contrast the three types of pneumonia.
■ Describe the conditions under which a lung abscess may occur.
■ Explain treatment modalities for pneumothorax.
■ Define pleurisy.

- Differentiate between transudate and exudate fluid.
- Name the most common chronic lung disease.
- List the predisposing factors of chronic bronchitis.
- Recall the signs and symptoms of emphysema.
- Discuss the prognosis for asthma.
- Explain the growth of the tuberculosis bacteria.
- Compare the four pneumoconioses.

INTRODUCTION

Respiration is essential for life. The body can survive a fair length of time without food, only days without water, but only minutes without air. Refer to Figure 7-1 for a review of the structure of the respiratory system.

There are two levels to the respiratory process—external and internal respiration. *External respiration* is the exchange of two gases within the lungs. Oxygen that is present in inhaled air is exchanged for carbon dioxide that diffuses across cell walls into the airspaces of the lungs from the blood. The carbon dioxide is then exhaled from the lungs. *Internal respiration* is the exchange of oxygen and carbon dioxide at the cellular level within the organs of the body. Carbon dioxide (CO_2) is a waste product when oxygen (O_2) and nutrients are metabolized within body cells.

EPISTAXIS (NOSEBLEED)

Description: *Epistaxis* is hemorrhage from the nose. This condition is more common in children than adults.

Etiology: Primary epistaxis is caused by trauma to the nose (including nose-picking). The condition may occur secondary to sinusitis, **rhinitis**, inhalation of irritating chemicals, hypertension, and various systemic infections or blood disorders. High altitudes or dry climates also may occasion epistaxis.

Signs and Symptoms: Bright red blood oozing from one or both nostrils is the common sign. If the blood is swallowed through the pharynx, the person may appear asymptomatic unless blood vomitus is evident. Bleeding is considered severe if it persists longer than 10 minutes. Prolonged epistaxis may cause significant blood loss.

Diagnostic Procedures: Casual observation may reveal epistaxis, but a more careful examination is necessary to locate the bleeding site. Any underlying causes of epistaxis require diagnosis and treatment.

Treatment: The person's head should be elevated and the soft portion of the nostrils pressed against the septum. Cold wet compresses also can be applied. A

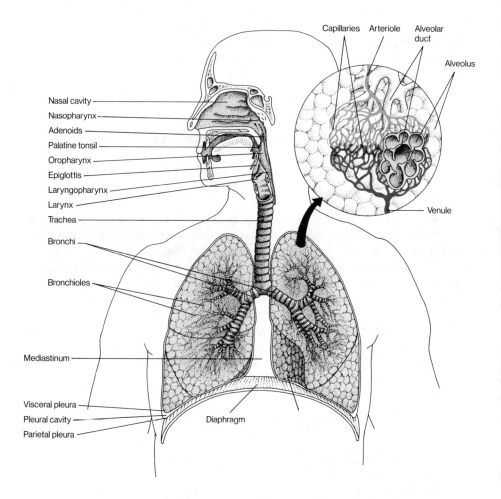

FIGURE 7–1. The respiratory system. (Modified from Gylys, B. A. and Wedding, M. E., *Medical Terminology: A Systems Approach,* ed. 2. F. A. Davis, Philadelphia, 1988, p. 123.)

vasoconstricting agent such as epinephrine may be applied to the bleeding site on a cotton ball. Cauterization or petrolatum gauze nasal packing may be needed. The patient may require **analgesics** for pain and antibiotics to prevent secondary infection.

Prognosis: The prognosis for most individuals with a nosebleed is good.

Prevention: Prevention includes keeping foreign objects out of the nose and refraining from picking the nose. The use of a humidifier may help persons living in dry climates or at high altitudes.

SINUSITIS

Description: *Sinusitis* is the inflammation of the paranasal sinus. The condition may be acute or chronic.

Etiology: Acute sinusitis is usually caused by pneumonococcal, streptococcal, or staphylococcal bacterial infections. The infection may spread to the sinuses during a cold, usually because of excessive nose blowing. Sinusitis also can result from swimming or diving, dental abscess or tooth extractions, or nasal allergies. Chronic sinusitis may be caused by the same etiologic factors as acute sinusitis, but more frequently its etiology cannot be determined.

Signs and Symptoms: An individual with acute or chronic sinusitis may exhibit the following symptoms: nasal congestion; pain; tenderness, redness, and swelling over the involved sinus; purulent nasal discharge; headache; **malaise**; and a nonproductive cough. A low-grade fever also may be present. Allergic sinusitis may be accompanied by watering eyes and sneezing.

Diagnostic Procedures: A nasal examination is commonly performed. A specimen of nasal secretions may be taken for culture in order to identify any infectious agent. A blood test may reveal an elevated white blood count. X-rays and **transillumination** may show clouding of the involved sinus.

Treatment: Analgesics for pain relief, vasoconstrictors to decrease nasal secretions, and antibiotics for control of infection are typically the treatments of choice. Bed rest may be recommended. Patients are to be encouraged to drink plenty of fluids to help liquefy secretions. The application of heat over the affected sinus may be helpful. Surgery to create an opening may be used to promote drainage if medicinal treatment fails.

Prognosis: The prognosis is excellent. Sinusitis is an uncomfortable condition, but usually it does not last long with proper care.

Prevention: Prevention involves prompt treatment of any respiratory tract infection.

ACUTE AND CHRONIC PHARYNGITIS

Description: *Pharyngitis* is inflammation of the pharynx.

Etiology: Acute pharyngitis can be caused by any of a number of bacterial or viral infections. *Streptococcus pyogenes* is the most common of many possible bacterial pathogens, whereas influenza virus and the common cold viruses are the most common viral pathogens causing the condition. Acute pharyngitis also may arise secondary to systemic viral infections such as measles or chickenpox. Noninfectious causes of the disease include trauma to the mucosa of the pharynx from heat, sharp objects, or chemical irritants. Chronic pharyngitis is more likely to have a noninfectious origin and is often associated with practices such as mouth breathing.

Signs and Symptoms: The hallmark of acute pharyngitis is sore throat. The pain may be mild or of such severity that swallowing becomes difficult. Accompanying symptoms may include malaise, fever, headache, and muscle and joint pain.

Diagnostic Procedures: Physical examination of the pharynx will typically reveal red, swollen mucous membranes. In severe cases, pustular ulcerations of the pharyngeal wall may be evident. A throat culture is usually performed in order to identify the infecting organism.

Treatment: Antibiotics are generally prescribed if the source of the infection is determined to be bacterial. Otherwise, treatment is symptomatic and may typically include the use of warm saline gargles, analgesics, and **antipyretics**. Bed rest and adequate fluid intake may be advised.

Prognosis: The prognosis for most forms of pharyngitis is generally good. Serious complications may result from streptococcal acute pharyngitis, including rheumatic fever and glomerulonephritis.

Prevention: There are no specific preventive measures for pharyngitis.

ACUTE AND CHRONIC LARYNGITIS

Description: *Laryngitis* is inflammation of the laryngeal mucosa and the vocal cords.

Etiology: Acute laryngitis may result from bacterial or viral infections, excessive use of the voice, or the inhalation of dust or chemical irritants. Acute laryngitis also may occur as a complication of acute rhinitis, pharyngitis, or influenza. Chronic laryngitis may arise from the acute form of the disease, but it is more frequently caused by prolonged irritation due to improper use of the voice or excessive smoking and drinking. Chronic laryngitis may arise secondary to other nose and throat diseases and may be a symptom of various benign or malignant neoplasms of the vocal cords.

Signs and Symptoms: Hoarseness or a complete lack of normal voice are the common signs. Also, there may be pain, dry cough, and malaise.

Diagnostic Procedures: Laryngoscopy will typically reveal red, inflamed, and possibly hemorrhagic vocal cords.

Treatment: Resting the voice is necessary for successful treatment. Any underlying pathology must be diagnosed and treated. Antibiotic therapy may be necessary if a bacterial infection is causing the condition. Heat applied to the neck, steam inhalations, analgesics, and cough suppressants may provide symptomatic relief.

Prognosis: The prognosis for acute laryngitis is good with proper treatment. The prognosis for chronic laryngitis varies according to the underlying cause.

Prevention: Preventive measures for acute or chronic laryngitis includes avoiding misusing or overusing the voice and avoiding irritants such as cigarette smoke, alcohol, and extremes of air temperature.

INFECTIOUS MONONUCLEOSIS

Description: *Infectious mononucleosis* is an acute upper respiratory tract infection characterized by sore throat, fever, and swollen cervical lymph glands. The disease primarily affects adolescents and young adults.

Etiology: Infectious mononucleosis is caused by the Epstein-Barr virus (EBV). This virus is shed in the saliva of infected individuals and is usually transmitted during kissing. Once in the body, EBV infects B-lymphocytes, which are a type of white cell found in the lymph, blood, and connective tissue and constitute one component of the body's immune system. The virus has an incubation period of 4 to 8 weeks.

Signs and Symptoms: Initial symptoms are usually vague, but they may include malaise, anorexia, and chills. Later symptoms include sore throat, fever, and swollen lymph glands in the throat and neck.

Diagnostic Procedures: A thorough patient history and physical examination are essential to rule out closely related disorders. A blood test is necessary for confirming the diagnosis and will show increased numbers of atypical lymphocytes and antibodies to EBV.

Treatment: Treatment is supportive. Bed rest may be indicated during the acute phase, although patients may still need to lessen their activities and get adequate rest until the disease completely subsides. Aspirin may be recommended for headache and sore throat. Warm saline gargles are also helpful.

Prognosis: The prognosis is good, but recovery may take several weeks or months.

Prevention: The best prevention is to avoid oropharyngeal contact with an EBV-infected person.

PNEUMONIA

Description: *Pneumonia* is inflammation of the respiratory bronchioles, alveolar ducts, alveolar sacs, and **alveoli** of the lung. The inflammation may be either unilateral or bilateral and involve all or a portion of the affected lung. Pneumonia is the fifth leading cause of death in the United States.

Etiology: As Table 7–1 illustrates, pneumonia may be caused by microorganisms such as bacteria, viruses, fungi, protozoans, or rickettsiae. The disease also may arise secondary to other systemic diseases or be induced by a variety of noninfectious agents such as chemicals and dusts. Most of the microbial and noninfectious agents that cause pneumonia are either inhaled from the air or aspirated from the naso- and oropharynx. The term *aspiration pneumonia*, however, is usually reserved for pneumonia caused by irritation from large quantities of foreign matter, especially gastric contents, drawn into the lungs.

TABLE 7–1. Pneumonias*

Specific Microbial Causes	Disease That May Be Accompanied by Pneumonia	Pneumonia Not Caused by Infections
Viruses:	Tularemia	Oil aspiration
Adenoviruses	Brucillosis	Radiation
Influenza viruses	Rheumatic fever	Chemicals
Rhinoviruses	Syphilis	Vegetable dusts
Respirosyncytial	Typhus	Silo-filler's disease
Coxsackie	Typhoid	
Coronaviruses	Rocky Mountain fever	
Mycoplasmas:	Q fever	
Mycoplasma pneumoniae	Acute viral respiratory disease	
Cocci:	Infectious mononucleosis	
Pneumococcus	Trichiniasis	
Staphylococcus	Acquired immune deficiency syndrome	
Hemolytic streptococcus	Psittacosis	
Protozoan (probable):	Plague	
Pneumocystis carinii	Legionnaires' disease	
Bacilli:	Rickettsial diseases	
Hemophilus influenzae		
Mycobacterium tuberculosis		
Klebsiella pneumoniae		
Gram-negative bacilli		
Chlamydiae:		
Chlamydia trachomatis		
Chlamydia psittaci		
Fungi:		
Histoplasma capsulatum		
Coccidioides immitis		
Rickettsiae:		
Rickettsia rickettsii		
Rickettsia burnetii		

*Adapted from Thomas, C. L. (ed.), *Taber's Cyclopedic Dictionary,* Ed. 15, F. A. Davis, Philadelphia, 1985, p. 1325, with permission.

The pneumococcus bacterium and the influenza viruses are the leading causes of pneumonia. The likelihood of contracting any form of pneumonia, however, is greatly influenced by one's age, immunologic status, and environment. Certain pneumonias, for example, are far more likely to be acquired during hospitalization, whereas others occur more frequently in school environments and still others in military settings.

Signs and Symptoms: The main symptoms are coughing, **sputum** production, stabbing chest pain, shaking chills, and high- or low-grade fever. Accompanying symptoms may include **rales**, **dyspnea**, **cyanosis**, and generalized weakness.

Diagnostic Procedures: A chest x-ray, taken in most suspected cases of pneumonia, will typically indicate the presence of infiltrates. Sputum smears and blood cultures will usually be made to isolate the suspected microorganism.

Treatment: The treatment procedure followed will necessarily vary with the etiology. Antibiotics will be prescribed for bacterial pneumonia. Supportive therapy for most types of pneumonia may include oxygen therapy, mechanical ventilation, a high-calorie diet, increased fluid intake, bed rest, analgesics, and **postural drainage**.

Prognosis: The prognosis for penumonia is always guarded, but it varies with etiology. If the pneumonia is secondary to another disease or if the patient is already debilitated, the prognosis is generally poor. A similar prognosis exists for influenza-caused penumonia, especially among the aged. A frequent complication of influenza-caused pneumonia is lung abscess.

Prevention: Persons who are high risk, such as the aged, should have annual influenza innoculations.

LEGIONELLA INFECTIONS
(LEGIONNAIRES' DISEASE)

Description: A *Legionella infection* is an acute respiratory disease producing severe pneumonia-like symptoms. The disease is commonly called *legionnaires' disease,* named after an epidemic outbreak of the illness that killed 34 people and sickened more than 200 attending an American Legion convention in Philadelphia in July of 1976. The disease may be mild and self-limiting or produce a pneumonia severe enough to be fatal.

Etiology: Legionnaires' disease is caused by the gram-negative bacillus *Legionella pneumophilia*. Other closely related bacteria within the genus *Legionella* also can produce outbreaks of the disease that are clinically indistinguishable from classic legionnaires' disease. The *Legionella* bacteria thrive in warm aquatic environments. They become problematic when they infect the cooling towers of air-conditioning systems and the hot water plumbing of buildings. The bacteria are then inhaled into the lungs from aerosol water droplets. Legionnaires' disease has an incubation period of about 1 week. Predisposing factors include smoking and prior physical debilitation, especially among those with chronic obstructive pulmonary disease or alcoholism.

Signs and Symptoms: The symptoms of legionnaires' disease are indistinguishable from those of pneumonia and may include malaise, headache, and cough, followed by the rapid onset of fever and chills, myalgia, chest pain, dyspnea, vomiting, diarrhea, and anorexia.

Diagnostic Procedures: Laboratory studies may show elevated leukocytes,

ESR, and liver enzymes. Special tests to isolate *Legionella* bacillae from respiratory secretions are necessary for confirmation of the diagnosis.

Treatment: Antibiotic therapy is typically started even before the disease is definitely diagnosed. Antipyretics and oxygen may be used.

Prognosis: The prognosis is usually good if treatment is initiated early in the course of the disease. Even so, response to treatment is usually slow. Complications may include delirium, heart failure, and shock. The latter usually is fatal.

Prevention: Prevention includes detecting and eradicating *Legionella* bacteria from environments in which they may potentially infect people.

LUNG ABSCESS

Description: A *lung abscess* is an area of necrotized lung tissue containing **purulent** material. Abscesses are more frequent in the lower dependent portions of the lungs and in the right lung, which has a more vertical bronchus.

Etiology: Lung abscesses caused by infectious organisms frequently arise as a complication of pneumonia. The major determinant in developing a lung abscess, as opposed to just developing pneumonia, is the causative microorganism's ability to necrotize lung tissue. A lung abscess also may be produced by a **septic** embolism being carried to the lung in the pulmonary circulation. Neoplasms, trauma from foreign objects lodged in lung tissue, or bronchial **stenosis** also may cause lung abscesses to form.

Signs and Symptoms: Lung abscesses produce a cough accompanied by bloody, purulent, or foul-smelling sputum and breath. Chest pain, sweating, chills, headache, fever, and dyspnea often are present.

Diagnostic Procedures: Chest **auscultation** reveals decreased breath sounds. A chest x-ray is necessary to localize the affected portions of the lung. Sputum culture also is used to detect possible infectious microorganisms. Blood culture may be used to assist in the diagnosis.

Treatment: Antibiotic therapy of fairly long duration is the treatment of choice until the abscess is gone. Surgical resection of the lesion may be required if antibiotic therapy is unsuccessful.

Prognosis: The prognosis is good with proper care and follow-up. A complication may be the development of a brain abscess if infected materials are carried by the blood into the brain.

Prevention: Postoperative patients should be monitored carefully to guard against aspiration of infected materials.

PNEUMOTHORAX

Description: A *pneumothorax* is a collection of air in the pleural cavity, typically resulting in the complete or partial collapse of the lung (atelectasis). One or both lungs may be affected. The condition is characterized as either spontaneous or secondary.

Etiology: Spontaneous pneumothorax is caused by the rupturing of small blebs along the surface of the lung. What causes these blebs to form is not known, but they tend to form near the apex (bottom tip) of each lung. Pneumothorax also may be secondary to other lung diseases, such as asthma, emphysema, lung abscess, or lung cancer. Other secondary causes include chest trauma such as a knife wound or fractured rib. A perforated esophagus or mechanical ventilators also can cause pneumothorax.

Signs and Symptoms: Classic symptoms are sudden, sharp chest pains that worsen with chest movement, coughing, or breathing. There may be shortness of breath and cyanosis. Profound respiratory distress accompanied by **pallor**, weak and rapid pulse, and anxiety also may occur.

Diagnostic Procedures: Physical examination may reveal asymmetrical expansion of the chest during inspiration. Auscultation typically reveals diminished breathing sounds on the affected side. A chest x-ray will usually provide confirmation.

Treatment: In spontaneous pneumothorax with no signs of increased pleural pressure, dyspnea, or a lung collapse of less than 30 percent, the treatment of choice is bed rest and careful monitoring of vital signs. In traumatic pneumothorax, a medical emergency exists. A chest tube may be inserted for drainage and to allow reexpansion of the collapsed lung. Recurring pneumothorax may require **thoracotomy** and **pleurectomy**.

Prognosis: The prognosis for pneumothorax is generally good with effective treatment. Spontaneous pneumothorax, however, tends to be a recurrent condition. A large pneumothorax can impair cardiac function.

Prevention: Individuals with a history of spontaneous pneumothorax should not subject themselves to extremes of atmospheric pressure such as would be encountered by flying in unpressurized aircraft or during scuba diving.

PLEURISY (PLEURITIS)

Description: *Pleurisy* is inflammation of the visceral (inner) and parietal (outer) pleural membranes that envelop each lung. The **pleura** of one or both lungs may be affected. The condition may be either primary or secondary.

Etiology: Primary pleurisy is caused by infection of the pleura by bacteria or viruses. The condition is frequently secondary to pneumonia, tuberculosis, pulmonary infarction, neoplasm, systemic lupus erythematosus, and chest trauma.

Signs and Symptoms: Symptoms may include coughing, fever and chills, and chest pain that is greater during inspiration. The pain can be quite severe. Dyspnea also may occur.

Diagnosis: Chest auscultation reveals pleural friction rub ("squeaky leather" or "grating" sounds) during respiration.

Treatment: Treatment is aimed at the underlying cause but is otherwise symptomatic. Such treatment may include the use of strong analgesics, the application of heat, or taping the chest to restrict its movement. Bed rest is usually indicated. Severe pain may require the use of a regional anesthetic in a procedure called an *intercostal nerve block*.

Prognosis: Prognosis is dependent on etiology. Pleural effusion, a collection of fluid in the pleural space, may develop.

Prevention: Early treatment of respiratory diseases is the best prevention.

PLEURAL EFFUSION

Description: *Pleural effusion* is an excess of fluid between the parietal and visceral pleural membranes enveloping each lung. The accumulating fluid may be characterized as **transudate**, with little or no protein, or **exudate**, protein-rich.

Etiology: Pleural effusion may occur with or without any pathologic process affecting the pleurae themselves. Transudative pleural effusions frequently result from congestive heart failure. Exudative pleural effusions more often are seen with tuberculosis, rheumatoid arthritis, pancreatitis, respiratory neoplasms, and bacterial pneumonia.

Signs and Symptoms: The person may be asymptomatic. When symptoms are manifested, they may include dyspnea and chest or shoulder pain. The symptoms of pleural effusion will typically accompany those of any underlying condition.

Diagnostic Procedures: Chest x-ray may demonstrate pleural effusion. Auscultation of the chest reveal decreased breath sounds. **Percussion** elicits dull sounds over the effused area. **Thoracentesis** and analysis of the extracted fluid are necessary to distinguish transudative from exudative effusions.

Treatment: Thoracentesis to alleviate fluid pressure may be necessary if the fluid is not reabsorbed. It is important, also, to treat the underlying cause of the pleural effusion.

Prognosis: The prognosis is dependent on the underlying disease.

Prevention: There is no specific prevention for pleural effusion other than prompt treatment and management of disorders that may lead to the condition.

CHRONIC OBSTRUCTIVE PULMONARY DISEASE (COPD)

Description: *Chronic obstructive pulmonary disease* is a functional diagnosis given to any pathologic process that decreases the ability of the lungs and bronchi to perform their function of ventilation. It is characterized by permanent changes in the structure of the lungs and bronchi. COPD is a common cause of death and disability in the United States.

Etiology: Diseases that may lead to COPD include emphysema, chronic bronchitis, chronic asthma, bronchiectasis, silicosis, and pulmonary tuberculosis. Smoking, prolonged exposure to polluted air, respiratory infections, and allergies are predisposing factors in this disease.

Signs and Symptoms: COPD tends to develop insidiously, so no symptoms may be present initially. Later, a person may tire easily while exercising or doing strenuous work. A productive cough follows. Dyspnea upon minimal exertion then develops.

Diagnostic Procedures: Physical examination, chest x-ray, pulmonary function tests, arterial blood gases, and ECG are the procedures used to diagnose COPD.

Treatment: Treatment is aimed at preventing further lung damage, relieving symptoms, and preventing complications. Persons diagnosed with COPD should be advised not to smoke. **Bronchodilators** may be used, and antibiotics may be prescribed in the event of respiratory infections. Also, an increase in fluid intake and maintaining a well-balanced diet can be helpful. Administration of oxygen may be necessary.

Prognosis: The prognosis for COPD is always guarded. The disease cannot be cured or lost pulmonary function restored. The degree of disability produced by COPD varies, but it tends to increase with time.

Prevention: Prevention includes not smoking, especially if family members have a history of the disease. Periodic physical examinations to evaluate chronic cough may be recommended.

CHRONIC BRONCHITIS

Description: *Chronic bronchitis* is imflammation of the bronchial mucous membranes. It is characterized by **hypertrophy** and **hyperplasia** of bronchial mucous glands, damage to bronchial **cilia**, and narrowing of the bronchial airways.

Etiology: Chronic bronchitis is strongly associated with long-term, heavy cigarette smoking. Occupational risk factors include exposure to textile dust fibers and certain petrochemicals. There is also evidence of a genetic predisposition to developing the disease.

Signs and Symptoms: A chronic cough with sputum production is the classic symptom. Weight gain due to **edema**, cyanosis, **tachypnea**, and wheezing also may be evident.

Diagnostic Procedures: A clinical diagnosis of chronic bronchitis requires that "productive cough be present on most days for a minimum of three months in the year in at least two consecutive years."[1]

Treatment: Individuals diagnosed with chronic bronchitis must be encouraged not to smoke. All precautions should be taken to avoid respiratory infections. Bronchodilators may be of assistance, as is increased fluid intake. **Diuretics** may be prescribed for edema. Oxygen therapy may be necessary.

Prognosis: The prognosis is guarded. In the most serious cases, there typically is progressive deterioration of pulmonary function with increasing episodes of respiratory failure. Chronic bronchitis frequently leads to COPD (see COPD). There is a high mortality rate from complicating respiratory infections. Right ventricular failure also may develop as a complication of chronic bronchitis.

Prevention: Avoiding known risk factors, such as smoking, is the best means of preventing chronic bronchitis.

CHRONIC PULMONARY EMPHYSEMA

Description: *Chronic pulmonary emphysema* is the permanent enlargement of the air spaces beyond the terminal bronchioles resulting from destruction of alveolar walls. As a consequence of this destruction, the lungs slowly lose their normal elasticity.

Etiology: The exact cause of chronic pulmonary emphysema is not known. It is intimately associated with chronic bronchitis but does not necessarily result from that disorder. Known risk factors of emphysema include smoking and long-term exposure to air pollution and other respiratory tract irritants. Evidence suggests that some forms of the disease may be hereditary. In less common instances, the disease is associated with a deficiency of $alpha_1$-antitrypsin, a protein that plays a role in maintaining lung elasticity.

Signs and Symptoms: The onset of the disease is insidious. Chronic pulmonary emphysema is generally characterized by progressive dyspnea on exertion. There may be a chronic cough. A characteristic "barrel chest" is often seen.

Diagnostic Procedures: Physical examination, chest x-ray, pulmonary function tests, arterial blood gases, ECG, and blood tests are used to diagnose emphysema.

Treatment: There is no effective treatment for emphysema other than management of the symptoms. Cigarette smoking and other toxic inhalants are to be avoided. Respiratory infections that do occur should be treated aggressively. Home oxygen and bronchodilators may be prescribed.

Prognosis: The prognosis is poor. Emphysema generally leads to COPD, with progressive diminution of pulmonary function and respiratory failure accounting for most deaths.

Prevention: Although there is no specific prevention, discouraging smoking may certainly help.

ASTHMA

Description: *Asthma* is a respiratory condition marked by recurrent attacks of labored breathing accompanied by wheezing. Asthma is the consequence of spasms of the bronchial tubes or swelling of their mucous membranes.

Etiology: The etiology of asthma is uncertain. There is often a family history of allergy and an individual history of hypersensitivity. Upper respiratory infection, exercise, and anxiety can bring on an attack.

Signs and Symptoms: During an acute episode, there will be pronounced wheezing due to difficulty in exhaling air from the lungs. Dyspnea, tachypnea, and chest tightness also may occur. The person experiencing an asthmatic attack also may perspire profusely.

Diagnostic Procedures: Physical examination, chest x-ray during an attack, sputum analysis, pulmonary function tests, arterial blood gases, and ECG may suggest the diagnosis. Skin tests may identify suspected allergens.

Treatment: Aerosol or oral bronchodilators and nasal decongestants may be helpful for relief of symptoms. Emergency treatment may include the administration of oxygen and antibiotics and intravenous therapy.

Prognosis: Prognosis is good with proper attention and care. Many asthmatic children become asymptomatic after reaching adulthood, but asthmatics with onset of symptoms after age 15 typically have persistent disease in adulthood.

Prevention: Among those with the condition, the frequency of asthmatic attacks may be reduced by avoiding known allergens and emotional distress as much as possible. Medications for the ailment should be taken as directed.

PULMONARY TUBERCULOSIS

Description: *Pulmonary tuberculosis* (TB) is a slowly developing bacterial lung infection characterized by progressive necrosis of lung tissue.

Etiology: Pulmonary tuberculosis is caused by *Mycobacterium tuberculosis*. The infected individual's immune system usually is able to wall the bacteria into a tubercle or tiny nodule. The bacteria can lie dormant for years and then reactivate and spread when conditions are favorable. The disease is transmitted in aerosol droplets exhaled by infected individuals.

Note: Although the lungs are the organs most commonly infected, the bacteria can infect other parts of the body as well.

Signs and Symptoms: Pulmonary tuberculosis may be asymptomatic. When symptoms are present, they are often vague and may include lassitude, malaise, fatigability, anorexia, afternoon fever, weight loss, cough, **hemoptysis**, and pleuritic chest pain. Advanced symptoms include wheezes, rales, and deviation of the trachea.

Diagnostic Procedures: A thorough physical examination, chest x-ray, and positive tuberculin test will confirm the diagnosis. The tuberculin test of choice is the Mantoux text, which consists of an intradermal injection of a purified protein derivative (PPD) of the tuberculin bacillus. Sputum studies are helpful, too. Pulmonary and pleural biopsies may be ordered.

Treatment: Drug therapy is indicated in every case of TB. However, there are many TB drugs, and these can be used in a number of different ways. Bed rest and isolation are indicated until the person is strong enough to resume activities or until the person is no longer deemed contagious. Surgery is used only in selected cases, such as in the event of bronchial stenosis or when drug therapy is not working.

Prognosis: The prognosis for an individual with active pulmonary tuberculosis is good if the disease is detected early.

Prevention: Preventive measures involve isolation of infected persons, tuberculin testing of persons known to have been in close contact with infected persons, and treatment of tuberculin reactors. Use of the bacille Calmette-Guérin (BCG) vaccination offers some protection for tuberculin-negative persons.

PNEUMOCONIOSIS

Pneumoconiosis is a disease of the respiratory tract caused by inhaling inorganic dust particles over a prolonged period. It is an occupational disorder associated with mining or stone cutting. Four varieties of pneumoconiosis will be considered: silicosis, asbestosis, berylliosis, and anthracosis.

Silicosis

Description: *Silicosis* is a form of pneumoconiosis resulting from the inhalation of silica (quartz) dust. Silicosis is characterized by the formation of small, discrete, silicotic nodules in the lung tissue. As the disease advances, a dense fibrosis of the lungs and emphysema with respiratory impairment may result. The disease is chronic and progressive.

Etiology: The occupations most prone to silica exposure are mining, drilling, blasting, grinding, and abrasive manufacturing. Required exposure varies from 2 to 30 years.

Signs and Symptoms: The disease may be asymptomatic, even though x-rays exhibit evidence of nodule formation. Dyspnea on exertion generally is the first symptom. A dry cough which later turns productive, tachypnea, pulmonary hypertension, and malaise may result.

Diagnostic Procedures: A thorough patient history is essential. Chest x-rays are not always diagnostic but are used, especially in advanced silicosis. Arterial blood gases and pulmonary function tests confirm the diagnosis.

Treatment: Treatment is symptomatic, especially for the cough and wheezing. A common complication, TB, must be aggressively treated.

Prognosis: The prognosis for an individual with silicosis is guarded at best. The disease can be rapidly fatal depending on the quantity and quality of the silica entering the lungs. Silicosis is always life-shortening.

Prevention: Prevention involves minimizing exposure to silica dust in the work environment.

Asbestosis

Description: *Asbestosis* is a form of pneumoconiosis due to exposure to asbestos fibers. The disease is characterized by a slow, progressive, diffuse fibrosis of the lung tissue. Despite recent health and safety regulations limiting workplace exposure to asbestos, asbestosis remains the most frequently occurring form of pneumoconiosis.

Etiology: Those at greatest risk of asbestosis include people who fabricate asbestos fibers, remove asbestos insulation from plumbing and buildings, or live within the area of an industry that discharges the fibers into the air. Family members of asbestos workers are also at risk of the disease if they handle the worker's clothing. Ten years of moderate exposure to asbestos dust usually is required before the characteristic lesions of the disease become evident.

Signs and Symptoms: The first symptom is dyspnea upon exertion, which worsens until dyspnea occurs even while at rest. Pleuritic chest pain, dry cough, and recurrent respiratory infections are common.

Diagnostic Procedures: A thorough patient history and physical examination are essential. Chest x-rays, pulmonary function studies, and arterial blood gases will confirm the diagnosis.

Treatment: As with all pneumoconioses, treatment is symptomatic and supportive.

Prognosis: The prognosis is poor, especially if the affected person is a smoker. There is increased incidence of bronchogenic carcinoma even after brief exposure.

Prevention: Prevention involves avoidance of the dust.

Berylliosis

Description: *Berylliosis* is beryllium poisoning, usually of the lungs. The skin and other bodily organs also may be affected. The acute form of the disease is characterized by the onset of pneumonia-like symptoms and other upper respiratory tract disorders. The more common chronic form is characterized by **granuloma** formation and diffuse interstitial pneumonitis.

Etiology: Those at risk of berylliosis include workers in the specialty metals, semiconductor, and ceramics industries. The metal may be either inhaled or directly absorbed through the skin in the form of dusts, salts, or fumes. As in asbestosis, berylliosis can affect family members who are exposed to dusts in the worker's clothing.

Signs and Symptoms: After exposure, nasal mucosal swelling and ulceration and dry cough occur. As the condition worsens, substernal pain, tachycardia, and dyspnea, weight loss, and pulmonary insufficiency result.

Diagnostic Procedures: A thorough patient history and physical examination are essential. Chest x-ray, pulmonary function studies, arterial blood gases, and a positive beryllium patch test confirm the diagnosis.

Treatment: Skin ulcers need to be excised. Corticosteroid therapy may be initiated. Oxygen, bronchodilators, and chest physical therapy methods may be required.

Prognosis: The prognosis is guarded. Individuals must modify their lifestyle. The disease is progressive.

Prevention: The best prevention is avoidance of beryllium fumes or dusts.

Anthracosis

Description: *Anthracosis*, also called *black lung disease* or *miner's asthma,* is a form of pneumonoconiosis caused by the accumulation of carbon deposits in the lungs. The disease is characterized by symptoms resembling those of chronic bronchitis.

Etiology: Anthracosis results from inhaling smoke or coal dust. Workers in the coal mining industry are those most likely to develop the disease. The effects of the disease are greatly compounded by smoking. Anthracosis frequently occurs with silicosis. Required exposure is usually 15 years or longer.

Signs and Symptoms: Exertional dyspnea, productive cough with inky-black sputum, and recurrent respiratory infections are common symptoms.

Diagnostic Procedures: A thorough patient history and physical examination are essential and may reveal a barrel chest, rales, **rhonchi**, and wheezes. Chest x-rays, pulmonary function studies, and blood gases will confirm the diagnosis.

Treatment: Treatment is strictly symptomatic and typically includes the use of bronchodilating and corticosteroid drugs, chest physical therapy to help remove secretions, and management of respiratory complications such as TB.

Prognosis: The prognosis is guarded. The disease is chronic and progressive. Complications worsen the prognosis.

Prevention: Prevention involves avoidance of coal dust.

RESPIRATORY MYCOSES

Description: *Mycoses,* fungal infections, are classified as either superficial or deep. Superficial mycoses affect only the skin and are considered in Chapter 12. Deep mycoses are systemic and may complicate other illnesses. The mycoses considered here are deep, systemic fungal infections that extensively affect the lungs. They are histoplasmosis, coccidioidomycosis, and blastomycosis.

Etiology: *Histoplasmosis, Ohio Valley disease,* is caused by *Histoplasma capsulatum.* The fungus is found in soil, especially soil contaminated by bird and chicken droppings. The disease is transmitted by fungal spores that are inhaled or that penetrate the skin following injury. The primary lesion is in the lungs.

Coccidioidomycosis, valley fever, is caused by *coccidioides immitis,* a fungus common in the dry desert soils of California and Arizona. The disease is transmitted by inhalation of fungal spores and commonly affects migrant farm laborers.

Blastomycosis, specifically *North American blastomycosis,* is caused by *Blastomyces dermatitidis.* It can cause a cutaneous infection, but usually it affects the lungs. In rare instances, a serious progressive systemic infection may occur.

Signs and Symptoms: The symptoms of all three diseases may be mild and similar to those of a common cold. More severe symptoms include malaise, fever, myalgia, headache, cough, and chest pain. In coccidioidomycosis, however, the only symptom may be a persistent fever of several weeks' duration. In blastomycosis, nonpruritic and painless papules or macules may appear on exposed body surfaces.

Diagnostic Procedures: In histoplasmosis, a positive *Histoplasma* skin test, sputum culture, or special stainings of biopsied tissue confirm the diagnosis. In coccidioidomycosis, a positive coccidioidin skin test, chest x-ray, and special serologic tests are necessary for confirmation. In blastomycosis, cultures to isolate the fungus from sputum or skin lesions are necessary. Tissue biopsy from the skin or lungs may be ordered.

Treatment: High-dose, long-term antifungal medications and supportive treatment for respiratory symptoms are used to treat histoplasmosis and blastomycosis. Coccidioidomycosis may heal spontaneously within a few weeks. Bed rest and symptomatic treatment may be all that are necessary. In some cases, surgery may be necessary to remove lung lesions.

Prognosis: The prognosis for an individual with histoplasmosis or coccidioidomycosis is usually excellent. Blastomycosis in its primary, acute form is self-limiting. If it progresses to a systemic infection, however, the prognosis is guarded.

Prevention: Prevention includes following proper sanitary measures, wearing a face mask during exposure to potentially contaminated soil, and protecting exposed skin from invasion by the spores.

PULMONARY EDEMA

Description: *Pulmonary edema* is a diffuse extravascular accumulation of fluid in the pulmonary tissues and air spaces. The condition is considered a medical emergency.

Etiology: Most commonly, pulmonary edema is the product of cardiac disease processes such as atherosclerosis, hypertension, or valvular disease. The condition is usually a direct consequence of left ventricular failure. More blood is added to the pulmonary circulation than can be adequately removed. Noncardiogenic causes may include narcotic overdose, toxic inhalants, renal failure, CVA, skull fracture, and exposure to high altitudes.

Signs and Symptoms: The onset of pulmonary edema frequently occurs at night after the person has been lying down for awhile. Dyspnea, coughing, and **orthopnea** are common symptoms. **Tachycardia**, tachypnea, diffuse rales, and frothy, bloody sputum also may occur. A decrease in blood pressure, **thready pulse**, and cold, clammy skin occur as cardiac output fails.

Diagnostic Procedures: Arterial blood gases and chest x-rays are useful in diagnosing this condition. Pulmonary artery catheterization may be used to confirm left ventricular failure.

Treatment: Oxygen is typically administered along with bronchodilators and diuretics. Digitalis may be administered to stimulate heart action. Medication may be prescribed to relieve anxiety, too. Fluid intake may be limited, and mechanical ventilation may be necessary.

Prognosis: The prognosis for an individual with pulmonary edema is guarded. When symptoms develop rapidly, the condition can be fatal.

Prevention: There is no known prevention.

COR PULMONALE

Description: *Cor pulmonale* is hypertrophy and failure of the right ventricle of the heart.

Etiology: Cor pulmonale is caused by various disorders of the lungs, the pulmonary vessels, or the chest wall that impede pulmonary circulation. Disorders that may lead to cor pulmonale include COPD, chronic bronchitis, bronchiectasis, pulmonary hypertension, **kyphoscoliosis**, multiple pulmonary emboli, and living at high altitudes. The condition may be acute, but is more commonly chronic.

Signs and Symptoms: Symptoms include a productive, chronic cough, exertional dyspnea, fatigability, and wheezing respirations. Tachypnea, orthopnea, dependent edema, cyanosis, **clubbing**, and distended neck veins may occur as the condition worsens.

Diagnostic Procedures: Chest x-rays, ECG, and pulmonary function studies are useful diagnostic tools. Echocardiography or angiography and arterial blood gases confirm the diagnosis.

Treatment: Cor pulmonale is frequently treated with medications such as digitalis to stimulate heart action, antibiotics for secondary respiratory infections, or pulmonary artery dilators, diuretics, and anticoagulants. Oxygen may be necessary. Restriction of salt and fluid may be advised.

Prognosis: The prognosis is typically poor for an individual with cor pulmonale, but it depends on the underlying cause of the condition.

Prevention: There is no known prevention.

PULMONARY EMBOLISM

Description: A *pulmonary embolism* is a mass of undissolved matter in the pulmonary artery or one of its branches.

Etiology: A pulmonary embolism generally originates in the pelvic veins or deep lower extremity veins and travels through the circulatory system until it blocks a pulmonary artery. At high risk for pulmonary emboli are individuals immobilized with chronic diseases, those in body casts, persons with congestive heart failure or neoplasms, or post-operative patients. Pregnant women, individuals with venous diseases such as **polycythemia vera, thrombocytosis,** or varicose veins, or women on oral contraceptives are also at risk.

Signs and Symptoms: Signs and symptoms depend on the size and location of the embolus. Acute symptoms may include dyspnea, anxiety, and substernal pain. Less severe symptoms are cough, pleuritic pain, and low-grade fever.

Diagnostic Procedures: Diagnosing this condition is frequently difficult, but an ECG may reveal tachycardia and a chest x-ray may indicate the location of the embolus. Lung scintiscan, pulmonary angiography, or ultrasound may help in the diagnosis.

Treatment: Treatment typically involves the use of anticoagulants such as heparin and warfarin to prevent clot formation and fibrinolytic therapy to dissolve the embolus. Surgical management may be indicated in exceptional cases, and this involves removing the embolus or **ligating** or **plicating** the vena cava to prevent the migration of new emboli into the pulmonary circulation.

Prognosis: The prognosis is guarded if the embolism is massive enough to trigger a **pulmonary infarction** (occurring in about 10 percent of cases).

Prevention: Prevention includes early postoperative ambulation or initiating prophylactic anticoagulant therapy for patients deemed to be at risk.

RESPIRATORY ACIDOSIS (HYPERCAPNIA)

Description: *Respiratory acidosis* is excessive acidity of body fluids attributable to inadequate removal of carbon dioxide (CO_2) by the lungs. Whenever CO_2 cannot be adequately ventilated, the CO_2 dissolved in the blood rapidly increases. As this level of CO_2—called the *partial pressure of CO_2,* or PCO_2—rises, it combines with water to form carbonic acid. Consequently, the **pH** of the blood decreases. The condition may be acute or chronic.

Etiology: Acute respiratory acidosis occurs whenever there is a sudden impairment of ventilation resulting from airway obstruction. This may be due to causes such as a foreign object blocking the airway or to the effects of certian drugs, neuromuscular diseases, or cardiac arrest. Chronic respiratory acidosis is caused by pulmonary diseases that change the characterisitics of lung tissue, impairing their ability to release CO_2. Examples of such diseases include emphysema, bronchitis, and chronic obstructive pulmonary disease. Chronic respiratory acidosis also may be a consequence of extreme obesity.

Signs and Symptoms: Symptoms vary with the etiology, but typically they include weakness, shallow respirations, confusion, muscle tremors, and tachycardia.

Diagnostic Procedures: Diagnosis of respiratory acidosis is usually evident from the clinical situation. Arterial blood gas testing to confirm elevated P_{CO_2} levels is required to confirm the diagnosis.

Treatment: The only useful treatment for respiratory acidosis involves measures to correct the underlying cause.

Prognosis: The prognosis for an individual with respiratory acidosis varies with the cause.

Prevention: There is no specific prevention.

RESPIRATORY ALKALOSIS (HYPOCAPNIA)

Description: *Respiratory alkalosis* is excessive alkalinity of body fluids attributable to the excessive removal of CO_2 by the lungs. When excessive amounts of CO_2 are ventilated by the lungs, the partial pressure of CO_2 (P_{CO_2}) in the blood decreases, initiating a series of chemical and metabolic changes that act to reduce the level of serum bicarbonate. Consequently, the pH of the blood increases. The condition may be acute or chronic.

Etiology: Respiratory alkalosis is caused by acute or chronic hyperventilation. Acute respiratory alkalosis may result from hyperventilation induced by anxiety or psychologic trauma, fever, pain, salicylate poisoning, excessive exercise, or excessive use of mechanical ventilators. It is also associated with **hypoxia** due to pneumonia, asthma, or pulmonary edema. Chronic respiratory alkalosis from hyperventilation is typically associated with hypoxia due to chronic cardiopulmonary diseases or high altitudes.

Signs and Symptoms: Symptoms vary with etiology, but they may include numbness or tingling of the extremities, light-headedness, and muscle spasms.

Diagnostic Procedures: Diagnosis of respiratory alkalosis usually is based on the clinical evidence presented, but it must be confirmed through a blood test revealing decreased levels of serum bicarbonate or decreased P_{CO_2} levels.

Treatment: Treatment is aimed at correcting the underlying cause. Short-term measures may involve having the person breathe into a bag or administering a sedative to relieve hyperventilation in very anxious patients.

Prognosis: The prognosis of an individual with respiratory alkalosis varies with etiology but is generally good.

Prevention: There are no specific preventive measures.

ATELECTASIS

Description: *Atelectasis* is a collapsed or airless condition of all or part of a lung. The condition may be acute or chronic.

Etiolgy: The condition may be caused by obstruction of the lung by foreign matter, mucous plugs, or excessive secretion. Compression of the lung by tumors, aneurysms, enlarged lymph nodes, or pneumothorax also may cause lung colapse (see Pneumothorax). Atelectasis is sometimes a complication of abdominal surgery or a general consequence of postoperative immobilization.

Signs and Symptoms: Symptoms of acute atelectasis typically include marked dyspnea, cyanosis, fever, tachycardia, anxiety, and **diaphoresis**. There may be a decrease in chest motion on the affected side. Chronic atelectasis may only be marked by the gradual onset of dyspnea.

Diagnostic Procedures: A thorough patient history, physical examination, and chest x-ray are essential for diagnosis. Percussion may be dull, and auscultation will reveal decreased breath sounds.

Treatment: Postural drainage, spirometry, chest percussion, and frequent coughing and deep breathing are advised. Bronchoscopy may be used to remove excessive secretions, although the procedure is controversial. Early postoperative ambulation is recommended. Broncodilators may be prescribed.

Prognosis: The prognosis in postoperative atelectasis usually is good, although death may result if it is untreated. In all other types of atelectasis, the prognosis is dependent on the cause.

Prevention: Prevention includes postoperative exercise and prompt treatment of any pulmonary problems.

BRONCHIECTASIS

Description: *Bronchiectasis* is the permanent abnormal dilation of small and medium-sized bronchi resulting from the destruction of muscular and elastic components of the bronchial walls. The condition usually is bilateral, involving the lower lobes of the lungs.

Etiology: Bronchiectasis may be caused by pulmonary diseases such as pneumonia or tuberculosis, by bronchial obstruction, or by inhalation of corrosive gas. Bronchiectasis is also a frequent, life-threatening complication of cystic fibrosis.

Signs and Symptoms: Affected individuals frequently have a chronic cough and expectorate large amounts of purulent, foul-smelling sputum, especially the first thing in the morning. Hemoptysis may occur to the extent that it frightens the patient. Dyspnea, wheezing, fever, and malaise may ensue as the condition progresses.

Diagnostic Procedures: Diagnosis of bronchiectasis may be difficult, especially initially when symptoms are vague. Chest x-rays and bronchography are the most valuable tools for diagnosis. Sputum culture and pulmonary function studies are helpful.

Treatment: Environmental irritants such as smoke, dust, and fumes should be avoided. Postural drainage, bronchodilators, and antibiotics may be ordered. Surgery may be performed if the condition is severe.

Prognosis: The condition is irreversible, and the prognosis is guarded.

Prevention: Prevention includes avoiding pulmonary irritants and smoking and seeking prompt treatment of any pulmonary ailments.

LUNG CANCER

Description: *Lung cancer* is any of various malignant neoplasms that may appear in the trachea, bronchi, or air sacs of the lungs. It is the leading cause of cancer deaths in the United States.

Etiology: Although the precise triggering mechanisms is not known, most lung cancers are caused either directly or indirectly by smoking. Tobacco smoke contains a number of chemicals known to be carcinogenic. Long-term exposure to atmospheric pollution and airborne pulmonary irritants is also associated with increased incidences of lung cancer.

Signs and Symptoms: Early-stage lung cancer usually produces no symptoms. When symptoms appear, they may include smoker's cough, wheezing, sputum streaked with blood, chest pain, dyspnea, and hemoptysis.

Diagnostic Procedures: Chest x-ray, a sputum cytology test, and fiberoptic bronchoscopy are useful in diagnosing lung cancer. Tissue biopsy is required for definitive diagnosis.

Treatment: Treatment most often involves a combination of surgery, radiation therapy, and chemotherapy, since lung cancer often metastasizes to other tissues by the time it is diagnosed.

Prognosis: The prognosis is poor. According to the American Cancer Society, only 9 percent of lung cancer patients live more than 5 years.

Prevention: Lung cancer is largely preventable if individuals avoid smoking and toxic inhalants.

COMMON SYMPTOMS OF LUNG DISEASES

Individuals may present with the following common symptoms which deserve attention from health professionals:

■ Pain anywhere in the respiratory tract, especially sore throat
■ Cough, either productive or nonproductive, chronic or acute
■ Breathing irregularities such as dyspnea, wheezing, tachypnea, or rales
■ Fever
■ Malaise
■ Headache
■ Cyanosis

REFERENCE

1. Krupp, M. A., and M. J. Chatton (Eds.), *Current Medical Diagnosis and Treatment*, Lange Medical Publications, Los Altos, Calif., 1984, p. 147.

REVIEW QUESTIONS

Matching
Match the following terms with their correct definitions.

_____ 1. Air in pleural cavity
_____ 2. Chronic obstructive pulmonary disease
_____ 3. Sore throat
_____ 4. Caused by Epstein-Barr virus
_____ 5. Excess fluid in pleural space
_____ 6. Black lung disease
_____ 7. Nosebleed
_____ 8. Lungs lose normal elasticity
_____ 9. Inflammation of pleura
_____ 10. Hoarseness or loss of voice

a. Epistaxis
b. Pharyngitis
c. Laryngitis
d. Infectious mononucleosis
e. Pneumothorax
f. Pleurisy
g. Pleural effusion
h. COPD
i. Emphysema
j. Anthracosis
k. Asthma
l. Cor pulmonale

Short Answer
1. List the four major causes of sinusitis.
   a.
   b.
   c.
   d.
2. Treatment of acute tonsillitis and adenoid hyperplasia is apt to be _____.
3. Identify the four causes of pneumonia:
   a.
   b.
   c.
   d.

4. From the preceding list, identify the most common form of pneumonia: _____ .
5. Identify a complication which may result from a lung abscess: _____ .
6. A diagnosis of chronic bronchitis has a requirement. Identify: _____ .
7. Identify the classic symptoms of asthma:
   a.
   b.
8. The diagnostic test of choice to confirm tuberculosis is _____ .
9. The best prevention for any of the four pneumoconioses is _____ .
10. Mycoses are _____ infections.

True/False

T F   1. Coccidioidomycosis is common in the Ohio Valley.
T F   2. Legionnaires' disease affects only Legion members.
T F   3. Cor pulmonale is left atrial hypertrophy.
T F   4. Immobile patients may be high-risk for pulmonary embolism.
T F   5. Respiratory acidosis is hypoventilation and CO_2 retention.
T F   6. Respiratory alkalosis is hyperventilation and CO_2 elimination.
T F   7. Bronchiectasis is collapse of part or all of a lung.
T F   8. Atelectasis is abnormal dilation of bronchi.
T F   9. Early-stage lung cancer usually produces no symptoms.
T F 10. The body can survive only minutes without air.

ANSWERS

Matching
1. e
2. h
3. b
4. d
5. g

6. j
7. a
8. i
9. f
10. c

Short Answer
1. a. Bacterial infection
   b. Swimming or diving
   c. Dental abscess or extractions
   d. Nasal allergies

2. T&A (tonsillectomy and adenoidectomy)

3. a. Viral
   b. Bacterial
   c. Aspiration
   d. Viral and bacterial

4. Bacterial pneumonia

5. Development of brain abscess

6. Productive cough on most days for a minimum of 3 months in the year in at least 2 consecutive years

7. Marked wheezing and difficulty in expiration

8. PPD—purified protein derivative tuberculin test

9. Avoidance of dust

10. Fungal

True/False
1. False
2. False
3. False
4. True
5. True
6. True
7. False
8. False
9. True
10. True

GLOSSARY

ALVEOLI (PULMONARY):   The microscopic air sacs in the lungs, through whose walls the exchange of carbon dioxide and oxygen occurs.

ANALGESIC: A drug or agent that relieves pain.

ANTIPYRETIC: A drug or agent that reduces fever.

AUSCULTATION: Listening to sounds produced by the internal organs or other body parts for diagnostic purposes.

BRONCHODILATOR: A drug or other agent that relaxes and expands the air passages of the lungs.

CILIA (BRONCHIAL):   Microscopic, hairlike extensions of cells lining the interior of the bronchi, whose rhythmical beating moves fluids, mucus, and particulants out of the lungs.

CLUBBING: A condition characterized by bulbous swelling of the tips of the fingers and toes.

CYANOSIS: A bluish discoloration of the skin and mucous membranes due to an increased proportion of unoxygenated hemoglobin in the blood.

DIAPHORESIS: Sweating, especially when profuse or medically induced.

DIURETIC: A drug or agent that promotes the secretion of urine.

DYSPNEA: Labored or difficult breathing, generally indicating an insufficient amount of oxygen in the blood.

EDEMA: Excessive accumulation of fluid in bodily tissues. May be localized or general.

EXUDATE: Fluid discharged through vessel walls and collecting in adjacent tissue, having a high content of protein and cellular debris. (Compare with *transudate*.)

GRANULOMA: One of a variety of growths of inflamed, granular-appearing tissue.

HEMOPTYSIS: The coughing and spitting up of blood due to bleeding in any portion of the respiratory tract.

HYPERPLASIA: Excessive proliferation of normal cells.

HYPERTROPHY: An increase in size or volume of an organ or other body structure produced entirely by an increase in the size of existing cells, not by an increase in number of cells.

HYPOXIA: Denoting a condition or state of diminished oxygen availability to the body tissues.

KYPHOSCOLIOSIS: Abnormal backward and lateral curvature of the spine.

LIGATION: Process of tying off blood vessels or constricting other body tissues for therapeutic purposes.

MALAISE: A generalized feeling of illness, discomfort, or depression indicative of some underlying disease or disorder.

ORTHOPNEA: Respiratory condition in which there is discomfort in breathing in any but erect standing or sitting positions.

PALLOR: Loss of color; paleness, as of the skin.

PERCUSSION: A diagnostic technique in which various surfaces of the body are tapped, the resulting sounds indicating the size, position, and general condition of the underlying organs or structures.

pH: The degree of acidity or alkalinity of a solution, expressed in numbers from 0 to 14. Increasing acidity is expressed as a number less than 7 and increasing alkalinity as a number greater than 7. Maximum acidity is pH 0 and maximum alkalinity pH14. A pH of 7 is neutral.

PLEURA: The saclike membrane enveloping each lung and lining the adjacent portion of the thoracic cavity, the two layers forming a potential space, the pleural cavity.

PLEURECTOMY: Surgical excision of a portion of the pleura.

PLICATION: Surgical procedure in which folds in the wall of an organ are stitched together to reduce its size.

POLYCYTHEMIA VERA: A chronic, life-shortening disorder of the blood-cell-producing tissue in the bone marrow, primarily characterized by abnormally high number of circulating red blood cells.

POSTURAL DRAINAGE: A therapeutic technique in which a patient is directed to assume a variety of positions that facilitate the drainage of secretions in the lobes of the lungs or the bronchial passages.

PULMONARY INFARCTION: The death of a localized area of lung tissue resulting from an interruption of blood flow to that area. Generally caused by a pulmonary embolism.

PURULENT: Containing pus.

RALES: An abnormal respiratory sound heard on auscultation of the lungs produced by the movement of air through secretion-filled or constricted bronchial passages.

RHINITIS: Inflammation of the nasal mucous membranes.

RHONCHUS: A rale or rattling in the throat, especially when it resembles snoring.

SEPTIC: Pertaining to disease-causing organisms or their toxins.

SPUTUM: Substance expelled by coughing or clearing the throat.

STENOSIS: Abnormal constriction or narrowing in an opening or passageway of an organ or body part.

TACHYCARDIA: An abnormally rapid heart beat, generally defined as exceeding 100 beats per minute.

TACHYPNEA: Abnormal, very rapid breathing.

THREADY PULSE: A fine, barely perceptible pulse.

THORACENTESIS: Surgical puncture of the chest wall to remove fluid from either of the pleural cavities.

THORACOTOMY: Surgical incision in the wall of the chest.

THROMBOCYTOSIS: An increase in the number of blood platelets.

TRANSILLUMINATION: Visual inspection of a body structure or organ by passing a light through its walls.

TRANSUDATE: A fluid discharged through a membrane or vessel wall. In contrast to an exudate a transudate has a low content of protein or cellular debris.

Chapter 8

Circulatory System Diseases

LEARNING OBJECTIVES

Upon successful completion of this chapter, you will
■ Describe the infectious heart diseases.
■ Identify the valvular heart diseases.
■ Identify individuals at high risk of developing hypertension.
■ Recall the safe time duration of angina pectoris.
■ List the classic signs and symptoms of myocardial infarction.
■ Describe congestive heart failure.
■ List the causes of heart murmurs.
■ Contrast three types of aneurysms.
■ Compare atherosclerosis to arteriosclerosis.
■ Discuss the prevention of thrombophlebitis.

- Define varicose veins.
- Compare five anemias.
- Discuss the various treatments of leukemia.
- Define lymphedema.
- Compare lymphosarcoma to Hodgkin's disease.
- List at least four common symptoms indicating cardiovascular disease.

INTRODUCTION

The circulatory system is comprised of the heart and blood vessels (the cardiovascular system) and the lymphatic system. The heart and blood vessels function to transport oxygen, nutrients, and hormones to cells and remove waste products and carbon dioxide from cells. The heart and blood vessels work together to pump and circulate the equivalent of 7200 quarts of blood through the heart in 24 hours. The heart, about the size of a human fist, is made of muscle and valves. (Figures 8–1

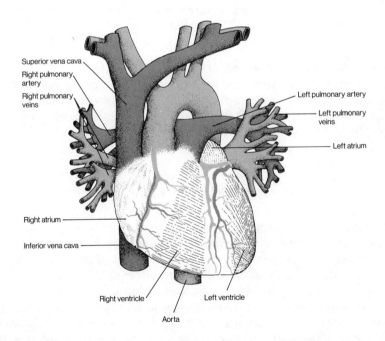

Figure 8–1. The heart (surface view). (From Gylys, B. A. and Wedding, M. E., *Medical Terminology: A Systems Approach,* ed. 2. F. A. Davis, Philadelphia, 1988, p. 148, with permission.)

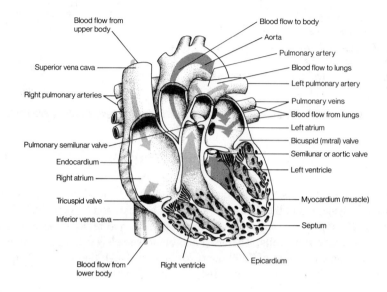

Figure 8–2. The heart (interior view). Arrows indicate direction of blood flow. (Modified from Gylys, B. A. and Wedding, M. E., *Medical Terminology: A Systems Approach,* ed. 2. F. A. Davis, Philadelphia, 1988, p. 149.)

and 8–2). The blood vessel network of the body is composed of arteries, arterioles, veins, venules, and capillaries, the latter linking the arteries and veins. The lymphatic system is composed of lymph capillaries, lacteals, nodes, vessels, and ducts. The lymphatic system transports fluids, nutrients, and wastes exuded from tissues back to the bloodstream through connections with major veins.

RHEUMATIC FEVER

Description: *Rheumatic fever* is a systemic inflammatory disease affecting the joints, heart, central nervous system, skin, and other body tissues. Despite a name that highlights the joint involvement characteristic of the disease, rheumatic fever is important because of the serious, irreparable damage it can cause to the heart in the form of acute carditis or rheumatic heart disease, a condition due to permanent scarring of the heart valves. Rheumatic fever usually strikes children and adolescents from 5 to 15 years of age, although it may occur at other ages as well.

Etiology: Rheumatic fever follows as a consequence of a pharyngeal infection from certain group A streptococci. Despite this association, the exact mechanism of the disease is not known. Indeed, the onset of rheumatic fever often occurs after group A streptococci are no longer detectable in the affected individual. The most popular theory of the etiology of rheumatic fever is that the disease is a bacterial-induced autoimmune disorder; that is, one in which the antibodies produced to fight the initial streptococcal infection begin to attack body tissue. Genetic risk factors also may be involved in rheumatic fever, possibly accounting for why only a small percentage of those individuals who experience a pharyngeal group A streptococcal infection ever actually contract the disease.

Signs and Symptoms: Rheumatic fever is characterized by a specific cluster of symptoms that include fever, polyarthritis, carditis, **chorea**, subcutaneous nodules, and erythema. These characteristic symptoms may occur in any combination and with varying degrees of severity.

■ *Polyarthritis.* This classic symptom of rheumatic fever is characterized by pain, redness, and swelling of the major joints of the extremities. The arthritic symptoms are often "migratory" in that as one joint begins to heal, another becomes inflamed.

■ *Carditis.* Since any or all layers of the heart—endocardium, myocardium, and pericardium—may be involved, the symptoms of carditis associated with rheumatic fever may vary. The most typical symptoms include heart murmur and **tachycardia**.

■ *Chorea.* Usually a late symptom of rheumatic fever, chorea is characterized by sudden, jerking, involuntary movements accompanied by general muscle weakness. Agitation and emotional disturbance almost always accompany the muscular spasms.

■ *Subcutaneous nodules.* These are painless, pea-sized swellings that form over bone surfaces, usually on the hands, elbows, and feet.

■ *Erythema.* The erythema associated with rheumatic fever is mild and diffuse, rapidly forming and then subsiding over areas of the trunk and extremities.

Diagnostic Procedures: A patient history revealing a recent pharyngeal streptococcal infection should immediately suggest the possibility of rheumatic fever. An antistreptolysin O (ASO) test will almost always be performed to detect the presence of streptococcal antibodies. Other laboratory data may show elevated white blood count (WBC), erythrocyte sedimentation rate (ESR), and cardiac enzymes. Physical examination will typically reveal one or more of the symptoms characteristic of the disease.

Treatment: There is no treatment that will alter the progress of the disease once it has started. Treatment is largely symptomatic and supportive. In most cases, though, treatment with antibiotics is begun to ensure that group A streptococci are no longer present in the body. Salicylates are helpful in reducing fever and joint pain and swelling. Bed rest is required. Because rheumatic fever may require long-term care, patient education is an important part of the treatment process.

Prognosis: The short-term prognosis for rheumatic fever varies according to the severity of the particular case, but it is best characterized as guarded. Death may result from acute carditis. Most cases subside within 6 to 12 weeks. The long-term prognosis for the disease depends on the degree of scarring and deformity that may have occurred to the heart valves. Rheumatic fever tends to be recurrent, especially within 5 years of the initial attack and especially among those who experience heart damage.

Prevention: Rheumatic fever is preventable through prompt treatment of any pharyngeal streptococcal infection. Recurrences are preventable through a continuous course of antibiotic therapy—a practice especially recommended for those who suffered heart damage as a consequence of an initial case of the disease.

CARDITIS

Pericarditis

Description: *Pericarditis* is inflammation of the pericardium, the saclike membrane that surrounds and protects the heart muscle. The disease can be acute or chronic.

Etiology: Pericarditis is usually caused by bacterial infection of the pericardium. The disease also may be caused by neoplasms metastasized from other organs, viruses, rheumatic fever, uremia, or a coronary thrombosis. Trauma or any injury that causes blood to leak into the pericardial sac also may incite pericarditis. Chronic pericarditis may develop from the acute form of the disease, but it is often idiopathic.

Signs and Symptoms: The classic symptom of pericarditis is pleuritic pain that increases with deep inspiration. The fluctuating nature of pericardial pain clearly differentiates it from the pain produced by a myocardial infarction (heart attack). If pericardial **effusion** occurs in acute pericarditis, **orthopnea, dyspnea**, and tachycardia typically result. If the fluid accumulates rapidly, the pressure against the heart may result in clammy skin, pallor, and a decrease in blood pressure. **Hepatomegaly** and **ascites** may occur in chronic pericarditis.

Diagnostic Procedures: Auscultation may indicate pericardial friction rub (a grating sound heard as the heart beats). Laboratory data may show elevated WBC, ESR, and cardiac enzymes. An ECG may detect cardiac **arrhythmias**.

Treatment: Underlying causes of the pericarditis must be treated and symptomatic relief provided. Bed rest with the upper body elevated and **analgesics** may be prescribed. If the case of pericarditis is bacterial in origin, antibiotic therapy may be started. **Pericardiocentesis** to promote drainage may be part of the treatment course, too.

Prognosis: The prognosis is determined by the etiology of the particular case, but generally it is good.

Prevention: The best prevention is the avoidance of infections; otherwise, none is known.

Myocarditis

Description: *Myocarditis* is inflammation of the cardiac muscle. The condition may be either acute or chronic.

Etiology: Myocarditis may be caused by viral or bacterial infections or be a consequence of systemic diseases such as rheumatic fever. Myocardial inflammation also may be caused by chronic alcoholism, various toxins, or as a side effect of certain drugs or radiation therapy. In many cases the disease is idiopathic.

Signs and Symptoms: The symptoms of myocarditis are often nonspecific, but they may include dyspnea, heart palpitations, fever, and fatigue.

Diagnostic Procedures: A patient history may reveal a recent upper respiratory infection, but an ECG provides the best diagnosis. Laboratory tests confirming the diagnosis may show elevated cardiac enzymes, WBC, and ESR.

Treatment: Bed rest is helpful, and antibiotics may be needed if a bacterial infection is determined to be the cause of the myocarditis. Oxygen therapy and sodium restriction may be recommended. If congestive heart failure occurs, diuretics and digitalis may be prescribed.

Prognosis: The prognosis for an individual with uncomplicated myocarditis is usually good. Complications may include left or right ventricular failure.

Prevention: There is no specific prevention.

Endocarditis

Description: *Endocarditis* is inflammation of the membrane lining the valves and chambers of the heart. The disease is characterized by the formation of abnormal growths called *vegetations* on or within the membrane.

Etiology: Endocarditis is most frequently caused by infection from streptococcal bacteria. The disease also may be caused by fungal infections, syphilis, and tuberculosis. It also may arise as a consequence of systemic diseases such as rheumatic fever or lupus erythematosus. Infecting organisms more readily establish themselves on the endocardium of a heart already damaged by congenital or acquired defects, although healthy endocardial tissue may be infected as well. A vegetation forms as the infected tissue is covered by a layer of platelets and fibrin.

Signs and Symptoms: Symptoms vary according to etiology and the portion of the heart affected. There may be weakness and fatigue, night sweats, and an intermittent fever which persists for weeks. A heart murmur may be heard that was not previously detected. Additional symptoms may arise if the vegetations break off into the bloodstream forming embolisms that lodge in other organs. Paralysis can occur if a large embolus lodges in the brain. If an embolus obstructs circulation in the kidney, there may be blood in the urine. If tiny vegetations lodge in the small vessels of the skin, subcutaneous ruptures called **petechiae** may appear.

Diagnostic Procedures: The patient history may reveal predisposing factors of endocarditis. An echocardiogram may reveal the presence of vegetative growths. Blood testing typically reveals leukocytosis and high concentrations of bacterial antibodies. Repeated blood cultures will usually result in positive identification of the causative microorganism.

Treatment: It is important to eliminate the infecting organism. Antibiotic therapy probably will continue over a number of weeks. Bed rest, analgesics, and increased fluid intake are helpful. Surgery may be necessary to repair severe valvular damage.

Prognosis: This disease is now curable when treated early with antibiotics. Before antibiotics, death was almost certain. Complications that may cause death include congestive heart failure and embolism damage to vital organs.

Prevention: Individuals at high risk should receive antibiotic therapy prior to undergoing surgery or certain dental procedures.

VALVULAR HEART DISEASE

Diseased heart valves may malfunction in two ways. The opening formed by a valve may be too large to close completely, allowing blood to leak back past the valve into the heart chamber from which it was pumped. Or the valve opening may be too narrow—a condition called valvular **stenosis**—impeding the flow of blood through the valve when it should be open and allowing blood to leak back when it should be closed. Either condition can cause heart failure.

Heart murmurs, periodic sounds heard during auscultation with a stethoscope, are generated by blood flow through the heart when there is an anomaly. Murmurs can be caused by blood leaking back through an incompetent or deformed valve, by blood forcing its way through a narrowed valve, from **dilatation** of the heart, or by a rapid diastolic flow. Exercise and tachycardia increase the intensity of any murmur.

Murmurs are graded on the basis of intensity, with Grade I the least intense and Grade VI the most intense. Detecting and interpreting heart murmurs is a useful tool in diagnosing and estimating the severity of valvular heart disease. Certain murmurs are consistently associated with severe heart dysfunctions. Conversely, other murmurs may be insignificant.

Mitral Insufficiency/Stenosis

Description: In *mitral insufficiency,* blood from the left ventricle flows back into the left atrium. In *mitral stenosis,* blood flow is obstructed from the left atrium to the left ventricle. In both cases, the result is an enlarged left atrium.

Etiology: Mitral insufficiency or stenosis most commonly results from rheumatic fever, but it also may be caused by mitral valve **prolapse** or myocardial infarction.

Signs and Symptoms: In both conditions, there may be dyspnea, fatigue, heart palpitations, peripheral edema, hepatomegaly, **rales**, orthopnea, and distension of the jugular veins.

Diagnostic Procedures: In both conditions, cardiac catheterization, x-ray, echocardiography, and ECG may establish the diagnosis.

Treatment: The treatment approach depends on the severity of the symptoms. Generally, the treatment of choice is **valvotomy** and valve reconstruction or valve replacement with an artificial valve.

Prognosis: The prognosis is good. The disease usually is not progressive, and many patients live a long time without surgery. Both mitral insufficiency and stenosis can lead to right ventricular **hypertrophy** and right ventricular failure.

Prevention: There is no known prevention other than the prevention of rheumatic fever and its complications.

Tricuspid Insufficiency/Stenosis

Description: In *tricuspid insufficiency,* blood flows back into the right atrium from the right ventricle, decreasing the blood flow to the left side of the heart. In *tricuspid stenosis,* the right atrium hypertrophies and increases pressure in the vena cava.

Etiology: Tricuspid insufficiency or stenosis may be caused by rheumatic fever. Tricuspid stenosis often is associated with mitral valve disease.

Signs and Symptoms: In both tricuspid insufficiency and stenosis, the most common symptoms are dyspnea and fatigue. Peripheral edema, distended jugular veins, hepatomegaly, and ascites may occur. **Syncope** may occur in tricuspid stenosis. A systolic murmur often occurs in tricuspid insufficiency, whereas a diastolic murmur may indicate tricuspid stenosis.

Diagnostic Procedures: Cardiac catheterization, x-ray, echocardiography, and ECG may establish the diagnosis.

Treatment: Treatment depends on the nature and severity of the condition. The condition may not be amenable to valvotomy. In some cases, the defective tricuspid valve may be replaced with a prosthetic valve (Figure 8–3). The disease may regress if the mitral valve is replaced.

Prognosis: The prognosis is good. Complications in the presence of either tricuspid insufficiency or stenosis can lead to heart failure.

Prevention: There is no known prevention.

Pulmonic Insufficiency/Stenosis

Description: With *pulmonic insufficiency,* blood flows back into the right ventricle causing right ventricular hypertrophy and eventual right ventricular failure. In *pulmonic stenosis,* blood flow is obstructed causing dilation of the right atrium and eventual right ventricular failure.

Etiology: Pulmonic insufficiency may result from pulmonary hypertension. Pulmonic stenosis may follow rheumatic heart disease. Both often are congenital in nature.

Signs and Symptoms: Individuals with either condition may exhibit dyspnea, fatigue, syncope, and chest pain. Peripheral edema, distended jugular veins,

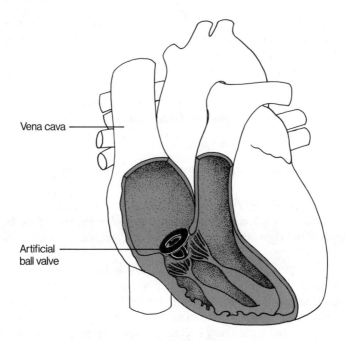

Figure 8–3. Artificial heart valve. In this example, a defective tricuspid valve has been replaced with an artificial ball valve. (From Gylys, B. A. and Wedding, M. E., *Medical Terminology: A Systems Approach,* ed. 2. F. A. Davis, Philadelphia, 1988, p. 156, with permission.)

and hepatomegaly also are possible. Pulmonic stenosis, however, may be asymptomatic. A diastolic murmur may be heard on auscultation in pulmonic insufficiency, whereas a systolic murmur may be heard in pulmonic stenosis.

Diagnostic Procedures: Cardiac catheterization and ECG are the most common diagnostic procedures for both conditions; however, x-ray may be used in pulmonic insufficiency.

Treatment: No treatment may be necessary if the person is able to live a normal life with the condition; if not, surgery is the treatment of choice.

Prognosis: With surgery, the prognosis generally is good. Infectious endocarditis is a possible complication.

Prevention: There is no known prevention.

Aortic Insufficiency/Stenosis

Description: *Aortic insufficiency* results in blood flowing back into the left ventricle, eventually causing left ventricular hypertrophy and failure. *Aortic steno-*

sis causes increased ventricular pressure as a result of a greater cardiac workload. Left ventricular failure may result.

Etiology: Either aortic insufficiency or stenosis can be caused by rheumatic fever. Syphilis, endocarditis, or hypertension can be the cause of aortic insufficiency. Congenital causes may give rise to aortic stenosis.

Signs and Symptoms: Dyspnea, fatigue, syncope, angina, and heart palpitations are the most common symptoms. Congestion in the pulmonary vein, congestive heart failure, and pulmonary edema may occur upon failure of the left ventricle. Auscultation may reveal a characteristic diastolic murmur in aortic insufficiency and a systolic murmur in aortic stenosis.

Diagnostic Procedures: As in most of the valvular heart diseases, common diagnostic procedures include cardiac catheterization, x-ray, echocardiography, and ECG.

Treatment: The person may only need to be assessed on a yearly basis by ECG, chest x-ray, and echocardiogram. Severe cases may require surgical replacement of the aortic valve.

Prognosis: The prognosis varies depending on the nature and severity of the disease. Complications include arrhythmias, ventricular **fibrillation**, and cardiac failure.

Prevention: There is no known prevention.

HYPERTENSIVE HEART DISEASE: ESSENTIAL HYPERTENSION

When the heart must work against increased resistance in the form of high blood pressure, hypertensive heart disease often results. What constitutes hypertension—high blood pressure—may be different for each person, but the medical community generally agrees that the condition exists if **systolic pressure** persists over 150 mmHg and **diastolic pressure** persists over 90 mmHg. Many persons with hypertension live long, vigorous lives. Others do not respond well to treatment and eventually die of heart failure, a cerebral vascular accident (CVA), or kidney dysfunction.

Description: *Essential hypertension* is persistently elevated blood pressure that develops without apparent cause.

Etiology: Although essential hypertension is idiopathic, some persons are at a higher risk than others. They include blacks, chronically stressed individuals, the obese, and those who favor a diet high in salt and saturated fats. The disease may be familial. Older persons, those with sedentary lifestyles, smokers, and those taking oral contraceptives also have a higher risk for hypertension.

Signs and Symptoms: Hypertension may remain asymptomatic for months or years. The person may exhibit vague symptoms, such as light-headedness, **tinnitus**, easy fatigability, and heart palpitations.

Diagnostic Procedures: Blood pressure readings taken on at least three separate occasions after the individual has rested will show pressure, greater than 150/90 mmHg. It is important that a history of blood pressure readings be kept for comparison because blood pressure can vary. Auscultation may reveal **bruits**. ECG and chest x-ray will help detect cardiovascular damage.

Treatment: Although there is no cure for essential hypertension, a change in lifestyle and diet and antihypertensive drug therapy can control the condition. A diet low in salt and fat, moderate exercise, and a reduction of stress are helpful. Diuretics or vasodilators also may be prescribed.

Prognosis: The prognosis is good if the person carefully follows the prescribed treatment regime. Complications may include cerebral vascular accident (CVA), heart failure, and kidney failure.

Prevention: Since the cause is idiopathic, there is no known prevention other than minimizing controllable risk factors.

CORONARY ARTERY DISEASE

Description: *Coronary artery disease* is the narrowing of the coronary arteries sufficient to prevent an adequate blood supply to portions of the myocardium, the heart muscle. As the **lumen** of the coronary artery narrows, gradual **ischemia** causes cells in the myocardium to weaken and die. These are then replaced with scar tissue.

Etiology: The leading cause of coronary artery disease is atherosclerosis, a condition in which the lumen of the coronary arteries is narrowed by fatty, fibrous plaques (see Atherosclerosis). Many factors seem to predispose this condition, including old age, heredity, obesity, diabetes mellitus, hypertension, smoking, and stress. The condition is more common in men.

Signs and Symptoms: An immediate result of inadequate blood supply to the myocardium is *angina,* a burning, squeezing, tightness in the chest that may radiate to the neck, the shoulder blade, and left arm. Nausea, vomiting, sweating, and a feeling of panic may accompany these symptoms. A complete discussion of angina pectoris follows.

Diagnostic Procedures: The patient history may reveal one or more of the risk factors for coronary artery disease and a pattern of angina. ECG changes during an angina attack may indicate the region of myocardial ischemia.

Treatment: The goal of treatment is to reduce angina by reducing myocardial oxygen demand or increasing oxygen supply. Nitroglycerin preparations are helpful in increasing the oxygen supply to the heart by dilating the coronary arteries. Coronary artery bypass surgery may be necessary to bridge obstructive lesions. There may be an attempt to compress the fatty plaque deposits in the coronary arteries by cardiac catheterization. Dietary restrictions may be necessary, and persons should be encouraged to refrain from smoking.

Prognosis: The prognosis varies greatly depending on the amount of arterial blockage and the extent of damage to the heart muscle. The annual mortality rate for individuals with coronary artery disease is 2.2 percent when one vessel is involved, 6.8 percent for two-vessel disease, and 11.4 percent for three-vessel disease.[1] The patient can die instantly of myocardial infarction (see Myocardial Infarction).

Prevention: The best prevention of coronary artery disease is to minimize controllable risk factors.

ANGINA PECTORIS

Description: *Angina pectoris* is chest pain resulting from ischemia to a part of the myocardium.

Etiology: Angina pectoris is usually a clinical syndrome accompanying arteriosclerotic heart disease. Less frequently, it may be produced by a coronary spasm and severe aortic stenosis or aortic insufficiency. Angina attacks are frequently triggered in susceptible individuals by any condition which increases myocardial oxygen demand, such as stress, eating, exertion, or even extremes of temperature and humidity.

Signs and Symptoms: The classic signs of an angina attack are burning, squeezing, and tightness in the chest that may radiate to the neck and the left arm and shoulder blade. Sometimes there is nausea and vomiting. Acute anxiety may accompany angina, especially in the person who is already aware of a heart problem and is worried whether this episode of angina is a precursor to a myocardial infarction. An angina attack usually lasts less than 15 minutes and not more than 30 minutes.

Diagnostic Procedures: ECG during the angina may indicate ischemia, and a patient history usually reveals a history of angina.

Treatment: Nitroglycerine preparations taken either sublingually or applied topically usually relieve anginal pain. Sedatives or tranquilizers may be prescribed. Coronary diseases causing disabling angina pectoris that does not respond to treatment may require coronary bypass procedures or **percutaneous transluminal coronary angioplasty**. In coronary bypass procedures, one to five bypass grafts can be made in the patient. In angioplasty, a balloon-tipped catheter is passed through a systemic artery to the occluded coronary artery and inflated, dilating the vessel. This procedure is performed under local anesthesia.

Prognosis: The prognosis is guarded. Angina pectoris usually is considered a warning to the person to lessen exertion and stress which might bring on myocardial infarction and heart failure. If the pain persists longer than 30 minutes, the individual should see a physician immediately.

Prevention: Prevention includes avoidance of stress and overexertion in the presence of ongoing coronary artery disease.

MYOCARDIAL INFARCTION (HEART ATTACK)

Description: *Myocardial infarction* (MI) is a life-threatening condition caused by the occlusion of one or more coronary arteries and the subsequent necrosis of a section of the heart muscle tissue served by those arteries (Figure 8–4). Myocardial infarction is a medical emergency requiring immediate attention.

Etiology: The predisposing factors of MI are the same as those for many other cardiovascular diseases. They include heredity, obesity, aging, hypertension, smoking, diabetes mellitus, a sedentary lifestyle, chronic stress, or "type A" behavior (competitive, aggressive behavior). Men are more susceptible than women.

Signs and Symptoms: The classic symptom is crushing chest pain that may radiate to the left arm, neck, and jaw. The pain may be similar to anginal pain but usually is severe and not relieved by the same measures which relieve angina. Some individuals, however, may exhibit few symptoms or confuse the pain with indigestion. Individuals with coronary heart disease should be suspicious if angina occurs with increasing frequency and duration. For some, an MI is preceded by vague feelings of discomfort, fear, nausea, and vomiting.

Diagnostic Procedures: A patient history revealing coronary artery disease and episodes of chest pain will help in the diagnosis. ECG and radioisotope studies may be performed. Blood tests for elevated cardiac enzyme levels—CPK, LDH, and SGOT—are useful in estimating the extent of myocardial damage.

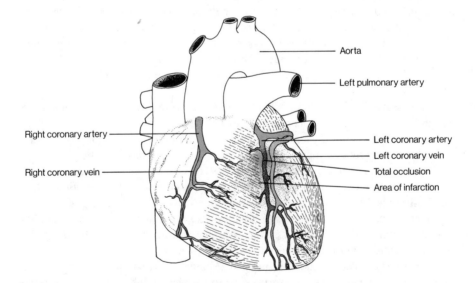

Figure 8–4. Myocardial Infarction. The shaded area beneath the left coronary artery represents an area of necrotized myocardial tissue. (From Gylys, B. A. and Wedding, M.E., *Medical Terminology: A Systems Approach,* ed. 2. F. A. Davis, Philadelphia, 1988, p. 155, with permission.)

Treatment: Immediate hospitalization is important to relieve pain, stabilize heart rhythm, and reduce cardiac workload. Complete bed rest with sedation and analgesia is typically instituted, and the person is apt to be placed on a cardiac monitor to detect cardiac arrhythmias, a common problem during the first 48 hours following an attack. If cardiac arrest occurs, cardiopulmonary resuscitation (CPR) efforts are begun immediately.

Prognosis: The prognosis of an individual experiencing MI depends on the extent of damage to the myocardium. The prognosis is guarded at best. The mortality rate is approximately 35 percent, with most deaths occurring within the first 12 hours. Complications of myocardial infarction include arrhythmias, congestive heart failure, **cardiogenic shock**, **mitral regurgitation**, **ventricular septal rupture**, pericarditis, and ventricular **aneurysm**.

Prevention: Prevention includes avoidance of any predisposing factors such as smoking, obesity, and stress.

CONGESTIVE HEART FAILURE

Description: *Congestive heart failure* (CHF) is a condition in which the pumping ability of the heart is progressively impaired to the point that it no longer meets bodily needs. Circulatory congestion may occur in the systemic venous circulation resulting in peripheral edema. Or the congestion may occur in the pulmonary circulation causing pulmonary edema, an acute, life-threatening condition.

Etiology: Either the left or right ventricles, alone or together, may be the sources of the inadequate pumping action. Chronic congestive heart failure is the product of many cardiac and pulmonary disease processes. Acute congestive heart failure most often results from a myocardial infarction.

Signs and Symptoms: Left ventricular failure may be manifested as dyspnea and fatigue. Right ventricular failure may cause distended neck veins and hepatomegaly. Symptoms of advanced CHF may include tachypnea, heart palpitations, edema, **diaphoresis**, and **cyanosis**. As the disease progresses, there may be **hemoptysis**, cyanosis, and **pitting edema** of the ankle.

Diagnostic Procedures: ECG, chest x-ray, and elevated central venous pressure will indicate the diagnosis.

Treatment: Treatment may involve the use of diuretics to reduce circulatory congestion by reducing total blood volume. Bed rest may be recommended. Drug therapy may include the prescription of vasodilators and digitalis to strengthen heart action. Dietary sodium may be restricted to combat edema.

Prognosis: Acute congestive heart failure usually responds quickly to therapeutic measures. The prognosis is good, although it is dependent on the cause. If the congestion is severe and chronic, the prognosis is poor. The person usually must continue medication indefinitely and be carefully supervised by a physician.

Prevention: Prevention is avoidance of any predisposing factors.

CARDIAC ARREST

Description: *Cardiac arrest* is the sudden, unexpected interruption of heart function. It is a medical emergency.

Etiology: Cardiac arrest may result from myocardial infarction, circulatory collapse due to various forms of shock, or ventricular fibrillation. Cardiac arrest also may result from drug reactions, electrocution, drowning, or other forms of accidental physical trauma.

Signs and Symptoms: Symptoms of impending cardiac arrest may include sudden tachycardia or **bradycardia**, a drop in blood pressure, respiratory failure, and changes in ECG patterns. An individual experiencing cardiac arrest usually loses consciousness and ceases to breathe.

Diagnostic Procedures: The diagnosis is based on the absence of respiration and pulse and accompanying loss of consciousness.

Treatment: Emergency first aid treatment may include establishing an airway, ventilating through artificial means, and giving external cardiac massage until the person can be transported to a hospital to receive more advanced life support.

Prognosis: The prognosis is guarded at best. However, persons may survive, especially if treatment begins within 3 minutes. Irreversible brain damage may occur after that time.

Prevention: The best prevention is to avoid any cardiac-related diseases and to carefully monitor any individual with heart disease.

BLOOD VESSEL DISEASES

Aneurysms: Abdominal, Thoracic, and Peripheral Arteries

Description: An *aneurysm* is a local dilation of an artery or chamber of the heart due to weakening of its walls. Aneurysms may be *saccular* (resembling a sac) or *fusiform* (a spindle-shaped enlargement). Aneurysms may cause **thrombus** formation, hemorrhage, or ischemia.[2] Three common types of aneurysms discussed here are abdominal, thoracic, and peripheral artery aneurysms.

Etiology: Aneurysms may be congenital or result from trauma, inflammation, and degeneration produced by atherosclerosis.

Signs and Symptoms: *Abdominal aneurysms* may be asymptomatic, but if the person is slender, a pulsating middle and upper abdominal mass may be detected on routine physical examination. Other symptoms may include mild to severe weakness, sweating, tachycardia, and hypotension.

Thoracic artery aneurysms may be asymptomatic, or the affected individual may exhibit signs of pressure on the trachea or superior vena cava. These signs include dyspnea, **stridor**, or edema in the neck and arms with distended neck veins. Pain may be present in the neck, back, or substernal areas.

In *peripheral artery aneurysms,* there may be no symptoms, or the person may have pain in the area of the aneurysm, edema, and venous distension. Severe ischemia caused by aneurysms in the foot or leg may result in gangrene.

Diagnostic Procedures: In abdominal aneurysms, an ECG and ultrasonography may be done. X-ray, ECG, aortography, and CT scans may be performed to detect thoracic aneurysms. Palpation, ultrasonography, and angiography may be used to detect peripheral artery aneurysms.

Treatment: The course of treatment chosen for any form of aneurysm depends on the size and site of the affected artery, the size of the aneurysm and the likelihood of its rupturing, as well as the general physical status of the individual. Most aneurysms are treated surgically. Small arteries may be clipped off before the aneurysm. Larger arteries may require surgical excision of the weakened portion of the vessel, arterial grafting, or arterial bypass.

Prognosis: The prognosis is guarded for most forms of aneurysm. Death may result from rupture of the aneurysm. A possible complication includes a thrombus forming along the wall of an aneurysm. A piece of the thrombus may break off, producing an **embolus** that may block the flow of blood to vital organs.

Prevention: There is no known prevention.

Arteriosclerosis and Atherosclerosis

Description: *Atherosclerosis* is a condition characterized by the accumulation of yellowish plaques of cholesterol, lipids, and cellular debris in the inner layers of the walls of large and medium-sized arteries (Figure 8-5). The vessel walls become thickened, fibrotic, and calcified, and the arterial lumen narrows. The most commonly affected vessels include the coronary and cerebral arteries. *Arteriosclerosis* is widespread thickening of the walls of small arteries and arterioles with a resulting loss of elasticity. Circulatory impairment is the consequence of both diseases; however, in atherosclerosis, the arteries are major and supply vital tissues. These arterial diseases are responsible for about 40 percent of the deaths in the United States.

Etiology: The etiology is unclear, but it may include trauma or the accumulation of lipids due to dietary excesses, faulty carbohydrate metabolism, or a genetic defect. Both diseases are seen with aging and often are associated with diabetes mellitus, hypertension, obesity, **nephrosclerosis**, and scleroderma.

Signs and Symptoms: Typical signs and symptoms include intermittent **claudication**, changes in skin temperature and color, bruits over the involved artery, headache, dizziness, and memory defects. Pain, especially at night, may be present due to sepsis or ischemia. Muscle cramping may occur.

Diagnostic Procedures: X-rays, arteriograms, and blood pressure measurements may be done for diagnosis.

Treatment: **Vasodilators**, exercise, and a diet low in saturated fats, cholesterol, and calories may be tried. Any infections, ulcers, or gangrene of the toes and

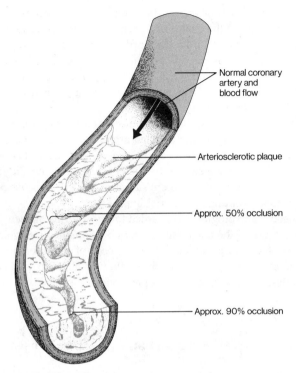

Normal coronary
artery and
blood flow

Arteriosclerotic plaque

Approx. 50% occlusion

Approx. 90% occlusion

Figure 8–5. Atherosclerosis. (From Gylys, B. A. and Wedding, M. E., *Medical Terminology: A Systems Approach,* ed. 2. F. A. Davis, Philadelphia, 1988, p. 154, with permission.)

foot need immediate attention. Surgery may be necessary in some cases and may involve arterial grafting, **thromboendarterectomy**, and **sympathectomy**.

Prognosis: The prognosis varies and is dependent on the site and amount of arterial occlusion and the person's overall physical condition. Complications include **gangrene**, infections, and coronary artery disease.

Prevention: Prevention includes adequate rest and exercise, avoidance of stress, and a diet low in cholesterol, calories, and saturated fats.

Thrombophlebitis

Description: *Thrombophlebitis* is inflammation of a vein in conjunction with the formation of a clot. The affected vein may be either partially or completely obstructed. The condition usually occurs in an extremity, most frequently in a leg, and can affect both superficial and deep veins.

Etiology: Thrombophlebitis may be caused by trauma, reduced blood flow, infection, chemical irritation, or prolonged immobility, or it may be idiopathic.

Signs and Symptoms: The person may be asymptomatic. Symptoms, however, will depend on the site of the affected vein and may include a dull aching and tight feeling at the site, **induration**, redness and tenderness along a superficial vein, and anxiety. Fever, chills, and malaise also may develop.

Diagnostic Procedures: Physical examination may reveal the inflammation. Phlebography, Doppler ultrasonography, and a radioactive fibrinogen uptake test may be used to diagnose thrombophlebitis.

Treatment: In superficial thrombophlebitis, the person may be advised to rest in bed, elevate the affected limb, and apply heat over the site of the affected vein. In deep-vein thrombophlebitis, the affected limb may be elevated and possibly wrapped with elastic bandages. Anticoagulant therapy may be prescribed. Surgical procedures such as vein ligation and femoral vein thrombectomy may be done for a case of deep-vein thrombophlebitis.

Prognosis: If only superficial veins are involved, the condition may be self-limiting, and the prognosis is good. When deep veins are involved, the prognosis is guarded. A serious complication of thrombophlebitis is the formation of a pulmonary embolism, a life-threatening condition.

Prevention: Individuals with a history of varicose veins or other conditions predisposing to thrombophlebitis should wear elastic hose. It may be advisable to allow for walking following long periods of sitting, such as when traveling or working.

Varicose Veins

Description: *Varicose veins* are enlarged, twisted, superficial veins. They may occur in almost any part of the body, but most frequently they occur in the lower legs, involving the greater and lesser saphenous veins.

Etiology: Varicose veins may be due to an inherited defect or venous diseases. They also may be produced by conditions that cause venostasis, such as pregnancy or jobs requiring prolonged standing or heavy lifting.

Signs and Symptoms: The person may be asymptomatic even though the varicose vein condition is severe. Quite frequently, however, the affected veins are visually evident. Characteristic symptoms of varicose veins of the legs include dull, aching heaviness or a feeling of fatigue after standing. Cramping may occur, followed by edema and stasis pigmentation.

Diagnostic Procedures: Trendelenberg's test and phlebography may be performed for diagnosis.

Treatment: The use of elastic stockings, a moderate exercise program, and avoidance of prolonged periods of standing or lifting may be recommended initially. Compression sclerotherapy may be done to collapse and produce permanent fibrosis of the affected veins. Severe varicose veins may require stripping and ligation.

Prognosis: The prognosis is good; however, further varicose veins may develop requiring treatment.

Prevention: Prevention includes avoidance of prolonged standing or lifting, avoidance of constrictive clothing, and elevation of the legs when possible.

ANEMIAS

Anemias are diseases characterized by a reduction in the number of circulating red cells or in the quantity of hemoglobin in the red cells. Five types of anemias discussed here are iron deficiency anemia, folic acid deficiency anemia, pernicious anemia, aplastic anemia, and sickle-cell anemia.

Iron Deficiency Anemia

Description: *Iron deficiency anemia* is characterized by inadequate reserves of iron in the body and the formation of unusually small, hemoglobin-poor red blood cells. Iron deficiency anemia occurs more frequently in premenopausal women and in adolescents. It is the most common chronic disease in the United States.

Etiology: Causes include excessive blood loss from conditions such as **menorrhagia**, gastrointestinal bleeding, or excessive blood donation. The condition also may result from poor diet, iron malabsorption, and pregnancy.

Signs and Symptoms: Common symptoms include pallor, lassitude, headache, and irritability. If the anemia progresses, symptoms become more severe, such as dyspnea, tachycardia, and brittle hair and nails.

Diagnostic Procedures: Blood testing typically indicates low hemoglobin and hematocrit values. Levels of serum iron and serum ferritin also may be low as well. The red blood count will typically reveal unusually high numbers of microcytic red cells. Bone marrow studies may be done to differentiate iron deficiency anemia from closely related blood disorders.

Treatment: Iron deficiency anemia may be treated with orally or **parenterally** administered iron supplements. Dietary modifications, however, are often sufficient to restore lost bodily iron reserves.

Prognosis: The prognosis for iron deficiency anemia is good if the underlying cause, such as unusual bleeding, is detected and treated. The condition may be chronic in some cases, however.

Prevention: Prevention includes a diet with adequate iron for daily needs and identification of high-risk individuals.

Folic Acid Deficiency Anemia

Description: *Folic acid deficiency anemia* is characterized by the appearance of large-sized, abnormal red blood cells (megaloblasts) owing to inadequate stores of folic acid within the body. Folic acid is one of the B-complex of vitamins.

Etiology: The cause of this anemia is often inadequate intake of folic acid due to poor diet or overcooking of vegetables or as a consequence of alcoholism. The disease also may arise from increased utilization of folic acid such as may occur during pregnancy, in infancy, or as a result of other blood disorders. Impaired absorption of folic acid by the body and drug-related folic imbalances also may produce the disease. The deficiency is more common in pregnant women, infants, children, and adolescents.

Signs and Symptoms: Symptoms may include weakness, fatigue, **anorexia**, pallor, forgetfulness, and irritability.

Diagnostic Procedures: Serum folate levels will typically be decreased. Bone marrow studies may be done to determine if there is a secondary cause of the disease.

Treatment: Folic acid supplements may be administered orally or parenterally if the person warrants more immediate effects.

Prognosis: The prognosis is dependent on the underlying cause of the folic acid deficiency. For most, the prognosis is good.

Prevention: Prevention includes a diet with adequate folic acid content such as found in beef liver, cooked collards, red beans, and asparagus spears.

Pernicious Anemia

Description: *Pernicious (megaloblastic) anemia* is characterized by the appearance of large-sized, abnormal red blood cells as a result of inadequate levels of vitamin B_{12} within the body. The disease is most common in persons of Scandinavian and northern European descent.

Etiology: Pernicious anemia is caused by failure of certain cells in the gastric mucosa to secrete adequate levels of a protein called *intrinsic factor* (IF). This protein is necessary for the absorption of dietary vitamin B_{12}, which is essential for red blood cell formation. Certain forms of the disease appear to be inherited, whereas other forms appear to be an autoimmune disorder. Persons with other autoimmune diseases are more likely to develop pernicious anemia.

Signs and Symptoms: The onset of symptoms is usually insidious but may eventually be manifested as fatigue, dyspnea, heart palpitations, sore tongue, and numbness and tingling of the extremities. Weakness, nausea, vomiting, **neuritis**, impaired coordination, altered vision, light-headedness, and tachycardia also may be present.

Diagnostic Procedures: A thorough patient history and physical examination are essential in the diagnosis of pernicious anemia. Laboratory studies may reveal decreased levels of hemoglobin and serum B_{12}. A Shilling test, specific for pernicious anemia, will confirm the diagnosis. Bone marrow aspiration and gastric analysis may be done.

Treatment: Parenteral administration of vitamin B_{12}, initially in high doses, is typically the first course of treatment. Then maintenance injections of vitamin B_{12} are necessary for life. Bed rest and transfusions may be necessary in extreme cases.

Prognosis: The damaged IF-secreting cells in the gastric mucosa will not regenerate, but if treated promptly and properly maintained, the person with pernicious anemia typically is able to lead a normal life.

Prevention: There is no known prevention.

Aplastic Anemia

Description: *Aplastic anemia* is characterized by insufficient or totally absent red blood cell production as a result of injury or destruction of the blood-forming tissue in the bone marrow. In over half the cases, aplastic anemia is idiopathic.

Etiology: Known causes include exposure to toxins such as chloramphenicol, cytotoxic agents, radiation, and the hepatitis virus.

Signs and Symptoms: Lassitude, pallor, **purpura**, bleeding, tachycardia, infections with high fever, dyspnea, headache, and congestive heart failure may be symptomatic of aplastic anemia. Pancytopenia, a decrease in all cellular components of the blood, may occur if the bone marrow is damaged to the point that healthy blood-forming tissues are replaced by fatty abnormal tissue.

Diagnostic Procedures: The RBC, WBC, and **reticulocyte** count will be low in the majority of cases. Bone marrow studies may show evidence of fatty tissue with **megakaryocytes**. The patient history may provide evidence of recent exposure to a toxin.

Treatment: Exposure to a known toxin must be discontinued. Bone marrow transplantation is the treatment of choice in young persons with severe aplastic anemia. Androgenic steroids or corticosteroids may be tried. Transfusions may be necessary.

Prognosis: The prognosis is poor for an individual with aplastic anemia. Death results in about 50 percent of cases. The remaining individuals may go into partial or complete remission or need to be treated with transfusions for years. Complications include infections, hemorrhage, or transfusion-related problems.

Prevention: Prevention includes avoidance of any chemcial or physical agents having the capacity to damage bone marrow.

Sickle-Cell Anemia

Description: *Sickle-cell anemia* is a hereditary, chronic anemia in which abnormal sickle- or crescent-shaped red blood cells are present. These abnormally shaped red blood cells tend to clump together within capillaries, impairing circulation, damaging blood vessels, and producing chronic organ damage. The incidence of sickle-cell anemia is highest among black individuals and those of Mediterranean ancestry.

Etiology: The condition is due to the presence of an abnormal form of **hemoglobin**, called *hemoglobin S,* within the red cells. The defective hemoglobin is synthesized as a result of inheriting homozygous hemoglobin S genes.

If the individual is heterozygous for the hemoglobin S gene, that individual is said to possess *sickle-cell trait*. This is a comparatively benign condition that typically produces no symptoms. However, the red blood cells of such individuals may sickle as a consequence of any condition that produces **hypoxia**. If two individuals with sickle-cell trait marry, their offspring have a 25 percent chance of inheriting sickle-cell anemia.

Signs and Symptoms: Signs and symptoms characteristic of sickle-cell anemia are episodic attacks of intense pain in the arms, legs, or abdomen. Recurrent bouts of fever, chronic fatigue, dyspnea, tachycardia, and pallor may be additional manifestations of the disease. Infections, stress, and extremes in temperature may trigger the painful crises.

Diagnostic Procedures: If parents are known carriers of the sickle-cell trait, the infant should be screened for the condition. A positive family history and a physical examination will confirm the diagnosis.

Treatment: Treatment of sickle-cell anemia is symptomatic and typically involves the prescription of analgesics and the maintenance of adequate hydration. Hospitalization may be required during attacks, and transfusions may be necessary.

Prognosis: The prognosis is highly variable. Sickle-cell anemia is a life-threatening disease. Many affected individuals die in childhood; however, because of improvements in the care of sickle-cell patients, some live into the middle years. Complications include leg ulcers, **cholelithiasis**, orthopedic disorders, cerebral hemorrhage, and shock.

Prevention: There is no prevention for sickle-cell anemia other than genetic counseling for those at risk.

LEUKEMIAS

Leukemias are progressive, malignant diseases of the blood-forming organs marked by the unrestrained growth of abnormal leukocytes and their percursors in the blood and bone marrow. Leukemia is classified according to the dominant abnormal cell type and the severity of the disease. Three types will be discussed: acute leukemia, chronic myelocytic leukemia, and chronic lymphatic leukemia.

Acute Leukemia

Description: *Acute leukemia* is a neoplasm characterized by the hyperproliferation of abnormal, immature white cell precursors called **blasts**. These abnormal cells accumulate in the blood, bone marrow, and body tissues. There are several forms of acute leukemia. The information that follows discusses the general characteristics of the disease.

Etiology: The cause of acute leukemia is unknown. Predisposing factors may include infection by certain viruses, abnormal exposure to radiation, and hereditary tendencies. Acute leukemia is more common in males, young children and those people living in industrialized and urban areas.

Signs and Symptoms: Symptoms may be sudden in onset. Initial symptoms may include weakness, malaise, bone and joint pain, and anorexia. These may be followed by pallor, fever, petechiae, and swollen lymph nodes. Unexplained bleeding and prolonged menses may also signal the onset of acute leukemia.

Diagnostic Procedures: Bone marrow aspiration and biopsy are necessary for diagnosis. Laboratory findings may include **thrombocytopenia** and **neutropenia**.

Treatment: A variety of chemotherapeutic agents are typically used in treating those with acute leukemias. Such treatments generally requires hospitalization. Bone marrow transplants may be used for some acute leukemias, especially in young persons during a period of remission who have a tissue-compatible sibling. Supportive care may include transfusion of whole blood or blood products and the use of antibiotics to prevent secondary infections.

Prognosis: The prognosis varies according to the form of acute leukemia and the age and general physical condition of the affected individual. If remission can be achieved, the individual typically has a life expectancy of 1 to 3 years, although longer survival periods occasionally occur.

Prevention: There is no known prevention.

Chronic Myelocytic Leukemia

Description: *Chronic myelocytic leukemia* (CML) is characterized by the proliferation of abnormal white cell precursors called *granulocytes* in the bone marrow. These abnormal granulocytes later enter the blood and invade other body tissues.

Etiology: Ninety percent of individuals with chronic myelocytic leukemia have what is termed the *Philadelphia chromosome,* an abnormality on chromosome 22. This abnormality is thought to be acquired rather than inherited. Factors that may cause this genetic abnormality include viruses, radiation, and carcinogenic chemicals. CML occurs more frequently in young and middle-age adults.

Signs and Symptoms: The symptoms occur in two phases. The first, an insidious chronic phase, lasts from 2 to 4 years and is followed by an acute phase, lasting 3 to 6 months. Symptoms include pallor, weakness, fever, purpura, skin nodules, sternal tenderness, headache, retinal hemorrhages, bleeding gums, nosebleeds, weight loss, and anorexia.

Diagnostic Procedures: Laboratory findings may reveal leukocytosis, neutropenia, and anemia. The Philadelphia chromosome can be detected through bone marrow or blood testing.

Treatment: Chemotherapy may be used to treat both the chronic and acute phases. Secondary infections must be treated immediately.

Prognosis: The disease is rapidly fatal after the onset of the acute phase.

Prevention: There is no known prevention.

Chronic Lymphocytic Leukemia

Description: *Chronic lymphocytic leukemia* (CLL) is characterized by the accumulation of immature, immunologically ineffective B-lymphocytes. These cells accumulate to enormous proportions in the lymphoid tissue, blood, and bone marrow. It is the most common form of leukemia in the United States, usually affecting people over the age of 50.

Etiology: The cause is unknown, but the disease is suspected to be genetic or immunologic in origin.

Signs and Symptoms: The onset is usually insidious. Symptoms eventually include pallor, weakness, lymph node enlargement, fatigue, fever, and weight loss. As the disease progresses, tachycardia, heart palpitations, and an increased incidence of infections are common.

Diagnostic Procedures: The disease often is found by accident during a routine physical examination. Laboratory findings indicating CLL include granulocytopenia, neutropenia, and anemia. The WBC often rises as the disease progresses. Bone marrow aspiration and biopsy confirm the diagnosis.

Treatment: Treatment may be withheld until the person manifests symptoms. When the person exhibits signs or symptoms or has anemia or thrombocytopenia, treatment with chemotherapy is usually initiated. Radiation therapy or corticosteroids may be tried, too. Complications such as anemia, hemorrhage, or secondary infections must be treated promptly.

Prognosis: With an asymptomatic leukemic person, the prognosis is good. If the person has anemia, the survival is less than 2 years. Various immunologic disorders may accompany CLL, worsening the prognosis.

Prevention: There is no known prevention.

LYMPHATIC DISEASES

Lymphedema

Description: *Lymphedema* is an abnormal accumulation of lymph, usually in the extremities.

Etiology: Lymphedema results from the inflammatory or mechanical obstruction of the lymph vessels or nodes (Figure 8–6). Such a condition may arise directly as a result of infections, neoplasms, allergic reactions, or thrombus formation. The condition also may arise secondary to surgery, trauma, burns, or radiation. Some forms of lymphedema are congenital. Young women seem more susceptible to developing lymphedema.

Signs and Symptoms: The affected limb, in part or whole, will typically be swollen and hypertrophied, with thickened and fibrotic skin. Lymphedema is usually painless, and it may be accompanied by episodes of lymphangitis and **cellulitis**. The edema may be either pitting or nonpitting.

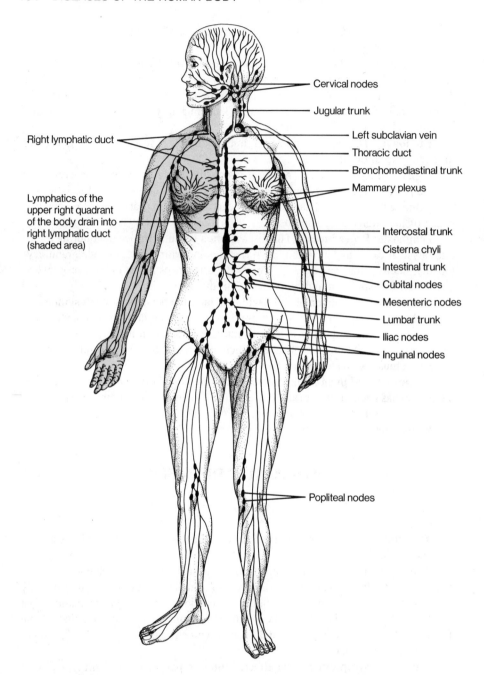

Figure 8–6. The lymphatic system. (From Gylys, B. A. and Wedding, M. E., *Medical Terminology: A Systems Approach,* ed. 2. F. A. Davis, Philadelphia, 1988, p. 181, with permission.)

Diagnostic Procedures: A thorough patient history and physical examination are necessary. Lymphangiography and radioactive isotope studies are helpful in detecting the site of lymphatic obstruction.

Treatment: Treatment is difficult but usually includes elevation of the affected part, especially at night, the use of special fitted elastic stockings put on prior to getting up and worn all day, and massaging the limb toward the trunk to "milk" the edema out of the extremity. **Diuretics** may be prescribed in some instances. Surgery to correct lymphatic obstruction and promote drainage is a last resort.

Prognosis: The prognosis for lymphedema is dependent on the cause. Infections worsen the prognosis.

Prevention: There is no known prevention.

Hodgkin's Disease

Description: *Hodgkin's disease* is a neoplastic malignancy of the lymphatic system characterized by painless enlargement of the lymph nodes, spleen, and other lymphatic tissues. It occurs more frequently in young and middle-aged adults.

Etiology: The exact cause of Hodgkin's disease is not known. There is even disagreement whether the disease is a true malignancy or an inflammatory immunologic disorder. Certain viruses are strongly suspected as etiologic agents.

Signs and Symptoms: The usual presenting symptom is enlarged, firm, nontender, painless regional lymph nodes. Fever, fatigue, weight loss, diaphoresis, and **pruritus** may follow. The disease is characterized by exacerbation and remission of symptoms.

Diagnostic Procedures: Laboratory findings may reveal **lymphocytopenia** and anemia. Definitive diagnosis is established by identifying the presence of Reed-Sternberg cells in lymphatic tissue. These are giant connective-tissue cells that usually possess two large nuclei. A lymph node biopsy, bone marrow biopsy, chest x-ray, lower extremity lymphangiogram, scintiscan of the liver and spleen, and liver function studies may be used to confirm the diagnosis. It is extremely important that the extent of the disease process be known and that it be staged prior to the initiation of therapy.

Treatment: Treatment is dependent on the stage of the disease, but radiation and/or chemotherapy generally is used.

Prognosis: The prognosis varies with the staging. In persons with Stage I and II disease, the prognosis is good if there are no manifestations for the first 5 years. About 50 percent of these persons have a 95 percent cure rate.[3]

Prevention: There is no known prevention.

Lymphosarcoma

Description: *Lymphosarcomas, or non-Hodgkin's lymphomas,* are a group of malignant diseases of the lymphatic system. They are categorized as follows:

(1) well-differentiated lymphatic, (2) poorly differentiated lymphocytic, (3) histio-cytic (formerly called *reticulum cell sarcoma*), (4) mixed lymphocytic and histio-cytic, and (5) undifferentiated or stem-cell malignant lymphoma.

Etiology: The cause is unknown, although viruses have been suggested as etiologic agents. Lymphosarcomas occur in all age groups but are more common in males.

Signs and Symptoms: Swollen lymph glands, especially enlarged tonsils and adenoids, are common presenting symptoms. Coughing, dyspnea, fatigue, sweat-ing, fever, and weight loss may follow.

Diagnostic Procedures: Diagnosis is by lymph node biopsy and/or bone marrow biopsy. Non-Hodgkin's lymphomas need to be distinguished from Hodgkin's disease.

Treatment: Treatment includes radiation therapy or chemotherapy. Staging is important prior to beginning any treatment. Refer to Chapter 2 for further informa-tion on staging.

Prognosis: The prognosis is good if the person is in remission; however, if a remission cannot be produced by treatment, the prognosis is poor.

Prevention: There is no known prevention.

COMMON SYMPTOMS OF CIRCULATORY SYSTEM DISEASES

Individuals with circulatory diseases may present with the following common complaints which deserve attention from health professionals:

- Fatigue
- Dyspnea
- Fever
- Weakness
- Tachycardia and heart palpitations
- Pallor
- Chest pain
- Unusual sweating, especially at night
- Edema
- Nausea, vomiting, or anorexia
- Anxiety
- Headache

REFERENCES

1. Huntington and Sheldon, *Boyd's Introduction to the Study of Disease,* Lea & Febiger, Philadelphia, 1984, p. 349.
2. Walters, J. B., *An Introduction to the Principles of Disease,* 2d Ed., W. B. Saunders Company, Philadelphia, 1982, p. 411.

3. Krupp, M. A., and M. J. Chatton (Eds.), *Current Medical Diagnosis and Treatment,* Lange Medical Publications, Los Altos, Calif., 1984, p. 331.

REVIEW QUESTIONS

Matching

Match the following infectious heart diseases with their definitions:

_____ 1. Inflammation of cardiac muscle   a. Endocarditis

_____ 2. Inflammation of the sac surrounding the
heart   b. Pericarditis

_____ 3. Inflammation of the heart valves and   c. Myocarditis
chambers

Match the following diseases with their correct definitions:

_____ 4. Heart suddenly ceases to pump   a. Thrombophlebitis

_____ 5. Local dilation of artery or chamber of heart   b. Cardiac arrest

_____ 6. Inflammation of vein with thrombus   c. Aneurysm
formation   d. Varicose veins

_____ 7. Dilated, tortuous veins   e. Aplastic anemia

     f. Lymphedema

True/False

T F 1. In pulmonic insufficiency, backflow of blood into the right ventricle causes ventricular hypertrophy.

T F 2. In aortic insufficiency, backflow of blood into the left ventricle causes ventricular hypertrophy.

T F 3. In tricuspid stenosis, backflow of blood into the right atrium causes atrial hypertrophy.

T F 4. In mitral stenosis, backflow of blood into the left atrium causes atrial hypertrophy.

Multiple Choice

1. Select all the high-risk individuals for hypertension:
a. Persons under great deal of stress
b. Persons who are black
c. Persons who are obese
d. Persons who eat food high in salt
e. Persons who lead sedentary lifestyles
f. Persons on oral contraceptives

Short Answers

1. Define the five types of anemias:
     a. Iron deficiency anemia:
     b. Folic acid deficiency anemia:
     c. Pernicious anemia:
     d. Aplastic anemia:
     e. Sickle-cell anemia:

2. Define the three types of leukemia:
   a. Acute leukemia:
   b. Chronic myelocytic leukemia:
   c. Chronic lymphocytic leukemia:
3. Define
   a. Atherosclerosis:
   b. Arteriosclerosis:
4. List the causes of heart murmurs:
   a.
   b.
   c.
   d.
5. Rheumatic fever, an inflammatory disease in children, generally follows _____ .
6. The classic symptom of myocardial infarction is _____ .
7. The medication taken sublingually or topically for angina pectoris is _____ .
8. Are lymphosarcoma and Hodgkin's disease similar? _____ Explain.

ANSWERS

Matching

1. c
2. b
3. a
4. b
5. c
6. a
7. d

True/False
1. T
2. T
3. T
4. T

Multiple Choice
1. All persons are high risk for hypertension.

Short Answers
1. a. Iron deficiency anemia: Inadequate supply of iron resulting in smaller blood cells.
   b. Folic acid deficiency anemia: Inadequate intake of folic acid, a nitrogenous acid found in some foods.
   c. Pernicious anemia: Failure of the gastric mucosa to secrete adequate intrinsic factor, resulting in malabsorption of vitamin B_{12}.
   d. Aplastic anemia: Absence of regeneration of red blood cells.
   e. Sickle-cell anemia: Genetically determined defect of hemoglobin synthesis occurring almost exclusively in Blacks.

2. a. Acute leukemia: A neoplasm of proliferating abnormal white cell blasts.
   b. Chronic myelocytic leukemia: Proliferation of abnormal white cells that invade the bone marrow, blood, and body tissue.
   c. Chronic lymphocytic leukemia: An abnormal accumulation of small lymphocytes that have lost the capacity to divide.
3. a. Atherosclerosis: A form of arteriosclerosis where the lumen of the coronary arteries is narrowed by fatty, fibrous plaques. Generally affects large and medium-sized arteries.
   b. Arteriosclerosis: Sclerosis and thickening of the walls of arterioles.
4. a. Blood leaking back through an incompetent or deformed valve.
   b. Blood forcing its way through a stenosed valve.
   c. Dilation of the heart.
   d. A rapid diastolic flow.
5. A streptococcal infection.
6. Crushing chest pain that may radiate to the left arm, neck, and jaw.
7. Nitrates, usualy nitroglycerin.
8. Yes and no. Lymphosarcoma is a non-Hodgkin's lymphoma. Both involve the lymph system, and signs and symptoms may be similar, as may the treatment; however, the prognoses differ.

GLOSSARY

ANALGESIC: A drug or agent that relieves pain.

ANEURYSM: An abnormal, saclike bulge in the wall of an artery, a vein, or the heart.

ANOREXIA: Loss of appetite for foods.

ARRHYTHMIA (CARDIAC): Any irregularity in the force of rhythm of heart action caused by disturbances in the discharge of cardiac impulses from the heart's sinoatrial node or their transmission through the heart's conductile tissue.

ASCITES: Abnormal accumulation of fluid in the peritoneal cavity.

BLAST: A precursor of the final, mature form of a cell.

BRADYCARDIA: Abnormally slow heartbeat, generally characterized by a pulse rate below 60 beats per minute.

BRUIT: An abnormal noise of venous or arterial origin heard during auscultation.

CARDIOGENIC SHOCK: Condition of acute circulatory failure caused by interruption of the heart's pumping action. Considered a medical emergency.

CELLULITIS: Inflammation of cellular or connective tissue.

CHOLELITHIASIS: The formation or presence of gallstones in the gallbladder or bile duct.

CHOREA: A nervous condition marked by involuntary muscular twitching of the limbs or facial muscles.

CLAUDICATION: Limping or lameness.

CYANOSIS: A bluish discoloration of the skin and mucous membranes due to an increased proportion of unoxygenated hemoglobin in the blood.

DIAPHORESIS: Sweating, especially when profuse or medically induced.

DIASTOLIC PRESSURE: The period of least pressure in the arterial blood vessels.

DILATATION: The expansion or enlargement of an organ or vessel.

DIURETIC: A drug or agent that promotes the secretion of urine.

DYSPNEA: Labored or difficult breathing, generally indicating an insufficient amount of oxygen in the blood.

EFFUSION: The seeping of fluid into a body cavity or part.

EMBOLUS: A clot or undissolved mass carried through the circulatory vessels by the blood or lymph flow. An embolus may be a blood clot, piece of tissue, fat globule, or air bubble. (Compare with *Thrombus.*)

FIBRILLATION (VENTRICULAR): A cardiac arrhythmia characterized by the rapid, incomplete, and uncoordinated contractions of the muscle fibers of ventricles of the heart. Can lead to cardiac arrest. (See *Arrhythmia.*)

GANGRENE: The death of masses of body tissue, followed by bacterial invasion and subsequent decay. Usually, but not exclusively, associated with the loss or interruption of blood supply to a tissue area.

HEMOGLOBIN: The oxygen-carrying pigment in red blood cells.

HEMOPTYSIS: The coughing and spitting up of blood due to bleeding in any portion of the respiratory tract.

HEPATOMEGALY: Enlargement of the liver.

HYPERTROPHY: An increase in size or volume of an organ or other body structure produced entirely by an increase in the size of existing cells, not by an increase in the number of cells.

HYPOXIA: Insufficient oxygenation of the blood.

INDURATION: An area of hardened tissue; the process of hardening.

ISCHEMIA: A temporary deficiency of blood in a body part due to a constriction or destruction of a blood vessel.

LYMPHOCYTOPENIA: The presence of abnormally small numbers of lymphocytes in the circulating blood.

LUMEN: The space within an artery, vein, intestine, or other tubular body structure.

MEGAKARYOCYTE: A large bone marrow cell with large or multiple nuclei. It gives rise to blood platelets.

MENORRHAGIA: Excessive bleeding at the time of the menstrual period.

MITRAL REGURGITATION: Backward flow of blood through the mitral valve of the heart.

NEPHROSCLEROSIS: Hardening of structures within the kidney, generally associated with hypertension or disease of the renal arterioles.

NEUTROPENIA: The presence of abnormally small numbers of neutrophils in the circulating blood.

NEURITIS: Inflammation of a nerve or nerves.

ORTHOPNEA: Respiratory condition in which there is discomfort in breathing in any but erect standing or sitting positions.

PARENTERAL: Taken into the body or administered by some route other than the digestive system, e.g., intravenous, subcutaneous, intramuscular, or mucosal.

PERCUTANEOUS TRANSLUMINAL CORONARY ANGIOPLASTY (PTCA): A method of treating localized arterial narrowing due to atherosclerosis. A balloon-tipped catheter is guided to the site of the narrowing and briefly inflated, resulting in dilation of the vessel.

PERICARDIOCENTESIS: Surgical puncture of the membranous sac surrounding the heart to draw out fluid.

PETECHIA: A small, reddish or purplish pinpoint spot on a body surface, such as the skin or mucous membranes, caused by a minute hemorrhage.

PITTING EDEMA: A form of tissue swelling beneath the skin which when pressed firmly with a finger will maintain the indentation produced by the finger for a few minutes.

PROLAPSE: A falling or dropping down of an organ or internal part.

PRURITUS: Severe itching.

PURPURA: A bleeding disorder with various manifestations and causes characterized by hemorrhages into the skin, mucous membranes, internal organs, and other tissues.

RALES: An abnormal respiratory sound heard on auscultation of the lungs, produced by the movement of air through secretion-filled or constricted bronchial passages.

RETICULOCYTE: An immature form of red blood cell, normally comprising about 1 percent of circulating red blood cells.

STENOSIS: An abnormal constriction or narrowing in an opening or passageway of the body.

STRIDOR: A harsh, high-pitched sound during respiration due to obstruction of air passages.

SYMPATHECTOMY: Surgical excision of a portion of a sympathetic nerve. The procedure causes dilation of the blood vessels affected by the interrupted nerve, resulting in improved blood supply to tissue supplied by those vessels.

SYNCOPE: A transient loss of consciousness due to inadequate blood flow to the brain.

SYSTOLIC PRESSURE: The period of maximum arterial blood pressure. (Compare with *Diastolic Pressure.*)

TACHYCARDIA: Abnormally rapid heart beat, generally defined as exceeding 100 beats per minute.

THROMBOCYTOPENIA: Abnormal decrease in the number of platelets in the circulating blood.

THROMBOENDARTERECTOMY: Surgical removal of a thrombus from an artery together with a portion of the inner lining of the artery.

THROMBUS: A blood clot formed along the wall of a blood vessel or in a cavity of the heart. It may be of sufficient size to obstruct blood flow, or all or a portion of it may break off becoming an embolus. (See *Embolus.*)

TINNITUS: A subjective, continuous ringing or buzzing sound in one or both ears.

VALVOTOMY: Surgical incision into a valve.

VASODILATOR: A drug or agent causing relaxation and expansion of the blood vessels.

VENTRICULAR SEPTAL RUPTURE: A breakage or tear in the septum between the left and right ventricles of the heart.

Nervous System Diseases

LEARNING OBJECTIVES

Upon successful completion of this chapter, you will
- Identify the three main divisions of the nervous system.
- Describe the basic unit of the nervous system and how it functions.
- List the causes for headache.
- Compare the prognoses for migraine and chronic headaches.
- Compare epidural to subdural hematomas.
- Contrast concussion to contusion.
- Recall four courses of treatment for spinal cord injuries.
- Distinguish the signs and symptoms of paraplegia and quadriplegia.
- Restate the noninjury cause of hemiplegia.
- Discuss the signs and symptoms of meningitis and encephalitis.
- Recall the prognosis for brain abscess.
- Identify at least three classifications of epilepsy.

■ Describe the disease process of peripheral neuritis.
■ Explain the characteristic symptoms of Bell's palsy.
■ Discuss cerebrovascular accident (CVA).
■ Review the causes and signs and symptoms for organic brain syndrome.
■ Recognize the signs and symptoms of Parkinson's disease.
■ Recall the etiology of multiple sclerosis.
■ Discuss appropriate treatment protocol for amyotrophic lateral sclerosis.
■ Describe the progression of brain tumors.
■ List at least four signs and symptoms characteristic of nervous system diseases.

INTRODUCTION

The body's nervous system is an elaborate, interlaced network of nerve cells of astonishing complexity and sophistication. This network is made up collectively of the brain, spinal cord, and nerves. The entire system functions to regulate and coordinate body activities and bring about responses by which the body adjusts to changes in its internal and external environment.

The nervous system is divided into two divisions. The *central nervous system* (CNS) includes the brain and spinal cord. The CNS processes and stores sensory information and includes the parts of the brain governing consciousness. The CNS interacts with the second division of the nervous system, the *peripheral nervous system* (PNS). The PNS is composed of all other nervous tissue outside the CNS and includes 12 pairs of cranial nerves, 31 pairs of spinal nerves, all sensory nerves, and the sympathetic and parasympathetic nerves. The sympathetic and parasympathetic nerves comprise the *autonomic nervous system* (ANS), which regulates involuntary muscle movements and the action of glands. Figure 9–1 illustrates the major subdivisions of the nervous system. Figure 9–2 illustrates the major sections of the brain.

The basic functional and structural unit of the nervous system is the *neuron,* a cell specialized to initiate or conduct electrochemical impulses. A neuron receives impulses through its rootlike system of dendrites. Impulses pass along one or more dendrites, through the cell body of the neuron, and out a long stalklike extension of the cell called an *axon.* Figure 9–3 illustrates the dendrites, cell body, and axon of sensory and motor neurons.

HEADACHE

Description: A *headache* is any diffuse pain occurring in different portions of the head. The condition may be acute or chronic. Headache is one of the most common maladies afflicting humans. In most cases, headache signals nothing more serious than fatigue or tension. Less frequently, but more important, headache may

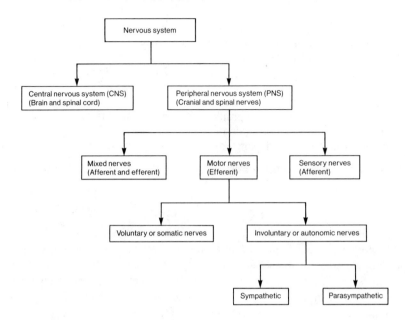

FIGURE 9–1. Subdivisions of the nervous system. (From Gylys, B. A. and Wedding, M. E., *Medical Terminology: A Systems Approach,* ed. 2. F. A. Davis, Philadelphia, 1988, p. 327, with permission.)

be the manifestation of an underlying disorder. For this reason, an individual's complaint of headache should not be minimized or unthinkingly treated with **analgesics** before the underlying cause has been determined.

Etiology: Headache is caused by irritation of one or more of the pain-sensitive structures or tissues in the head and neck. These structures include the cranial arteries and veins, the cranial and spinal nerves, the cranial and cervical muscles, and the **meninges.** (Curiously enough, most of the tissue of the brain itself is insensitive to pain.) Almost any disturbance of body function can lead to irritation of these structures and occasion a headache. Causes of headache can be grouped into organic, psychoneurologic, and environmental categories. Table 9–1 summarizes possible causes of acute and chronic headaches for each of these categories.

Signs and Symptoms: The character of headache pain varies markedly from individual to individual. It may be a dull, aching pain or an acute, almost unbearable pain. The pain may be intermittent and intense or throbbing. The pain may focus in the front, sides, or back of the head, or it may be confined to one side of the head or to a region over one or both eyes.

Diagnostic Procedures: If a medical history reveals a pattern of recurrent or unusually severe headaches, further medical testing is typically undertaken to try to detect an underlying cause. This may include a thorough physical examination and

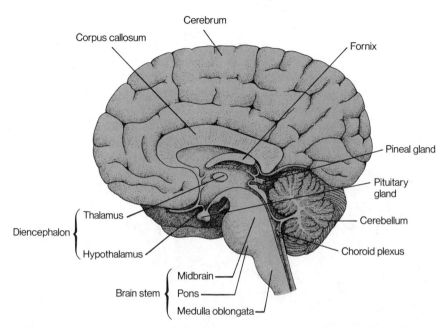

FIGURE 9–2. Sections of the brain. (From Gylys, B. A. and Wedding, M. E.: *Medical Terminology: A Systems Approach,* ed. 2. F. A. Davis, Philadelphia, 1988, p. 331, with permission.)

neurologic testing. Diagnostic tests may include cranial CT scans, electroencephalogram (EEG), x-rays of the skull and spine, and lumbar puncture to detect abnormalities in the **cerebrospinal fluid** (CSF).

Treatment: The course of treatment chosen is entirely determined by the cause of the headache. Analgesics are generally effective in providing temporary, symptomatic relief of headache pain. Ultimately, though, any underlying cause must be treated as well.

Prognosis: The prognosis for most acute headaches is good. The prognosis for chronic headaches is more variable and is usually determined by the nature and severity of the underlying cause.

Prevention: Prevention of acute and chronic headaches is dependent on the cause.

MIGRAINE HEADACHE

Description: A *migraine headache* is a recurrent, frequently incapacitating type of headache characterized by intense, throbbing pain often accompanied by

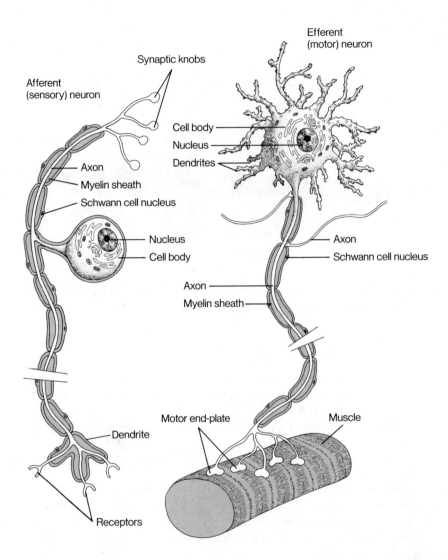

FIGURE 9–3. Illustration of sensory and motor neurons. Note dendrites, cell body, and axon of both forms of neurons. (From Gylys, B. A. and Wedding, M. E., *Medical Terminology: A Systems Approach,* ed. 2. F. A. Davis, Philadelphia, 1988, p. 329, with permission.)

TABLE 9–1 Etiologies of Acute and Chronic Headaches*

Organic:	Toxins: Drugs, alcohol, tobacco, poisonous gases, nitrites in foods, toxins produced by local or systemic bacterial infections
	Systemic diseases: Nephritis, diabetes mellitus, arthritis, blood diseases
	Gastrointestinal disturbances: Gastric hyper- or hypoacidity, constipation
	Cardiovascular diseases: Congestive heart failure
	Endocrine diseases: Tumors of the adrenal, pituitary, thyroid glands; ovarian tumors.
	Gynecologic disturbances: Menstruation, pregnancy, menopause, dysmenorrhea
	Respiratory disturbances: Infection or blockage in paranasal sinuses, adenoidal infection, deviated nasal septum
	Organic brain disease: Brain tumor, abscess, cyst, hydrocephalus, intracranial hemorrhage, embolus, thrombus, meningitis, encephalitis
	Sensory organ diseases: Glaucoma, conjunctivitis, iritis, otitis media.
Psychoneurologic:	Nervous tension or exhaustion Fatigue Worry Excitement Psychoneuroses
Environmental insults:	Head trauma Bright lights Noise Rapid altitude change Rapid temperature change Irritants: Smoke, dust, pollen Sunstroke Motion sickness

*Adapted from Thomas, C. L. (ed.): *Taber's Cyclopedic Medical Dictionary*, ed. 15. F. A. Davis, Philadelphia, 1985.

nausea and vomiting. Migraine headaches usually begin in adolescence or early adulthood and diminish slowly in frequency and intensity with advancing age. Women are affected more than twice as frequently as men.

Etiology: Migraine headaches are occasioned by changes in the cerebral blood flow, presumably due to vasoconstriction and subsequent vasodilation of cerebral-cranial arterioles. What initiates this process, however, is not known. Susceptibility to migraine headaches may be hereditary.

Signs and Symptoms: Prior to the onset of pain, many migraine sufferers report symptoms such as flashing lights before their eyes, photophobia, or tinnitus. Other symptoms occurring before the migraine attack (called *premonitory symptoms*) may include unusual thirst, craving for sweet foods, and alterations in mood or mental clarity. Once the pain of the attack begins, it is typically accompanied by nausea, vomiting, and photophobia.

Diagnostic Procedures: A patient history revealing a recurrent pattern of severe headaches preceded by any of the classic premonitory symptoms noted previously suggests the diagnosis of migraine headache.

Treatment: Drug therapy may include the use of ergot preparations, which have proven effective in some cases in forestalling an impending attack or in lessening the severity of an ongoing attack. Simple analgesics, however, may be all that are necessary. In some cases, no treatment is chosen other than bed rest in a quiet, darkened room for the duration of the attack. More recently, biofeedback and relaxation exercises have been used successfully in some cases to lessen the number of attacks.

Prognosis: The prognosis varies. No form of therapy has proved successful in permanently disrupting the cycle of migraine attacks. As noted earlier, migraine headaches tend to become less frequent and less severe with age.

Prevention: There is no specific prevention of migraine headaches.

HEAD TRAUMA

Head trauma usually results from an accident, a blow to the head, or a serious fall. Recovery may be rapid or extended, depending on the severity of the trauma. It is important to watch an individual who has suffered head trauma for any signs of dizziness, nausea, severe headache, and loss of consciousness. Forms of head trauma considered here are hematomas, concussions, and contusions.

Epidural and Subdural Hematoma (Acute)

Description: An *epidural hematoma* is a mass of blood (usually clotted) formed between the skull and the outer membrane covering the brain, the *dura mater.* In a *subdural hematoma,* the blood collects between the dura mater and the second membrane covering the brain, the *arachnoid membrane.* In both cases, pressure from the mass of blood can be sufficient to impair brain function.

Etiology: Both epidural and subdural hematomas are caused by blood seeping from ruptured vessels above or below the dural membrane. The blood vessel damage occasioning an epidural hematoma is usually the result of a blow to the head, whereas a subdural hematoma is more often caused by the head striking an immovable object. Skull fractures are almost always accompanied by cerebral hematomas.

Signs and Symptoms: The symptoms of epidural hematoma typically include an initial loss of consciousness followed by an intervening period of consciousness that may last from a few minutes to several hours. As the condition worsens, there may be **hemiparesis**, severe headache, and dilated pupils. These symptoms may occur within a short period of time or over a period of days, depending on the rate that blood accumulates. Subdural hematomas generally exhibit similar symptoms but with a delayed onset because the blood typically accumulates more slowly. Loss of consciousness will occur, however, as well as weakness on one or both sides of the body. Nausea, vomiting, dizziness, and convulsions also may occur.

Diagnostic Procedures: The individual's clinical picture and a medical history revealing head trauma should suggest a potential diagnosis of epidural or subdural hematoma. Skull x-rays or CT scans and cerebral angiography may be ordered to pinpoint the position of the hematoma.

Treatment: It may be necessary to perform a **craniotomy** to aspirate the accumulated blood and control further bleeding. Surgery may be performed on an emergency basis if rising intracranial pressure proves life-threatening.

Prognosis: The prognosis for both epidural and subdural hematomas is always guarded. Barring any complications, a person can recover with few, if any, residual effects. Irreversible brain damage, however, may result in serious cases.

Prevention: The best prevention is to minimize the risk of head trauma.

Cerebral Concussion

Description: A *cerebral concussion* is an immediate loss of consciousness, typically lasting from a few seconds to a few minutes, followed by a short period of amnesia. The reaction of a boxer who has just been "knocked out" is a classic example of cerebral concussion.

Etiology: This condition is usually caused by a blunt impact to the head of sufficient force to cause the brain to strike and rebound from the skull. The loss of consciousness, subsequent amnesia, and other bodily symptoms of cerebral concussion are due to disruption of normal electrical activity in the brain. The brain tissue itself is usually not injured.

Signs and Symptoms: Primary symptoms are temporary loss of consciousness with shallow respirations, depressed pulse rate, and flaccid muscle tone. After regaining consciousness, there is usually a variable period of amnesia that may be accompanied by **bradycardia**, faintness, pallor, **hypotension**, and photophobia. Delayed symptoms may include headache, nausea, vomiting, and blurred vision.

Diagnostic Procedures: A careful neurologic assessment will typically be performed. Cranial CT scans will usually reveal no evidence of brain tissue damage (compare with Cerebral Contusion).

Treatment: Treatment usually involves nothing more than quiet bed rest. The affected individual should be closely watched for any behavioral changes that may indicate progressive brain injury.

Prognosis: If the individual remains alert with only one or two symptoms such as headache, nausea, a brief episode of vomiting, impaired concentration, or slightly blurred vision, the prognosis is usually good, with a low risk of subsequent complications. Brain edema is a life-threatening complication most often seen in child and adolescent concussion victims.

Prevention: Prevention of concussions includes following safety measures that minimize the risk of head injury, such as the use of approved head protection when playing sports and the use of seat belts while driving.

Cerebral Contusion

Description: A *cerebral contusion* is a serious injury which involves bruising the tissue along or just beneath the surface of the brain. Blood from broken vessels usually accumulates in the surrounding brain tissue.

Etiology: Cerebral contusions are produced by a blow to the head or the impact of the head against a surface that causes the hemispheres of the brain to twist against or slide along the inner surface of the skull. The twisting or shearing force may be sufficient to damage deep structures in the brain as well.

Signs and Symptoms: The signs and symptoms of cerebral contusions vary according to the location and extent of the tissue injury to the brain. Symptoms may range from transient loss of consciousness to coma. When conscious, an individual may exhibit hemiparesis, severe headache, and a variety of behavioral disturbances such as lethargy, apathy, and drowsiness on the one hand or hostility and combativeness on the other.

Diagnostic Procedures: A thorough neurologic assessment is required. Cranial CT scans will typically reveal the location and extent of tissue damage produced by a cerebral contusion.

Treatment: The treatment required varies according to the location and severity of the contusion. Contusion victims need to be hospitalized so that their vital signs can be monitored and rapid medical intervention can take place should it be required.

Prognosis: The prognosis for cerebral contusion is always guarded, ultimately depending on the extent of the brain injury. Sudden, progressive edema of the brain with a consequent escalation of intracranial pressure is a serious, life-threatening complication of cerebral contusion. Other complications include cerebral hemorrhage and epidural or subdural hematoma. Permanent neurologic deficits may result from contusions, including epilepsy caused by scar tissue formation at the site of the contusion.

Prevention: See preventive measures for cerebral concussion.

HEMIPLEGIA

Description: *Hemiplegia* is the loss of voluntary muscular control and sensation on one side of the body only.

Etiology: Hemiplegia is most frequently caused by disease processes such as cerebrovascular accident (CVA) that disrupt the blood supply to the brain and brain stem. The condition also may result from cerebral contusion and epidural or subdural hematoma resulting from head trauma. Damage to the right side of the brain causes left-sided paralysis, and vice versa.

Signs and Symptoms: Symptoms of hemiplegia include paralysis or weakness of the arm, leg, and (usually) face on one side of the body. The condition often is accompanied by communication disorders such as **aphasia**, **agnosia**, **apraxia**, **agraphia**, and **alexia**. The onset of these symptoms may be sudden, as in the case of CVA, or may occur more gradually, as in the case of a tumor.

Diagnostic Procedures: A thorough neurologic assessment is necessary. Cranial CT scans, complete blood analysis, and EEG may be performed as well.

Treatment: Treatment is directed at the cause of the hemiplegia. Otherwise, treatment measures are largely supportive. Physical rehabilitation should begin as soon as possible.

Prognosis: The extent of neurologic damage determines, in part, the prognosis. Physical rehabilitation, always an arduous process, is the hemiplegic's best hope for recovering lost motor and sensory function.

Prevention: There are no specific preventive measures for hemiplegia.

SPINAL CORD INJURIES: PARAPLEGIA AND QUADRIPLEGIA

Description: Spinal cord injuries often are characterized by the degree of motor and sensory disability they occasion. *Paraplegia* is the loss of voluntary motion or sensation (paralysis) of the trunk and lower extremities. *Quadriplegia* is paralysis of all four extremities and, usually, the trunk.

Etiology: In general, spinal cord injury resulting in paraplegia or quadriplegia is a consequence of fracture, dislocation, or both, of the vertebral column. The location of the spinal cord injury, the type of trauma inflicted on the cord, and the severity of that trauma determines whether paraplegia or quadriplegia may result. Refer to Figure 9–4 while reading the remaining discussion for a better understanding of the location of spinal cord injuries resulting in paraplegia or quadriplegia.

Spinal cord injury resulting in paraplegia is usually due to trauma to the thoracic and lumbar portions of the vertebral column (T1 or lower). Trauma that produces vertical compression and twisting (flexion) of this portion of the spinal cord is the usual mechanism of injury.

Spinal cord trauma at or above C5 on the cervical portion of the vertebral column may result in quadriplegia. Injuries between C5 and C7 may result in varying degrees of motor and sensory weakness to the arms and shoulders. Injuries above C3 usually result in death. Trauma that produces stretching (hyperextension) or flexion of this portion of the spinal cord is the usual mechanism of injury.

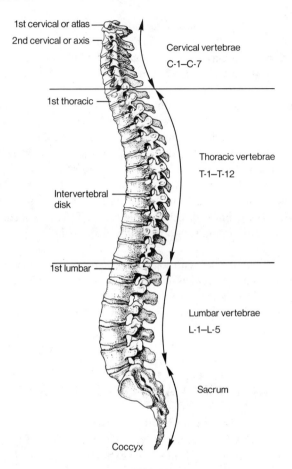

1st cervical or atlas

2nd cervical or axis

Cervical vertebrae
C-1–C-7

1st thoracic

Thoracic vertebrae
T-1–T-12

Intervertebral
disk

1st lumbar

Lumbar vertebrae
L-1–L-5

Sacrum

Coccyx

FIGURE 9–4. The vertebrae. Injuries of the thoracic and lumbar portions of the spine may cause paraplegia; injuries of the cervical vertebrae may cause quadriplegia. (Modified from Gylys, B. A. and Wedding, M. E., *Medical Terminology: A Systems Approach,* ed. 2. F. A. Davis, Philadelphia, 1988, p. 205, with permission.)

Signs and Symptoms: Loss of motor and sensory functions in the legs and trunk are the symptoms of paraplegia. Bowel, bladder, and sexual function also may be lost.

The symptoms of quadriplegia are those of paraplegia and total or partial loss of motor and sensory functions in the upper limbs and trunk. These symptoms also may be accompanied by falling blood pressure and body temperature, bradycardia, and respiratory difficulties. In some cases, unassisted respiration may cease.

Diagnostic Procedures: A thorough neurologic assessment is necessary. Spinal x-rays, spinal CT scans, and magnetic resonance imaging (MRI) will typically be performed to gauge the nature of the spinal cord injury, as well as to detect possible spinal ischemia, edema, and blockage of the flow of cerebrospinal fluid.

Treatment: The treatment goals for all spinal cord injuries include (1) restoration of normal alignment of the spine, (2) early insurance of complete stability of the injured spinal area, (3) decompression of compressed neurologic structures, and (4) early rehabilitation to an active, productive life.[1] Much of the early treatment effort is directed at preventing progressive spinal cord tissue damage that may occur following the initial trauma. This may involve surgery, the use of specialized drugs, or cooling the affected portion of the spine.

Prognosis: The prognosis for individuals with spinal cord injuries is always guarded. It may take several months to adequately assess the extent of the paralysis. If the damage to the spinal cord is complete, there is little hope of regaining lost motor and sensory functions. In general, though, the sooner treatment procedures are begun following an incident of spinal cord trauma, the better is the prognosis.

Prevention: Preventing paraplegia and quadriplegia involves following safety measures that minimize the risk of spinal cord injury. Such measures include wearing seat belts while driving, checking the water depth before diving into any body of water, and wearing protective gear when participating in contact sports.

INFECTIONS OF THE CENTRAL NERVOUS SYSTEM

Infections of the CNS can be caused by almost any bacterial or viral agent. Certain symptoms of CNS infections are fairly common. These include headache, fever, sensory disturbances, neck and back stiffness, positive **Kernig** and **Brudzinski** signs, and CSF abnormalities. Such infections usually constitute a medical emergency, and immediate steps must be taken to diagnose and treat the condition.

Acute Bacterial Meningitis

Description: *Acute bacterial meningitis* is inflammation of the three-layer membrane called the *meninges* that surrounds the brain and spinal cord. This disease is considered a medical emergency.

Etiology: The principal bacterial agents causing this disease are *Hemophilus influenzae* type B, *Neisseria meningitidis,* and *Streptococcus pneumoniae.* Many other bacteria also may cause the condition. The disease often arises as a complication of other bacterial infections elsewhere in the body, such as pneumonia, osteomyelitis, endocarditis, and otitis media. The disease also may follow in the wake of head trauma.

Signs and Symptoms: In addition to the common signs noted above, acute bacterial meningitis is usually marked by the sudden onset of severe headache, vomiting, and seizures. **Nuchal rigidity**, particularly upon bending the neck forward, is a classic sign of acute bacterial meningitis. Initial drowsiness may progress to **stupor** or **coma**.

Diagnostic Procedures: A thorough medical history and physical examination are essential. The diagnosis is usually established by performing a lumbar puncture to confirm elevated cerebrospinal fluid pressure and to analyze the CSF for the presence of bacteria and elevated levels of proteins and leukocytes. Blood, urine, and throat cultures also may be useful in isolating the infectious agent. Chest, skull, and sinus x-rays and an EEG may be ordered.

Treatment: An aggressive, sustained course of antibiotic therapy is usually begun as soon as possible. Supportive therapy includes measures to lessen brain swelling and prevent blockage of movement of cerebrospinal fluid. Isolation may be required. The patient should maintain good nutrition and adequate fluid intake.

Prognosis: Acute bacterial meningitis can prove fatal, especially among infants and the elderly. The prognosis is good, however, in the event of prompt diagnosis and effective treatment. Meningitis can cause lasting neurologic damage in children, particularly hearing loss, retardation, and epilepsy.

Prevention: There is no known prevention, but careful handling of excretions and proper handwashing techniques help prevent the spread of the disease.

Encephalitis

Description: *Encephalitis* is inflammation of the brain, especially of the cerebral hemisphere, cerebellum, and brain stem. The disease sometimes occurs in epidemic outbreaks.

Etiology: The disease can be caused by any one of a group of four arboviruses (arthropod-borne viruses). As their name implies, these viruses are often spread by insects, principally mosquitoes. Less frequently, encephalitis arises following measles, varicella, rubella, herpesvirus infection, and complications of vaccination.

Signs and Symptoms: Symptoms of encephalitis vary with age. The disease is frequently manifested in infants by the sudden onset of fever and convulsions. Children may experience headache, fever, and drowsiness followed by nausea, vomiting, muscular pain, and stiff neck. Adults typically experience an abrupt onset of fever, nausea, and vomiting, accompanied by a severe headache. Varying degrees of mental confusion and disorientation are a hallmark of encephalitis in adults. Other symptoms may include diffuse muscle aching and photophobia.

Diagnostic Procedures: A careful medical history is necessary. Lumbar puncture and analysis of the cerebrospinal fluid is the most important diagnostic tool. Detection of a virus or its antibody in the CSF or blood serum will confirm the diagnosis. The fluid also may show evidence of increased leukocyte counts and high protein levels. EEGs, cranial CT scans, or MRI may prove useful in isolating a focal point of the infection.

Treatment: Treatment is mostly supportive. Drug therapy may be employed to control convulsions and reduce inflammation and edema. It is important for the patient to receive adequate rest, nutrition, and fluid intake.

Prognosis: The prognosis varies according to the infecting species of virus, but it is generally guarded. Certain forms of the disease have high mortality rates. Severe bouts of the disease can leave survivors with lasting neurologic impairments.

Prevention: Control of insects known to be arbovirus carriers is the major form of prevention of encephalitis.

Brain Abscess

Description: *Brain abscess* is a collection of pus, usually found in the cerebellum or the frontal or temporal lobes of the cerebrum. The pus accumulation may be free or encapsulated, vary in size, and may occur at single or multiple sites.

Etiology: Generally, a brain abscess is secondary to some other infection, such as otitis media, sinusitis, or mastoiditis. Other causes include **bacteremia**, pulmonary infections, cranial trauma, or congenital heart disease.

Signs and Symptoms: Signs and symptoms may include headache (which is usually worse in the morning), nausea, vomiting, disturbances in vision, hemiplegia, slowed pulse and respiration, fever, pallor, and drowsiness.

Diagnostic Procedures: A patient history revealing a recent or ongoing infection in the sinuses, ears, or respiratory tract and the clinical symptoms mentioned should suggest a diagnosis of brain abscess. Skull x-rays, EEG, cranial CT scans, and cerebral angiography may help to localize the site of the infection. Lumbar puncture may confirm increased intracranial pressure.

Treatment: Elimination of the abscess is the goal of treatment. **Antibiotics** are used in the treatment of the underlying infections. The pus needs to be drained, but surgery will not be attempted unless the pus is encapsulated.

Prognosis: A brain abscess is usually fatal if untreated. With treatment, the prognosis is guarded owing to potential brain tissue damage.

Prevention: The only known prevention is prompt treatment of any infections.

EPILEPSY

Description: *Epilepsy* is a chronic brain disorder characterized by recurring attacks of abnormal sensory, motor, and psychological activity. During these attacks, the individual may or may not lose consciousness. Each attack or epileptic episode is called a *seizure*. Not all seizures are epilepsy, though. Only a chronic pattern of seizures that exhibit similar characteristics with each recurrence is epilepsy. Epilepsy represents a disruption of the normal pattern of electrical activity within the brain. During an epileptic seizure, neurons within the brain discharge in a random, intense manner. This hyperactivity may be focused within a small section of the brain or involve several areas of the brain at once. Epilepsy can begin at any time of life.

The International Classification of Epileptic Seizures categorizes seizures as partial, generalized, or unclassified. *Partial* seizures are focal in origin; that is, they affect only one part of the brain. *Generalized* seizures are nonfocal in origin and may affect the entire brain. *Unclassified* seizures are identified thus because of insufficient information about the nature of these seizures.[2]

Etiology: Most cases of epilepsy are idiopathic. Epilepsies may follow birth trauma, congenital malformations of the brain, head trauma, CVA, CNS infections such as meningitis and encephalitis, or neoplasms. Other causes may include brain tissue damage produced by chemicals, drugs, and toxins or degenerative brain disorders and structure defects of the brain.

Signs and Symptoms: Individuals may experience a warning or "aura" of the impending seizure or no warning at all. Symptoms of the seizure may be a simple uncontrollable twitch of the finger, hand, or mouth. The person may be dizzy and experience unusual or unpleasant sights, sounds, or odors, all without losing consciousness. Some individuals experience sudden loss of consciousness and intense rigidity of the body, with alternating relaxation and contraction of muscles. A characteristic cry may be uttered. Cyanosis, inhibited respiration, incontinence, and chewing of the tongue may occur. After the seizure has passed, amnesia, headache, and drowsiness are common occurrences. Some may sleep for hours following a seizure; others may not return to normal for days.

Diagnostic Procedures: A thorough medical history is essential. Recurrent seizures or a family history of epilepsy should suggest the diagnosis. Epilepsy is also indicated in the presence of seizures following head trauma, CNS infections, or CVA. Because many individuals with epilepsy exhibit abnormalities in brain-wave patterns, even between seizures, EEGs are very helpful in diagnosis. Cranial CT scans also are useful in pinpointing brain lesions that may be triggering seizures.

Treatment: An array of anticonvulsant drugs exists that have proved effective in controlling epileptic seizures. Because certain drugs are more effective in controlling specific forms of seizures, the patient and the physician may have to engage in a process of trial and error before settling on one drug that best controls the individual's seizures with the fewest side effects. Neurosurgery may be attempted in some cases when a severe case of epilepsy can be traced to the presence of a specific, accessible brain lesion. Educating and counseling the person with epilepsy about the nature of the disease are an essential part of the treatment process.

Prognosis: The prognosis varies from case to case. The prognosis is good if a course of drug therapy can be found that effectively suppresses the seizures. An individual in these circumstances can generally expect to live a normal life. The prognosis is not so favorable if seizures cannot be controlled. Such individuals may have to lead a comparatively restricted existence.

Prevention: Only certain forms of epilepsy are preventable. Preventive measures involve avoiding head injuries, prompt treatment of brain infections, and avoiding the abuse of drugs and alcohol.

PERIPHERAL NERVE DISEASES

Peripheral Neuritis

Description: *Peripheral neuritis* is a degeneration of the nerves supplying the muscles of the extremities. The syndrome is noninflammatory, more frequently affecting men between 30 and 50 years of age.

Etiology: Causes include chronic alcohol intoxication or toxicity from poisons, drugs, or heavy metals. Infections such as meningitis, pneumonia, and tuberculosis may induce peripheral neuritis, as may metabolic disorders such as gout, diabetes mellitus, and lupus erythematosus. Additional causes include nutritional deficiencies and tumors.

Signs and Symptoms: The onset is slow in most cases and may be marked by progressive muscular weakness, paresthesia, tenderness and pain, usually in the distal portions of the extremities. Physical wasting, loss of reflexes, and clumsiness may result.

Diagnostic Procedures: A thorough history and physical examination to determine motor and sensory deficits are necessary. Electromyography may be ordered.

Treatment: The treatment is dependent on the cause. Toxins must be neutralized, infections and metabolic diseases treated, and nutritional deficiencies corrected. Analgesics and bed rest, especially of the affected limb, are essential. Physical therapy may be required to recover function of the affected limb or limbs.

Prognosis: The prognosis depends on how successfully the underlying cause can be treated and the extent of existing nerve damage.

Prevention: Prevention includes prompt treatment of nutritional deficiencies, infections, and metabolic diseases. Avoidance of toxins is essential for prevention, too.

Bell's Palsy

Description: *Bell's palsy* is a disease of the facial nerve (the seventh cranial nerve) causing paralysis of the muscles on one side of the face. It is more common in persons between 20 and 50 years of age.

Etiology: Bell's palsy is idiopathic, although possible causes may be vascular ischemia, autoimmune disease, or viral disease.

Signs and Symptoms: Symptoms include facial weakness and characteristic drooping mouth. The sense of taste may be disrupted. Pain in the jaw or behind the ear may precede or accompany the paralysis. *Bell's phenomenon* is a symptom of the disease resulting when the eye cannot close completely. When the patient attempts to close the eye, it rolls upward and may tear excessively.

Diagnostic Procedures: The clinical picture of the sudden, unexplained onset of facial paralysis suggests the diagnosis.

Treatment: The affected portion of the face, particularly the eye, must be protected from trauma, wind, or temperature extremes. Electrical stimulation, massage, and heat may be prescribed. Corticosteroid drugs may be prescribed in some instances.

Prognosis: The prognosis is good in the majority of cases. In most patients, the palsy disappears spontaneously within 1 to 8 weeks. If the palsy remains, facial **contractures** may develop.

Prevention: There is no known prevention for Bell's palsy.

CEREBROVASCULAR ACCIDENT (STROKE)

Description: *Cerebrovascular accident* (CVA) is a clinical syndrome marked by the sudden impairment of consciousness and subsequent paralysis due to occlusion or hemorrhaging of blood vessels supplying a portion of the brain. Deprived of adequate blood supply, the tissue in the affected portion of the brain becomes necrotic. The condition is commonly known as a *stroke*.

Etiology: Three mechanisms may produce a stroke. These include cerebral hemorrhage and **thrombosis** or **embolism** of cerebral arteries. These processes are chiefly a consequence of atherosclerotic disease. They also may result from a variety of blood disorders, hypertension, cardiac **arrhythmias**, systemic diseases such as diabetes mellitus or syphilis, head trauma, cerebral aneurysms, or rheumatic heart disease. Contributing factors include smoking, lack of exercise, poor diet, a family history of atherosclerotic disease, or the use of oral contraceptives.

Signs and Symptoms: The signs and symptoms of CVA reflect the portion of the brain involved in the attack and whether the attack is caused by a thrombus, an embolus, or a hemorrhage. The symptoms of strokes caused by an embolus or a hemorrhage are often sudden in onset, whereas those caused by a thrombus may appear more gradually. Common symptoms include impaired consciousness ranging from stupor to coma, **Cheyne-Stokes respiration**, full and slow pulse, and hemiparesis. Other symptoms include **dysphasia**, numbness, sensory disturbances, **diplopia**, poor coordination, confusion, and dizziness.

Diagnostic Procedures: Lumbar puncture and analysis of CSF, cerebral angiography, and EEGs are useful in confirming the diagnosis. Cranial CT scans and MRI often prove useful in pinpointing the affected portion of the brain and in determining the mechanism that produced the stroke.

Treatment: Treatment of CVA depends on the severity of the event and whether it was hemorrhagic, thrombotic, or embolic in origin. General treatment protocols may include drug therapy (anticoagulant or antiplatelet agents) or surgery to improve cerebral circulation or to remove clots. Other therapeutic procedures may include measures to guard against or to control brain edema. Physical rehabilitation is necessary for most stroke patients and needs to be started early and continued until patients are able to do as much for themselves as possible.

Prognosis: The prognosis for an individual experiencing a CVA is determined by the extent of damage to the affected portion of the brain. In general, the greater the delay in recovery following the event, the poorer is the ultimate prognosis.

Prevention: Prevention includes prompt treatment of cardiac and circulatory problems and avoidance of predisposing factors such as smoking and lack of exercise.

TRANSIENT ISCHEMIC ATTACKS

Description: *Transient ischemic attacks* (TIAs) are temporary, often recurrent episodes of impaired neurologic activity resulting from insufficient blood flow to a part of the brain. These "little strokes" may last for seconds or hours, after which the symptoms gradually subside. TIAs share a common pathophysiology with strokes and may serve as a warning of an impending CVA.

Etiology: TIAs are caused by the temporary obstruction of cerebral arterioles by very small emboli or by ischemia of a small portion of brain tissue due to arterial narrowing in that region. These processes are usually the result of atherosclerotic disease. See Cerebrovascular Accident (Stroke) for other potential causes and risk factors.

Signs and Symptoms: The particular combination of symptoms during a TIA, like those for a CVA, depend on which portion of the brain is affected. Symptoms may include the sudden onset of muscle weakness in the arm, leg, or foot on one side of the body. Other symptoms may include transient blindness in one eye, speech difficulties, dizziness, and mild impairment of consciousness. TIAs generally do not result in unconsciousness.

Diagnostic Procedures: EEGs, cranial CT scans, and cranial MRIs are helpful in isolating the area of ischemia within the brain.

Treatment: The course of treatment selected depends on the location of the area of ischemia and the underlying cause. Antiplatelet and anticoagulant drugs are typically used to treat an ongoing attack and minimize the chance of another. Surgery to promote blood flow to the affected area may be attempted in certain cases.

Prognosis: The prognosis for an individual experiencing transient ischemic attacks is guarded. Although the symptoms subside, TIAs tend to be recurrent and may signal an impending cerebrovascular accident.

Prevention: See preventive measures for cerebrovascular accident.

DEGENERATIVE DISEASES

Organic Brain Syndrome

Description: *Organic brain syndrome* is irreversible, diffuse brain damage characterized by progressive **dementia** and **delirium**. The syndrome generally is progressive even when the cause is treatable.

Etiology: The causes of organic brain syndrome are varied and include chronic alcohol intoxication, drug withdrawal, CNS infections, metabolic disturbances, nutritional deficiencies, head trauma, or neoplasms.

Signs and Symptoms: Common symptoms include a variety of cognitive, emotional, and behavioral disturbances. The patient frequently has no regard for personal appearance, suffers memory lapses, and may be depressed, irritable, or aggressive. Delirium, dementia, and hallucinations may result.

Diagnostic Procedures: A complete patient history and physical examination, including a neurologic assessment, are paramount. Cranial CT scans, lumbar puncture and analysis of the cerebrospinal fluid, and electrolyte analyses may be done to assist in the diagnosis of organic brain syndrome.

Treatment: The individual needs to have a safe, comfortable, and nonthreatening environment. Everything needs to be done to reorient the person. The underlying cause must be treated, if possible.

Prognosis: The prognosis is poor if the syndrome has progressed and cerebral deterioration has occurred.

Prevention: Prevention is dependent on the cause.

Alzheimer's Disease

Description: *Alzheimer's disease,* formerly called *presenile dementia,* is a type of chronic organic brain syndrome characterized by the death of neurons in the cerebral cortex and their replacement by microscopic "plaques." The result is progressive intellectual impairment. The disease affects mainly people between 50 and 60 years old.

Etiology: The cause of Alzheimer's disease is unknown, but hereditary factors, autoimmune reactions, and cellular changes of viral origin have all been proposed.

Signs and Symptoms: The disease progresses through three distinct stages. The first stage exhibits mild mental impairment. In the second stage, there is increased forgetfulness, agitation, irritability, and extreme restlessness. In the third and final stage, patients are unable to care for themselves, are incontinent, and are unable to communicate. The rate at which a patient progresses through each stage varies.

Diagnostic Procedures: The goal of diagnosis is to rule out other degenerative brain diseases producing similar symptoms. An EEG and cranial CT and MRI scans may be performed, the latter two to detect the characteristic lesions of the disease.

Treatment: Treatment is merely palliative and directed toward maintaining nutrition, hydration, and safety. Emotional support of family members is important, too.

Prognosis: The prognosis is poor, with the disease progressing over a period of 5 to 10 years. Death may occur from secondary causes such as septic **decubitus ulcers** or pneumonia.

Prevention: There is no known prevention.

Parkinson's Disease

Description: Parkinson's disease is a chronic nervous disease characterized by progressive muscle rigidity and involuntary tremors. Parkinson's is a common crippling disease in the United States, affecting more men than women, usually in their fifties and sixties.

Etiology: The cause is unknown, but the condition may be related to a deficiency within the brain of a neurotransmitter chemical called *dopamine.* Dopamine is necessary for brain cell functioning.

Signs and Symptoms: The onset of Parkinson's is slow and insidious. Symptoms eventually may include muscle weakness, progressively rigid extremities, and "pill-rolling" tremors beginning in the fingers. The individual's facial expression may appear fixed. Stress, fatigue, and anxiety tend to aggravate the tremors. The patient's intellect typically remains unaffected.

Diagnostic Procedures: Diagnosis is made on the basis of the unique set of physical symptoms characteristic of Parkinson's. The tremors and rigidity must be differentiated from other diseases. A urinalysis may be done to check the level of dopamine.

Treatment: Treatment of Parkinsons' disease is strictly palliative. Medical measures are usually withheld until the patient has trouble with the activities of daily living. Then **anticholinergic drugs** or antiviral agents may be prescribed. Levodopa, a dopamine replacement, may be used. Physical therapy and psychological support and reassurance are necessary, too. If drug therapy is unsuccessful, certain surgical techniques may be attempted that destroy part of the thalamus and limit involuntary movement.

Prognosis: Although the disease is slowly progressive and debilitating, because of effective treatment strategies, many individuals with Parkinson's can live comparatively normal lives for many years. Dementia may ultimately result in a third of all cases.

Prevention: There is no known prevention.

Multiple Sclerosis

Description: *Multiple sclerosis* (MS) is a chronic, progressive nervous disease characterized by the destruction of the lipid and protein layer called the *myelin* *sheath* that insulates and protects the axons of certain nerve cells. The demyelination process occurs at scattered sites throughout the CNS and results in progressive physical disability. The onset of MS is usually during early adulthood. Women account for the majority of cases. The disease is a common cause of chronic disability.

Etiology: The cause of MS is unknown, although immunologic, viral, and genetic etiologies have been proposed.

Signs and Symptoms: Symptoms may include sudden, transient motor and sensory disturbances, impaired vision, muscle weakness, paralysis, incontinence, and mood swings such as euphoria or depression. The initial onset of symptoms, and later relapses, may occur following acute infection, trauma, serum injections, pregnancy, or stress. The symptoms usually come and go with no pattern or warning. They may last hours or weeks.

Diagnostic Procedures: A neurologic examination, CSF analysis, and cranial CT and MRI scans may be useful in the diagnosis of MS. The disease is difficult to diagnose, however, because the onset may be mild and take years to progress. Periodic testing and observation are usually necessary.

Treatment: There is no specific treatment for MS. Treatment efforts are directed at relieving symptoms and forestalling future attacks. Medications such as **ACTH**, corticosteroids, and mood-altering drugs may be prescribed. Avoidance of temperature extremes and stress is important. Psychological counseling and physical therapy are essential for most patients.

Prognosis: Because the course of the disease is varied and unpredictable, the prognosis is guarded. Individuals with MS experience remissions and exacerbations of symptoms, but as the disease progresses, remissions usually are incomplete and are shorter in duration.

Prevention: There is no known prevention for MS.

Amyotrophic Lateral Sclerosis (ALS)

Description: *Amyotrophic lateral sclerosis,* commonly known as *Lou Gehrig's disease,* is a disease of motor neurons that results in progressive muscular atrophy and weakness. The disease is more common in men and generally occurs between 40 and 60 years of age.

Etiology: The cause is unknown.

Signs and Symptoms: Symptoms of ALS include involuntary muscular contractions and muscular atrophy, weakness, and twitching, especially in the muscles of the extremities. The individual may have problems with speech, chewing, swallowing, and even breathing if the brain stem is affected.

Diagnostic Procedures: The disease may be diagnosed on the basis of the presenting signs and symptoms. Electromyography and muscle biopsy will help identify nerve rather than muscle disease. It is necesary to rule out several other disorders that may produce similar symptoms, such as multiple sclerosis, spinal cord neoplasm, and myasthenia gravis.

Treatment: There is no effective treatment for ALS. Treatment is symptomatic and may include emotional as well as physical support. Persons afflicted with the disease are likely to become confined to a wheelchair or a bed, need to be taught to suction themselves to prevent choking, require assistance with personal hygiene, and need a great deal of emotional support.

Prognosis: The prognosis is dependent on the area involved and the speed at which the disease progresses. ALS is usually fatal within 2 to 5 years after onset. Death most often results from respiratory failure or aspiration pneumonia.

Prevention: There is no known prevention.

TUMORS OF THE BRAIN

Description: *Primary brain tumors* are benign or malignant neoplasms originating within the brain. *Secondary brain tumors* are the result of metastasis of neoplasms from elsewhere in the body. This latter category of tumors accounts for the majority of cases. Tumors cause neurologic deterioration by replacing healthy brain tissue, by compressing brain tissue, or by blocking the blood supply or the flow of cerebrospinal fluid to a portion of the brain.

Etiology: The cause is unknown.

Signs and Symptoms: Brain tumors may be difficult to diagnose because of vague symptoms and their slow onset. The location of the growth in the brain will partially dictate the symptoms. Headache, vomiting, defective memory, mood changes, seizures, visual distrubances, motor impairment, and personality changes may occur.

Diagnostic Procedures: A complete history and physical examination, including neurologic assessment, are essential. Skull x-rays, lumbar puncture, EEG, cranial CT and MRI scans, or biopsy of the lesion will confirm the diagnosis. Further studies may be done to locate the primary site of a metastatic brain tumor.

Treatment: Surgery, radiation therapy, or chemotherapy—individually or in combination—may be used to remove the tumor. Medications may be ordered for symptomatic treatment of seizures, edema, and headache.

Prognosis: The prognosis is dependent on the size, location, and type of tumor.

Prevention: There is no known prevention.

COMMON SYMPTOMS OF NERVOUS SYSTEM DISEASES

Individuals may present with the following common symptoms, which deserve attention from health professionals:

■ Headache
■ Weakness
■ Nausea and vomiting
■ Motor disturbances such as stiff neck or back, rigid muscles, seizures, convulsions, or paralysis
■ Sensory disturbances of any kind, especially vision or speech
■ Drowsiness, stupor, or coma
■ Mood swings
■ Fever

REFERENCES

1. *Diseases,* Nursing '83 Books, Intermed Communications, Inc., Springhouse, Pa., 1983, Culp, H. P., and R. D. Lemerman, p. 628.
2. Brunner, L. S., et al., *Textbook of Medical-Surgical Nursing,* 6th ed., J. B. Lippincott, Philadelphia, 1988, p. 1491.

REVIEW QUESTIONS

Matching
_____ 1. Sensory loss in lower extremities   a. Quadriplegia
_____ 2. Sensory loss in all extremities   b. Paraplegia
_____ 3. Unilateral sensory loss   c. Hemiplegia

Short Answer
1. List at least four common signs and symptoms of CNS infections:
   a.
   b.
   c.
   d.
2. Name and define the three classifications of seizures:
   a.
   b.
   c.
3. Another term for *cerebrovascular accident* is _____
4. What are TIAs?
5. What is the difference between organic brain syndrome and Alzheimer's disease?
6. Can a brain abscess exhibit signs and symptoms similar to a brain tumor? Explain.
7. Name the disease:
   a. _____ is progressive demyelination of patches of white matter.
   b. _____ is progressive muscle rigidity and involuntary tremors.

True/False

T F 1. Peripheral neuritis is an inflammatory degeneration of peripheral nerves.

T F 2. The onset of peripheral neuritis is rapid in most cases.

T F 3. Bell's palsy is a disease of a facial nerve, the fifth cranial nerve.

T F 4. The prognosis of Bell's palsy is good.

ANSWERS

Matching

1. b
2. a
3. c

Short Answer

1. Headache, fever, sensory disturbances, neck and back stiffness, positive Kernig and Brudzinski signs, and cerebrospinal fluid abnormalities.
2. a. Partial seizures—focal in origin; affect only part of brain.
   b. Generalized seizures—nonspecific in origin; affect entire brain.
   c. Unclassified—identified thus because of incomplete data.
3. Stroke.
4. TIAs are transient ischemic attacks; recurrent episodes of neurologic deficit resulting from lack of blood flow to a part of the brain; "little strokes."
5. Organic brain syndrome is a disorder associated with impairment of brain tissue and some degree of cognitive impairment. The prognosis is good if in the acute stage. Alzheimer's disease is a type of chronic organic brain syndrome where there is progressive cerebral degeneration which can occur in all areas of the cortex or the brain causing intellectual impairment. It is sometimes called *presenile dementia*. The prognosis is poor.
6. Yes, the signs and symptoms of a brain tumor and abscess may be similar, i.e., headache, nausea, vomiting, decreased vision, hemiparesis, slowed pulse and respiration, fever, pallor, and drowsiness. Both apply pressure; both are abnormal.
7. a. Multiple sclerosis
   b. Parkinson's disease

True/False

1. F
2. F
3. F
4. T

GLOSSARY

ACTH: Adrenocorticotropic hormone. Normally produced by the pituitary gland, it stimulates hormone production by the cortex of the adrenal gland. Sometimes administered as a therapeutic agent due to its anti-inflammatory properties.

AGNOSIA: Loss of ability to understand or interpret auditory, visual, or other forms of sensory information even though the respective sensory organs are functioning properly.

AGRAPHIA: Loss of ability to convert thought into writing.

ALEXIA: Loss of ability to understand written language.

ANALGESICS: Drugs or other agents that relieve pain.

ANTIBIOTICS: Any of a variety of natural or synthetic substances that inhibit the growth of or destroy microorganisms. Used in the treatment of infectious diseases.

ANTICHOLINERGIC (DRUG): Drug or agent that inhibits the action of the neurotransmitter chemical acetylcholine, blocking parasympathetic nerve impulses, with consequent reduction of smooth-muscle contractions and various bodily secretions.

APHASIA: Loss or impairment of the ability to communicate through speech, writing, or signs due to dysfunction of brain centers.

APRAXIA: Loss or impairment of ability to perform coordinated movements, especially impairment of the ability to use common objects for their intended purposes.

ARRHYTHMIAS (CARDIAC): Irregularities in the force or rhythm of heart action caused by disturbances in the discharge of cardiac impulses from the heart's sinoatrial node or their transmission through the heart's conductile tissue.

BACTEREMIA: Bacteria in the blood.

BRADYCARDIA: Abnormally slow heart beat, generally characterized by a pulse rate below 60 beats per minute.

BRUDZINSKI'S SIGN: A diagnostic indicator of meningitis, characterized by the involuntary flexion of the hips and knees in response to the forward flexion of the neck.

CEREBROSPINAL FLUID (CSF): The clear fluid that bathes the ventricles of the brain and the central cavity of the spinal cord.

CHEYNE-STOKES RESPIRATION: A breathing pattern disturbance characterized by a period of deep, rapid respirations followed by a period of shallow respirations or no respirations at all. The cycle rhythmically repeats every 45 seconds to 3 minutes.

COMA: A state of profound unconsciousness occurring in illness, as a result of it, or due to an injury. The affected individual cannot be aroused by external stimuli.

CONTRACTURE: Permanent shortening or contraction of a muscle, often producing physical distortion or deformity.

CRANIOTOMY: Surgical incision through the cranium.

DECUBITUS ULCER: An open sore or skin lesion resulting from impaired circulation to a portion of the body surface caused by prolonged pressure from a bed or chair. Commonly called a *bedsore.*

DELIRIUM: A state of temporary mental confusion and impaired consciousness resulting from fever, shock, exhaustion, metabolic disorders, or drug or alcohol intoxication. Characterized by anxiety, excitement, hallucinations, and incoherence.

DEMENTIA: Irreversibly deteriorating mental state characterized by impaired memory, judgment, and ability to think caused by cerebral damage due to an organic brain disease.

DIPLOPIA: Double vision.

DYSPHASIA: Impairment of speech resulting from a brain lesion.

EMBOLISM: Obstruction of a blood vessel by foreign substances or a blood clot.

HEMIPARESIS: Paralysis affecting only one side of the body.

HYPOTENSION: Persistently low systolic and diastolic blood pressure.

KERNIG'S SIGN: A diagnostic indicator of meningitis, characterized by the inability to straighten the knee while the hip is flexed.

MENINGES: The three membranes enclosing the brain and spinal cord.

NUCHAL RIGIDITY: Stiff neck.

STUPOR: A condition of unconsciousness or lethargy.

THROMBOSIS: The formation or presence of a blood clot within a blood vessel.

Chapter 10

Endocrine System Diseases

LEARNING OBJECTIVES

Upon successful completion of this chapter, you will
- Describe the two forms of hyperpituitarism.
- Discuss the signs and symptoms of hypopituitarism.
- Identify the classic symptoms of diabetes insipidus.
- Recall the cause of simple goiter.
- Explain the treatment for Hashimoto's thyroiditis.
- Recognize the signs and symptoms of hyperthyroidism.
- Compare cretinism with myxedema.
- Relate hypercalcemia to hyperparathyroidism.
- Relate hypocalcemia to hypoparathyroidism.
- Review the classic symptoms of Cushing's syndrome.
- Recall the etiology of diabetes mellitus.
- Report the treatment of diabetes mellitus.
- Describe the complications of diabetes mellitus.
- List at least four common symptoms of endocrine diseases.

INTRODUCTION

The endocrine system is a network of ductless glands that acts to regulate many of the body's physiologic processes. Each type of endocrine gland produces one or more secretions that are discharged into the blood or lymph and circulated to all parts of the body. These secretions are called *hormones*. A hormone is a chemical substance that produces a specific effect on a particular type of tissue, on an organ, or on the body as a whole.

The principal organs of the endocrine system include the pituitary gland, the thyroid gland, the parathyroid glands, the adrenal glands, and the pineal body (the function of this gland is not known). In addition to their other roles, the pancreas and the testes or ovaries also have important endocrine functions. Figure 10–1 illustrates the location of the endocrine glands within the body. Table 10–1 lists the hormones produced by the principal endocrine glands and summarizes their major effects on the body.

The secretion of hormones by the endocrine system is governed by an amazingly intricate interrelationship between the glands themselves, the nervous system, and the levels of various substances in the blood. Dysfunction of an endocrine gland may result in either too little secretion of its hormone *(hyposecretion)* or too much *(hypersecretion)*. Because of the effect this system has on the entire body, many disease conditions result from or are associated with endocrine dysfunction.

PITUITARY GLAND DISEASES

Hyperpituitarism (Gigantism, Acromegaly)

Description: *Hyperpituitarism* is the hypersecretion of growth hormone (GH) by a portion of the pituitary gland. Two distinct conditions may result from hyperpituitarism, depending on the time of life this dysfunction begins. *Gigantism* results from the hypersecretion of GH during an individual's growing years, especially prior to puberty (Figure 10–2). The person with gigantism grows abnormally tall, although the relative proportions of the body parts and sexual development remain unaffected. When GH hypersecretion occurs during adulthood, *acromegaly* results. Acromegaly is a chronic, disfiguring, life-shortening disease characterized by the overgrowth of bones and soft tissues (Figure 10–3).

Etiology: The hypersecretion of GH that produces gigantism and acromegaly is typically due to benign, slow-growing adenomas in the anterior pituitary. Not subject to normal control, these neoplastic cells release abnormally high levels of GH.

Signs and Symptoms: The principal symptom of gigantism is excessive growth of the long bones of the body. This results in an abnormal increase in height. A child with the condition may grow as much as 6 inches a year.

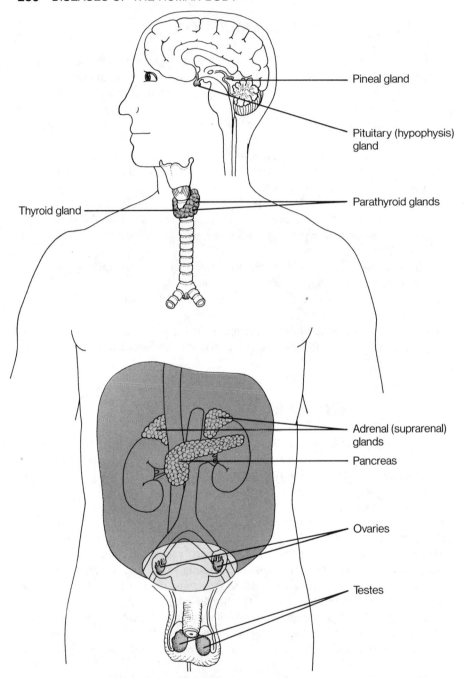

FIGURE 10–1. Glands of the endocrine system. (Modified from Gylys, B. A. and Wedding, M. E., *Medical Terminology: A Systems Approach,* ed. 2. F. A. Davis, Philadelphia, 1988, p. 300, with permission.)

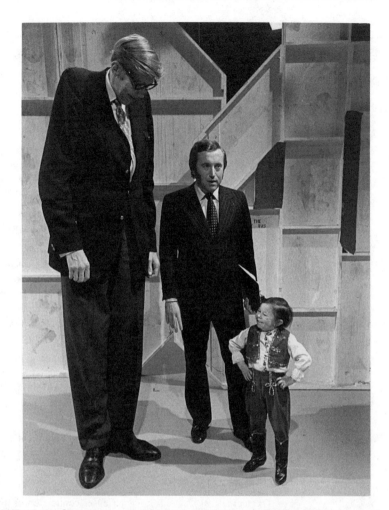

FIGURE 10–2. Gigantism and dwarfism, caused respectively by the overproduction or underproduction of growth hormone (GH) during childhood and adolescence. (Photo by Michael Serino/The Picture Cube.)

The symptoms of acromegaly generally appear very gradually, causing the deformation and coarsening of facial features and enlargement of the hands, feet, head, and tongue. Serious physiologic symptoms also may appear, such as increased sweating, oily skin, and chronic sinus congestion. The person with acromegaly will often complain of headaches, weakness, paresthesia, joint pain, and vision disorders.

Diagnostic Procedures: The clinical picture of symptoms will suggest the diagnosis. A glucose suppression test is the standard method for confirming ele-

TABLE 10–1. Endocrine System Hormones*

Gland	Hormone	Major Effects
Pituitary	Growth hormone (GH)	Stimulates bone and body growth
	Thyroid-stimulating hormone (TSH)	Controls secretions of hormones from the thyroid gland
	Prolactin	Promotes growth of breast tissue; stimulates milk production after birth
	Adrenocorticotropic hormone (ACTH)	Stimulates secretions by the adrenal cortex, especially cortisol
	Gonadotropin: follicle-stimulating hormone (FSH)	Stimulates development of eggs in the ovaries; stimulates secretions of estrogens in females; stimulates production of sperm in the testes
	Luteinizing hormone (LH), or interstitial cell-stimulating hormone (ICSH) in males	Promotes secretion of sex hormones in both males and females; plays a role in the release of the egg cell in females
	Antidiuretic hormone (ADH), or vasopressin	Decreases volume of urine excreted; increases volume of water reabsorbed in the kidney
	Oxytocin	Causes contraction of the uterus during labor; stimulates milk secretion
Thyroid	Triiodothyroxine (T_4), triiodothyronine (T_3)	Increases oxygen consumption and metabolism of all cells
	Calcitonin	Lowers calcium level in blood by inhibiting release of calcium from bones
Parathyroids	Parathyroid hormone (PTH)	Regulates the metabolism of calcium; stimulates formation of new bone cells

TABLE 10–1. *Continued*

Gland	Hormone	Major Effects
Adrenals	Mineralocorticoids (aldosterone)	Regulates the amount of salts in the body
	Glucocorticoids (cortisol)	Regulates the metabolism of carbohydrates, proteins, and fats
	Gonadocorticoids (androgens, estrogens, and progestins)	Maintain secondary sex characteristics
	Epinephrine	Vasodilator, cardiac stimulant
	Norepinephrine	Vasoconstrictor
Pancreas	Insulin	Promotes the movement of glucose through cell membranes (lowering the blood glucose level)
	Glucagon	Stimulates the liver to convert glycogen to glucose (raising the blood glucose level)

*Adapted from Gylys, B. A., and M. E. Wedding, *Medical Terminology: A Systems Approach,* ed. 2. F. A. Davis, Philadelphia, 1988, pp. 302–305, with permission.

vated GH levels. Conventional skull x-rays or cranial CT and MRI scans are useful in pinpointing the location and estimating the extent of the pituitary tumor.

Treatment: Treatment goals involve lowering GH levels to normal and stabilizing or removing the tumor while minimizing damage to the pituitary gland itself. Surgery may be attempted depending on the size and location of the tumor. Otherwise, radiation therapy or drug therapy may be used.

Prognosis: The prognosis for an individual with either gigantism or acromegaly depends on how far the condition has advanced before successful treatment. Gigantism is generally not life-threatening, and the prognosis is usually good. An individual with advanced acromegaly, however, may suffer serious complications such as congestive heart failure, diabetes mellitus, respiratory diseases, or cerebrovascular diseases. Even if successfully treated, the pituitary tumors may recur. Hypopituitarism may be an unintended consequence of treatment for either condition.

Prevention: There is no specific prevention for hyperpituitarism.

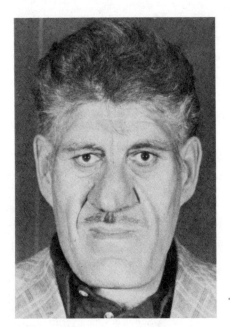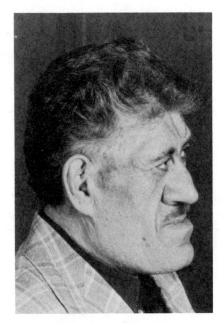

FIGURE 10–3. Acromegaly in a 56-year-old man. (From Martin, J. B., Reichlin, S., and Brown, G. M., *Clinical Neuroendocrinology.* Contemporary Neurology Series, #14. F. A. Davis, Philadelphia, 1977, p. 353, with permission.)

Hypopituitarism

Description: *Hypopituitarism* is an endocrine deficiency in which any of the hormones produced by the anterior portion of the pituitary gland are secreted at insufficient levels or are absent. Growth hormone (GH) and gonadotropin are the most commonly deficient hormones in hypopituitarism. Less frequently, adrenocorticotropic hormone (ACTH) and thyroid-stimulating hormone (TSH) are deficient. When all the anterior pituitary's hormones are affected, the condition is called *panhypopituitarism.* As Table 10–1 indicates, the major effect of some anterior pituitary hormones is the stimulation of hormone production by other endocrine glands. For this reason, hypopituitarism may have a cascading effect, resulting in hyposecretion of essential hormones by the "target" glands and producing symptoms that may mimic disorders of these glands.

Etiology: Hypopituitarism is often caused by damage from pituitary tumors or from tumors of the hypothalamus. Infection and inflammation of these structures is a less frequent etiology. Other significant causes include pituitary vascular diseases, especially postpartum hemorrhage of the pituitary gland. Head injuries and iatrogenic damage from surgery and radiation therapy also may result in hypopituitarism.

Signs and Symptoms: The symptoms of hypopituitarism depend on the age and sex of the affected individual and on the specific hormones that are deficient. In children, GH deficiency will produce dwarfism, whereas gonadotropin deficiency may interfere with the emergence of secondary sexual characteristics. Gonadotropin deficiency in adult women may cause ammenorhea and infertility or cause testosterone deficiencies, decreased libido, and loss of body and facial hair in men. ACTH and TSH deficiencies may produce generalized symptoms such as fatigue, anorexia, weight loss, loss of skin pigmentation, low tolerance to cold, and a poor response to stress. Naturally enough, panhypopituitarism may result in all the preceding symptoms as well as mental and physiologic abnormalities.

Diagnostic Procedures: The individual's clinical history of symptoms will suggest the diagnosis. A battery of laboratory tests to measure the levels of each of the principal pituitary hormones will typically be run to confirm the diagnosis. It is essential that laboratory tests also be run to measure the normal output of "target" glands (e.g., cortisol production by the adrenal glands), since deficiencies of these secretions may prove life-threatening. Conventional skull x-rays and cranial CT and MRI scans are useful in pinpointing pituitary tumors or lesions.

Treatment: Hormone replacement therapy, both of pituitary hormones and of those secreted by the target glands, is the typical course of treatment. A newly bioengineered GH preparation is effective for treating GH-deficient growth abnormalities in children. Because hormonal balances normally change during growth and development, constant monitoring is necessary during hormone replacement therapy to make certain that appropriate hormonal levels are maintained. Surgical management of pituitary neoplasms may be required.

Prognosis: Despite the fact that lost pituitary function generally cannot be restored, the prognosis can be good if hormone replacement therapy is effective. Total loss of all hormonal secretions from the anterior pituitary may result in fatal complications.

Prevention: There is no specific prevention for hypopituitarism.

Diabetes Insipidus

Description: Diabetes insipidus is **polyuria** and excessive thirst resulting from insufficient secretion of **vasopressin** by the posterior portion of the pituitary gland. Vasopressin, also known as *antidiuretic hormone* (ADH), helps regulate the amount of fluid the kidneys release as urine. Other things being equal, the higher the level of vasopressin, the greater is the fluid reabsorption by the kidneys. Diabetes insipidus usually starts in childhood or early adulthood and affects males more commonly than females.

Etiology: Most cases of diabetes insipidus are idiopathic, especially those cases arising during childhood. Other causes include primary tumors of the pituitary gland and hypothalamus and damage to the posterior portion of the pituitary gland as a result of severe head injuries or from surgery.

Signs and Symptoms: The classic symptom is polyuria. As much as 1 to 16 gallons of dilute urine may be produced in 24 hours. This makes the person extremely thirsty because of the need to replace the fluids lost from the body. Consequently, there may be signs of dehydration such as weakness, fever, mental confusion, and prostration.

Diagnostic Procedures: Urinalysis will reveal a colorless urine with low osmolality (i.e., containing low levels of dissolved wastes). In order to differentiate diabetes insipidus from other diseases causing polyuria, a "dehydration test" will typically be run. In this test, the person will be denied fluids, and hourly measurements will be made of urine osmolality, body weight, and blood pressure. After a period of several hours, the individual will be given a vasopressin medication. If the person has diabetes insipidus, the vasopressin will decrease the urine output and increase the urine's osmolality.

Treatment: Hormone replacement therapy using various vasopressin medications is the most common treatment protocol for diabetes insipidus.

Prognosis: The prognosis of an individual with diabetes insipidus depends on the underlying cause of the condition. If the underlying cause is difficult to treat, such as cancer, the prognosis is guarded. In other cases, though, with effective vasopressin replacement therapy, the individual should typically be able to lead a normal life.

Prevention: There is no specific prevention for diabetes insipidus.

THYROID GLAND DISEASES

Simple Goiter

Description: A *goiter* is enlargement (**hyperplasia**) of the thyroid gland. A *simple goiter* is any thyroid enlargement that is not caused by an infection or neoplasm and that does not result from another hypo- or hyperthyroid disorder. In certain parts of the world, simple goiter is an *endemic* condition (affecting many people in a given area). In the United States, however, simple goiter is now a *sporadic* condition (affecting only a few).

Etiology: The thyroid gland hyperplasia that characterizes a goiter occurs when the thyroid gland cannot secrete sufficient levels of two iodine-rich hormones: triiodothyroxine (T_4) and triiodothyronine (T_3). The thyroid gland tissue enlarges in order to compensate for the deficiency. In simple goiter, the inadequate secretion of these thyroid hormones may be caused by a dietary iodine deficiency, the ingestion of substances known to induce goiter (**goitrogens**), or some error in the hormone formation process within the thyroid gland. In many cases, though, the condition is idiopathic.

Signs and Symptoms: The extent of thyroid enlargement will vary from case to case. A simple goiter may display as a small nodule, or it can be quite massive, presenting a conspicuous swollen mass at the front of the neck, just above the sternum. The goiter may compress the esophagus or trachea, producing **dysphagia**, dizziness, and **syncope**.

Diagnostic Procedures: Diagnosis of simple goiter is made on the basis of thyroid gland enlargement in the presence of normal levels of T_3 and T_4 hormones. A T_3 and T_4 radioimmunoassay test will accurately measure the levels of these two hormones.

Treatment: The treatment goal is to reduce the size of the goiter. How this is accomplished will depend in part on the underlying cause of the condition. Treatment procedures may include dietary supplements of iodine or T_3 and T_4 hormone replacement therapy. In the case of idiopathic simple goiter, treatment may involve thyroid suppression therapy, i.e., the use of certain drugs that slow thyroid gland activity. A large goiter that is unresponsive to therapy may require excision.

Prognosis: The prognosis is generally good following effective treatment. Complications from severe cases of simple goiter include hemorrhage of thyroid gland blood vessels or hypo- or hyperthyroid conditions.

Prevention: Prevention of simple goiter includes adequate dietary intake of iodine and avoidance of substances known to cause goiter.

Hashimoto's Thyroiditis

Description: *Hashimoto's thyroiditis* is an inflammatory autoimmune disease of the thyroid gland. It is a leading cause of nonsimple goiter and hypothyroidism. The disease is characterized by the infiltration of the thyroid gland with lymphocytes and by elevated blood serum levels of immunoglobulins and antibodies against thyroid tissue. Fibrous tissue slowly replaces healthy tissue within the thyroid gland as the disease progresses. This disease is more common in middle-age women and in children. It sometimes accompanies other autoimmune diseases.

Etiology: The cause of Hashimoto's thyroiditis is not known, but genetic factors are strongly suspected.

Signs and Symptoms: Goiter is the principal symptom of Hashimoto's thyroiditis. As the disease advances, the individual typically begins to show symptoms of hypothyroidism.

Diagnostic Procedures: Blood testing will typically reveal elevated immunoglobulin levels and the presence of antibodies that react with thyroid tissue. These findings in the presence of goiter suggest a diagnosis of Hashimoto's thyroiditis. A needle biopsy of thyroid tisssue also may be performed to examine the tissue for changes that are characteristic of the disease. A radioactive iodine uptake (RAIU) test may be run to measure thyroid function.

Treatment: Thyroid hormone replacement therapy is a standard form of treatment. The therapy usually must be continued for life.

Prognosis: The condition is chronic, but the prognosis is good if thyroid hormone replacement therapy is effective.

Prevention: There is no known prevention for Hashimoto's thyroiditis.

Hyperthyroidism (Graves' Disease)

Description: *Hyperthyroidism* is a condition caused by the oversecretion of hormones by the thyroid gland. As Table 10–1 reveals, thyroid hormones such as triiodothyroxine (T_4) and triiodothyronine (T_3) influence the metabolism of cells throughout the body. Consequently, when levels of these hormones are constantly elevated, as occurs in hyperthyroidism, profound changes can occur in the body's normal physiologic processes. These changes frequently produce a cluster of symptoms called *thyrotoxicosis*. The symptoms of thyrotoxicosis will be discussed below.

A hyperthyroid state can result from a number of conditions and diseases. The most important of these, though, is Graves' disease. Graves' is an autoimmune disease marked by hypothyroidism with goiter, characteristic changes in the structure of the eyes (ophthalmopathy), and characteristic skin lesions (dermopathy). The immune system of an individual affected by this disease produces immunoglobulins that attack the regulating mechanism of the thyroid gland, stimulating the excess production of thyroid hormones. This disease affects more women than men, and it typically appears between the ages of 30 and 50. The remaining portions of this discussion will focus on Graves' disease.

Etiology: The cause of Graves' disease is not known, although a familial predisposition to the disease has led researchers to strongly suspect a genetic etiology.

Signs and Symptoms: The classic manifestations of Graves' disease are goiter, symptoms of thyrotoxicosis, ophthalmopathy, and dermopathy. These symptoms may appear independently of one another and go through cycles of remission and exacerbation.

The symptoms of thyrotoxicosis include nervousness, loss of sleep, excessive perspiration, and heat intolerance. Wasting of muscle and decalcification of the skeleton may lead to persistent weight loss and fatigue. The symptoms of thyrotoxicosis also may include a host of cardiac manifestations such as tachycardia, arrythmias, heart murmurs, and cardiomegaly.

The ophthalmopathy characteristic of Graves' disease includes **exophthalmos** (Figure 10–4), protruding eyeballs that give the affected individual a "frightened" appearance. Inflammation of the muscles surrounding the eye may interfere with normal eye movements, including blinking. The dermopathy associated with Graves' disease is marked by the appearance of thickened patches of skin, usually on the feet or legs, having an "orange skin" texture and uneven pigmentation.

Diagnostic Procedures: Diagnosis is based largely on the characteristic physical manifestations of the disease. A radioimmunoassay will confirm increased serum levels of T_4 and T_3, and a thyroid radioactive iodine uptake (RAIU) test will confirm thyroid hyperactivity. Blood tests indicating elevated levels of certain antithyroid immunoglobulins also strongly suggest a diagnosis of Graves' disease.

Treatment: The course of treatment chosen depends on the affected individual's age and sex and on the severity of the case. One approach involves the use of

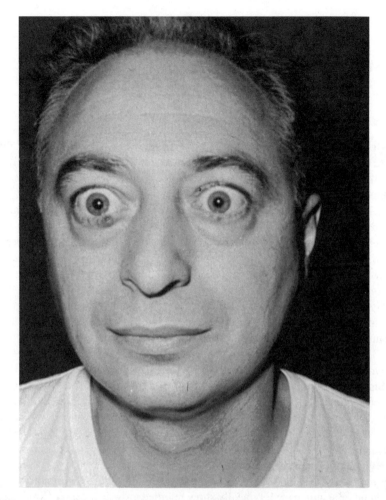

FIGURE 10–4. Exophthalmos caused by hyperthyroidism (Graves' disease). (Photo by Lester V. Bergman, N.Y..)

antithyroid agents, i.e., drugs that block hormone synthesis within the thyroid gland. Another approach involves altering the structure of the thyroid gland itself, through either surgery or radioactive iodine therapy. Short-term control of the hyperthyroidism of Graves' disease also may be obtained by administration of iodide compounds.

Prognosis: The prognosis of Graves' disease varies from case to case. If the course of treatment results in the remission of symptoms and the disappearance of immunoglobulins associated with the disease, then the prognosis for a complete recovery without recurrence is good. A potentially fatal complication of Graves' disease is *thyroid storm,* a severe episode of thyrotoxicosis. It is marked by the rapid onset of fever, sweating, tachycardia, pulmonary edema, and congestive heart failure. This condition requires emergency medical intervention.

Prevention: There is no specific prevention for Graves' disease.

Hypothyroidism (Cretinism, Myxedema)

Description: *Hypothyroidism* is undersecretion of hormones by the thyroid gland. Hypothyroidism is called *cretinism* when it appears as a congenital condition, and it is called *myxedema* when it is acquired later in childhood or during adulthood.

Etiology: Hypothyroidism may be caused by either an insufficient quantity of thyroid tissue or the loss of functional thyroid tissue. The former condition may be iatrogenic, resulting from thyroid surgery, radioactive iodine therapy performed to treat another thyroid disease, or a congenital thyroid abnormality. The progressive loss of functional thyroid tissue is generally idiopathic, but it shows strong evidence of being an autoimmune disorder.

Hashimoto's disease is a leading cause of hypothyroidism with goiter (see Hashimoto's Disease). Other forms of hypothyroidism accompanied by goiter may be caused by dietary or metabolic iodine deficiencies or be induced by certain drugs. Hypothyroidism also may arise secondarily from diseases of the anterior pituitary that result in hyposecretion of thyroid-stimulating hormone (TSH).

Signs and Symptoms: Since the thyroid hormones triiodothyroxine (T_4) and triiodothyronine (T_3) influence the metabolism of cells throughout the body, the persistently low levels of these hormones in hypothyroidism can result in a host of symptoms. The assortment of symptoms will vary with the age of the affected individual.

Hypothyroid newborns may exhibit constipation and feeding problems, may sleep too much, and may have a hoarse cry. Children with the condition (either congenital or acquired) will typically show retarded growth, a delayed emergence of secondary sexual characteristics, impaired intelligence, and one or more of the adult symptoms of hypothyroidism.

The onset of hypothyroidism during adulthood is often insidious. Initial symptoms may include fatigue, constipation, intolerance to cold, muscle cramps, and **menorrhagia**. Later symptoms may include mental clouding, diminished appetite, and weight gain. The skin may become dry, and the hair and nails may become brittle. In advanced forms of the disease, the affected individual may have an expressionless face and sparse hair. Other systemic conditions such as cardiomegaly and megacolon also may occur late in the disease.

Diagnostic Procedures: The composite picture of presenting signs and symptoms may suggest the diagnosis. Radioimmunoassay will typically show depressed levels of T_4 and T_3. A similar test will usually reveal elevated levels of thyroid-stimulating hormone (TSH), except for hypothyroidism arising from pituitary gland dysfunction, in which case TSH levels may range from undetectable to near normal. ECGs may reveal abnormalities in heart action.

Treatment: Treatment for hypothyroidism involves hormone replacement therapy with synthetic or animal-derived thyroid hormones. In the case of infants and children, therapy should begin as soon as possible to avoid or minimize intellectual impairment.

Prognosis: With effective thyroid hormone replacement therapy, the prognosis for an individual with hypothyroidism is good. A life-threatening complication of hypothyroidism is *myxedema coma*. This condition is marked by the onset of hypothermia and stupor, and it requires immediate medical attention.

Prevention: Only hypothyroidism due to dietary iodine deficiency or drug-induced forms of the disease are preventable.

PARATHYROID GLAND DISEASES

Hyperparathyroidism (Hypercalcemia)

Description: *Hyperparathyroidism* is a general disorder of calcium and phosphate metabolism caused by excessive secretion of parathyroid hormone (PTH) by the parathyroid glands. The persistently high level of PTH typically depresses the concentration of phosphates in the extracellular fluid (*hypophosphatemia*) and elevates the concentration of calcium (*hypercalcemia*). It is hypercalcemia that creates most of the troubling effects associated with hyperparathyroidism. The disease is far more common than once suspected, and it affects women twice as frequently as men.

Etiology: Hyperparathyroidism may have either a primary or a secondary etiology. The most common primary etiology is an adenoma on one of the parathyroid glands. Less commonly, the parathyroid glands may be affected by one of various forms of inherited endocrine system disorders. The condition also may be iatrogenic, appearing in those receiving lithium therapy for certain psychiatric disorders.

Secondary etiologies of hyperparathyroidism are those which act to reduce levels of circulating calcium, causing the parathyroid glands to hypersecrete in an effort to counteract the shortage of serum calcium. Such etiologies include chronic renal failure, dietary insufficiency of calcium, or calcium malabsorption disorders.

Signs and Symptoms: The onset of hyperparathyroidism is usually very gradual, with over half the affected individuals remaining asymptomatic for extended periods of time. Symptoms are usually related to hypercalcemia and may include weak, brittle bones and joint pain or the presence of kidney stones. Other hypercalcemic symptoms include CNS disturbances such as personality disorders or intellectual impairment or gastrointestinal disturbances such as duodenal ulcers, nausea, and vomiting. Additional symptoms may include muscle weakness or atrophy, chronic fatigue, and cardiac disturbances.

Diagnostic Procedures: Radioimmunoassay will typically reveal elevated concentrations of PTH. Blood testing will usually reveal abnormally high serum calcium levels in primary forms of the disease and diminished or nearly normal levels for secondary forms. Urinalysis may reveal elevated calcium. Conventional x-rays or CT scans of bone may reveal evidence of demineralization or increased bone turnover (i.e., newly formed bone mass balancing the reabsorption of older bone mass).

Treatment: The treatment of hyperparathyroidism varies with etiology. In primary forms of the disease, the goal is to reduce the level of circulating calcium. This may be accomplished surgically by removing the neoplastic or hypertrophic parathyroid glands. Increased hydration and sodium intake also may be used to lower serum calcium levels. In some cases, drugs that increase the excretion of calcium by the kidneys or inhibit the reabsorption of calcium from bone may be employed. Secondary forms of hyperparathyroidism can only be corrected by treating the underlying cause.

Prognosis: The prognosis for an individual with hyperparathyroidism is generally good, given successful treatment. Complications may result from organ damage due to chronic hypercalcemia. Coma and cardiac arrest may result in instances of severe hypercalcemia.

Prevention: There is no known prevention.

Hypoparathyroidism (Hypocalcemia)

Description: *Hypoparathyroidism* is undersecretion of parathyroid hormone (PTH) by the parathyroid glands. Consequently, circulating concentrations of calcium are reduced, resulting in hypocalcemia.

Etiology: Some cases of hypoparathyroidism are caused by hereditary disorders that result in underdevelopment of parathyroid tissue. Far more frequently, however, hyperparathyroidism is iatrogenic, usually resulting from the deliberate or inadvertent removal of parathyroid tissue during attempts to cure other endocrine disorders.

Signs and Symptoms: The signs and symptoms of hypoparathyroidism are generally dependent on the degree of hypocalcemia. Symptoms may include numbness and tingling of the extremities and muscle cramps. CNS symptoms may include general irritability and depression. **Tetany** also may occur, leading to laryngospasm, **cyanosis**, and grand mal seizures in severe cases. The affected individual may have brittle fingernails and hair loss.

Diagnostic Procedures: Radioimmunoassay revealing decreased PTH and serum calcium levels will suggest the diagnosis. Serum phosphorus will typically be increased. ECGs may indicate cardiac waveform abnormalities. X-rays may indicate decreased bone density.

Treatment: Treatment usually consists of lifelong vitamin D and calcium supplementation. Serum calcium levels should be tested regularly.

Prognosis: Although the condition is chronic, with successful treatment, the individual with hypoparathyroidism can lead a relatively normal life.

Prevention: There is no known prevention.

ADRENAL GLAND DISEASE: CUSHING'S SYNDROME

Description: *Cushing's syndrome* is hypersecretion of the adrenal cortex of the adrenal glands, resulting in the excess production of cortisol.

Etiology: One cause of Cushing's syndrome is bilateral hyperplasia of the adrenal glands due to elevated serum levels of adrenocorticotropic hormone (ACTH). Elevated concentrations of ACTH may result from overproduction of this hormone by a malfunctioning pituitary gland or from ACTH-secreting neoplasms elsewhere in the body. In either case, the result is overstimulation of the cortices of the adrenal gland and hypersecretion of cortisol. Another cause of Cushing's syndrome is benign or malignant neoplasms of an adrenal cortex. Finally, the disease is frequently iatrogenic, produced as a side effect of the long-term administration of steroid drugs used to treat other diseases.

Signs and Symptoms: The classic symptom of Cushing's syndrome is a round, "moon-shaped" face with acne. The head and trunk often are grossly exaggerated, with pencil-thin arms and legs. There may be impaired glucose tolerance, muscle weakness, stretch marks on the skin, a "buffalo" hump on the upper back, peptic ulcer, emotional changes, hypertension, and increased susceptibility to infection. The person also may have diabetes mellitus.

Diagnostic Procedures: The diagnostic procedures employed are chosen to establish a diagnosis of Cushing's syndrome and to pinpoint its etiology—a frequently difficult task. A 24-hour urine will typically exhibit elevated free cortisol levels. It is important to determine both serum and urine steroid levels. Pituitary and abdominal CT scans may be helpful in locating tumors.

Treatment: The treatment goal in each case is to restore the concentration of serum cortisol to normal levels. The approach chosen, however, will necessarily vary according to the etiology. In the case of adrenal hyperplasia due to elevated ACTH levels, surgery is usually performed to remove tumors on the pituitary gland or at ectopic sites. In some cases, drug therapy or radiation therapy may be attempted to suppress ACTH secretion. Occasionally, total adrenalectomy is the treatment of choice, but with the subsequent requirement for lifelong cortisol replacement therapy. Surgery is again the treatment of choice when Cushing's syndrome is caused by tumors of the adrenal cortex. Chemotherapy also may be attempted in such cases.

Prognosis: The prognosis for Cushing's syndrome depends on the etiology of the case and on how far the disease has progressed before the institution of treatment. The prognosis is poor for an individual with Cushing's syndrome caused by a carcinoma of the adrenal cortex. The prognosis is generally good if the condition is caused by a localized adenoma of the pituitary gland.

Prevention: Iatrogenic forms of Cushing's syndrome are preventable. Individuals receiving glucocorticoid steroids or ACTH preparations to treat other diseases should be carefully monitored for symptoms of Cushing's disease.

ENDOCRINE DYSFUNCTION OF THE PANCREAS: DIABETES MELLITUS

Description: *Diabetes mellitus* is a chronic disorder of carbohydrate metabolism resulting from insufficient production of insulin or from inadequate utilization of this hormone by the body's cells. Insulin is produced by the beta cells within structures called the *islets of Langerhans* scattered throughout the pancreas. As Table 10–1 reveals, insulin acts to lower the levels of glucose in the blood by enabling glucose absorption by body cells. When the beta cells cannot produce sufficient levels of insulin, the glucose concentration in the blood rises to abnormally high levels, a condition called *hyperglycemia.* Deprived of glucose, their principal fuel, the body cells begin to metabolize fats and proteins, depositing unusually high levels of wastes called *ketones* in the blood, causing a condition called *ketosis.* These two conditions, hyperglycemia and ketosis, are responsible for the host of troubling and often life-threatening symptoms of diabetes mellitus. The disease is distinguished by two primary forms:

■ *Insulin-dependent diabetes mellitus (IDDM, type I).* This form of the disease has an abrupt onset, usually appearing before the age of 25. Type I diabetes mellitus is frequently marked by the complete absence of insulin secretion, making this form of the disease quite difficult to regulate. Another common name for this form of the disease is *juvenile-onset diabetes.*

■ *Non-insulin-dependent diabetes mellitus (NIDDM, type II).* This more common form of the disease typically has a gradual onset, usually appearing in adults over the age of 40. The pancreas of the type II diabetic generally retains some insulin-secreting ability, making management of this disease less problematic than type I diabetes mellitus. (Despite its name, a few type II diabetics are insulin-dependent.)

Etiology: The cause of type I and type II diabetes mellitus is still not known. The type I form of the disease, however, seems to be an autoimmune disorder. Individuals who develop this form of diabetes mellitus inherit a defective gene that renders them susceptible to the disease. At some point early in life, a triggering event occurs in these individuals—perhaps a viral infection—that initiates a process resulting in the production of antibodies that destroy the beta cells. Type II diabetes mellitus also seems to be genetically linked, but little else is known about how this form of the disease arises.

Diabetes mellitus also may occur secondary to other diseases or conditions. Etiologies of this variety include chronic pancreatitis, pancreatic neoplasms, or drug-induced suppression of insulin production. Other endocrine disorders, such as Cushing's syndrome, also may induce diabetes mellitus. The disease also may be caused by genetic abnormalities that render the body's cells insensitive to insulin.

Signs and Symptoms: The classic symptoms of most cases of diabetes mellitus are polyuria, **glycosuria**, and **polydipsia**. In addition to these symptoms, type I diabetics usually experience weight loss and **polyphagia**, and they are susceptible to **ketoacidosis**. Type II diabetics, on the other hand, are usually overweight and may experience symptoms such as **pruritus**. Other generalized symptoms of both forms of the disease may include muscle weakness and fatigue. Because type II diabetes has such a gradual onset, individuals with this form of the disease often are still asymptomatic when the disease is discovered during routine screening.

Diagnostic Procedures: The individual's presenting symptoms may suggest a diagnosis of diabetes mellitus. Even if the individual is asymptomatic, a positive glucose tolerance test confirms the diagnosis.

Treatment: A combination of diet, insulin, and exercise is used to treat most forms of diabetes mellitus. Type I diabetics typically need to follow a consistent dietary pattern that is closely linked to the injection of insulin. A consistent routine of exercise will lessen the need for insulin. Type II diabetics usually require a diet that restricts their caloric intake. Diet therapy alone may be all that is necessary to control their symptoms. If not, hypoglycemic drugs may be prescribed. These drugs act to stimulate insulin production or make body cells more sensitive to insulin. In some instances, type II diabetics also may require injected insulin. Self-management of the disease is the treatment goal for both forms of diabetes mellitus.

Prognosis: The prognosis for an individual with diabetes mellitus is uncertain. Even a well-motivated individual following a carefully balanced treatment regimen may eventually fall victim to one or more of the life-threatening late complications of the disease. In general, though, if diabetes mellitus is detected early and the affected individual's glucose levels can be stabilized near normal levels, the diabetic can reasonably expect to live for many years with few complications. Patient motivation and knowledge of the disease process contribute significantly to the outcome of the disease. The complications affecting the prognosis may be classified as acute or late.

The *acute* complications of diabetes mellitus are metabolic crises resulting from swings in the level of blood glucose or blood pH. One such complication is *diabetic coma*. This condition may be triggered by skipping or delaying an insulin injection or consuming too much food. It also may be occasioned by a period of emotional or physical stress. Whatever the precipitating event, the physiologic process is the same. Severe hyperglycemia induces polyuria and subsequent dehydration, while severe ketosis raises blood acidity. The affected individual may experience intense thirst, abdominal pain with nausea or vomiting, and become lethargic and drowsy. From that point, the individual may lapse into coma. A person in a diabetic coma will typically exhibit deep, slow breathing, have a "fruity" breath odor (from ketones in the blood transpiring through the lungs), and exhibit red, dry skin and a dry tongue. Individuals in a diabetic coma require emergency medical treatment consisting of a large dose of insulin and IV administration of fluids and salts.

Another acute complication is *insulin shock.* This situation may be occasioned by injecting too much insulin, inadequate food intake, or excessive exercise. As a result, blood glucose levels drop below normal (hypoglycemia). The affected person may begin feeling faint, shaky, and begin to perspire. Speech disturbances, double vision, and clouded consciousness may follow. From this point, the individual may become comatose. Regrettably, coma produced by insulin shock is often difficult to distinguish from diabetic coma. A few distinguishing features of insulin-induced coma include short, shallow breathing with no characteristic breath odor and moist, clammy skin. Individuals experiencing insulin shock require emergency medical treatment consisting of intravenous administration of glucose.

The *late* complications of diabetes mellitus typically appear only after many years or even decades. Over time, the lipids that are released into the blood as a consequence of ketosis may cause arteriosclerotic disease. The subsequent impairment of blood flow in the extremities may produce intermittent claudication or even tissue necrosis and gangrene, especially in the feet and lower legs. Other arteriosclerotic complications may include coronary artery disease, cerebrovascular accident, and organic impotence in men.

The vascular system is not the only system subject to damage, though. Diabetes mellitus is a leading cause of kidney disease and renal failure, while diabetes-induced **retinopathy** is a leading cause of blindness. The nervous system also may be affected over time. CNS damage may produce numbness, paresthesias, and intermittent but severe bouts of pain. Autonomic nervous system damage may produce difficulties in swallowing, constipation or diarrhea, and neurogenic bladder problems. Diabetes mellitus also may hamper an individual's immune response, causing slow wound healing and leaving the person open to frequent infections.

Prevention: There are currently no specific measures to prevent any form of diabetes mellitus.

COMMON SYMPTOMS
OF ENDOCRINE SYSTEM DISEASES

Individuals may present with the following common symptoms, which deserve attention from health professionals:
- Mental abnormalities
- Unusual change in energy level
- Changes in skin
- Muscle atrophy

REVIEW QUESTIONS

Matching

_____ 1. Gigantism	a. Most common form of hyperthyroidism
_____ 2. Acromegaly	b. Usually caused by tumor of anterior pituitary
_____ 3. Hypopituitarism	c. Thyroid enlargement
_____ 4. Diabetes insipidus	d. Hypothyroidism in adults
_____ 5. Simple goiter	e. Hyperfunction of GH before puberty
_____ 6. Graves' disease	f. Disorder caused by insulin lack or resistance
_____ 7. Myxedema	g. Hypocalcemia
_____ 8. Hypoparathyroidism	h. Hyperfunction of GH after puberty
_____ 9. Diabetes mellitus	i. Classic symptom is polyuria
	j. Caused by excessive glucocorticosteroid hormones
	k. Hypothyroidism in children

Fill in the Blanks

1. A test likely to be ordered in a number of endocrine-related diseases which will help determine hormone levels in blood serum is _____ .
2. An inadequate dietary intake of iodine may cause _____ .
3. Thyroid crisis or "storm" is a medical emergency. Describe the symptoms.
4. An infant who sleeps too much, shows signs of apathy, stupor, dry skin, constipation, and slow talking, and has a large tongue and pot belly may suffer from _____ .
5. Classic symptoms of round, moon-shaped face with acne are an indication of _____ .

Discussion Question

Discuss the inner-relatedness of the endocrine diseases and why hyper/hypo function of one gland often affects the other endocrine glands.

ANSWERS

Matching

1. e
2. h
3. b
4. i
5. c
6. a
7. d
8. g
9. f

Fill in the Blanks

1. Radioimmunoassay

2. Endemic goiter
3. High fever, tachycardia, delirium
4. Cretinism
5. Cushing's syndrome

Discussion Question

Answers will vary.

GLOSSARY

CYANOSIS: A bluish discoloration of the skin and mucous membranes due to an increased proportion of unoxygenated hemoglobin in the blood.

DYSPHAGIA: Difficulty in swallowing or inability to swallow.

EXOPHTHALMOS: Abnormal protrusion of the eyeball.

GLYCOSURIA: The presence of sugar, particularly glucose, in the urine.

GOITROGENS: Substances that cause goiters. These occur in nature in certain foods, including turnips, rutabagas, and cabbage.

HYPERPLASIA: Excessive proliferation of normal cells.

KETOACIDOSIS: Abnormally high concentrations in the blood or tissues of organic compounds called *ketone bodies:* beta-hydroxybutyric acid, acetoacidic acid, and acetone. A condition frequently associated with diabetes mellitus.

MENORRHAGIA: Excessive menstrual flow, either in duration, quantity, or both.

POLYDIPSIA: Excessive thirst.

POLYPHAGIA: Eating abnormally large amounts of food at a meal.

POLYURIA: Excessive formation and discharge of urine.

PRURITUS: Severe itching.

RETINOPATHY: Any disease of the retina of the eye.

SYNCOPE: Temporary loss of consciousness due to inadequate blood flow to the brain; fainting.

TETANY: A nervous condition characterized by sharp, painful, periodic muscle contractions, particularly those of the extremities.

VASOPRESSIN: A hormone secreted by the hypothalamus that raises blood pressure, increases peristalsis, and promotes resorption of water by the kidney. Synthetic or prepared extracts are administered as antidiuretics. Also known as *antidiuretic hormone* (ADH).

Chapter 11
Musculoskeletal Diseases

LEARNING OBJECTIVES

Upon successful completion of this chapter, you will
- Describe three spine deformities.
- Identify the common cause for intervertebral disk herniation.
- Compare osteoporosis to osteomalacia.
- Recall the description for osteomyelitis.
- List at least three diagnostic procedures used specifically for determining bone disorders
- Illustrate at least four kinds of fractures with a simple drawing.
- Compare and contrast osteoarthritis and rheumatoid arthritis.
- Describe the treatment process for bursitis and tendinitis.
- Discuss signs and symptoms of Duchenne's muscular dystrophy.
- Identify the etiology of myasthenia gravis.
- Recall the signs and symptoms of polymyositis.
- Describe the prognosis for systemic lupus erythematosus.

INTRODUCTION

The musculoskeletal system consists of bones, joints, bursae, muscles, tendons, and ligaments. The musculoskeletal system provides physical support and protection for the organs of the body. The action of muscles and bones allows physical movement, and the marrow within the bones produces blood cells. Figure 11-1 depicts the bones of the skeleton. Figures 11-2 and 11-3 illustrate the major muscles of the body. Any pathology of this system greatly affects activities of daily living.

BONES

Deformities of the Spine: Lordosis, Kyphosis, Scoliosis

Description: *Lordosis* is an abnormal inward curvature of a portion of the spine, commonly called swayback. *Kyphosis* is an abnormal outward curvature of the spine, commonly known as *humpback* or *hunchback*. *Scoliosis* is an abnormal sideward curvature of the spine either to the left or right. Some rotation of a portion of the vertebral column also may occur. Scoliosis often occurs in combination with kyphosis and lordosis. These three spinal deformities may affect children as well as adults.

Etiology: Lordosis, kyphosis, or scoliosis may be caused by a variety of problems, including congenital spinal defects, poor posture, and disorders that cause overly rapid growth. These deformities also may result from tumors, trauma, osteoarthritis, tuberculosis, muscle diseases, and degeneration of the spine associated with aging. Lordosis, kyphosis, and scoliosis also may be idiopathic.

Signs and Symptoms: The onset of lordosis, kyphosis, and scoliosis frequently is insidious. Symptoms may eventually include chronic fatigue and backache. Scoliosis is often detected by individuals when they notice that their clothing seems longer in length on one side than the other. Or they may notice when looking in a mirror that the height of their hips and shoulders appears uneven.

Diagnostic Procedures: Physical examination and x-rays of the spine are the most commonly used procedures to detect these spinal deformities.

Treatment: Treatment will vary according to the nature and the severity of the spinal curvature and will depend on the underlying cause of the disorder. Physical therapy, exercise, and back braces may all play a role in the treatment of these conditions. Surgery may be the treatment of choice in cases of adolescent scoliosis if the curvature seriously interferes with mobility or breathing. New surgical procedures are being employed to correct back deformities by implanting metal rods to straighten the spine. Analgesics may be prescribed to alleviate the pain that frequently accompanies these disorders.

Prognosis: The prognosis of an individual with lordosis, kyphosis, or scoliosis depends on the underlying cause of the particular disease, how early it is de-

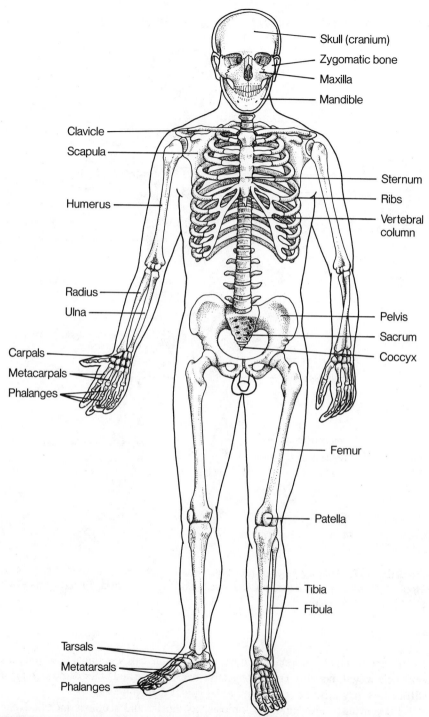

FIGURE 11–1. Bones of the human skeleton. (From Gylys, B. A. and Wedding, M. E., *Medical Terminology: A Systems Approach,* ed. 2. F. A. Davis, Philadelphia, 1988, p. 204, with permission.)

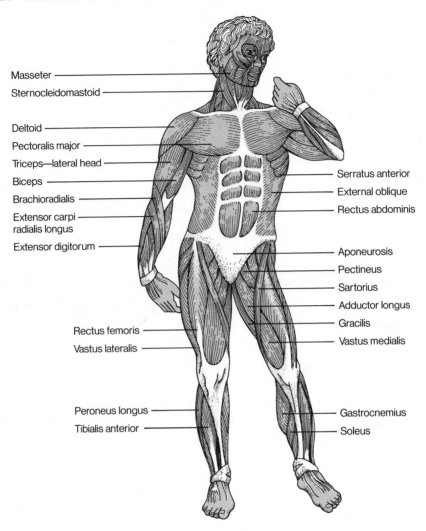

Masseter
Sternocleidomastoid

Deltoid
Pectoralis major
Triceps—lateral head
Biceps
Brachioradialis
Extensor carpi radialis longus
Extensor digitorum

Serratus anterior
External oblique
Rectus abdominis

Aponeurosis
Pectineus
Sartorius
Adductor longus
Gracilis
Vastus medialis

Rectus femoris
Vastus lateralis

Peroneus longus
Tibialis anterior

Gastrocnemius
Soleus

FIGURE 11–2. Anterior view of muscles. (From Gylys, B. A. and Wedding, M. E., *Medical Terminology: A Systems Approach,* ed. 2. F. A. Davis, Philadelphia, 1988, p. 210, with permission.)

tected, and whether it responds to treatment. In some cases, a spinal deformity may only be arrested, not corrected. Congestive heart failure and other cardiopulmonary difficulties may arise as complications of spinal deformities.

Prevention: Prevention of lordosis, kyphosis, and scoliosis includes maintaining good posture. Scoliosis screening is mandated by law in public schools in some states.

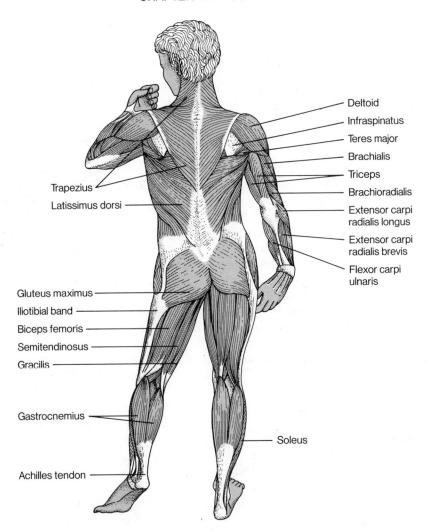

FIGURE 11–3. Posterior view of muscles. (From Gylys, B. A. and Wedding, M. E., *Medical Terminology: A Systems Approach,* ed. 2. F. A. Davis, Philadelphia, 1988, p. 211, with permission.)

Herniated Intervertebral Disk

Description: An *intervertebral disk* is a saclike mass of cartilage. One is found between each of the 33 vertebrae. Within each intervertebral disk is the nucleus pulposus, a soft, gelatinous mass that helps each disk cushion the movements of the vertebrae. A *herniated intervertebral disk* is the rupture of the nucleus pulposus through the wall of the disk and into the spinal canal where it may press on spinal nerves causing pain and disability. The condition is commonly called a *slipped disk*. The most common sites for herniated disks are between the fourth and fifth lumbar vertebrae or the fifth lumbar and the first sacral vertebrae. The condition is more common in males.

Etiology: A herniated intervertebral disk usually is caused by spinal trauma from a fall, straining, or heavy lifting. The herniation may occur at the time of the trauma or sometime later.

Signs and Symptoms: Symptoms depend on the particular site of herniation, but severe back pain that worsens with motion is common. **Paresthesia** and restricted mobility of the neck often occur. The sciatic nerve may be painful upon pressure.

Diagnostic Procedures: A thorough patient history is important to eliminate other causes of back pain. The diagnosis is confirmed if the individual complains of "sciatic pain" when a straight-leg-raising test is performed. Spinal x-rays and CT scans may be ordered, too. Myelography may show the point of spinal compression caused by the herniated disk.

Treatment: Bed rest, heat applied to the affected portion of the spine, and **salicylate analgesics** may be prescribed. Traction of the lower extremities and a back brace may be beneficial in the event of a herniated lumbosacral disk. A cervical halter or a cervical collar may be used to treat a slipped cervical disk. If conservative treatment is not successful, surgical removal of the herniated disk may be necessary.

Prognosis: With surgery, the prognosis is improved.

Prevention: Following proper lifting techniques may help prevent herniated intervertebral disks.

Osteoporosis

Description: *Osteoporosis* is a metabolic bone disease affecting 5 to 10 million Americans. This disease especially affects women who are 50 years of age or older, postmenopausal, small-boned, or who come from a Northern European, especially Scandinavian, background. The total bone mass for someone affected by osteoporosis is less than expected for their age and sex. The proportion of bone mineral to bone matrix is normal, however, and there usually is no detectable abnormality of bone composition.

Etiology: Osteoporosis may be (1) idiopathic, which is infrequent and does not respond well to therapy, (2) senile, postmenopausal or involutional, which is usually due to lack of estrogen and is the most common form of osteoporosis, and (3) juvenile, which is a rare form, with its onset in puberty.[1]

Signs and Symptoms: Symptoms include bone pain, especially in the lower back and in the weight-bearing bones; spontaneous fractures, especially vertebrae at the midthoracic level or thoracolumbar junction; and loss of height.

Diagnostic Procedures: Blood tests are run to measure levels of phosphorus, alkaline phosphatase, total protein, albumin, and creatine. Excretion of calcium, phosphate, creatinine, and hydroxyproline also may be monitored through urinalysis. X-rays are helpful but may be difficult to interpret in cases of osteoporosis because the density of skeletal parts may appear to be similar to soft tissue. A bone scintiscan and bone biopsy may be ordered if more specific diagnostic data are necessary.

Treatment: The treatment varies depending on the cause. Increased dietary calcium, phosphate supplements, and multivitamins may be prescribed. In postmenopausal osteoporosis, estrogen therapy may be attempted. Exercise may help minimize osteoporosis by slowing loss of mineral calcium, but if the bones have become brittle, exercise of any kind may be prohibited. Analgesics and muscle relaxants may be needed if pain or muscle spasms are a problem. Frequent rest periods are advised if bone pain is severe.

Prognosis: The prognosis is mostly dictated by the cause. Osteoporosis can cause permanent disability if not arrested.

Prevention: Prevention includes a calcium-rich diet. A person at risk may need to take more calcium, a multivitamin, and exercise daily.

Osteomalacia and Rickets

Description: *Osteomalacia* is a disease in which there is defective mineralization of the bone-forming tissue. The disease is characterized by increasing softness of the bones, so that they become flexible and brittle, causing deformities. When the disease occurs in children, it is called *rickets*.

Etiology: Osteomalacia is caused by insufficient bodily stores or ineffective utilization of vitamin D, a substance that plays a central role in the physiologic process of bone formation. Inadequate dietary intake of vitamin D may cause the disorder, as may inadequate exposure to sunlight, so that the body cannot synthesize its own vitamin D. Other causes include intestinal malabsorption of vitamin D or defective metabolism of the substance. Conditions such as chronic acidosis, chronic renal failure, and other renal diseases or certain drugs and toxins also may cause osteomalacia.

Signs and Symptoms: Symptoms may include mild, aching bone pain, loss of height, and muscular weakness. Bending, flattening, or deformation of bones is common in osteomalacia.

Diagnostic Procedures: Laboratory tests include blood analysis of phosphate, alkaline phosphatase, total protein, 25-hydroxyvitamin D_3, albumin, and creatinine. Urinalysis to determine levels of urine calcium, phosphorus, and creatinine may be performed. Skeletal x-rays will typically reveal zones of decalcification, called *pseudofractures,* appearing along the surface of certain bones, especially on the scapula, the rim of the pelvis, or the neck of the femur. Ultimately, a bone biopsy may be needed.

Treatment: The treatment is dependent on the cause. Treatment may consist of vitamin D supplementation, possibly in conjunction with phosphorus supplementation, and a diet high in calcium. Analgesics may be prescribed to alleviate pain. Because the bones may be soft, the patient may need to sit or lie down more frequently. If the disease is caused by deficient absorption or metabolism of vitamin D, treatment of the underlying problem must accompany vitamin D supplementation.

Prognosis: Although osteomalacia is potentially curable, the underlying cause influences the prognosis.

Prevention: Ensuring an adequate dietary vitamin D intake is necessary for prevention of osteomalacia.

Osteomyelitis

Description: *Osteomyelitis* is infection of the bone-forming tissue. Such infections are characterized by inflammation, edema, and circulatory congestion of the bone marrow. As the infection progresses, pus may form and sustained inflammatory pressure may cause fracturing of small pieces of bone. Osteomyelitis usually begins as an acute infection, but it may evolve into a chronic condition. The disease is more common in children.

Etiology: Osteomyelitis is most often caused by bacterial infection, particularly by *Staphylococcus aureus,* although other viruses and fungi also may cause the condition. The infectious microorganisms may reach the bone marrow through the blood, by spreading from infected adjacent tissue, or be introduced directly into the bone tissue following physical trauma or surgery. Diabetes mellitus may predispose an individual to osteomyelitis, as may the presence of prosthetic hardware (screws, plates, rods) within the bone.

Signs and Symptoms: Specific symptoms depend on which bone or bones are affected and the virulence of the infecting microorganisms. Generalized symptoms may include the sudden onset of fever, chills, malaise, sweating, pain, and tenderness and swelling over the affected bone. Both the acute and chronic forms of osteomyelitis may exhibit the same clinical picture, although the chronic form may persist for years before it is detected following a flareup due to minor trauma.

Diagnostic Procedures: Blood cultures or aspiration and culture of fluid from the infection site are essential to isolate the causative microorganism. X-rays may prove helpful in determining the site and extent of the infection.

Treatment: Bed rest and parenterally administered antibiotics often suffice. If not, surgical drainage to remove pus and dead bone may be necessary. Immobilization of the affected part and analgesics may be required.

Prognosis: With today's therapeutic options, osteomyelitis frequently resolves favorably. If the acute form of the disease progresses to a chronic form, the prognosis is poor.

Prevention: Contamination during surgery or following trauma must be prevented so that the disease does not have a chance to develop.

Paget's Disease (Osteitis Deformans)

Description: *Paget's disease* is a chronic skeletal disease. It is characterized by an initial phase marked by a high rate of bone turnover. Bone is rapidly resorbed and replaced with bone of a course, irregular consistency. Consequently, the affected bone becomes thicker but softer. A later phase of the disease is characterized by the replacement of normal bone marrow with highly vascular fibrous tissue. The disease may occur in only one bone or at numerous sites throughout the skeletal system. The disease usually appears in individuals over 40 years of age, and it becomes increasingly common with advancing age.

Etiology: The cause of Paget's disease is not known.

Signs and Symptoms: Many individuals with Paget's disease are asymptomatic. The nature of symptoms that do appear depends on the extent of the disease and which bone or bones are affected. Some individuals may first notice a swelling or other deformity in one of the long bones of the body or a need to increase their hat size if the bones of the skull are involved. The gradual onset of dull but persistent pain around the area of the affected bone may be the first symptom in some. The pain may become severe enough to be disabling, however. Gradual hearing loss may occur in the event of involvement of the ossicles or nearby skull bones.

Diagnostic Procedures: X-rays, bone scintiscans, and bone marrow biopsies may help diagnose the disease. Blood analysis indicating a high serum concentration of alkaline phosphatase and urinalysis revealing a high concentration of hydroxyproline indicate the high rate of bone turnover that is characteristic of the disease.

Treatment: A mild, asymptomatic case of Paget's disease may require no treatment. Treatment for more severe cases may include a high-protein, high-calcium diet and vitamin D supplementation. Aspirin may be prescribed for pain relief and to suppress the level of activity of the disease. Treatment with certain anti-inflammatory drugs and cytotoxic agents may be attempted. The use of calcitonins, hormone derivatives that prevent bone loss, also has been beneficial in many cases.

Prognosis: If the disease is mild, the prognosis is good. For more severe forms, however, the prognosis is poor. Complications may include frequent fractures, hypercalcemia, kidney stones, deafness, blindness, and spinal cord injuries. An especially deadly complication is bone sarcoma.

Prevention: There are no preventive measures for Paget's disease.

Fractures

Description: A *fracture* is a break or crack in a bone. Types of fractures include the following:

■ *Closed fracture*. A break in the bone with no external wound to the skin.

- *Open or compound fracture.* A break in the bone in which there is an open wound leading down to the site of the fracture or in which a piece of broken bone protrudes through the skin.
- *Greenstick fracture.* One in which the bone is partially bent and split, as a green stick or twig does when bent. This type of fracture occurs most frequently in children or among adults with soft bones.
- *Comminuted fracture.* One in which the bone is broken or splintered into pieces, often with fragments embedded in surrounding tissue.
- *Impacted fracture.* One in which the bone is broken with one end forced into the interior of the other.

Figure 11–4 illustrates major forms of fractures.

Etiology: Bone fractures are usually caused by physical trauma. A host of pathologic processes, though, may occasion a bone fracture after only minimal trauma or following normal muscular contractions. Examples of diseases or conditions that may induce fractures include bone neoplasms, osteoporosis, Paget's disease, osteomalacia, osteomyelitis, and nutritional and vitamin deficiency disorders.

Signs and Symptoms: Common symptoms of fractures include acute pain at the affected site, muscle spasm, and perhaps hemorrhage and shock. Bone may protrude through the skin.

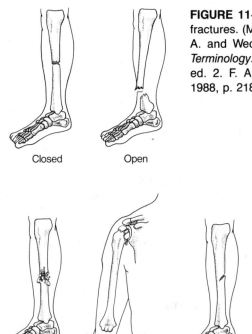

Closed   Open

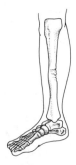

FIGURE 11–4. Common types of fractures. (Modified from Gylys, B. A. and Wedding, M. E., *Medical Terminology: A Systems Approach,* ed. 2. F. A. Davis, Philadelphia, 1988, p. 218.)

Comminuted   Impacted   Incomplete   Greenstick

Diagnostic Procedures: X-rays are used to locate the fracture and determine its severity. A bone scintiscan may be ordered to detect hairline fractures.

Treatment: Immobilization of the affected parts and control of any bleeding are paramount. Open or closed reduction may be needed to place the parts in their normal position for proper healing. *Open reduction* is accomplished by surgery, followed by external fixation such as casting, or by internal fixation with the use of metal plates, screws, or rods. *Closed reduction* is manipulation and casting without a surgical incision. Traction may be used, especially for fractures of the leg bones until healing takes place or until internal fixation can be performed. Rib fractures may require no treatment, or the chest may be bandaged or taped for support and pain control. Analgesics or muscle relaxants may be ordered to ease the pain accompanying many types of fractures.

Prognosis: The prognosis depends on the severity of the fracture and the age of the individual. The existence of an underlying pathologic process worsens the prognosis by complicating the healing process. Complications can occur in any type of fracture and may include embolism, infection, delayed union, or nonunion of the fracture or complications resulting from immobilization.

Prevention: The best prevention of fractures is conscientious adherence to safety at work and in play.

JOINTS

Osteoarthritis

Description: *Osteoarthritis* is a chronic inflammatory process of the joints and bones resulting in degeneration of joint cartilage and subsequent **hypertrophy** of the surrounding bone. The disease may affect any joint in the body but especially weight-bearing ones such as the knee and hip. It is the most common form of arthritis, and it occurs with equal frequency in both sexes, especially among the elderly.

Etiology: The cause of osteoarthritis is not known, but autoimmune factors may play a role.

Signs and Symptoms: The onset of osteoarthritis typically is insidious. The first symptom may include joint pain that usually is relieved by rest. There may be stiffness, especially in the morning, and aching during weather changes. There usually is minimal inflammation. **Crepitation** may be heard on joint movement. Deformity may be minimal in some cases, but bony enlargement can occur.

Diagnostic Procedures: Skeletal x-rays from various angles may be necessary to diagnose the changes in the joint and bone.

Treatment: Because osteoarthritis cannot be cured, the goal of treatment is to minimize pain and inflammation and to maintain joint function. Various analgesics and anti-inflammatory drugs may be prescribed. Physical activity restrictions, rest, and the use of crutches or a cane may be necessary. Local heat, paraffin application of the hands, and weight reduction may be helpful. If the condition is severe, various forms of orthopedic surgery may help to relieve pain and improve joint function. The replacement of hip and knee joints with prosthetic devices also may be attempted.

Prognosis: Prognosis depends on the site affected and the severity of the disease. Disability can range from minor to severe. The progression of osteoarthritis varies.

Prevention: There is no known prevention.

Rheumatoid Arthritis

Description: *Rheumatoid arthritis* (RA) is a chronic, systemic, inflammatory disease affecting the synovial membranes of multiple joints. The disease has the capacity to destroy cartilage, erode bone, and deform joints. The course of the disease is characterized by spontaneous remissions and unpredictable exacerbations. It occurs most frequently in females, with the prevalence of the disease increasing with advancing age.

Etiology: The cause of RA is not known. Research suggests that some may be genetically predisposed to acquiring the disease.

Signs and Symptoms: RA develops insidiously among most affected individuals. The earliest signs and symptoms may include malaise, persistent low-grade fever, fatigue, and weight loss. Joint pain and stiffness gradually emerge as the principal symptoms, usually affecting the joints of the fingers, wrists, knees, ankles, and toes in a symmetrical pattern. The pain is characteristically aggravated by movement of the affected joints. In advanced cases of RA affecting the hands, the interphalangeal joints are swollen, edematous, and have a characteristic tapered appearance.

Diagnostic Procedures: A positive rheumatoid factor blood test is diagnostic in most cases. Other useful laboratory tests include antinuclear antibody, lupus erythematosus cell, serum protein electrophoresis, ESR, CBC, and synovial fluid analysis. X-rays are useful, too.

Treatment: The primary objectives of treatment are reduction of inflammation and pain, preservation of joint function, and prevention of joint deformity.[2] Rest, salicylates (particularly aspirin), and physical therapy generally are prescribed. Advanced rheumatoid arthritis may require surgical repair of the hip, knee, or hand joints.

Prognosis: The course of the disease is generally unpredictable. Permanent spontaneous remission may occur with return to normal function or less disability than previously. However, the disease generally is progressive with some degree of consequent deformity. Only a small percentage suffer total disability.

Prevention: There is no known prevention.

Gout

Description: *Gout* is a chronic disorder of uric acid metabolism. It is manifested as acute, episodic attacks of a form of arthritis in which crystals of uric acid compounds appear in the synovial fluid of joints. The disease also is marked by deposits of other urate compounds called *tophi* in and around the joints of the extremities, a situation that frequently leads to joint deformity and disability. Gout is also characterized by hyperuricemia, renal dysfunction, and kidney stones. The disease affects more men than women, usually appearing after the age of 30. Among women, gout usually appears after menopause.

Etiology: The cause of gout may be metabolic, renal, or both. *Metabolic gout* is inherited, and several possible genetic factors have the potential to produce the condition. In this form of gout, the body produces more uric acid than can be cleared by the kidneys into the urine. *Renal gout* is caused by one of many possible renal dysfunctions. In this form of gout, the body may produce normal levels of uric acid, but the action of the kidneys is insufficient to clear the compound from the blood.

Signs and Symptoms: The classic manifestation of gout is the sudden onset of excruciating joint pain, usually affecting the joints of the big toe. Other joints may be involved as well, especially those of the feet, ankles, and knees. The pain generally reaches a peak after several hours and then gradually subsides. An acute attack also may be accompanied by mild fever and chills. The individual is characteristically free of any symptoms between attacks. As the disease progresses, the interval between acute attacks diminishes, and tophi may appear around the affected joints or at other points of the body.

Diagnostic Procedures: Identification of urate crystals in joint fluid or the presence of tophi in and around joints is indicative of gout. Urinalysis will almost always reveal hyperuricemia. Other laboratory tests include ESR and WBC. Skeletal x-rays may be used to assess the degree of damage to the affected joints.

Treatment: Treatment of an acute attack may involve bed rest, immobilization of the affected part, local applications of heat or cold, and analgesics. Anti-inflammatory agents such as colchicine may be prescribed to alleviate the symptoms of an acute attack or to lessen the likelihood of a recurrence. Management of gout also may involve attempts to control the rate of uric acid formation by having the individual follow a low-purine diet. (Purines are end products of protein metabolism and are broken down to form uric acid.) In order to promote uric acid clearance by the kidneys, individuals with gout will usually be encouraged to take fluids frequently and also may have to take various antihyperuricemic agents.

Prognosis: Because of modern treatment procedures, gout is seldom as permanently disabling as it once was. Treatment measures may need to be maintained indefinitely. Complications include hypertension, kidney stones, and renal damage.

Prevention: There are not specific preventative measures for gout, but a low-purine diet and maintaining adequate hydration may lessen the chance of the disease occurring among those known to be at risk.

MUSCLES AND CONNECTIVE TISSUE

Sprains and Strains

Description: A *sprain* is the tearing or stretching of a ligament surrounding a joint. A *strain* is a tearing or stretching of a tendon or a muscle.

Etiology: Sprains and strains may be caused by trauma or result from excessive use of a body part.

Signs and Symptoms: Symptoms are localized pain and inflammation, discoloration at the site of the injury, and loss of mobility. Sprains and strains caused by chronic overuse of a ligament, muscle, or tendon will typically cause stiffness, soreness, and tenderness, whereas a sharp, transient pain may result when either condition is acute.

Diagnostic Procedures: A medical history revealing recent physical activities with the potential for causing sprains or strains may suggest the diagnosis. X-rays to rule out the possibility of a fracture may be necessary.

Treatment: Sprains and strains usually require elevating and resting the injured part. Cold compresses may be applied to the affected site to lessen swelling. Depending on the severity of the injury, immobilization of the affected part may be attempted by applying an elastic wrap or soft cast. Analgesics may be necessary to control pain or discomfort. Surgical repair may be indicated if the injury heals improperly or if a rupture results.

Prognosis: With proper treatment, healing of a strain or sprain generally occurs within 2 to 4 weeks.

Prevention: Prevention of these injuries includes warming up when preparing for exercise or physical activity, following safety precautions, and recognizing personal physical limitations.

Bursitis

Description: *Bursitis* is inflammation of a bursa, a thin-walled sac lined with synovial tissue which facilitates movement of tendons and muscles over bony prominences. Common forms of bursitis include subacromial (shoulder); subdeltoid (arm); olecranon (elbow), which is commonly referred to as *miner's* or *tennis elbow;* prepatellar (knee), which is referred to as *housemaid's knee;* and ischial (pelvis), which is commonly referred to as *weaver's bottom.*

Etiology: Bursitis may be caused by excessive frictional forces, trauma, systemic diseases such as gout or rheumatoid arthritis, or infection.

Signs and Symptoms: The classic symptom is tenderness or pain, especially on movement of the affected part. Restricted movement, swelling, and edema at the site are common.

Diagnostic Procedures: The patient's clinical picture and a medical history may be all that are necessary for diagnosis. X-rays occasionally may show calcific deposits at the affected site.

Treatment: Treatment may include local heat, immobilization of the affected part, analgesics, nonsteroidal anti-inflammatory agents, and local steroid injections. Active mobilization to prevent adhesions will prove helpful after the acute pain subsides.

Prognosis: The prognosis is good if the bursitis is treated as soon as possible. Bursitis may become chronic, in which case activity restrictions may be required or surgical intervention may be attempted to remove calcification. If infection results, surgical drainage or aspiration may be necessary, followed by antibiotic therapy.

Prevention: Prevention of bursitis includes avoiding trauma and strenuous exercise that might stress or pressure a joint.

Tendonitis

Description: *Tendonitis* is inflammation of a tendon or the tendon-muscle attachments to bone, usually in the shoulder rotator cuff, hip, Achilles tendon, or hamstring. The condition is characterized by inflammation, fibrosis and tears in the tendon.

Etiology: Tendonitis generally results from trauma, another musculoskeletal disease such as rheumatoid arthritis, postural misalignment, or hypermobility.

Signs and Symptoms: Symptoms usually include dull aching in the affected tendon area and severe pain when the area is moved. At night, the pain often interferes with sleep.

Diagnostic Procedures: A medical history indicating physical strain or injury and the patient's clinical picture generally are sufficient for diagnosis. X-rays may be normal or show bony fragments or calcium deposits. An arthrogram may establish the diagnosis.

Treatment: Treatment of tendonitis may include rest or immobilization of the affected area, nonsteroid anti-inflammatory drugs, local steroid injections, and physical therapy.

Prognosis: Tendonitis usually responds to medical treatment and a change in physical activities. If untreated, it can become disabling. Chronic tendonitis may require surgical intervention to remove calcium deposits.

Prevention: Prevention of tendonitis includes avoidance of strenuous exercise and trauma that would stress or pressure a tendon.

Duchenne's Muscular Dystrophy

Description: *Duchenne's muscular dystrophy* is a congenital disorder characterized by progressive bilateral wasting of skeletal muscles, but it does not include neural or sensory defects. It affects males exclusively, about 4 in 100,000.[3]

Etiology: The disease is the result of a genetic defect that is usually inherited, but it may be due to a newly acquired mutation. The exact mechanism by which the genetic defect produces muscle wasting is not known.

Signs and Symptoms: Manifestations of Duchenne's muscular dystrophy begin between the ages of 3 and 5 years. The disease first affects the leg and pelvic muscles before spreading to involuntary muscles. The affected child may have a characteristic waddling gait, engage in toe-walking, and may suffer from lordosis or other spinal deformities. The child may have difficulty running and climbing stairs and may tend to fall easily. Muscle deterioration is progressive, and **contractures** typically develop. Children with this disease are frequently mentally impaired.

Diagnostic Procedures: A family history of the disease together with the clinical picture of characteristic symptoms suggests the diagnosis. A muscle biopsy showing characteristic connective tissue and fat deposits will confirm the diagnosis. Electromyography can rule out muscle atrophy that is neurologic in origin. Tests of urine creatinine and serum levels of CPK, LDH, and transaminase will usually be ordered.

Treatment: No known treatment is successful in curing Duchenne's muscular dystrophy, but procedures to correct or preserve mobility are helpful. These include orthopedic appliances, exercise, physical therapy, and surgery.

Prognosis: The prognosis is poor for a child with Duchenne's muscular dystrophy. Children with this condition are usually confined to a wheelchair by the ages of 9 to 12. Within 10 to 15 years of the onset of the disease, death commonly results from cardiac or respiratory complications or infections.

Prevention: Carriers of the genetic defect known to cause muscular dystrophy may want to receive genetic counseling regarding the risks of transmitting the disease.

Myasthenia Gravis

Description: *Myasthenia gravis* is a chronic, progressive neuromuscular disease. Curiously enough, neither the motor nerves nor the muscles themselves are directly affected by this disease. Rather, myasthenia gravis is due to the disappearance of receptors for the neurotransmitter **acetylcholine**, the substance that transfers a nerve impulse from the nerve ending across to the muscle fiber itself. The condition occurs more frequently in women than in men and has its highest incidence between the ages of 20 and 40. *Thymomas*, i.e., tumors of the thymus gland, accompany myasthenia gravis in approximately 15 percent of cases.

Etiology: The cause of this disease is not known, but it appears to be an acquired autoimmune disorder in which antibodies are produced that destroy the acetylcholine receptors.

Signs and Symptoms: Onset may be sudden and most affected individuals will notice drooping eyelids and double vision as the first signs that something is wrong. Since muscles innervated by the cranial nerves mostly are affected (face, lips, tongue, neck, and throat), a blank expression, nasal regurgitation of fluids, difficulty swallowing, **ptosis**, and a bobbing head may result.

Skeletal muscle weakness and fatigability occur. Muscle weakness typically occurs later in the day or after strenuous exercise. Although short rest periods characteristically restore muscle function, the muscle weakness is progressive in myasthenia gravis, and more muscles will be affected until paralysis occurs. Menses, emotional stress, prolonged exposure to sunlight or cold, and infections will heighten the symptoms. Respiratory muscle weakness or myasthenic crisis (sudden inability to swallow and respiratory distress) may be severe enough to require mechanical ventilation.

Diagnostic Procedures: The improvement of muscle strength after resting or following injection of anticholinesterase drugs strongly suggests the diagnosis. Electromyography with repeated neural stimulation may be used to confirm the diagnosis. Serologic tests to detect the presence of antibodies characteristically present in myasthenia gravis also may be performed.

Treatment: Treatment is symptomatic and supportive. Anticholinesterase drugs are effective against fatigue and muscle weakness, but they become less effective as the disease progresses. Thymectomy is being used with some success. Corticosteroids may be beneficial. It is important to guard against myasthenic crisis and to treat it with emergency measures should it occur.

Prognosis: Unexplained, spontaneous remissions may occur, but usually the disease is a lifelong condition with periodic remissions, exacerbations, and day-to-day fluctuations.

Prevention: There is no known prevention.

Polymyositis

Description: *Polymyositis* is a chronic, progressive disease of connective tissue characterized by edema, inflammation, and degeneration of skeletal muscles. When the disease occurs with skin involvement, it is called *dermatomyositis*. Polymyositis appears twice as frequently in women as in men, usually occurring between the ages of 30 and 60.

Etiology: Polymyositis is an idiopathic disease. Viral and autoimmune etiologies have been proposed but not confirmed. Nearly a third of cases are associated with other connective-tissue disorders such as rheumatoid arthritis and systemic lupus erythematosus. Other cases, particularly among the elderly, are associated with malignancies.

Signs and Symptoms: Polymyositis usually develops insidiously over a period of a few months to a few years. The most frequent initial manifestation of the disease is muscle weakness in the hips and thighs. Consequently, the affected individual will often report difficulty in ascending or descending stairs or difficulty in rising from a sitting or kneeling position. Occasionally, the disease will localize in specific muscle groups, weakening only the neck, shoulder, or quadricep muscles. Later symptoms include dysphagia and respiratory difficulties. In rare instances, the disease may appear as an acute condition, with the rapid onset and development of the symptoms noted.

When the disease develops as dermatomyositis, the previously mentioned symptoms may be preceded or accompanied by characteristic dermatologic changes. These include the appearance of a telltale lilac-colored rash on the eyelids, the bridge of the nose, and the cheeks, forehead, chest, elbows, and knees. The rash-covered portions of the body may itch severely. Dermatomyositis also may be accompanied by edema around the eye sockets.

Diagnostic Procedures: A muscle biopsy may reveal tissue changes characteristic of polymyositis, such as muscle fiber necrosis, infiltration of the muscle tissue with inflammatory cells (leukocytes), and patterns of tissue degeneration and regeneration. Blood testing will typically indicate increased serum levels of enzymes normally present in skeletal muscles, such as CPK, SGOT, LDH, and SGPT. The ESR also will usually be elevated. Evidence of muscle destruction includes the presence of myoglobin in the urine. ECG may indicate cardiac abnormalities.

Treatment: High doses of corticosteroid drugs are often administered to bring the disease under control, followed by lower maintainence doses over a period of years. Cytotoxic drugs also may be used to lower the number of inflammatory cells affecting the muscles. Physiotherapy and physical rehabilitation to regain muscle function are important components of the treatment process.

Prognosis: The prognosis is variable. Roughly half of those affected by polymyositis recover within 5 years and can discontinue therapy. Others must remain on drug therapy indefinitely. Still others die from acute cardiac, pulmonary, or renal complications.

Prevention: There is no specific prevention for polymyositis.

Systemic Lupus Erythematosus (SLE)

Description: *Systemic lupus erythematosus* (SLE) is a chronic, inflammatory connective-tissue disorder in which cells and tissues throughout the body are damaged by a variety of autoantibodies and immune complexes. The disease affects women in 90 percent of cases.

Etiology: The cause of the autoimmune response that characterizes SLE is not known. Genetic factors may predispose an individual to the disease, as well as environmental and hormonal factors. Stress, overexposure to ultraviolet light, immunization reactions, and pregnancy are events that may precipitate the condition. Certain drugs also have the capacity to induce an SLE-like syndrome.

Signs and Symptoms: Because SLE can affect any part of the body, a host of symptoms are possible. The most common and striking manifestation of the disease, however, is the "butterfly rash" (Figure 11–5), which may be found on the face, neck, and scalp. Similar rashes may appear on other body surfaces, especially on exposed areas. There also may be photosensitivity of the skin, joint and muscle pain, joint deformities, malaise, fever, anorexia, and weight loss. Other signs and symptoms include oral or nasopharyngeal ulcerations, **alopecia**, pleuritis or pericarditis, and **Raynaud's phenomenon**.

Diagnostic Procedures: CBC with differential, platelet count, ESR, serum electrophoresis, antinuclear antibody, anti-DNA, and lupus erythematosus (LE)

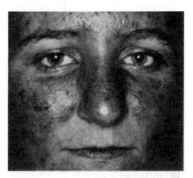

FIGURE 11-5. Butterfly rash of SLE. (From Lazarus, G. S. and Goldsmith, L. A., *Diagnosis of Skin Disease.* F. A. Davis, Philadelphia, 1980, p. 164, with permission.)

tests may be done. LE cells (polymorphonuclear leukocytes) often will be found in the bone marrow. The anti-DNA test, which detects a particular autoantibody, is the most specific test for SLE, but it must be performed while the disease is in its active stage.

Treatment: The mild stage of the disease requires only anti-inflammatory agents, including aspirin. Skin lesions will require topical treatment such as corticosteroid creams. Corticosteroid drugs remain the treatment of choice to control SLE, either for acute generalized exacerbations or for exacerbations of the disease localized to vital organ systems. Photosensitive patients should wear protective clothing when in the sun and use an effective sunscreen agent.

Prognosis: The prognosis improves with early detection and careful treatment, but it remains poor for patients who develop cardiovascular, renal, or neurologic complications or serious bacterial infections. There is a high death rate, usually within 5 years of onset.

Prevention: There are no specific preventive measures for SLE.

Neoplasms

Primary neoplasms of the musculoskeletal system are uncommon, but when they do occur, the prognosis usually is poor. Primary malignancy may arise from osseous tissue. These tumors include the following: (1) osteogenic sarcoma, which primarily affects the long bones of the body; (2) chondrosarcoma, which also affects the long bones but which tends to metastasize more slowly than osteogenic sarcoma; and (3) malignant giant-cell tumor, which is common at the ends of long bones, especially near the knee and lower radius.

Nonosseous tumors include fibrosarcoma, chondroma, and Ewing's sarcoma, a malignant tumor originating from bone marrow, usually in long bones or the pelvis.

Bone pain is the classic symptom. The pain is dull, localized, and may be more intense at night. A bone biopsy, bone x-ray, and bone scintiscan may be necessary for diagnosis. The treatments of choice are radiation and surgery, which usually involves amputation. With any amputation, rehabilitation therapy is necessary.

COMMON SYMPTOMS
OF MUSCULOSKELETAL DISEASES

Individuals may present with the following common symptoms, which deserve attention from health professionals:

- Pain
- Tenderness and swelling
- Malaise, weakness, and fatigue
- Fever
- Obvious bone deformation, including spontaneous fractures
- Inflammation
- Stiffness
- Weight loss

REFERENCES

1. Mundy, C. R., Differential Diagnosis of Osteopenia, *Hospital Practice*, November 1978, pp. 65–66.
2. Krupp, M. A., and M. J. Cnatton (eds.), *Current Medical Diagnosis and Treatment, 1984,* Lange Medical Publications, Los Altos, Calif., 1984, p. 502.
3. D'Agostino, J., T. F. Dagi, and L. Pelczynski, *Diseases,* Nursing '83 Books. Intermed Communications, Inc., Springhouse, Pa., 1983, p. 681.

REVIEW QUESTIONS

Matching

_____ 1. Posterior angulation of spine; roundback   a. Lordosis

_____ 2. Lateral curvature of spine   b. Kyphosis

_____ 3. Spinal curvature with a forward convexity;   c. Scoliosis
      swayback   d. Herniated intervertebral

_____ 4. Ruptured or slipped disk   disk

True/False

T F 1. Osteomyelitis is a pyogenic infection.

T F 2. Osteomyelitis involves both the bone marrow cavity and the bone itself.

T F 3. Paget's disease is a metabolic bone disease.

T F 4. Paget's disease is also called osteitis deformans.

T F 5. Osteoarthritis is an acute degeneration and deterioration of joint cartilage.

T F 6. Rheumatoid arthritis is a chronic, systemic inflammatory disease affecting joints.

T F 7. Gouty arthritis is a metabolic disease affecting more men than women.

Short Answer

1. Name and define five types of fractures:
   a.
   b.
   c.
   d.
   e.
2. What is the difference between a sprain and a strain?
3. Compare and contrast osteoporosis and osteomalacia.

Multiple Choice

Circle all the correct responses.

1. Duchenne's muscular dystrophy is
   a. identified with a poor prognosis.
   b. progressive bilateral wasting of skeletal muscles.
   c. a disease which first affects leg and pelvic muscles.
   d. diagnosed by muscle biopsy.

2. Myasthenia gravis is
   a. a failure in transmission of muscle impulses at the neuromuscular junction.
   b. a condition in which there is too much acetylcholine released at the junction.
   c. diagnosed by muscle biopsy.
   d. a disease that can be cured and prevented.

ANSWERS

Matching

1. b
2. c
3. a
4. d

True/False

1. T
2. T
3. F
4. T
5. F
6. T
7. T

Short Answer

1. a. Closed fracture: break in the bone that does not break the skin.
   b. Compound or open fracture: more than one break in bone with a break in the skin.
   c. Greenstick fracture: an incomplete break in the bone where the bone bends and splits like green wood.

    d. Comminuted fracture: broken or crushed in small pieces and fragments may be embedded in surrounding tissue.

    e. Impacted fracture: one bone fragment is forced into another.

2. A sprain is a tear or stretching of a ligament, whereas a strain is a tear or stretching of a tendon or a muscle.

3. Both are metabolic bone diseases; both have similiar diagnostic tests to include serum calcium, phosphate, alkaline phosphatase, total protein, urine calcium, phosphorus, and creatinine. X-rays and bone scintiscans may be ordered. Osteoporosis: Affects mostly women, 50 years or older, postmenopausal, small-boned; northern European. Total bone mass is less than expected. Proportion of bone mineral to bone matrix is normal with no detectable abnormality of bone composition. Causes are idiopathic, senile, or juvenile. Bone pain, especially low back; spontaneous fractures; loss of height. Osteomalacia: Vitamin D deficiency; often familial. Osteoid tissue increases; calcification does not occur. Mild, aching bone pain; loss of height; muscular weakness; pseudofractures.

Multiple Choice

1. All are correct.
2. All are incorrect.

GLOSSARY

ACETYLCHOLINE: A neurotransmitter substance that transfers nerve impulses across neuromuscular junctions, stimulating contraction of muscle fibers.

ALOPECIA: Absence or loss of hair, especially on the head.

ANALGESIC: A drug or agent that relieves pain.

CREPITATION: A crackling sound, such as that produced by the grating of ends of a broken bone.

CONTRACTURE: Permanent shortening or contracting of a muscle, often producing physical distortion or deformity.

HYPERTROPHY: An increase in the volume or size of an organ or other body structure produced entirely by an increase in the size of existing cells, not by an increase in the number of cells.

PARESTHESIA: Sensation of numbness, prickling, or tingling.

PTOSIS: Draping or drooping of an organ or part, such as the upper eyelid from paralysis or the visceral organs from weakness of the abdominal muscles.

RAYNAUD'S PHENOMENON: Intermittent interruptions of blood supply to the fingers, toes, and sometimes ears, marked by severe pallor of these parts and accompanied by numbness, tingling, or severe pain.

SALICYLATE: Any of the salts of salicylic acid used for their pain-relieving, fever-reducing, and anti-inflammatory properties. The most widely used salicylate is aspirin (acetylsalicylic acid).

Chapter 12

Skin Diseases

LEARNING OBJECTIVES

Upon successful completion of this chapter, you will
- Compare and contrast seborrheic dermatitis and psoriasis.
- Identify the etiology of contact and atopic dermatitis.
- Compare the life of a normal skin cell to that of a psoriatic skin cell.
- Identify the signs and symptoms of urticaria.
- Discuss the progression which occurs when a comedo becomes an acne pustule or papule.
- List at least five causes of alopecia.
- Recall the sources of infection of herpes simplex.
- Describe the etiologic process of herpes zoster.
- Restate the prognosis and prevention for impetigo.
- Compare and contrast furuncle and carbuncle.
- List the three common locations for pediculosis.
- Discuss the prevention of decubitus ulcers.
- Recall the five areas where dermatophytosis is likely to occur.
- Recall the treatment for corns and calluses.
- Identify the etiology of warts.
- Describe the signs and symptoms of discoid lupus erythematosus.
- Restate the prognosis for scleroderma.

271

■ Name the two most common types of skin cancers.
■ Identify the four types of malignant melanomas.
■ List at least four common symptoms of skin diseases.

INTRODUCTION

The integumentary system, comprising the skin and its accessory organs, provides protection for the body against infection, trauma, and toxic compounds. Skin contains the receptors for touch and other sensations that are important to our individual well-being from birth to death. The skin helps regulate body temperature and even synthesizes vitamin D when exposed to sunlight. Figure 12–1 illustrates the structure of the skin.

The three layers of the skin are the epidermis, the dermis, and the subcutaneous layer of tissue. The *epidermis,* or outer layer, produces **keratin** and the pigment **melanin** that give the skin its color. The *dermis,* or middle layer, consists of fibrous proteins that give the skin strength and elasticity. The *subcutaneous layer* is mostly fat, providing insulation against heat loss. Nails, hair, sebaceous (oil) glands, and sudiferous (sweat) glands are part of the integumentary system, also.

Skin diseases are freuqently manifested by alterations in the skin surface called *lesions.* Because most skin diseases produce a specific type of lesion or set of lesions, diagnoses are often made on the basis of the appearance of the lesions. Figure 12–2 illustrates nine basic types of skin lesions. Refer to this figure as you study the signs and symptoms of the various skin diseases discussed in this chapter.

DERMATITIS

Dermatitis is inflammation of the skin manifested by itching, redness, and the appearance of various skin lesions. The disease may be acute, subacute, or chronic. This chapter will consider the following forms of dermatitis: seborrheic dermatitis, contact dermatitis, and atopic dermatitis.

Seborrheic Dermatitis

Description: *Seborrheic dermatitis* is a chronic functional disease of the sebaceous glands marked by an increase in the amount and often alteration in the quality of the sebaceous secretion.

Etiology: Seborrheic dermatitis is an idiopathic disease. Heredity may predispose an individual to develop the condition, whereas emotional stress may precipitate it.

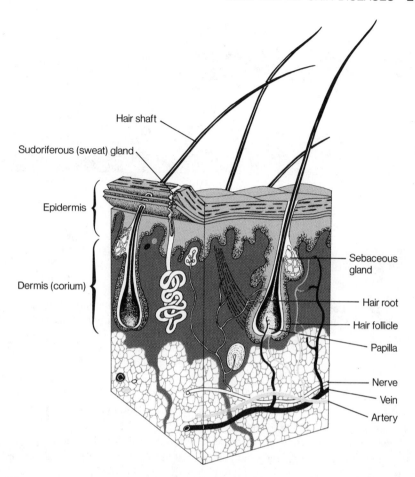

FIGURE 12–1. Cross section of the skin and its accessory organs. (Modified from Gylys, B. A. and Wedding, M. E., *Medical Terminology: A Systems Approach,* ed. 2. F. A. Davis, Philadelphia, 1988, p. 66.)

Signs and Symptoms: The disease is characterized by skin eruptions on areas of the scalp, face, or trunk that produce dry, moist, or greasy scales. Such scaling produced by the scalp is commonly called *dandruff*. The affected area of the skin frequently itches and may appear reddened.

Diagnostic Procedures: The diagnosis is usually made on the basis of the patient history and observation of the characteristic lesions. The disease must be differentiated from psoriasis (see Psoriasis).

Treatment: Shampoos containing selenium sulfide or zinc pyrithione are often helpful in controlling the scaling. Hydrocortisone creams may be prescribed to

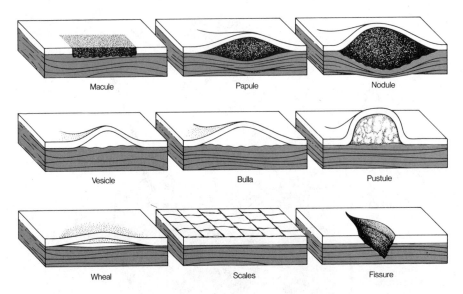

FIGURE 12–2. Lesions of the skin. (From Gylys, B. A. and Wedding, M. E., *Medical Terminology: A Systems Approach,* ed. 2. F. A. Davis, Philadelphia, 1988, p. 71, with permission.)

relieve redness and itching. Generalized seborrheic dermatitis requires careful attention, including scrupulous skin hygiene and keeping the skin as dry as possible.

Prognosis: Seborrheic dermatitis is a chronic condition, but the prognosis is good given effective treatment. The presence of secondary infections may complicate treatment.

Prevention: Adequate diet and sleep, regular exercise, sensible work habits, and a reduction of stress may help prevent the disease in those who are susceptible.

Contact Dermatitis

Description: *Contact dermatitis* is any acute skin inflammation caused by the direct action of various irritants on the surface of the skin or by contact with a substance to which an individual is allergic or sensitive.

Etiology: A wide variety of animal, vegetable, or mineral substances may induce contact dermatitis. These may include drugs, acids, alkalies, or resins from plants such as poison ivy, poison oak, or poison sumac. The dyes used in colored toilet or facial tissue or in some soaps also may cause the condition. Some individuals are even sensitive to the composition of certain metals and may experience contact dermatitis as a consequence of wearing jewelry.

Signs and Symptoms: The symptoms include **erythema** and the appearance of small skin **vesicles** that ooze, scale, itch, burn, or sting. The affected area may be hot and swollen.

Diagnostic Procedures: Diagnosis is usually made on the basis of the appearance of the inflamed area of skin. A medical history revealing prior outbreaks of the condition and the location of the affected area of skin may help in isolating the specific irritant or allergen.

Treatment: The skin surface must be thoroughly cleansed of the suspected irritant. Lotions or creams may be the treatment of choice.

Prognosis: Contact dermatitis is generally self-limiting. The problem will tend to recur if the individual is reexposed to the particular irritant or allergen.

Prevention: The best prevention is avoidance of known allergens or irritants.

Atopic Dermatitis (Eczema)

Description: *Atopic dermatitis* is an inflammation of the skin of unknown etiology in an individual with inherently irritable skin. The disease is common among infants, but it may occur at any time of life.

Etiology: Although the condition is idiopathic, it appears to have allergic, hereditary, or psychologic components. In about 70 percent of cases there is a family history of the disease. An allergic component is nearly always present, since the symptoms are frequently exacerbated by contact with wool, soaps, or oils and marked by an allergic sensitivity to certain foods.

Signs and Symptoms: There will be **pruritus** and often severe characteristic lesions on the face, neck, upper trunk, and the bends of the knees and elbows. Atopic dermatitis may cause vesicular and exudative eruptions in children and dry, leathery vesicles in adults.

Diagnostic Procedures: Observation of the skin and a medical history revealing a family tendency toward developing atopic dermatitis assist in diagnosing the condition. Serum IgE levels may be elevated.

Treatment: Local and systemic agents may be prescribed to prevent itching. Careful daily skin care and total avoidance of known irritants are important. Creams and ointments may be prescribed, too.

Prognosis: The prognosis is good, but the disorder is often frustrating to control and may have to be dealt with throughout most of the individual's lifetime.

Prevention: The best prevention is avoidance of known irritants.

PSORIASIS

Description: *Psoriasis* is a chronic skin disease marked by the appearance of discrete pink or dull-red skin lesions surmounted by a characteristic silvery scaling. The disease may begin at any age and is noninfectious.

Etiology: The cause of psoriasis is not known, but it appears to be genetically determined. The disease may be an autoimmune disorder. Precipitating factors may include hormonal changes such as those occurring during pregnancy, emotional stress, or even changes in climate.

Signs and Symptoms: A high rate of skin cell turnover produces the thick, flaky scaling that is characteristic of psoriasis. The affected areas of skin typically appear dry, cracked, and encrusted. These lesions may appear on the scalp, chest, buttocks, and extremities. In some individuals, psoriasis spreads to the nail beds, causing thickened, crumbling nails which separate from the skin.

Diagnostic Procedures: Observation of the skin, a careful patient history, or a skin biopsy may suggest the diagnosis.

Treatment: There is no cure for the disease, and the treatment is only palliative. The scales may be removed after they are softened. Exposure to ultraviolet light may retard the cell reproduction, and coal tar preparations may be applied to affected areas. Steroid creams, low-dosage antihistamines, oatmeal baths, and open, wet dressings may be ordered. Careful skin hygiene is important.

Prognosis: Psoriasis is controllable, but remissions and exacerbations frequently occur. The unsightly lesions that characterize the disease may cause psychological distress.

Prevention: There is no known prevention.

URTICARIA (HIVES)

Description: *Urticaria (hives)* is an inflammatory reaction of the capillaries beneath a localized area of the skin.

Etiology: Urticaria most frequently results following ingestion of certain foods such as shellfish or berries. The condition also may result from allergic reactions to insect stings or some inhalants, such as animal dander. Heat, cold, water, and sunlight may be predisposing factors of urticaria.

Signs and Symptoms: The condition is characterized by the eruption of pale raised **wheals** on the skin, possibly surrounded by erythema. The lesions usually form and then resolve quite rapidly, often moving from one portion of the body to another. This vascular reaction usually is accompanied by intense itching.

Diagnostic Procedures: The medical history should cover topics such as medications used, frequently ingested foods, environmental factors, and psychological status. The appearance of the inflamed area and this history should help pinpoint a diagnosis of urticaria. Sensitization testing may help to identify the causative agent.

Treatment: When the offending stimulus is removed, urticaria usually subsides. Antihistamines are often useful in controlling an ongoing attack. Epinephrine may be injected to control severe reactions. Hydrocortisone creams or lotions are helpful in providing symptomatic relief from itching.

Prognosis: The prognosis for an individual with this uncomfortable disorder is good.

Prevention: Avoiding the causative agent is the best means of preventing urticaria.

ACNE VULGARIS

Description: *Acne vulgaris* is an inflammatory disease of the sebaceous glands and hair follicles characterized by the apperance of **comedos, papules,** and **pustules**. It is more common in adolescents, but the lesions can appear at an earlier or later age, too.

Etiology: The cause of acne vulgaris is not known. Predisposing factors include hereditary tendencies and disturbances in hormonal balances affecting the activity of the sebaceous glands. Precipitating factors may include food allergies, endocrine disorders, the use of steroid drugs, or psychogenic factors. The fact that bacteria are important in the disease process is indicated by successful results following antibiotic therapy.

Signs and Symptoms: The acne plug often appears first as a comedo (whitehead) or a closed comedo (blackhcad). The color in the blackhead is caused by the melanin produced by the hair follicle, not by dirt. Eventually, an enlarged plug may rupture or leak, spreading its contents to the dermis. This results in inflammation and acne pustules or papules. Scars can develop if chronic irritation continues over a period of time.

Diagnostic Procedures: A patient history and observation of the characteristic lesions confirm the diagnosis.

Treatment: Therapy may include the use of a strong antibacterial solution applied to the skin, orally administered antibiotics, or both. Topically applied cleansing and peeling (**keratolytic**) agents may prove useful to some, but in general, the skin should be kept as clean and dry as possible.

Prognosis: Acne vulgaris is a persistent, often emotionally upsetting problem usually requiring prolonged treatment before it subsides. The ultimate prognosis for most acne sufferers is good. For a few, though, the disease can produce permanent scarring and disfigurement.

Prevention: There is no known prevention.

ALOPECIA

Description: *Alopecia* is the absence or loss of hair, especially on the head.

Etiology: Alopecia may result as a consequence of certain systemic illnesses, endocrine disorders, nutritional problems, and certain forms of dermatitis. It may be caused by the use of certain drugs or occur as a consequence of chemotherapy or radiation therapy. More frequently, though, alopecia is not related to any specific pathologic process. Among men, alopecia seems to be part of the aging process. This form of the condition, called *male pattern baldness,* seems to be related to levels of the hormone androgen and may be genetically determined. In infants, alopecia is a common, temporary physiologic condition.

Signs and Symptoms: Alopecia may occur gradually with advancing age, or it may be more sudden, occurring all at once or in patchy spots.

Diagnostic Procedures: The visual examination may be all that is necessary, but the cause must be determined, too.

Treatment: Treatment varies with the cause of alopecia. For scarring alopecia, there is no treatment. In nonscarring alopecia, spontaneous regrowth may occur, requiring no treatment. If the cause is a change in androgen levels, medications may be ordered. Minoxidil preparations have recently been approved to treat male pattern baldness.

Prognosis: The prognosis is dependent upon the cause. Alopecia due to scarring is permanent.

Prevention: There is no known prevention for some forms of alopecia. For others, early treatment of any disease known to cause alopecia is essential.

HERPES-RELATED SKIN LESIONS

Cold Sores and Fever Blisters

Description: *Cold sores* and *fever blisters* are skin eruptions occurring about the perimeter of the mouth, lips, and nose or on the mucous membranes within the mouth. The condition is common in children, but it affects people of any age.

Etiology: These lesions are produced by the herpes simplex virus type 1 (HSV-1). This virus may lie dormant within the body for extended periods, reactivating during periods of lowered resistance or emotional and physical stress. Cold sores may erupt following a rise in body temperature such as may occur during a common cold or even preceding menstruation. In some instances, however, they may occur prior to the onset of illness or for no apparent reason at all.

Signs and Symptoms: The characteristic lesions are small, pale vesicles appearing individually or in clusters, especially on the lips or about the mouth. The affected area may burn and sting. The lesions may eventually break, forming ulcers or crusts.

Diagnostic Procedures: The diagnosis is made on the basis of the individual's characteristic lesions. The virus may need to be isolated by histologic examination of scrapings, too.

Treatment: Treatment is strictly symptomatic. The lesions should be kept as dry and clean as possible and protected from trauma. Topical analgesics or ointments may be applied to relieve burning and itching. Antibiotic ointments may be recommended to prevent secondary infection of open lesions.

Prognosis: Cold sores and fever blisters usually resolve within 1 to 3 weeks. The herpes simplex virus resumes dormancy, however, and may reappear again given favorable conditions.

Prevention: There is no specific prevention other than avoiding contact with persons with visible cold sores.

Herpes Zoster (Shingles)

Description: *Herpes zoster (shingles)* is an acute inflammatory eruption of highly painful vesicles on the trunk of the body or occasionally on the face. Adults past the age of 50 are primarily affected.

Etiology: Shingles is caused by reactivation of the herpes zoster virus, the same virus that causes chickenpox. What triggers this reactivation is not known. The lesions occur on a segment of skin lying above the course of a nerve which has been infected by the virus.

Signs and Symptoms: The first symptom is pain along the course of the affected nerve, usually occurring 1 to 3 days prior to the appearance of the lesions. The skin eruption begins as an erythematous maculopapular rash that develops quite rapidly into vesicles. The site of these lesions is usually on one side of the trunk of the body, but if nerves supplying the face are involved, lesions also may appear on one side of the face, mouth, or tongue or around one eye. The region around the affected site is often intensely painful.

Diagnostic Procedures: The condition is diagnosed by its characteristic pattern of painful lesions. Confirmation of the diagnosis can be made by isolating the virus in cell cultures grown from scrapings of the lesions or by detecting varicella-zoster antibodies in the blood.

Treatment: Sedatives, analgesics, and **antipruritics** may be prescribed. If the vesicles are infected, antibiotics may be given to prevent secondary infection.

Prognosis: The prognosis is usually good; shingles runs its course within 7 to 10 days. However, recurrent bouts of severe pain may persist for weeks or months after the lesions have resolved. The disease may cause serious damage to the structure of the eye if nerves supplying the eye are involved. Unlike cold sores or fever blisters, shingles will not recur.

Prevention: There is no specific prevention for shingles.

IMPETIGO

Description: *Impetigo* is a contagious superficial skin infection marked by vesicles or **bullae** that become pustular, rupture, and form yellow crusts.

Etiology: The disease is usually caused by *Streptococcus* or *Staphylococcus* bacteria. Predisposing factors include poor hygiene, malnutrition, and anemia. Impetigo occurs more frequently in warm weather.

Signs and Symptoms: The lesions of impetigo begin as **macules**, vesicles, and pustules, usually accompanied by pruritus. A thick, yellow crust eventually forms over the infected site. Satellite lesions may appear as a result of autoinoculation. Erythema with ulcerations and scarring may result.

Diagnostic Procedures: The characteristic lesions assist in the diagnosis. A Gram's stain and a Tzanck smear may be useful in differentiating impetigo from other skin diseases.

Treatment: Antibiotics are essential. Thorough cleansing of the lesions is necessary two to three times daily.

Prognosis: The prognosis is good.

Prevention: Prevention includes good hygiene and avoidance of infected persons.

FURUNCLES AND CARBUNCLES

Description: A *furuncle,* or boil, is an abscess involving the entire hair follicle and adjacent subcutaneous tissue. A *carbuncle* is several furuncles developing in adjoining hair follicles with multiple drainage sinuses. The most common sites of these lesions are hairy parts of the body exposed to irritation, pressure, friction, or moisture.

Etiology: Infection by *Staphylococcus* bacteria is the most common cause. Predisposing factors include diabetes mellitus, **nephritis**, debilitation, or infected wound elsewhere in the body.

Signs and Symptoms: The affected portion of skin may be extremely tender, painful, and swollen. The abscess may eventually enlarge, soften, and open, discharging pus and necrotic material. Erythema and edema may persist at the site for days or weeks. A mild fever may accompany this condition.

Diagnostic Procedures: Diagnosis is made on the basis of the appearance of the characteristic lesion. There may be slight **leukocytosis**. A wound culture may be done to isolate the causative organism.

Treatment: The infected area must be cleansed with soap and water, and hot, wet compresses should be applied. Antibiotic agents are frequently prescribed. Surgical incision and drainage may be necessary after the lesion is mature.

Prognosis: The condition may recur for months or years. Complications from carbuncles may include **bacteremia**.

Prevention: Prevention includes good personal hygiene and prevention of any infectious process.

PEDICULOSIS

Description: *Pediculosis* is skin infestation with lice, a parasitic insect. The body (pediculosis corporis), the scalp (pediculosis capitis), or the pubic area (pediculosis pubis) are the most common sites for infestation to occur.

Etiology: The lice feed on human blood and lay their eggs, or nits, in body hair or clothing, and the eggs hatch, feed, and mature in 2 to 3 weeks. The louse bite injects a toxin in the skin. Pediculosis is more common in people who live in overcrowded places with inadequate facilities and poor personal hygiene. Pediculosis can be transmitted from infected clothing, hats, combs, bed sheets, and towels. Pubic lice may be acquired through sexual intercourse with an infested person.

Signs and Symptoms: Intense pruritus and evidence of nits (eggs) on hair shafts or lice on clothing or on skin are the most common signs and symptoms. There may be gross excoriation of patches of skin and **pyoderma**. Rashes or wheals may develop.

Diagnostic Procedures: Visual examination usually is all that is necessary. Nits can be found on the hair, body, or clothing.

Treatment: For scalp lice, a special shampoo must be used, followed by the use of fine-tooth comb to remove lice and nits. Body lice must be washed with soap and water, although the same special shampoo used for head lice may be prescribed for the body lice. All clothing and bedding must be washed or dry cleaned. Pubic lice may be treated with creams, lotions, or shampoos.

Prognosis: The prognosis is excellent with treatment.

Prevention: Prevention includes good hygiene and avoiding contact with infested persons.

DECUBITUS ULCERS

Description: A *decubitus ulcer* is a localized area of dead skin and subcutaneous tissue.

Etiology: These lesions are caused by impairment of the blood supply to the affected area as a result of persistent pressure against the skin surface. The condition is most frequently a consequence of prolonged immobilization and is often seen in the debilitated, the unconscious, or those who are paralyzed. Those with weak circulation, especially the elderly, are at greatest risk of developing decubitus ulcers.

Signs and Symptoms: Early signs of decubitus ulcer include shiny, reddened skin, usually appearing over a bony prominence. Small blisters, erosions, necrosis, and ulceration eventually occur. If the ulcer becomes infected, it will be foul-smelling and purulent. Pain may or may not accompany the lesion.

Diagnostic Procedures: Visual examination of the lesion usually is enough to establish the diagnosis. Wound culture and sensitivity testing may be done to isolate the causative organism if infection is suspected.

Treatment: Skin pressure must be alleviated and excellent skin hygiene provided. The affected area must be kept clean and dry. Topical antibiotic powders may be prescribed. Surgery may be necessary in severe cases.

Prognosis: The sooner the decubitus ulcer is diagnosed and treated, the better is the prognosis. The healing process generally is slow and tedious.

Prevention: Prevention includes frequent repositioning of patients who are immobilized and gentle massage to pressure areas to increase circulation.

DERMATOPHYTOSES

Description: *Dermatophytosis* is a chronic superficial fungal infection. Dermatophytoses can occur in the scalp (tinea capitis), body (tinea corporis), nails (tinea unguium), feet (tinea pedis), or groin (tinea cruris).

Etiology: Dermatophytosis is caused by several species of fungus that have the ability to invade the keratinous structures of the body. The infection is transmitted by direct contact with the fungus or its spores. Infection is more likely if the skin is traumatized or **abraded** or in cases of poor hygiene.

Signs and Symptoms:

- *Tinea capitis* is a persistent, contagious, often epidemic infection occurring most frequently in children. The child may be asymptomatic or have slight itching of the scalp. The characteristic lesions are round, gray, and scaly.
- *Tinea corporis,* or ringworm, occurs on exposed skin surfaces in persons with a history of exposure to infected domestic animals, especially cats. The lesions are ringed and scaled with small vesicles.
- *Tinea unguium* is usually asymptomatic. The infection frequently starts at the tip of one or more toenails, with the affected nail appearing lusterless, brittle, and hypertrophic.
- *Tinea pedia,* or athltete's foot, causes intense, persistent itching as its most common presenting symptom. Burning, stinging, and pain may result. The entire sole may become inflamed and dry with exfoliation and fissuring.
- *Tinea cruris,* or jock itch, may be associated with tinea pedis and often occurs among male athletes. It is characterized by red, raised, sharply defined, itching lesions in the groin.

Diagnostic Procedures: Diagnosis is dependent on the location and appearance of the skin lesion. The suspected lesions may be cultured to isolate the fungus. Skin tests or a Wood's light (a special ultraviolet light source) may be used to detect the lesions.

Treatment: It may be necessary to treat the lesions by applying a topical fungicidal medication. Extreme caution is necessary when applying such preparations because they are strong irritants. Some medications may be prescribed orally, but these must be taken with caution, too, because of their side effects. The affected area of skin must be kept as dry and clean as possible. Loose-fitting clothing should be worn, and it should be changed frequently. Exercise and activity may need to be limited for a time to prevent excessive perspiration.

Prognosis: All forms of dermatophytoses tend to be chronic and persistent. Scrupulous management is required to resolve the condition. Even so, recurrences may be common.

Prevention: Following proper hygiene practices is the best means of preventing dermatophytoses.

CORNS AND CALLUSES

Description: *Corns* are horny **indurations** and thickenings of the **stratum corneum** of the skin. *Calluses* are localized hyperplasia of the stratum corneum.

Etiology: Both conditions may be caused by pressure or friction from ill-fitting shoes, orthopedic deformities, or faulty weight-bearing. Persons who expose their skin to repeated trauma, such as manual laborers or string instrument players, are prone to calluses. Also, diabetics and individuals with impaired circulation are more apt to develop corns and calluses.

Signs and Symptoms: Tenderness and pain after the corns or calluses are seen are common symptoms. Corns have a glassy core, are smaller and more clearly defined, and are more painful than calluses.

Diagnostic Procedures: A physical examination of the affected area and medical history are usually sufficient for diagnosis.

Treatment: Treatment consists of relieving pressure or friction points along the skin as soon as possible. Surgical **debridement** under local anesthetic may be necessary. Local injections of corticosteroids to relieve pain may be tried. Metatarsal and corn pads may be worn.

Prognosis: The prognosis is good if the causative factor is removed.

Prevention: Prevention includes wearing well-fitting shoes and avoiding any trauma to the feet or hands.

WARTS

Description: *Warts* (verrucae) are circumscribed, elevated skin lesions resulting from hypertrophy of the epidermis. Warts may be solitary or clustered, occurring most often on the exposed surfaces of the fingers and hands. Children are affected most frequently.

Etiology: Warts are caused by infection from one of five possible papilloma viruses, each tending to infect different parts of the body.

Signs and Symptoms: The size, shape, and appearance of warts will vary widely. Tenderness and itching may accompany the lesions.

Diagnostic Procedures: Visual examination of the wart usually is sufficient for diagnosis.

Treatment: The wart may be removed by surgical excision, cryosurgery, or the use of keratolytic (peeling) agents. Immunotherapy may be tried for resistant warts. Treatment can be tedious and often is painful.

Prognosis: Spontaneous cures occur in about 50 percent of cases, but warts may resist any treatment, and recurrences are frequent.

Prevention: Because warts can be transmitted by direct contact, avoidance of warts is important for prevention.

DISCOID LUPUS ERYTHEMATOSUS

Description: *Discoid lupus erythematosus* (DLE) is a connective-tissue disorder characterized by a superficial, localized inflammation of the skin occurring most frequently on exposed skin surfaces. (The systemic form of the disease is discussed in Chapter 11.)

Etiology: The cause of lupus is unknown. It affects women more frequently than men.

Signs and Symptoms: Macules, papules, **plaques**, plugged follicles, and atrophic areas are evident, usually on the face, neck, and upper extremities. The lesions are dusky red, well-localized, and covered by dry, horny, adherent scales.

Diagnostic Procedures: There is no specific test for discoid lupus erythematosus, but the disease may be differentiated from the systemic form by means of an antinuclear antibody test. Laboratory tests may include CBC, ESR, and urinalysis (UA).

Treatment: The skin lesions may be treated with a topical corticosteroid cream or injected with the medication. Systemic drugs may be tried if topical forms do not work. The individual may be advised to avoid extreme fatigue and stress, as well as overexposure to sunlight.

Prognosis: DLE is a chronic condition, but it can be successfully controlled. The prognosis is good if the disease does not develop into a systemic condition.

Prevention: There is no known prevention.

SCLERODERMA

Description: *Scleroderma* is a progressive, chronic, systemic disease characterized by diffuse fibrosis of the skin and internal organs. It may appear in two forms: morphea and systemic scleroderma. *Morphea* is purely a cutaneous disease, in which the skin becomes thickened and densely fibrous. *Systemic scleroderma* is a form in which both skin and internal organs are involved. Parts of the gastrointestinal tract may become fibrotic and may exhibit impaired peristalsis.

Etiology: The cause is unknown, but scleroderma appears to be an autoimmune disorder. Women are more frequently affected, especially those 30 to 50 years old.

Signs and Symptoms: **Raynaud's phenomenon** generally is the first symptom, followed by pain, stiffness, and swelling of the fingers and joints. The skin becomes thick, shiny, and taut. **Contractures** eventually develop. Gastrointestinal symptoms include heartburn, reflux, diarrhea, constipation, weight loss, **dysphagia**, malabsorption, and mild anemia.

Diagnostic Procedures: The typical cutaneous clinical picture will help pinpoint the disease. Hand, chest, and gastrointestinal x-rays may show systemic changes. Urinalysis may indicate renal involvement. A skin biopsy may be done.

Treatment: Treatment is palliative. Chemotherapy with immunosuppressive drugs may be tried. Raynaud's phenomenon may be treated with vasodilators and antihypertensive drugs. Any digital ulcerations require immediate treatment. Physical therapy may be prescribed to promote muscle function.

Prognosis: The prognosis is poor, with death usually resulting from renal, cardiac, or pulmonary failure.

Prevention: There is no known prevention, except for complications of the disease. The patient is to avoid cold, stress, and trauma.

SKIN CARCINOMAS

Description: The most common skin cancers are basal cell carcinoma and squamous cell carcinoma. *Basal cell carcinomas* arise from the basal cell layer of the epidermis or hair follicles, are locally invasive, but very rarely metastasize. *Squamous cell carcinomas* also arise from the epidermis and produce keratin. Squamous cell carcinomas also arise from the epidermis and produce keratin. Squamous cell carcinoma is the more serious of the two because of its tendency to metastasize.

Etiology: Repeated overexposure to the sun's ultraviolet rays is the most important etiologic factor in skin carcinomas.

Signs and Symptoms: Cancerous skin lesions may appear any place on the body, but the common sites are sun-exposed areas of the body, such as the face, chest, back, ears, forearms, and the back of hands. Initially, both forms are painless. Basal cell carcinoma appears as a smooth, small, waxy nodule that appears translucent. Squamous cell carcinoma is a firm, red nodule with visible scales. Both carcinomas often ulcerate and form a crust.

Diagnostic Procedures: A medical history, careful observation of the skin revealing characteristic lesions, and biopsy of the lesions are necessary for diagnosis.

Treatment: The goal of treatment is to completely eradicate the lesions. The size, shape, location, and invasiveness of the carcinoma will determine treatment. Preferred treatment of basal cell carcinoma is excision, currettage, and **electrodesiccation** or cryosurgery. Treatment of squamous cell carcinoma may involve local application of chemotherapeutic agents or cryosurgery.

Prognosis: The prognosis for carcinomas of the skin is good, with a 90 percent cure rate if detected and treated in the early stage. While basal cell carcinomas rarely metastasize, untreated they may result in the loss of an ear, nose, or lip.

Because squamous cell carcinomas may metastasize, individuals should be followed closely for a minimum of 5 years to detect new lesions or metastasis.

Prevention: The best prevention is to avoid overexposure to the sun. Sun damage to the skin is cumulative, so sunscreens and protective measures should be used throughout life.

Malignant Melanoma

Description: A *malignant melanoma* is a neoplasm composed of abnormal melanocytes appearing in both the epidermis and dermis. Malignant melanoma appears in one of four forms: *superficial spreading melanoma* occurs on any body site and is the most common form of melanoma; *lentigomaligna melanoma* occurs on exposed skin areas, especially the head and neck, and is a slowly evolving pigmented lesion; *nodular melanoma* occurs on any site and directly invades tissue below the dermis; *acral-lentiginous melanoma* occurs where hair follicles are absent (palms of hands, soles of feet, nail beds) and appears as irregular pigmented macules which develop into nodules and become invasive early. The incidence of malignant melanoma is increasing and has doubled in the past 10 years. It causes more deaths than all other skin diseases.

Etiology: While ultraviolet rays are suspect, the etiology is unknown. The persons at greatest risk have fair complexions, blue eyes, red or blonde hair, and freckles.

Signs and Symptoms: Malignant melanomas are characterized by lesions having irregular borders and a diversity of colors. The lesion of *superficial spreading* melanoma tends to be circular, flat and visibly or palpably elevated. Color variations include tan, brown, black mixed with gray, bluish black, or white. There may be a whitish pink color in a small area within the lesion. The *lentigomaligna* melanoma appears as a brown or black, flat lesion that undergoes changes in size and color with time. The *nodular* melanoma is generally blue-black in color, resembling a "blood blister" that fails to resolve. The lesion is spherical with a relatively smooth surface. The *acral-lentiginous* melanoma appears as a dark brown, flat lesion or a blue-black or brown-black, raised lesion.

Diagnostic Procedures: Suspicious skin lesions must be biopsied to determine the diagnosis.

Treatment: The level of invasion and measure of the melanoma's thickness will determine the appropriate treatment. Surgical excision of the lesion is the most common treatment modality. Chemotherapy may be recommended.

Prognosis: The prognosis is related to the level of the dermal invasion and the thickness of the lesion. The prognosis is poorer if the melanoma grows vertically rather than horizontally. If metastasis occurs, it can affect every organ of the body. If the melanoma is detected and treated early, there is a 5-year survival rate of 90 percent.

Prevention: Avoiding overexposure to the sun and ultraviolet rays and seeking prompt treatment for any suspected lesions are the best prevention.

COMMON SYMPTOMS OF SKIN DISEASES

Individuals may present with the following common complaints, which deserve attention from health professionals:

- Skin eruptions
- Pruritus
- Erythema
- Pain
- Swelling
- Inflammation

REVIEW QUESTIONS

Matching

_____ 1. Seborrheic dermatitis
_____ 2. Contact dermatitis
_____ 3. Atopic dermatitis
_____ 4. Psoriasis
_____ 5. Urticaria
_____ 6. Acne vulgaris
_____ 7. Alopecia
_____ 8. Herpes simplex I
_____ 9. Herpes zoster
_____ 10. Impetigo

a. Shingles
b. Hives
c. Inflammatory disease of sebaceous follicles
d. Appears to have allergic, hereditary, or psychologic components
e. Produces dry, moist or greasy scaling
f. Characterized by high rate of skin turnover
g. Cold or fever sores
h. Baldness
i. Contagious strep. or staph. skin infection
j. Causes erythema and small skin vesicles
k. Boil or abscess
l. Bedsore

Fill in the Blanks

1. A _____ or boil is an abscess involving the hair follicle and subcutaneous tissue. A _____ is several furuncles developing in adjoining hair follicles with multiple drainage sinuses.
2. Pediculosis is skin infestation with _____ .
3. Dermatophytosis is caused by _____ infections of the skin.
4. A skin disorder you might find on a person who is elderly, debilitated, or paralyzed is _____ .
5. Warts or verrucae are caused by the _____ .
6. Describe the classic symptom of discoid lupus erythematosus.
7. Name three skin cancers:
   a. _____
   b. _____
   c. _____
8. Name one important factor in skin cancers: _____ .

Discussion Question

Discuss the health problems which may occur from tanning booths.

ANSWERS

Matching

1. e
2. j
3. d
4. f
5. b
6. c
7. h
8. g
9. a
10. i

Fill in the Blanks

1. Furuncle, carbuncle
2. Lice
3. Fungal
4. Decubitus ulcer
5. Papilloma viruses
6. Dusky red, butterfly-patterned lesion over the nose and cheeks
7. a. Basal cell carcinoma
   b. Squamous cell carcinoma
   c. Malignant melanoma
8. Excessive exposure to sunlight

Discussion Question

Answers will vary.

GLOSSARY

ABRADE: To chafe; to roughen or remove by friction.

ANTIPRURITIC: An agent that prevents or relieves itching.

BACTEREMIA: Presence of bacteria in the blood.

BULLA: A large (generally greater than 0.5 cm) fluid-filled blister.

COMEDO: A plug of dried, discolored fatty matter clogging a pore of the skin. Commonly called a *blackhead*.

CONTRACTURE: Permanent shortening or contraction of a muscle, often producing physical distortion or deformity.

DEBRIDEMENT: The removal of dead or damaged tissue or other matter, especially from a wound.

DYSPHAGIA: Difficulty in swallowing or inability to swallow.

ELECTRODESICCATION: A method of electrosurgery in which tissue is destroyed by dehydration by application of a probe generating a series of short, high-frequency electric sparks.

ERYTHEMA: Diffuse redness of the skin due to dilation of the superficial capillaries.

INDURATION: An area of hardened tissue; the process of hardening.

KERATIN: A hard, fibrous protein that is the primary constituent of hair and nails.

KERATOLYTIC: An agent used to loosen and remove the outer layer of the epidermis.

LEUKOCYTOSIS: A temporary increase in number of white cells in the blood, typically, but not exclusively, caused by the presence of infection.

MACULE: A discolored spot of skin that is neither elevated above nor depressed below the surrounding skin surface.

MELANIN: A dark pigment that gives color to skin and hair.

NEPHRITIS: Any form of inflammation of the kidney, acute or chronic.

PAPULE: A solid, red, elevated skin lesion.

PLAQUE: As used here, a solid, elevated patch of skin. Often formed from the combination of numerous, closely spaced papules (see *Papule*).

PRURITUS: Severe itching.

PUSTULE: A circumscribed, raised skin lesion filled with pus.

PYODERMA: Any acute, pus-causing, inflammatory skin disease.

RAYNAUD'S   PHENOMENON: Intermittent interruptions of blood supply to the fingers, toes, and sometimes the ears, marked by severe pallor of these parts and accompanied by numbness, tingling, or severe pain.

STRATUM   CORNEUM: The outermost or horny layer of the epidermis.

VESICLE: A small (generally less than 0.5 cm), fluid-filled blister.

WHEAL: A generally round, transient elevation of the skin, white in the center, with pale red edges, often accompanied by itching.

Chapter 13
Eye and Ear Diseases

LEARNING OBJECTIVES

Upon successful completion of this chapter, you will
- Describe four common refractive errors.
- Identify the signs and symptoms of nystagmus.
- Recall the treatment for stye.
- Discuss the prognosis of corneal abrasions.
- List the various causes of cataracts.
- Restate the prognosis and prevention for glaucoma.
- Describe the process which causes retinal detachment.
- Identify the signs and symptoms of conjunctivitis.
- Describe the two common forms of uveitis.
- Recall the signs and symptoms of blepharitis.
- Restate the etiology of keratitis.
- Describe treatment for impacted cerumen.
- Identify the etiology of external otitis or swimmer's ear.
- Compare and contrast serous otitis media to suppurative otitis media.
- Define otosclerosis.
- Discuss the treatment for motion sickness.
- Recall the etiology for hearing loss.

290

■ Restate the treatment for Meniere's disease.
■ List at least three common symptoms of both eye and ear diseases.

INTRODUCTION

Our most important sensory receptors are the eyes and the ears. The eye is the primary organ for sight, and the ear is the primary organ for sound and equilibrium. Obviously, any impairment of either of these sensory receptors can be a traumatic experience as well as cause serious disability.

When studying the material in this chapter, it will be helpful to refer to Figures 13–1 and 13–2, which indicate the major parts of the eye and ear.

EYE DISEASES

Refractive Errors

Description: *Refractive errors* are defects in visual acuity resulting from the inability of the eye to effectively focus light on the surface of the retina. Four common refractive errors are

■ *Hyperopia.* This condition occurs when light entering the eye comes to a focus behind the retina so that vision is better for distant objects. For this reason, the condition is commonly referred to as *farsightedness*. Hyperopia often results when the globe of the eye is abnormally short in length from front to back.

■ *Presbyopia.* This refractive error is a form of farsightedness. Unlike hyperopia, however, presbyopia results from a loss of elasticity in the crystalline lens of the eye. When the eye focuses on a distant object, muscles encircling the lens contract, stretch or flatten it. When the eye focuses on a nearby object, the muscles relax, allowing the lens to resume a more spherical shape. In presbyopia, however, the lens remains in a comparatively flattened position after the muscles have relaxed. This condition is a consequence of advancing age.

■ *Myopia.* This condition occurs when light entering the eye comes to a focus in front of the retina so that vision is better for nearby objects. Consequently, the condition is commonly called *nearsightedness*. Myopia often results when the eyeball is abnormally long from front to back.

■ *Astigmatism.* This refractive error occurs when light entering the eye is focused unevenly or diffusely across the retina so that some of the visual field appears properly focused while some does not. The condition is caused by variations in the curvature over certain portions of the lens or cornea of the eye.

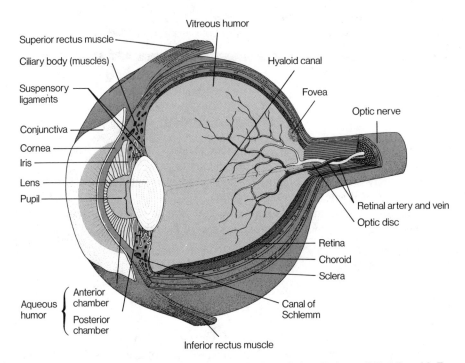

FIGURE 13–1. Structures of the eye. (Modified from Gylys, B. A. and Wedding, M. E., *Medical Terminology: A Systems Approach,* ed. 2. F. A. Davis, Philadelphia, 1988, p. 353.)

Etiology: It is not known what causes some individuals to develop these visual defects while others do not. Some types of refractive errors, however, show a strong familial pattern, suggesting a genetic predisposition to acquiring them.

Signs and Symptoms: In addition to the characteristic visual deficits just described, general symptoms of refractive errors may include squinting, headaches, and frequent rubbing of the eyes.

Diagnostic Procedures: The diagnosis of refractive errors usually involves testing for visual acuity using the Snelling eye chart, ophthalmoscopic examination of the interior of the eye, and tests to detect eye muscle function.

Treatment: Treatment of refractive errors involves the prescription and fitting of corrective lenses, either in the form of eyeglasses or contact lenses. **Radial keratotomy** is a surgical procedure now in use to correct myopia and astigmatism. While the procedure is effective for many people, some ophthalmologists are still concerned about potentially adverse long-term effects.

Prognosis: The prognosis is good with corrective lenses in all four refractive errors.

Prevention: There are no specific preventive measures for any of these refractive errors.

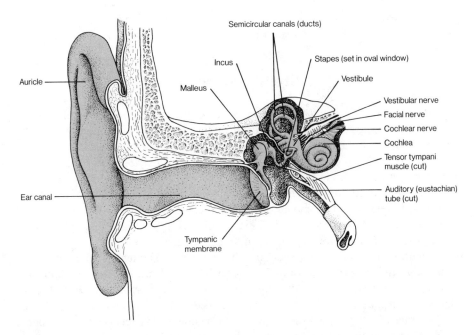

FIGURE 13–2. Structures of the ear. (Modified from Gylys, B. A. and Wedding, M. E., *Medical Terminology: A Systems Approach,* ed. 2. F. A. Davis, Philadelphia, 1988, p. 355.)

Nystagmus

Description: *Nystagmus* is repetitive involuntary movement of the eye. The condition is classified into various subcategories according to the characteristic pattern of eye movements that occurs. One or both eyes may be affected.

Etiology: Nystagmus may be either congenital or acquired. Acquired nystagmus results from disease processes that produce lesions in the portions of the brain or the structures within the ears that help govern eye movement. Diseases that may cause nystagmus include Meniere's disease and multiple sclerosis (see Meniere's Disease). Chronic visual impairment, certain drugs, or alcohol abuse also may produce this condition.

Signs and Symptoms: The symptoms of nystagmus are continuous horizontal, vertical, or circular eye movements (or a combination of these). The individual also may report blurred vision.

Diagnostic Procedures: A number of tests to assess eye movement such as an opticokinetic drum test may be performed to help in determining which structures within the ear or CNS may be causing the nystagmus.

Treatment: Treatment must be directed at the underlying cause of the nystagmus.

Prognosis: The prognosis is dependent on the underlying cause.
Prevention: There is no specific prevention for nystagmus.

Stye (Hordeolum)

Description: A *stye* (*hordeolum*) is a localized, purulent, inflammatory infection of one or more of the sebaceous glands of the eyelid. Styes commonly occur on the skin surface at the edge of the lid or on the surface of the **conjunctiva**.

Etiology: Styes usually result from infection by *Staphylococcus* bacteria. Often an eyelash is found in the center of the stye.

Signs and Symptoms: The chief symptom is pain and tenderness of an intensity directly related to the amount of swelling. There is redness at the site.

Diagnostic Procedures: Visual examination is all that is necessary in most cases. However, a culture may be taken to isolate *Staphylococcus*.

Treatment: Warm compresses may be prescribed to hasten the pointing of the abscess. Antibiotic eye drops or ointment may be used. If the infection warrants it, oral antibiotics may be ordered. Removal of the eyelash may be followed by pus drainage. An incision of the abscess may be necessary.

Prognosis: The prognosis is good with treatment, but recurrences are common. A complication of a stye is **cellulitis** of the eyelid.

Prevention: Prevention includes cleanliness and proper eye care.

Corneal Abrasion

Description: A *corneal abrasion* is a scratch on the transparent anterior cellular layer of the eye.

Etiology: Corneal abrasions may be produced by foreign bodies such as dirt, dust, or metal particles trapped between the cornea and the eyelid. A scratch also may result from fingernail contact with the cornea or from wearing poorly fitting or scratched contact lenses.

Signs and Symptoms: Pain, redness, and tearing are common symptoms. The person may experience a sensation that something is constantly in the eye. Visual acuity may be impaired.

Diagnostic Procedures: A medical history and visual examination may be all that is necessary to suggest the diagnosis. Instilling the affected eye with a fluorescein stain may help highlight the presence of any corneal lesion. This technique may be used alone or in conjunction with a slit-lamp examination.

Treatment: If a foreign body is indeed present in the eye, irrigation of the corneal surface may be attempted or a topical anesthetic administered and the object removed. Once the eye surface is clear of debris, an antibiotic ophthalmic ointment will often be prescribed, followed by the application of an eye bandage to reduce movement of the eyelid across the cornea.

Prognosis: The prognosis is good with treatment. Complications of untreated corneal abrasion include ulceration of the cornea and permanent vision loss.

Prevention: Prevention of corneal abrasions includes wearing protective eyewear when engaging in hazardous occupations or sports and following recommendations for cleaning and wearing contact lenses.

Cataract

Description: A *cataract* is an opacity or clouding of the crystalline lens of the eye or its surrounding membrane. The condition may be unilateral or bilateral.

Etiology: Cataracts may be congenital or due to trauma, aging, drug toxicity, systemic disease, or a complication of another eye condition such as glaucoma or uveitis.

Signs and Symptoms: A gradual loss or blurring of vision is the common symptom. Some patients report seeing halos around lights, and some have problems driving at night because of glare from the lights of oncoming cars. As a cataract matures, the pupil of the eye may appear white to an observer. The condition is painless.

Diagnostic Procedures: Ophthalmoscopy, pen-light examination, or slit-lamp examination will be used to confirm the diagnosis.

Treatment: Treatment is dependent on the degree of visual impairment and the age, general health, and occupation of the affected individual. Most cataracts require surgical extraction of the defective lens followed by refractive correction using eyeglasses, contact lenses, or surgically implanted artificial lenses.

Prognosis: The prognosis is good with surgery, improving visual acuity in 95 percent of cases.

Prevention: There is no known prevention for most cataracts.

Glaucoma

Description: *Glaucoma* is a condition in which accumulating fluid pressure within the eye damages the retina and optic nerve, often causing blindness. The buildup of pressure occurs because more fluid, called *aqueous humor,* is produced than can be drained from the eye. The most common form of this condition, called *open-angle glaucoma,* results from obstruction of passages within the eye called the *trabecular meshwork,* which drains the aqueous humor into the lymphatic system. Glaucoma is a leading cause of blindness and affects more women than men. The condition may be unilateral or bilateral.

Etiology: Primary forms of the condition, such as open-angle glaucoma, are idiopathic. However, a strong familial tendency toward developing this condition suggests that unknown genetic factors may be involved. Glaucoma also may arise secondary to a wide variety of other diseases or be induced by certain drugs or toxins.

Signs and Symptoms: The most common forms of glaucoma develop asymptomatically and are often not detected until irreparable damage has already occurred to the retinas or optic nerves. When symptoms appear late in the course of the disease, they may include mild aching in the eyes and visual disturbances such as seeing halos around lights or a noticeable loss of peripheral vision.

Diagnostic Procedures: A positive family history for the disease should suggest a potential diagnosis of glaucoma. One of various types of tonometers will be used to detect elevated intraocular pressure. Ophthalmoscopic inspection of the retinal surface is essential to determine whether retinal damage has occurred.

Treatment: Drug therapy is the standard course of treatment for glaucoma and may take one or two forms. Certain types of drugs may be applied to the surface of the eye to decrease intraocular pressure. Other drugs may be prescribed that act to decrease the production of aqueous humor. Severe cases of glaucoma may be treated using a new laser surgery technique that promotes drainage of aqueous humor through the trabecular meshwork.

Prognosis: The prognosis usually is good with early treatment. Drug therapy must be maintained for life.

Prevention: It is important for all persons 20 years of age and older to have ophthalmoscopic examinations that include a test for glaucoma every 3 to 5 years.

Retinal Detachment

Description: *Retinal detachment* is the complete or partial separation of the retina from the choroid layer of the eye (Figure 13–3), leading to the loss of retinal function and blindness. The condition occurs as a result of a hole or break in the retina that allows fluid, the *vitreous humor,* to accumulate between the two layers.

Etiology: Retinal detachment usually is caused by head trauma. Hemorrhages or tumors of the outer (choroid) layer also may cause the condition. Certain systemic diseases such as diabetes mellitus may predispose to the condition. Spontaneous retinal detachments also may occur among the elderly.

Signs and Symptoms: An individual with retinal detachment may report seeing floating spots or flashes of light. As more of the retina detaches from the choroid surface, there will be a progressive loss of vision. The condition is painless.

Diagnostic Procedures: Ophthalmoscopic examination while the pupils are fully dilated reveals the detached portion of the retina suspended in the vitreous humor of the eye.

Treatment: Treatment depends on the location and extent of the detachment, but generally it involves restriction of eye movement through sedation, bed rest, or the use of an eye patch. Surgery, often using newly developed laser techniques, may be required to reattach the floating portion of the retina to the choroid surface.

Prognosis: The prognosis is good, with successful surgical repair in about 80 percent of cases. The prognosis is worse if the portion of the retina that produces the

RETINAL DETACHMENT

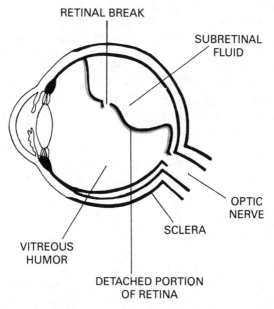

FIGURE 13–3. Retinal detachment. (From Thomas, C. L. [ed.], *Taber's Cyclopedic Medical Dictionary,* ed. 15. F. A. Davis, Philadelphia, 1985, p. 1483, with permission.)

sharpest vision (the *mucula lutea*) is detached. Without treatment, retinal detachment may become total in a few months.

Prevention: There is no specific prevention for retinal detachment other than following safety measures that minimize the risk of head trauma.

Eye Inflammation

Conjunctivitis

Description: *Conjunctivitis* is inflammation of the conjunctiva, the mucous membrane structure that lines the inner surface of the eyelids and the anterior portion of the eyeball. The condition may be unilateral or bilateral.

Etiology: Acute, sometimes epidemic, outbreaks of conjunctivitis are caused by infection from certain viruses or bacteria. These highly infectious forms of the disease commonly are referred to as *pinkeye.* Conjunctivitis also may be caused by irritation from heat, cold, chemicals, allergies, or exposure to ultraviolet light.

Signs and Symptoms: Conjunctivitis is marked by red, swollen conjunctivae, that may itch or burn or cause pain, especially when blinking. The eyes may tear excessively and may be overly sensitive to light.

Diagnostic Procedures: Physical examination will reveal inflammation of the conjunctivae. Stained smears of conjunctival scrapings may include monocytes, polymorphonuclear leukocytes, and macrophages. Culture and sensitivity tests will identify the specific causative organism and indicate appropriate treatment.

Treatment: Treatment varies depending on the causative agent, but antibiotic therapy may take the form of eyedrops on systemic medication. Often, warm compresses applied to the eye three to four times a day for 10 to 15 minutes are recommended.

Prognosis: The prognosis is good if degeneration or corneal damage does not occur. The disease normally is benign and self-limiting.

Prevention: Prevention involves careful hygiene, proper hand washing, and the use of clean washcloths to prevent infection.

Uveitis

Description: *Uveitis* is inflammation of the uveal tract (iris, ciliary body, choroid). The condition is usually unilateral. Uveitis may be classified as *granulomatous,* involving any portion of the uveal tract, or *nongranulomatous,* involving the iris, ciliary body, or anterior portion of the eye.

Etiology: Granulomatous uveitis may be caused by microbial infections or debilitating diseases such as tuberculosis, toxoplasmosis, and histoplasmosis. Nongranulomatous uveitis results from improperly healed corneal abrasions.

Signs and Symptoms: Symptoms include pain, **photophobia**, blurred vision, redness, and constricted pupils. Nongranulomatous uveitis characteristically produces more pain and photophobia than the granulomatous form.

Diagnostic Procedures: A slit-lamp examination is necessary for diagnosis. Skin tests for tuberculosis, toxoplasmosis, and histoplasmosis may be helpful in detecting granulomatous forms of the disease.

Treatment: Treatment is specific to the particular type of uveitis. For granulomatous uveitis, **atropine** is used to reduce the likelihood of adhesions. Anti-infective chemotherapy and corticosteroid drugs may be necessary. Analgesics may be prescribed, and intraocular pressure must be monitored. Nongranulomatous uveitis is also treated with atropine so that the pupil remains dilated. Steroids may be required.

Prognosis: Nongranulomatous uveitis usually subsides in a few weeks with treatment. Granulomatous uveitis may persist despite treatment. Adhesions may develop that can cause glaucoma, cataracts, or even retinal detachment.

Prevention: There is no known prevention other than prompt treatment of infections and the debilitating diseases mentioned.

Blepharitis

Description: *Blepharitis* is the ulcerative or nonulcerative inflammation of the edges of the eyelids involving hair follicles and glands that open onto the surface. It is a condition commonly seen in children.

Etiology: Ulcerative forms of blepharitis usually result from infection by *Staphylococcus* bacteria. Nonulcerative forms may be due to allergy or exposure to dust, smoke, or chemical irritants. The condition also may arise secondary to **seborrhea** of the sebaceous glands of the eyelids or pediculosis of the eyelashes or eyebrows.

Signs and Symptoms: The affected individual may experience burning and itching or the feeling of a foreign body in the eye. The eyes usually appear red-rimmed. Both dry and oily scales may be present on the eyelid margins.

Diagnostic Procedures: The characteristic symptoms, a bacterial culture which may reveal *Staphylococcus,* or examination of the eyelashes for nits will suggest the diagnosis.

Treatment: Seborrheic blepharitis requires daily shampooing to remove the scales. An antibiotic ointment will be prescribed for blepharitis caused by *Staphylococcus.* Pediculosis blepharitis requires the removal of nits and treatment with an ointment.

Prognosis: The prognosis is good with proper treatment and care, but some forms of the disease tend to recur and become chronic.

Prevention: The best prevention is cleanliness and proper eye care.

Keratitis

Description: *Keratitis* is inflammation of the cornea. The condition usually is unilateral.

Etiology: Keratitis is most frequently due to infection of the cornea by herpes virus type I or certain bacteria or fungi. The condition also may arise secondary to syphilis and, rarely, tuberculosis. Noninfectious keratitis may be caused by prolonged exposure to dry air or intense light or may result from corneal trauma.

Signs and Symptoms: Symptoms of keratitis include irritation, tearing, and photophobia. When the cause is herpes simplex virus type 1, an upper respiratory infection with facial cold sores may be the precursor. When exposure is the cause, the symptoms exhibit about 12 hours later. The patient experiences severe photophobia.

Diagnostic Procedures: Slit-lamp examination of the corneal surface confirms the diagnosis. Vision testing may indicate decreased visual acuity, and the medical history may reveal a recent upper respiratory infection.

Treatment: Topical treatment with eyedrops and ointment is likely to be prescribed. A broad-spectrum antibiotic may prevent secondary infection. An eye patch may be recommended for a period of time.

Prognosis: The prognosis is good when the condition is properly treated, but untreated keratitis may lead to blindness.

Prevention: The best prevention is proper eye care.

COMMON SYMPTOMS OF EYE DISEASES

Individuals may present with the following common symptoms which deserve attention from health professionals:

■ Any visual disturbance
■ Pain or burning in the eye and any of its structures
■ Eye redness

EAR DISEASES

Impacted Cerumen

Description: *Cerumen* is the soft, brown, waxlike secretion found in the external canal of the ear. The abnormal accumulation and eventual impaction of this substance within the ear canal can cause temporary hearing loss.

Etiology: Abnormal cerumen accumulation may be due to dryness and scaling of the skin or excessive hair in the ear canal. Individuals with narrow or tortuous ear canals may be predisposed to the condition.

Signs and Symptoms: There may be a gradual loss of hearing, and the patient may notice a feeling of fullness in the ear or exerience **tinnitus**.

Diagnostic Procedures: An otologic examination will reveal a soft or hard wax mass.

Treatment: A dull ring **curet** put through a speculum may be all that is necessary to remove the wax. If the impaction adheres to the wall of the canal, it may be softened by repeated instillations of oily ear drops or hydrogen peroxide and then irrigated with water.

Prognosis: The prognosis is good with removal of the wax; however, it may recur.

Prevention: There is no known prevention.

External Otitis (Swimmer's Ear)

Description: *External otitis (swimmer's ear)* is inflammation of the external ear canal.

Etiology: The inflammation may be caused by a bacterial or fungal infection or a dermatologic condition such as seborrhea or psoriasis. Predisposing factors include swimming or bathing in contaminated water or trauma to the ear canal from attempts to clean or scratch the ear. The frequent use of earphones, earplugs, or earmuffs may create a favorable environment within the ear canal in which bacteria and fungi may propagate.

Signs and Symptoms: Pain and **pruritus** are common presenting symptoms. Drainage from the ear may be either purulent or watery. Fever and hearing loss may result.

Diagnostic Procedures: An otologic examination will confirm the diagnosis. WBC may be normal or elevated. A bacterial culture of ear canal scrapings and sensitivity tests may be done if an infection is suspected.

Treatment: Antibiotics and analgesics may be prescribed. The ear must be kept dry and clean, and it should be protected from trauma. Ear drops or ointments may be instilled.

Prognosis: External otitis tends to recur and become chronic.

Prevention: Prevention includes wearing earplugs when swimming, bathing, or showering and avoiding cleaning the ear with any foreign objects to minimize the risk of trauma to the ear canal.

Otitis Media

Description: *Otitis media* is an accumulation of fluid within the structure of the middle ear. The condition is subclassified into either serous or **suppurative** categories according to the composition of the accumulating fluid. In serious otitis media, the fluid is comparatively clear and sterile, secreted from the membranes lining the inner ear. In suppurative otitis media, the fluid is the product of pus-producing bacteria. The pressure from the accumulating fluid in either form of the condition may be enough to occasion temporary hearing loss. Both serous and suppurative forms of the disease may occur as acute or chronic conditions. Otitis media is most common among children.

Etiology: Acute serous otitis media may occur spontaneously or following an upper respiratory tract infection. It also may be occasioned by rapid changes in atmospheric pressure, such as occur during flying, or by allergic reactions. The chronic form of serous otitis media may develop from the acute condition or result from the overgrowth of adenoidal tissue or chronic sinus infections.

Suppurative otitis media is caused by the introduction of pyogenic microorganisms into the middle ear, usually *H. influenzae, Streptococcus, Pneumococcus,* or *Staphylococcus.* The condition often follows the mumps, flu, or colds and may be induced by overly forceful nose blowing. Swimming in contaminated water also may result in a middle ear infection.

Irrespective of the particular form of the condition, or its ultimate cause, variations in the structure or function of the eustachian tube may strongly predispose an individual to developing otitis media. Narrowing or constriction of the eustachian tubes may interfere with the normal drainage of secretions from the middle ear.

Conversely, those with eustachian tubes that are shorter, wider, or more horizontally placed than normal may be more prone to infectious forms of otitis media.

Signs and Symptoms: A person with serous otitis media usually only experiences a sensation of fullness or pressure in the affected ear, along with varying degrees of hearing impairment. Suppurative otitis media, on the other hand, is usually manifested by pain in the affected ear and is often accompanied by general symptoms of infection such as fever and chills, nausea, and vomiting. Both conditions may occasion dizziness.

Diagnostic Procedures: Examination of the affected ear with an otoscope will reveal bulging of the ear drum. Fluid bubbles may be discernible behind the ear drum. The individual's WBC is typically elevated in cases of suppurative otitis media.

Treatment: Antibiotics will be ordered to control suppurative otitis media and analgesics may be prescribed to relieve pain and discomfort of either form. Decongestants may be ordered to promote drainage. In severe cases, drainage may be accomplished by myringotomy or needle aspiration. For chronic forms of otitis media, the acute attacks must be treated as previously described, but further surgery may be necessary, such as myringoplasty and tympanoplasty.

Prognosis: The prognosis of an individual with either form of acute otitis media usually is good, given prompt treatment. Chronic otitis media, however, may lead to scarring, adhesions, and severe ear damage with hearing loss. Complications are possible, ranging from either acute or chronic forms of suppurative otitis media to brain abscess, meningitis, or mastoiditis.

Prevention: Prompt treatment of any upper respiratory tract infection and otitis media.

Otosclerosis

Description: *Otosclerosis* is the formation of spongy bone, especially around the oval window, with resulting immobilization of the stapes. The condition is characterized by chronic, progressive deafness. The disease occurs primarily among women, usually appearing between the ages of 15 and 30 years.

Etiology: Otosclerosis is an idiopathic condition, but because the disease shows a familial pattern, genetic factors are suspected. The condition is often aggravated by pregnancy.

Signs and Symptoms: A gradual bilateral hearing loss of low tones or soft sounds is the first sign. Tinnitus may accompany the condition.

Diagnostic Procedures: A Rinne test is diagnostic of otosclerosis. An audiogram may reveal a moderate to severe hearing loss.

Treatment: The ear that is most affected may undergo **stapedectomy** with a prosthesis inserted. The other ear will have the same surgery later. If surgery is not an option, a hearing aid may be tried.

Prognosis: The prognosis improves following surgery, although some degree of lasting hearing impairment is characteristic of the disease.

Prevention: There is no known prevention.

Motion Sickness

Description: *Motion sickness* is nausea, vomiting, and **vertigo** induced by irregular or rhythmic movements, such as may occur during airplane, boat, or automobile travel.

Etiology: This disorder is caused by any motion capable of disturbing the equilibrium of the organs of balance in the inner ear (the semicircular canals). Strong emotions such as fear and grief, digestive upset, or offensive odors, may trigger or exacerbate the problem.

Signs and Symptoms: An individual affected by motion sickness may experience loss of equilibrium, nausea, vomiting, dizziness, **diaphoresis**, headache, and anorexia. Symptoms may disappear almost immediately after the inciting motion has ceased, or they may persist for hours or days.

Diagnostic Procedures: Diagnosis is by patient history and complaints.

Treatment: Ongoing attacks of motion sickness usually are successfully treated with antihistamines, antiemetics, or sedatives.

Prognosis: While the condition may be severe enough to be debilitating for some, the symptoms of motion sickness usually disappear with the restoration of equilibrium.

Prevention: Certain **anticholinergic drug** preparations taken prior to traveling are quite useful in preventing the onset of symptoms in susceptible individuals.

Meniere's Disease

Description: *Meniere's disease* is a chronic inner ear syndrome marked by attacks of vertigo, progressive deafness, tinnitus, and a sensation of fullness in the ears. The condition usually appears between the ages of 40 and 50 years.

Etiology: The cause of Meniere's disease is not known, but the disease process appears to destroy the hair cells within the cochlea. Head trauma, middle ear infection, autonomic nervous system dysfunction, and premenstrual edema may be predisposing factors.

Signs and Symptoms: The classic symptoms are severe vertigo, tinnitus, and sensorineural hearing loss. An acute attack of vertigo may cause nausea, vomiting, sweating, and loss of balance. These attacks may occur several times a year, but remissions also can last several years.

Diagnostic Procedures: When all three symptoms are present, the diagnosis is not difficult. Further testing using audiometry and x-rays of the internal meatus of the ear may be necessary.

Treatment: A salt-free diet, diuretics, antihistamines, and mild sedatives are helpful in long-term care. Severe attacks may require epinephrine. If the disease persists and causes debilitating vertigo, surgical destruction of the affected labyrinth may be necessary. This relieves symptoms but causes irreversible hearing loss.

Prognosis: The prognosis varies, but usually multiple attacks over several years lead to residual tinnitus and hearing loss.

Prevention: There is no known prevention.

COMMON SYMPTOMS OF EAR DISEASE

Individuals may present with the following common symptoms, which deserve attention from health professionals:

- Hearing loss
- Tinnitus
- Ear pressure
- Nausea and vomiting
- Pain
- Dizziness

REVIEW QUESTIONS

True/False

T F 1. Hyperopia or farsightedness is the most common refractive error.

T F 2. Myopia is nearsightedness.

T F 3. Presbyopia is an elliptical curvature of the cornea.

T F 4. *Nystagmus* is the medical term for stye.

T F 5. Complications of corneal abrasion are ulceration and permanent vision loss.

T F 6. In a mature cataract, the pupil of the eye becomes white.

T F 7. A common sign of a cataract is eye pain.

T F 8. Adults should be tested for glaucoma every 3 to 5 years.

T F 9. An uncommon eye disorder is conjunctivitis.

T F 10. Blepharitis may be caused by a *Staphylococcus* infection.

T F 11. *Photophobia* is the term to describe the eye's sensitivity to light.

T F 12. Exposure keratitis may be caused by "snow blindness."

MATCHING

_____ 1. Cerumen

_____ 2. External otitis

_____ 3. Otitis media

_____ 4. Otosclerosis

_____ 5. Tinnitus

_____ 6. Meniere's disease

_____ 7. Uveitis

a. Ear ache or inflammation of middle ear

b. Noise or ringing in ear

c. Causes severe vertigo

d. Swimmer's ear

e. Hearing loss due to aging

f. Ear wax

g. Spongy bone in labyrinth's capsule

h. Inflammation of the uveal tract

i. Inflammation of the cornea

Discussion Question

Determine what a physician looks for in a physical examination of the eye and the ear.

Answers

True/False

1. T
2. T
3. F
4. F
5. T
6. T
7. F
8. T
9. F
10. T
11. T
12. T

Matching

1. f
2. d
3. a
4. g
5. b
6. c
7. h

Discussion Question

Answers will vary.

GLOSSARY

ANTICHOLINERGIC (DRUG): Drug or agent that inhibits the action of the neuro-transmitting chemical acetylcholine, blocking parasympathetic nerve impulses, with consequent reduction of smooth-muscle contractions and various bodily secretions.

ATROPINE: Anticholinergic agent that counteracts effects of parasympathetic stimulation.

CELLULITIS: Inflammation of cellular or connective tissue.

CONJUNCTIVA: The mucous membrane structure that lines the inner surface of the eyelids and that is reflected onto the anterior portion of the eyeball.

CURET: Surgical instrument shaped like a spoon or scoop for scraping and removing material from a cavity.

DIAPHORESIS: Sweating, especially when profuse or medically induced.

PHOTOPHOBIA: Unusual intolerance of light.

PRURITUS: Severe itching.

RADIAL KERATOTOMY: A surgical procedure in which a series of spokelike incisions are made in the surface of the cornea. Intraocular pressure stretches the incisions, slightly flattening the curvature of the cornea. Used to correct certain refractive errors.

SEBORRHEA: Functional disease of the sabaceous glands marked by an increase in the amount, and often an alteration of the quality, of the sebacous secretion.

STAPEDECTOMY: Excision of the stapes in the ear in order to improve hearing, especially in cases of otosclerosis. The stapes is replaced by a prosthesis.

SUPPURATIVE: Producing or generating pus.

TINNITUS: A subjective, continuous ringing or buzzing sound in one or both ears.

VERTIGO: A sensation of spinning around in space or of having objects spin around the person.

Chapter 14

Childhood Diseases

LEARNING OBJECTIVES

Upon successful completion of this chapter, you will
- Identify reasons for the decrease in communicable diseases.
- Compare and contrast rubella and rubeola.
- Recall the prognosis and prevention for mumps.
- Describe the signs and symptoms of varicella.
- Define diphtheria, pertussis, and tetanus.
- Recognize the signs and symptoms of influenza.
- Review the etiology of SIDS.
- Recall the most common disease causing time loss from work and school.
- Report the treatment of choice for chronic tonsillitis and adenoid hyperplasia.

307

- Describe the signs and symptoms of croup.
- Identify the etiology of epiglottitis.
- Discuss the etiology of colic.
- Compare and contrast acute and chronic diarrhea.
- Explain the treatment of vomiting.
- List the most common nutritional allergens.
- Compare and constrast roundworm and pinworm infestations.
- Restate the etiology of Reye's syndrome.
- Explain the treatment of diaper rash.
- Review the prognosis and prevention of strabismus.

INTRODUCTION

An infant acquires limited natural immunity to disease from its mother and through the activity of its thymus gland. But the immature physiologic systems of infants predispose them to illness, and when a child reaches school age, the incidence of disease increases manyfold. Childhood has its own particular set of medical problems which require special care and attention. There is nothing quite so heartrending as a child who is unable to participate in the daily activities of life because of illness or disease.

> Children feel their hearts a burning.
> Let them live their natural yearning.[1]

COMMUNICABLE DISEASES OF CHILDHOOD AND ADOLESCENCE

The incidence of certain communicable diseases in the United States has steadily decreased over recent decades. Children and adolescents are no longer the routine victims of many diseases thanks to advances in medical knowledge, general improvements in living conditions, and government-mandated immunization programs. Poliomyelitis, for example, once endemic in the United States, is now considered rare since the advent of the Salk vaccine.

Caution cannot be thrown to the wind, however. A serious outbreak of rubeola occurred recently on a college campus where a substantial number of students had not been vaccinated against the disease owing to their religious beliefs. In the absence of the effective immunization provided by vaccines, communicable disease can still cause major epidemics.

A *vaccine* is a suspension of infectious agents or some part of them. It is given for the purpose of establishing resistance to an infectious disease. There are four general classes of vaccines:

- Those containing living infectious organisms. The organisms are either disabled or otherwise nonvirulent strains.
- Those containing infectious agents killed by physical or chemical means.
- Those containing solutions of toxins from microorganisms. The toxins may be used directly, but usually they are treated to neutralize their toxic potential.
- Those containing substances extracted from a portion of an infectious agent. Effective antiviral vaccines often are made by extracting only a small portion of the virus's protein coat.

Whatever its class a vaccine stimulates the development of specific defensive mechanisms that result in more or less permanent protection from the disease. Table 14-1 highlights the vaccines that are either routinely or commonly administered during childhood and adolescence.

Measles (Rubeola)

Description: *Measles* is a highly communicable disease characterized by fever and the appearance of a characteristic rash. The disease is most common in school-age children, with outbreaks occurring in the winter and spring. Recently, though, the disease has occurred with increasing frequency among high school and college students.

Etiology: Measles is caused by the rubeola virus. The virus has an incubation period of from 10 to 20 days.

Signs and Symptoms: The onset of symptoms is usually gradual. Initial symptoms may include rhinitis, drowsiness, anorexia, and a slow but progressive rise in temperature to 101 to 103°F by the second day. **Koplik's spots** appear on the oral mucosa by the second or third day. **Photophobia** and cough soon follow. By about the fourth day, the fever usually reaches its maximum (as high as 104 to 106°F) and the characteristic rash appears. The rash first appears on the face as tiny maculopapular lesions. These rapidly enlarge and spread to other areas of the body. The lesions may be so densely clustered in certain areas that the skin surface appears generally swollen and red.

Diagnostic Procedures: The individual's clinical picture of symptoms is usually a sufficient basis for a diagnosis of measles. Blood testing may reveal **leukopenia**, and various tests are available to detect the presence of measles antibody.

Treatment: Treatment for measles is essentially symptomatic. Bed rest is indicated, usually in a darkened room to alleviate the discomfort of photophobia. **Antipyretics** and liquids may be recommended. The affected individual should be kept isolated until the rash disappears.

Prognosis: Measles is usually a benign disease, running its course in about 5 days after the rash appears. An attack of measles usually confers permanent immunity. Complications may arise, however, including croup, conjunctivitis, myocarditis, hepatitis, and opportunistic respiratory tract infections from *Staphylococcus*, Streptococcus, or *H. influenzae*. Measles infection during pregnancy may result in

**TABLE 14–1. Vaccines Commonly Administered
During Childhood***

Name	Age Administered	Booster Schedule	Comments
DTP (diphtheria, tetanus, pertussis)	Given routinely beginning as early as 3 months; a total of three inoculations at 4- to 6-week intervals; a fourth dose is given a year later	Repeat inoculation at time of entering school; after that, children need *only* tetanus and diphtheria immunization every 10 years	Tetanus booster may be required following a wound even though all routine and booster immunizations have been received; booster of diphtheria toxoid should be given if child under 6 is exposed to diphtheria
Hepatitis B	All ages of persons at risk of contracting the virus, e.g., dialysis patients	Every 6 to 12 months	The vaccine is expensive and should be given only to those at high risk of developing the disease who do not show evidence of immunity to the virus
Influenza (flu)	All ages	Variable depending on strain of virus predicted to cause the next influenza epidemic	Recommended for those who may become seriously ill if they develop flu, i.e., the elderly and those of any age who have chronic diseases of the heart or lungs or metabolic diseases such as diabetes
Measles (live attenuated rubeola)	15 months, but may be given as early as 6 months during an epidemic	If vaccinated before 10 months of age, should be revaccinated within a year	Vaccine will usually prevent measles if given within 2 days after a child has been exposed to the disease; not given to adults; contraindicated in those known to be hypersensitive to eggs, chicken, chicken feathers, or neomycin
Mumps	Any age after 15 months	Not indicated	Particularly valuable for children approaching puberty, adolescents, and adults who have never had mumps; contraindicated in those known to be hypersensitive to eggs, chicken, chicken feathers, or neomycin

TABLE 14–1. *Continued*

Name	Age Administered	Booster Schedule	Comments
Polio (live oral trivalent vaccine)	6 to 8 weeks for first dose; second given 6 weeks later; third, 2 months later; fourth at 15 to 18 months of age	At time of entering school	Administration postponed in those with persistent vomiting, diarrhea, or acute illness
Rubella (German measles)	No earlier than 1 year of age	Not indicated	Objective is to prevent infection of the fetus; because the major source of virus dissemination is from children in elementary school, all children regardless of their previous experience with rubella should be vaccinated *Caution:* Pregnant women should not be given rubella vaccine.

*Adapted from Thomas, C. L., (ed.): *Taber's Cyclopedic Medical Dictionary,* ed. 15. F. A. Davis, Philadelphia, Pa., 1985, pp. 1826–1628, with permission.

the death of the fetus, but it does not seem to produce birth defects, as does rubella (see Rubella).

Prevention: Measles can be prevented within 5 days after exposure by administration of **gamma globulin**. Active immunization can be produced by administration of measles vaccine, preferably containing the live attenuated virus.

Rubella (German Measles)

Description: *Rubella* is an acute infectious disease characterized by fever and rash. It closely resembles measles, but it differs in its short course, mild fever, and relative freedom from complications. Rubella is not as contagious as measles, and it now occurs more frequently among high school age children and young adults.

Etiology: The disease is caused by the rubella virus. This virus has an incubation period of from 14 to 21 days.

Signs and Symptoms: The onset of the disease is sometimes characterized by malaise, headache, slight fever, and sore throat. These symptoms may be entirely absent, however, especially among children. The rash typically appears the first or second day after onset. It may be composed of pale red, slightly elevated, discrete **papules,** or it may be highly diffuse and bright red. The rash begins on the face, spreads rapidly to other portions of the body, and usually fades so rapidly that the face may clear before the extremities are affected. Rash-covered portions of skin may itch or peel.

Diagnostic Procedures: Because rubella can be easily confused with other diseases, a definitive diagnosis can only be reached by isolating the virus or detecting its antibody.

Treatment: Treatment is nonspecific and symptomatic. Bed rest is indicated. Topical antipruritics or warm water baths may be recommended to relieve itching. Antipyretics may be prescribed.

Prognosis: The prognosis for an individual with rubella is usually good. The disease is benign, seldom produces complications, and runs its course in 3 days. Rubella is dangerous, however, when it occurs in pregnant women, especially during the first trimester of pregnancy. The virus is capable of producing severe fetal malformation.

Prevention: Administration of gamma globulin shortly after exposure may prevent development of the disease, but it still may not prevent transfer of the virus to the fetus if exposure occurs during pregnancy. Lasting immunization can be conferred through use of a live rubella vaccine. This vaccine must not be administered to pregnant women or to those who may become pregnant within 3 months after immunization.

Mumps

Description: *Mumps* is an acute contagious disease characterized by fever and inflammation of the parotid and salivary glands. The disease is most common among children and young adults.

Etiology: The disease is caused by the mumps virus, which has an incubation period of 18 days.

Signs and Symptoms: The classic symptoms of mumps are unilateral or bilateral swollen parotid glands. Headache, malaise, fever, and earache may occur. Other salivary glands may become swollen, too.

Diagnostic Procedures: The clinical picture of mumps and a history of recent exposure usually is sufficient for diagnosis.

Treatment: Analgesics, antipyretics, and adequate fluid intake may be recommended. Isolation of the affected individual is important during the contagious period.

Prognosis: The prognosis for an individual with mumps is good. Complications can occur, however, and include **epididymo-orchitis,** pancreatitis, and various CNS manifestations. Epididymo-orchitis, which causes swelling of the testes, is extremely uncomfortable but rarely causes sterility, as often is feared.

Prevention: The best prevention is to receive the mumps vaccine and avoid exposure to the disease during its period of communicability.

Varicella (Chickenpox)

Description: *Varicella (chickenpox)* is a highly contagious disease characterized by the appearance of a distinctive rash that passes through stages of macules, papules, **vesicles**, and crusts. The disease occurs most commonly among children and may occur in epidemic outbreaks in winter and spring.

Etiology: The disease is caused by the varicella-zoster virus (VZV). Its incubation period is from 2 to 3 weeks, usually between 13 and 17 days.

Signs and Symptoms: The signs of chickenpox are a pruritic rash which begins as erythematous macules that produce papules and then clear vesicles. The rash usually contains a combination of papules, vesicles, and scabs in all stages. Anorexia, malaise, and fever may accompany the rash.

Diagnostic Procedures: The clinical signs usually are sufficient for the diagnosis. A history which indicates recent exposure is helpful, too.

Treatment: Isolation is important during the infectious period—usually until all the scabs disappear. The only treatment necessary is to reduce the itching. Calamine lotion or cool bicarbonate of soda baths can be very helpful. It is best not to scratch the lesions. *Note:* Aspirin should *not* be used to treat fever in cases of chickenpox among children and adolescents because of its association with an increased incidence of Reye's syndrome (see Reye's Syndrome).

Prognosis: The prognosis for an individual with varicella is good. The disease runs its course in about 2 to 3 weeks. Complications may include secondary bacterial infections of the skin as a result of scratching open lesions.

Prevention: In certain situations, varicella-zoster immune globulin (VZIG) may be administered within 72 hours of exposure to stop development of the disease.

Diphtheria

Description: *Diphtheria* is an acute, life-threatening infectious disease. It is characterized by a membrane-like coating that forms over mucous membrane surfaces, particularly along the respiratory tract, and by a toxic reaction primarily affecting the heart and peripheral nerves. The disease may occasionally involve the skin. Most cases occur in children prior to age 10, but older children and adults also may be affected. Diphtheria used to be a frequent affliction of children in the United States, but thanks to diligent immunization efforts, the disease now appears only sporadically.

Etiology: Diphtheria is caused by *Corynebacterium diphtheriae*. The bacterium has an incubation period of from 2 to 5 days. *C. diphtheriae* has two principal pathogenic effects. As it multiplies along mucous membrane surfaces, the bacteria forms a distinctive, leathery, blue-white membrane composed of bacteria, necrotized tissue, inflammatory cells, and **fibrin**. This false membrane may enlarge to the extent that it impairs respiratory function. Most strains of *C. diphtheriae* also release a highly potent toxin capable of damaging the heart, kidneys, and peripheral nerves.

Signs and Symptoms: The specific symptoms vary with the site of infection. In typical cases, diphtheria may first present as a slight headache and malaise. A mild fever (100 to 101°F) may ensue, followed by the appearance of the characteristic membrane adhering to the tonsils or the walls of the pharynx. If the bacterium localizes in the nasal passages, fever may be more pronounced, and a steady, blood-tinged discharge may appear from the nostrils. There may be a strong, foul odor to the breath. Manifestations of myocarditis and neuritis commonly develop as late symptoms. Some individuals infected with *C. diphtheriae* remain asymptomatic but become carriers of the disease.

Diagnostic Procedures: The appearance of the characteristic membrane may be enough to establish a diagnosis of diphtheria. A definitive diagnosis can be made only by identifying the bacterium in smears or cultures.

Treatment: The only specific treatment is administration of sufficient quantities of diphtheria antitoxin as early in the course of the disease as possible. The affected individual must be isolated, and bed rest is required. A soft or liquid diet is recommended. Emergency measures may be required to maintain an airway or control cardiac complications. Carriers of diphtheria are usually treated with antibiotics.

Prognosis: The prognosis for an individual with diphtheria varies according to the severity of the disease. Mild cases of diphtheria resolve in 3 to 4 days, or a week in moderate cases. Even with effective antitoxin therapy, however, death may result from extension of the diphtherial membrane into the lower respiratory tract or from organ system damage produced by the diphtheria toxin.

Prevention: Diphtheria is highly preventable. Innoculation with diphtheria toxoid at the age of 3 months is normally routine. Booster doses should be administered at appropriate intervals during early childhood (see Table 14–1). Diphtheria toxoid is usually administered along with the vaccine for pertussis and the toxoid for tetanus (the DPT shot), since higher levels of antibodies are produced when all three are administered simultaneously rather than individually.

Pertussis (Whooping Cough)

Description: *Pertussis* is an acute, highly infectious respiratory tract disease characterized by a repetitious, paroxysmal cough and a prolonged, harsh or shrill sound during inspiration (the "whoop"). Prior to effective immunization, pertussis caused more deaths among infants and young children than any other communicable childhood disease. Pertussis still affects infants and children more frequently and more severely than it does adults, although the incidence of the disease among adults has recently increased.

Etiology: Most cases of pertussis are caused by *Bordetella pertussis*. This bacterium has an incubation period of 7 to 10 days. *B. pertussis* multiplies along the surfaces of airways, most often affecting the bronchi and bronchioles, less frequently affecting the trachea, larynx, and nasopharynx. The bacterium induces a mucopurulent secretion and hampers the natural ability of the respiratory tract to clear such secretions. Consequently, mucus accumulates in the airways and obstructs airflow. The bacterium also may produce a mild toxic reaction.

Signs and Symptoms: The signs and symptoms of pertussis can be divided into three stages. The *catarrhal stage* is marked by the gradual onset of coldlike symptoms: mild fever, running nose, dry cough, irritability, and anorexia. This stage lasts from 1 to 2 weeks. The *paroxysmal stage* is marked by the onset of the classic cough, consisting of a series of several short, severe coughs in rapid succession followed by a slow, strained inspiration, during which a "whoop" (**stridor**) may be heard. The coughing occurs in periodic attacks. This stage, lasting 3 to 4 weeks, may be accompanied by weight loss, dehydration, vomiting, epistaxis, and hypoxia. After several weeks, a period of *decline* begins, marked by the gradual diminishment of coughing.

Diagnostic Procedures: A history of exposure to another infected individual and the presence of the classic cough may be enough to establish the diagnosis. A very high white blood count is a further distinguishing feature of pertussis. A definitive diagnosis may depend on identifying the bacteria in respiratory secretions.

Treatment: Antibiotics administered during the catarrhal stage may check the development of the disease; if administration is delayed past this stage, antibiotics have little effect. The individual with pertussis requires meticulous care to ensure adequate nutrition, hydration, and clearance of mucous secretions.

Prognosis: The prognosis for an individual with pertussis varies from case to case. Uncomplicated pertussis may run its course in 12 weeks. Recovery may be considerably extended, however, particularly among infants. Death usually is caused by pneumonia, produced by *B. pertussis* itself or by a secondary infection.

Prevention: A child can be rendered less susceptible to pertussis by receiving a series of immunizations with pertussis vaccine, starting around the age of 3 months. Receiving the vaccine or having the disease, however, does not guarantee lasting immunity from pertussis. Furthermore, pertussis vaccine causes reactions of varying intensity in nearly half the individuals who receive it.

Tetanus (Lockjaw)

Description: *Tetanus* is an acute, life-threatening infectious disease characterized by persistent, painful contractions of skeletal muscles. The disease may affect any person at any time, but children are at greater risk because of their tendency to develop skin wounds as a result of play activities.

Etiology: The disease is caused by *Clostridium tetani,* a bacterium commonly found in soil. The bacillus becomes pathogenic when it breeds within human tissue. Wounds, burns, surgical incisions, and chronic skin ulcers may provide opportunities for infection with *C. tetani,* as may generalized conditions such as otitis media and dental infections. The microorganism produces a powerful toxin that attacks the central nervous system and that also acts directly on voluntary muscles to produce contraction.

Signs and Symptoms: The onset of symptoms may be either gradual or abrupt. Stiffness of the jaw, esophageal muscles, and some neck muscles is often the first sign of the disease. Later, in the most common manifestation of tetanus, the jaws become rigidly fixed (lockjaw), the voice is altered, and the facial muscles contract, contorting the individual's face into a grimace. Finally, the muscles of the back and the extremities may become rigid or the individual may experience extremely severe convulsive spasms of muscles. This final phase of the disease often is accompanied by high fever, profuse sweating, tachycardia, dysphagia, and intense pain.

Diagnostic Procedures: Tetanus is diagnosed on the basis of its classic symptomatology.

Treatment: The site of the wound or the point of infection must be thoroughly cleaned and debrided. Human tetanus immune globulin (TIG) often will be administered. Muscle relaxants may be prescribed. A tetanus patient requires meticulous care and support to maintain adequate nutrition and hydration and to avoid developing decubitus ulcers. Tracheostomy is routinely performed in moderate to severe cases of tetanus to prevent choking.

Prognosis: Despite effective treatment measures, tetanus is frequently fatal, especially among the elderly. Death may result from asphyxiation, a host of possible complications, and sometimes from sheer exhaustion. In cases of tetanus in which the individual survives, the disease usually runs its course in about 6 to 7 weeks, seldom producing any lasting disability.

Prevention: Surprisingly enough, having tetanus does not confer future immunity to the disease. Immunization with tetanus toxoid should be routinely started at 3 months of age. Boosters are required periodically throughout life. The risk of contracting tetanus also can be minimized by prompt cleansing and care of wounds and other skin lesions.

Influenza

Description: *Influenza (flu)* is an acute, contagious respiratory disease characterized by fever, chills, headache, and **myalgia**. The disease may affect anyone, but school-age children and the elderly are especially susceptible. Flu often occurs in epidemic outbreaks, particularly in the winter and spring.

Etiology: Flu is caused by viruses that are members of the Orthomyxoviridae family. For diagnostic and treatment purposes, the viruses are classified as either type A, B, or C based on their antigenic properties. Influenza viruses frequently mutate, creating new strains that easily infect populations that had acquired immunity to previous strains of the virus.

Signs and Symptoms: The onset generally is abrupt, with fever, chills, croup in children, malaise, muscular aching, headache, nasal congestion, laryngitis, and a cough.

Diagnostic Procedures: Because the signs and symptoms of flu resemble so many other illnesses, it is frequently difficult to diagnose solely on the basis of symptomatology unless there is an ongoing epidemic. A throat culture may be performed to isolate the virus, or various immunofluorescence techniques may be performed to detect viral antigens.

Treatment: Treatment consists of bed rest, maintaining adequate fluid intake and administering analgesics and antipyretics. *Note:* Aspirin should *not* be used to treat fever and muscle pain in children and adolescents with flu owing to its association with an increased incidence of Reye's syndrome (see Reye's Syndrome).

Prognosis: The prognosis is good with proper care. Complications include sinusitis, otitis media, bronchitis, and pneumonia.

Prevention: Influenza vaccines prepared from the most recent strains of A and B type viruses are useful in preventing flu. The vaccines may produce reactions in some, especially people who are allergic to egg products. The U.S. Public Health Service recommends inoculation against influenza for those with chronic cardiac and respiratory conditions, for those with serious systemic diseases, and for the elderly.

Common Cold

Description: The *common cold* is an acute infection causing inflammation of the upper respiratory tract. Colds occur more frequently in children and account for more lost time from work or school than any other cause. The highest incidence of colds is during the winter months.

Etiology: Colds are usually caused by viruses. Some colds, however, result from **Mycoplasma**. These microorganisms are transmitted by airborne respiratory droplets.

Signs and Symptoms: Common symptoms include nasal congestion, pharyngitis, headache, malaise, burning and watery eyes, and low-grade fever A productive or nonproductive cough may be present. The symptoms commonly last from 2 to 4 days, but nasal congestion may persist for an indefinite period. Reinfection is common, but complications are rare. The cold is contagious for 2 to 3 days after onset.

Diagnostic Procedures: There is no specific diagnostic test for the common cold. A throat culture may be done to rule out other diseases.

Treatment: Treatment of the cold is symptomatic and includes mild analgesics, ample fluid intake, and rest. Decongestants, nose drops, throat lozenges, and steam may be helpful. Dehydration must be prevented, if possible, or treated. If secondary bacterial infections are suspected, antibiotics may be prescribed.

Prognosis: The disease is self-limiting, but it can lead to secondary bacterial infection.

Prevention: There is no known prevention. Fatigue and exposure to drafts do increase susceptibility.

RESPIRATORY DISEASES

Sudden Infant Death Syndrome (SIDS)

Description: *Sudden infant death syndrome* (SIDS) is the completely unexpected and unexplained death of an apparently normal and healthy infant, usually 10 to 12 weeks old. Generally, the death occurs when the infant is sleeping. SIDS occurs more frequently in males than in females, in premature infants, and during the winter months.

Etiology: The cause is unknown, but several have been suggested, including mechanical suffocation, prolonged **apnea**, lack of **biotin** in the diet, an unknown virus, immunoglobin abnormalities, a defect in the respiratory mucosal defense, or an anatomically abnormal larynx.

Signs and Symptoms: There are no premonitory signs and symptoms. The infant generally does not cry out or show evidence of distress or struggle. When found, the infant is dead and may have mottled skin indicating cyanosis. There may be blood-tinged sputum. The infant's diaper is likely to be wet or filled with stool.

Diagnostic Procedures: A diagnosis of SIDS is exclusionary, i.e., made only after all other causes of death have been eliminated as possibilities.

Treatment: There is no treatment. There are SIDS support groups for parents.

Prognosis: It is currently believed that children are no longer at risk of SIDS by 1 year of age.

Prevention: Some home monitoring devices have been tried on infants who have experienced apneic periods, but their use remains controversial. Prevention of SIDS is largely aimed at trying to identify infants at risk.

Pneumonia

Pneumonia is inflammation of the lungs caused primarily by bacteria, viruses, and chemical irritants. Pneumonia in childhood occurs more frequently in infancy and young children. Viral pneumonias occur more frequently than bacterial pneumonias and often follow a viral upper respiratory infection.

The onset of pneumonia may be acute or insidious, with symptoms ranging from mild fever, slight cough, and malaise to high fever and severe cough. The prognosis generally is good, although a viral pneumonia can leave a child more susceptible to a secondary bacterial infection. For a further discussion of penumonia, see Chapter 7.

Acute Tonsillitis

Description: *Acute tonsillitis* is inflammation of a tonsil, especially one or both of the palatine tonsils that lie on either side of the opening of the throat.

Etiology: Acute tonsillitis is most frequently caused by infection by the bacteria *Streptococcus pyogenes* or *Stapholoccus aureus,* although a variety of infectious agents may possibly be involved. The condition is a common complication of pharyngitis.

Signs and Symptoms: Tonsillitis is typically manifested by the sudden onset of chills and a high-grade fever. Additional symptoms may include malaise, headache, sore throat, and dysphagia.

Diagnostic Procedures: Upon physical examination, the tonsils will appear red and swollen. In severe cases, abscesses may be visible on the affected tonsil's surface. Blood tests may reveal leukocytosis. A throat culture to detect bacteria will typically be performed.

Treatment: Antibiotic, especially penicillin, therapy is prescribed for bacterial tonsillitis in its early stages. Symptomatic relief includes saline gargles, analgesics, and antipyretics. Bed rest is usually indicated. Recurrent bouts of tonsillitis may require tonsillectomy.

Prognosis: The prognosis for acute tonsillitis is usually good. In severe cases, however, the tonsils may swell sufficiently to interfere with breathing. Serious complications include rheumatic fever, glomerulonephritis, and carditis. More localized complications may include otitis media, mastoiditis, and sinusitis.

Prevention: There is no specific prevention for acute tonsillitis except for prompt treatment of any pharyngeal infection.

Adenoid Hyperplasia

Description: *Adenoid hyperplasia* is the enlargement of the lymphoid tissue of the nasopharynx.

Etiology: The cause is essentially unknown. Circumstances which may cause the adenoids to continue to grow when they normally would atrophy (approximately ages 5 to 8) may include repeated infection and nasal congestion, chronic allergies, and heredity.

Signs and Symptoms: The most common symptoms are chronic mouth breathing, snoring, and frequent head colds.

Diagnostic Procedures: Diagnosis is usually made by visualizing the hyperplastic adenoidal tissue.

Treatment: The treatment of choice is adenoidectomy, often performed in conjunction with a tonsillectomy (T&A).

Prognosis: The prognosis is excellent with proper care and attention. If untreated, however, adenoid hyperplasia can lead to changes in facial features and complications such as otitis media with accompanying risk of hearing loss.

Prevention: There is no specific prevention for this condition.

Croup

Description: *Croup* is an acute viral infection of the respiratory tract occurring most frequently in infants 3 months to 3 years of age. It is more common in males.

Etiology: The condition may be caused by parainfluenza virus, adenoviruses, respiratory syncytial viruses, and influenza A and B viruses. Croup generally follows an upper respiratory tract infection.

Signs and Symptoms: Common symptoms include hoarseness, fever, a distinctive harsh, brassy, barklike cough, persistent stridor during inspiration, and respiratory distress.

Diagnostic Procedures: Cultures of the causative organism are done. Neck x-ray and laryngoscopy may be performed, too.

Treatment: Children are treated symptomatically at home in most cases with bed rest, liquids, and antipyretics. If dehydration is suspected, hospitalization may be necessary and antibiotic therapy and oxygen therapy may be started.

Prognosis: The prognosis is good with treatment.

Prevention: Prevention includes prompt treatment of any respiratory tract infections.

Acute Epiglottitis

Description: *Acute epiglottitis* is severe inflammation of the epiglottis. It primarily affects children between the ages of 2 and 12 years.

Etiology: The causative agent generally is *Hemophilus influenzae* type B. Pneumococci and group A streptococci also can cause epiglottitis.

Signs and Symptoms: Common symptoms include fever, swollen and erythematous epiglottis, sore throat, stridor, and croupy cough. If the epiglottis is swollen and inflamed enough, there could be total obstruction of the larynx. The child may sit with the neck hyperextended and the mouth open and tongue protruding in an attempt to "get more air."

Diagnostic Procedures: Physical examination may be all that is necessary to reveal the inflamed epiglottis. Neck x-rays and laryngoscopy may be done, too.

Treatment: The child will be hospitalized and possibly require emergency tracheostomy or endotracheal intubation. Oxgyen therapy, antibiotics, and close monitoring may be necessary.

Prognosis: The prognosis is good with prompt treatment.
Prevention: Prevention includes prompt treatment of any respiratory illness.

Asthma

Asthma is one of the leading causes of chronic illness in children. Prior to puberty, it occurs twice as often in boys as in girls, whereas during adolescence, both sexes are equally affected. The majority of cases have their onset before 7 years of age. Most childhood asthma is caused by an allergic reaction in the bronchi. Asthma tends to run in families, and sometimes the child may have a history of eczema in early childhood. Some children "outgrow" asthma at puberty. See Chapter 7 for a complete discussion of this condition.

GASTROINTESTINAL DISEASES

Infantile Colic

Description: *Infantile colic* is paroxysmal abdominal pain or cramping. The condition usually occurs during the first few months of life.
Etiology: Excessive fermentation and gas production in the intestines is thought to be the cause of colic. Other factors include too rapid feeding, overeating, swallowing air, or poor burping techniques. Many times the cause cannot be determined.
Signs and Symptoms: Loud crying and drawing the legs up to the abdomen are behaviors typical of an infant experiencing colic. The symptoms are more apt to occur late in the afternoon or in early evening.
Diagnostic Procedures: There is no specific diagnostic test for this disorder. Observing the parent and infant interacting may help in the diagnosis.
Treatment: The best treatment may be the availability of a calm setting for feeding time for both parent and child and gentle burping midway through the feeding and again at the end. Support of the parent is necessary, too. A vicious circle can occur if the parent's anxiety about the problem is sensed by the infant. At times, no form of treatment is effective.
Prognosis: The prognosis is good. The infant will continue to thrive and develop even with the colic. Colic usually disappears spontaneously after three months.
Prevention: The best prevention is frequent and smaller feedings and relaxed parents.

Note: Diarrhea and vomiting are not disease entities; rather, they are symptoms of a problem. Since they are so common in infants and children, the following material is provided.

Diarrhea

Acute diarrhea is a sudden change in the frequency and liquid content of the stool. *Chronic diarrhea* is the passage of loose stools with increased frequency for 2 weeks or more. The latter may be caused by anatomic defects, allergic reactions, or disorders of malabsorption. A variety of factors can cause either type of diarrhea in the infant and child. It may be caused by an inflammatory process of infectious origin or a toxic reaction to "dietary indiscretions" or ingestion of poisons.

Treatment of diarrhea is dependent on the cause and severity. Treatment includes reducing the child's activities and encouraging a diet of clear liquids for a few days. Severe diarrhea may require hospitalization to prevent dehydration.

Vomiting

Vomiting may be caused by overfeeding, gastrointestinal disorders, infections, increased intracranial pressure, and ingestion of toxic substances. The signs and symptoms range from mild regurgitation to projectile vomiting, such as occurs in pyloric stenosis. In diagnosis, the frequency and duration of vomiting will be considered as well as the character of the vomitus.

Treatment is dependent on the cause and severity of the vomiting and includes taking the child off solid foods and allowing the gastrointestinal tract to rest. Feeding smaller amounts more frequently may be helpful.

Food Allergies

Description: A *food allergy* is a hypersensitivity reaction to certain foods.

Etiology: Some of the more common food allergens are milk products, eggs, wheat, nuts, legumes, fish, chocolate, berries, citrus fruits, and nitrate-containing products such as weiners and bacon.

Signs and Symptoms: Symptoms may include inflammation and swelling in the face or around the lip, gastrointestinal disturbances, vomiting, and diarrhea.

Diagnostic Procedures: If food allergies are suspected, the child may be taken off the regular diet. Foods may then be added gradually, one at a time, until a reaction occurs. This may pinpoint an allergen.

Treatment: Once the allergen is determined, it should be avoided and not reintroduced into the diet for 6 months. It may be necessary to find alternatives for those foods which must be avoided yet are necessary to a balanced diet.

Prognosis: The prognosis is good with proper dietary management. Many children "outgrow" their food allergies.

Prevention: Food allergies sometimes can be prevented. If there is a strong family history of allergy to certain foods, these should be avoided during the child's first year.

Helminths (Worms)

Etiology: *Toxocariasis* is caused by the ingestion of roundworm larvae, often deposited by family dogs and cats. It is likely to occur when children eat dirt or sand which contains the ova of roundworms. The ova hatch in the intestine, mature, and migrate to the lymph vessels and other parts of the body.

Enterobiasis, infestation by pinworms, is caused by *Enterobius vermicularis,* which lives in the lower gut. The female worms deposit their eggs around the anus during the night and then die. Severe pruritus ani occurs, which causes children to scratch. The ova then are deposited on the hands and under the nails. As children put their fingers in their mouths, they swallow the ova, which develop into more mature worms in the intestine.

Signs and Symptoms: Roundworm infestation produces symptoms which correspond to the affected body part. General symptoms may include fever, cough, **hepatomegaly**, nausea, vomiting, and weight loss. Pruritus ani is the classic symptom of enterobiasis.

Diagnostic Procedures: Toxocariasis is diagnosed through a patient history and blood testing. Enterobiasis is diagnosed by a history of pruritus ani and the recovery of *Enterobius* ova from the perianal area.

Treatment: Treatment for toxocariasis usually is symptomatic. The disease is self-limiting. Enterobiasis requires drugs to destroy the parasites. Daily bathing of children (showers preferred) and regular changes of bed linens and nightclothes are necessary in proper management of enterobiasis. It is important in both conditions to test and treat the entire family.

Prognosis: The prognosis for both conditions is good no matter how unpleasant either may sound.

Prevention: The best prevention is to teach children proper personal hygiene, such as hand washing and keeping fingers out of the mouth. Worming of pets and proper disposal of animal feces are important in preventing toxocariasis.

BLOOD DISEASES

Leukemias

Leukemia is the most common form of cancer in children, occurring most frequently between the ages of 2 and 5 years. The acute forms of leukemia are more common in children. Great improvements have been made in the treatment of childhood leukemias; however, the disease still causes great physical, financial, and emotional stress among affected children and their families. See Chapter 8 for a complete discussion of leukemias.

Anemias

The most common types of anemia to occur in children are *iron deficiency anemia, folic acid anemia,* and *aplastic anemia.* Iron deficiency anemia is more common in adolescents, whereas folic acid anemia is more common in infants and adolescents. In addition, a congenital form of aplastic anemia may develop between birth and age 10. Aplastic anemia is associated with a large number of congenital anomalies. For both iron deficiency and folic acid anemias, the prognosis is good with treatment. However, in aplastic anemia, the prognosis is poor. See Chapter 8 for a complete discussion of anemias.

REYE'S SYNDROME

Description: *Reye's syndrome* is an acute illness that disrupts the body's urea cycle, resulting in the accumulation of ammonia in the blood, **hypoglycemia**, severe brain edema, and dangerously high intracranial pressure. The disease almost exclusively affects those under 18 years of age.

Etiology: The etiology is now known, but Reye's syndrome almost always follows an upper respiratory infection and is especially associated with type B influenza and varicella. The incidence of the disease also has been linked to the use of aspirin during influenza or varicella infections.

Signs and Symptoms: The symptoms of Reye's syndrome develop in five stages. They are Stage I, lethargy, vomiting, and hepatic dysfunction; Stage II, hyperventilation, delirium, and hyperactive reflexes; Stage III, coma, rigidity of organ cortices; Stage IV, deepening coma, large and fixed pupils, and loss of cerebral functions; and Stage V, seizures, loss of deep tendon reflexes, flaccidity, and respiratory arrest.

Diagnostic Procedures: A patient history of prior viral infection accompanied by any of the clinical features mentioned previously is strongly suggestive of Reye's syndrome. An increased level of ammonia in the blood confirms the diagnosis. SCOT, SGPT, liver biopsy, and cerebral spinal fluid analysis may be necessary.

Treatment: Reye's syndrome requires hospitalization and intensive treatment to restore blood sugar levels, control cerebral edema, and correct acid-base imbalances. Intracranial pressure must be decreased to prevent seizures. Endotracheal intubation and mechanical ventilation may be necessary.

Prognosis: The prognosis is largely dependent on the stage of progression of the disease. The mortality rate is high in children younger than 2 years old. However, recovery is rapid and complete for those who survive.

Prevention: The risk of developing Reye's syndrome as a consequence of influenza or varicella infection is lessened by avoiding the use of aspirin during the course of those diseases.

SKIN DISEASES

Atopic Dermatitis

Atopic dermatitis (see Chapter 12) is a common childhood skin disease that may be chronic and familial in nature. The condition is characterized by erythema and edema, with papules, vesicles, and crusts forming usually on the cheeks and then spreading to the neck and creases of the arms and legs. Generally, there is itching associated with the rash. The most common allergens producing atopic dermatitis in infancy are foods, especially cow's milk and egg albumin. Later, environmental inhalants and pollen become stronger allergens. While atopic dermatitis may be self-limiting in infancy, about half the affected infants develop asthma as children and hay fever or other allergies as adults. It is important to restrict the child from scratching to prevent secondary infection. The best prevention is removal of known offending agents.

Diaper Rash

Description: *Diaper rash* is a maculopapular and occasionally excoriated eruption in the diaper area of infants.

Etiology: The condition is caused by irritation from heat, moisture, feces, or ammonia produced by the bacterial decomposition of urine.

Signs and Symptoms: A rash in the diaper area will be evident. The infant may become irritable due to the discomfort of the rash.

Diagnostic Procedures: Observation of the characteristic rash is usually sufficient to establish the diagnosis.

Treatment: Exposing the affected area to air and applying a heat lamp may be effective in many cases. Topical antimicrobial medication may be necessary in the event of secondary infection.

Prognosis: The prognosis is good with treatment.

Prevention: Prevention includes frequent changing of diapers and keeping the perianal area dry and clean.

Pediculosis

Pediculosis is skin infestation with lice, a parasitic insect. It is more common in children, especially girls who share combs, brushes, and clothing. The prognosis is good with topical treatment. See Chapter 12 for a complete discussion of this condition.

Dermatophytosis

Dermatophytoses is a general term referring to superficial fungal infections of the skin. *Tinea capitis,* a fungal infection of the scalp, is a persistent, contagious, often epidemic infection occurring most frequently in children. *Tinea corporis,* a fungal infection of the body, occurs on exposed skin surfaces in persons with a history of exposure to domestic animals, especially cats. Both conditions can be treated by topical fungicidal medication. The prognosis is good for either condition. Both may clear spontaneously after puberty. See Chapter 12 for a full discussion of dermatophytoses.

EAR AND EYE DISEASES

Deafness

Deafness occurring during childhood may be congenital, transmitted as a dominant, autosomal dominant, autosomal recessive, or sex-linked recessive trait. It may be due to trauma, toxicity, or infection during pregnancy or delivery. The most common cause of sudden deafness in children is mumps. Other bacterial and viral infections, however, also can cause sudden deafness that may occasion permanent loss of hearing.

Otitis Media

Acute otitis media is common in children under 6 years of age. The most common organism causing the condition is *H. influenzae.* Predisposing factors in children include a shorter, wider, and more horizontal eustachian tube, as well as abundant lymphoid tissue of the pharynx which may cause obstruction of the nasopharynx. With prompt treatment, the prognosis is excellent. See Chapter 13 for a complete discussion of this condition.

Blepharitis

Blepharitis is a common eye inflammation in children. The cause may be a *Staphylococcus* infection or from pediculosis of the brows and lashes. The prognosis is good if there is no ocular involvement. See Chapter 13 for more information about this eye disease.

Strabismus

Description: *Strabismus* is a disorder in which the eyes cannot be directed to focus on the same object. The condition may affect one or both eyes.

Etiology: The most common cause in children is lazy eye, or **amblyopia**. Other causes include unequal occular muscle tone, farsightedness, central nervous system disturbances, or hereditary factors.

Signs and Symptoms: There may be **diplopia** and blurred vision.

Diagnostic Procedures: The affected eye will appear to wander. If both eyes are involved, they may appear crossed, giving the child a "walleyed" appearance. A complete ophthalmologic examination is necessary. A neurologic examination may be indicated as well.

Treatment: Treatment is dependent on the cause but often consists of covering the normal eye, forcing the child to use the deviating one. Eye exercises and corrective lenses may be ordered. Surgical correction may be necessary.

Prognosis: Generally, the earlier treatment is begun, the more rapid and effective it is. By the age of 6, the vision in the deviating eye usually has become so suppressed that treatment is not effective and visual loss is permanent.

Prevention: There is no known prevention.

REFERENCE

1. Rinder, W., *Love Is an Attitude,* Celestial Arts Publishing, Millbrae, Calif., 1970.

REVIEW QUESTIONS

Fill in the Blanks

1. Koplik's spots are characteristic of what childhood disease? _____ .
2. Another name for German measles is _____ .
3. Another name for regular measles is _____ .
4. The _____ virus causes mumps.
5. Another name for chickenpox is _____ . It is caused by the
_____ .
6. DPT stands for _____ , _____ , and _____ .
All are caused by _____ .
7. Flu is called _____ and is caused by the _____ .

Matching

_____ 1. Unexplained sudden death of infant
_____ 2. Acute viral URI
_____ 3. Inflammation of the tonsils
_____ 4. Enlargement of the lymphoid tissue of nasopharynx
_____ 5. Acute viral infection affecting 3 mo. to 3 year olds
_____ 6. Inflammation of the epiglottis
_____ 7. Caused by allergic reaction in bronchi

a. Asthma
b. Common cold
c. Epiglottitis
d. Croup
e. Tonsillitis
f. Adenoid hyperplasia
g. SIDS
h. Pneumonia
i. Polyps

Short Answer

1. Name and define three childhood GI disorders:
   a.
   b.
   c.
2. Name four of the more common food allergens:
   a.
   b.
   c.
   d.
3. Define
   a. *Toxocariasis:*
   b. *Enterobiasis:*
4. List and describe the five stages of Reye's syndrome:
   a.
   b.
   c.
   d.
   e.
5. Describe the treatment for diaper rash.
6. Describe the prognosis of strabismus.

ANSWERS

Fill in the Blanks

1. Rubella
2. Rubella
3. Rubeola
4. Paramyxovirus
5. Varicella; herpes virus
6. Diphtheria, pertussis, tetanus; bacteria.
7. Influenza; myxovirus influenzae.

Matching

1. g
2. b
3. e
4. f
5. d
6. c
7. a

Short Answer

1. a. Colic: Paroxysmal abdominal cramping accompanied by loud crying and drawing the legs up to the abdomen.
   b. Diarrhea: Change in frequency and liquid content of stool. May be acute or chronic.
   c. Vomiting: Spitting up; regurgitation; may be projectile.

2. a. Milk products
   b. Eggs
   c. Wheat
   d. Nuts
   e. Legumes
   f. Fish
   g. Chocolate
3. a. Toxocariasis: Caused by ingestion of roundworm larvae; ova hatch in intestine, mature, migrate to lymph vessels. Symptoms correspond to body part affected.
   b. Enterobiasis: Caused by pinworm ingestion; worms live in lower gut. Female deposits eggs around anus; child itches; child puts fingers in mouth and cycle begins again. Pruritus ani is classic symptom.
4. a. Stage I: Lethargy, vomiting, and hepatic dysfunction
   b. Stage II: Hyperventilation, delirium, hyperactive reflexes
   c. Stage III: Coma, rigidity of organ cortices
   d. Stage IV: Deepening coma, large and fixed pupils, loss of cerebral functions
   e. Stage V: Seizures, loss of deep tendon reflexes, flaccidity, respiratory arrest
5. Exposure of area to air; heat lamp; change diapers frequently; keep skin clean, dry, and cool.
6. Usually, the earlier treatment is begun, the more rapid and effective it is. By the age of 6, the deviating eye usually has become so suppressed that treatment is not effective and permanent visual loss has occurred.

GLOSSARY

AMBLYOPIA: Reduction or dimness of vision, especially that in which there is no apparent pathologic condition of the eye.

ANTIPYRETIC: A drug or agent that reduces fever.

APNEA: Temporary cessation in breathing.

BIOTIN: A component of the vitamin B complex required for life.

DIPLOPIA: Double vision.

EPIDIDYMO-ORCHITIS: Inflammation of the epididymis and testis.

FIBRIN: A whitish protein that is the basis for the clotting of blood.

GAMMA GLOBULIN: A protein formed in the blood. Ability to resist infection is related to concentration of such proteins.

HEPATOMEGALY: Abnormal enlargement of the liver.

HYPOGLYCEMIA: Abnormally low concentration of glucose in the blood.

LEUKOPENIA: An abnormal decrease in the number of circulating white blood cells.

KOPLIK'S SPOTS: Small red spots with bluish white centers on the oral mucosa, particularly in the region opposite the molars. A diagnostic sign in measles.

MYALGIA: Muscle pain or tenderness.

MYCOPLASMA: A group of fungal microorganisms.

PAPULE: A solid, red, elevated skin lesion.

PHOTOPHOBIA: Unusual intolerance of light.

STRIDOR: A harsh, high-pitched sound during respiration due to obstruction of air passages.

VESICLE: A small (generally less than 0.5 cm), fluid-filled blister.

Chapter 15
Pain and Its Management

LEARNING OBJECTIVES

Upon successful completion of this chapter you, will
- Define pain.
- List at least four factors which influence how we experience pain.
- Discuss the purpose of pain.
- Explain the gate control theory of pain.
- Describe the pain assessment tool.
- Compare and contrast acute pain and chronic pain.
- List and describe at least six types of treatment for pain.

INTRODUCTION

Pain affects each of us during our lifetime. Physiologic pain accompanies many diseases and disorders of the body. Psychological pain often is expressed as sorrow over losses such as death or divorce. Psychological pain may become physiologic pain, or the two may be concurrent. While pain may be sensed as having a negative effect on the body, it may be positive, also. For instance, if the pain could not be felt, you might not know you were burning your flesh on a hot stove.

Health professionals often are frustrated in their attempts to treat individuals who experience pain, especially when the cause of pain is not readily identifiable. Patients in pain may be frustrated and confused, too, and may find the pain unbearable.

What is pain? What purpose, if any, does it serve? What happens in the body when a person feels pain? How does the health professional assess pain? What are the differences between acute and chronic pain? Can pain be treated? If so, how? These are some of the questions that will be addressed in this chapter.

WHAT IS PAIN?

Definition of Pain

Webster defines *pain* as a sensation of hurting, or of strong discomfort, in some part of the body, caused by an injury, disease, or functional disorder and transmitted through the nervous system. *Pain* also may be defined as the distress or suffering (mental or physical) that is caused by great anxiety, anguish, grief, disappointment, or other pyschological or emotional stimuli. A nurse who has worked for more than 20 years with patients in pain defines *pain* as "whatever the experiencing person says it is, existing when he says it does."[1] This definition is, perhaps, the most useful, for it acknowledges the patient's complaint, recognizes the subjective nature of pain, and implicitly suggests that diverse measures may be undertaken to relieve pain.

How we experience pain is based in part, on our early experiences of pain, our cultural backgrounds, our anxiety level, our attention level, and any suggestions we have or are given at the time we experience the pain. As health care professionals, we too will be influenced by our past experience, our attitudes, and our beliefs regarding pain. Must there be an organic reason before pain is "real"? Who understands pain better—the patient experiencing the pain or the health professional? It has been shown that if a patient continues pain management for a lengthy time, the health care professional may be overly concerned about the patient becoming addicted or merely malingering.

Purpose of Pain

Pain is a warning that something is wrong in normal body functioning. It is one of the most common complaints of a person seeking medical attention. It warns of inflammation, tissue damage, infection, bodily injury, or trauma—physical or emotional—somewhere in the body.

Pathophysiology of Pain

What occurs at the cellular level when we experience pain? The "gate control theory of pain" offers a useful model of the physiologic process of pain. In gate control theory, "the experience of pain is the result of the summation of the action of both **neurotransmitters** and neuromodulators at each neural receptor site from the site of injury to the cortex. At each neuron **synapse**, if the amount of neurotransmitter (**histamine, acetylcholine**, etc.) exceeds the amount of neuromodulators (**endorphin**, etc.), then the impulse continues to the next synapse where similar interactions are in operation."[2] In other words, we experience pain whenever the substances that tend to propagate a pain impulse across each "gate" in a nerve pathway overpower the substances that tend to block such an impulse. No currrent theory of pain is entirely satisfactory, however. New theories will undoubtedly continue to be advanced and debated.

ASSESSMENT OF PAIN

Health care professionals may find the following tool useful for assessing a patient in pain:[3]

■ *P = place* (patient points with one finger to the pain's location).
■ *A = amount* (patient rates pain on a scale from 0, no pain, to 10, the worst pain possible).
■ *I = interactions* (patient describes what makes the pain worse).
■ *N = neutralizers* (patient describes what makes the pain less).

Further pain assessment skills include observing the patient's appearance and activity. Monitoring the patient's vital signs may be of value in assessing acute pain, but not necessarily chronic pain.

ACUTE VS. CHRONIC PAIN

Acute and chronic pain need to be differentiated prior to the beginning of treatment. *Acute pain* is recent in onset and occurs over a period lasting less than 6 months. Such pain may be manifested as an increase in heart rate, blood pressure, and muscle tension and a decrease in salivary flow and gut motility. Acute pain frequently serves as a warning sign of a disturbance in some physiologic process and usually is accompanied by anxiety.

Chronic pain may be either continuous or intermittent, occurring over a period longer than 6 months. Unlike the acute form, chronic pain may not serve as a warning of physiologic disturbance. It is frequently debilitating, exhausting an individual's physical and emotional resources. Many times the patient is depressed and preoccupied with self. Chronic pain may be associated with a decrease in sleep, libido, and appetite. Because the parasympathetic nervous system tends to adapt to a state of chronic pain, however, there may be few, if any, outward physiologic signs or behavioral changes noted in individuals experiencing such pain.

TREATMENT

Treatment of pain is diverse and difficult. The multidisciplinary approach to pain management is being attempted by many pain clinics across the United States with success. This team approach involves both medical and nonmedical personnel. Pain therapy may include any of the following.

Medications

Medications tend to be the treatment of choice for many patients experiencing acute pain. Analgesics, anesthetics, and anti-inflammatory agents may be prescribed to decrease or eliminate pain, but not eliminate the cause of pain. Analgesics can be **narcotic** or nonnarcotic, prescription or over-the-counter, strong or weak.

Surgery

Surgery may be attempted to block the transmission of pain or to remove the cause of pain. Surgery for relief of pain may include such procedures as **neurotomy**, **cordotomy**, and **hypophysectomy**, as well as the removal of any causative factor.

Biofeedback

Biofeedback is aimed at helping an individual gain voluntary control over normally involuntary physiologic functions. Various forms of electronic feedback produced by monitoring physiologic events may promote blood flow and reduce muscle tension, which, in turn, may reduce the concentration of neurotransmitters at the site of pain. Currently, biofeedback of four different types is being used to control chronic pain: (1) EEG feedback, (2) skin temperature feedback, (3) cephalic blood volume–pulse feedback, and (4) electromyographic feedback.

The Biofeedback Society of America recommends the use of biofeedback for controlling pain in six major areas: (1) vascular headache, (2) muscle contraction headache, (3) vasoconstrictive disorders, (4) psychophysiologic disorders, (5) gastrointestinal disorders, and (6) physical medicine and rehabilitation.

Relaxation

Relaxation therapy can be utilized to modify muscle tension believed to cause or exacerbate pain. The individual is taught a series of techniques for relaxation which are used any time pain occurs. Audiotapes are used in beginning practice sessions; then the person learns to relax without any assistance. Relaxation therapy is especially successful when used in conjunction with biofeedback and imagery.

Imagery

Imagery is therapy used by a person experiencing pain to produce relaxation and increase the production of endorphins. The person imagines and concentrates on a pleasant scene or experience and is taught to relax. To be effective, imagery necessitates a positive relationship to the image scene; otherwise, the imagery may only exacerbate the pain.

Autohypnosis

Hypnosis is a state that resembles sleep but is induced by a hypnotizer who makes readily accepted suggestions to the subject. *Autohypnosis,* self-induced hypnosis, is most effective when a person is motivated—and pain is a strong motivating force. The period of pain relief from autohypnosis is from 4 to 6 hours, and the time of relief is extended with repeated hypnotic reinforcement. Autohypnosis can be learned in a few hours.

Transcutaneous Electrical Nerve Stimulation (TENS)

Transecutaneous electrical nerve stimulation (TENS) is a therapeutic procedure in which an electrical impulse is induced in the large nerve fibers that carry non-painful information in order to block or reduce the transmission of painful impulses. The electrodes are connected by lead wires to a stimulator called a *TENS unit.* The electric current produced can be varied in frequency and intensity. Although still considered experimental by some, the use of TENS has proved effective for pain relief in some patients.

Massage

Massage is manipulation, methodical pressure, friction, and kneading of the body. A mentholated rub may be used to increase stimulation. Massage may be performed over or around an area of pain or at **trigger points**. This type of treatment stimulates blood flow, induces relaxation, and increases the production of endorphins.

Humor, Laughter, and Play

Norman Cousins, former editor of the *Saturday Review,* popularized the concept of making laughter and humor an antedote for pain. While quite ill in the hospital, he discovered he could go much longer without his pain medication when he had been doing a great deal of laughing. He watched comedy films and read humor books. Humor and laughter control pain in four ways: (1) by distracting attention, (2) by reducing tension, (3) by changing expectations, and (4) by increasing production of endorphins—the body's natural painkillers.[4]

Play is another activity which is helpful in reducing pain, even for the severely debilitated person. Play can be childlike or quite adult-like. Consider the following: Two toddlers, riding tricycles, approach the charge nurse on the floor of the burn unit in a major city hospital. The burns of both are obvious, but their "race" through the corridors has become part of their treatment. One child is quite concerned over the loss of his baseball hat—a gift to all the children from a major league team. The reason for the concern? All the children were leaving shortly to play ball with one of the therapists. Who can play ball without a cap? The tricycle race and following game focus the child's attention on play—not pain.

Music

Physicians and dentists have discovered that music will help alleviate pain. Dentists know that some patients are receptive enough to music to have their teeth extracted without anesthesia. Some hospitals allow music to be piped into their surgical rooms because it puts both patients and practitioners in a more relaxed state.

John Diamond, M.D., practices preventive medicine and psychiatry in Valley Cottage, New York, and has spent more than 25 years researching music and its therapeutic value and life-enhancing quality. His book, *The Life Energy in Music,*[5] would be particularly interesting to any person seeking more knowledge about music therapy and its healing powers.

CONCLUSION

Despite its multitude of forms and sometimes highly subjective qualities, pain is real. Pain needs to be understood and accepted in the terms of the person experiencing it. Each person experiences pain differently. Pain should be managed as aggressively as is its cause. The health professional and the person in pain should be willing to investigate many forms of pain management and seek the one or ones that best suit the individual's needs.

Finally, a useful attitude toward pain management is captured in the following statement by David Black in *The Laughter Prescription:* "Pain is an energy monster; we give it the power to hurt us. And we take that power away—depending on how we choose to view ourselves. All pain is real, but you can change your reality."[6]

REFERENCES

1. McCaffery, M., *Nursing Management of the Patient with Pain,* 2nd ed., J. B. Lippincott, Philadelphia, 1979.
2. Donova, M., "Cancer Pain: You Can Help!" *Nursing Clinics of North America* 17(4):713, 1982.
3. McGuire, L., "A Short, Simple Tool for Assessing Your Patient's Pain," *Nursing 81,* 11:48–49, 1981.
4. Peter, L. J., and Bill Dana. *The Laughter Prescription,* Ballantine Books, New York, 1982, p. 8.
5. Diamond, J., The Life Energy in Music, Vols. 1 and 2, Archaeus Press, Valley Cottage, New York, 1983.
6. Peter, op. cit., p. 8.

REVIEW QUESTIONS

1. Using the two definitions of pain given in the text, define pain in your own words, including *your* definition of pain.
2. Describe the purpose of pain.
3. Define the gate control theory of pain. What do you see as its limitations?
4. Give a short, simple tool for assessing pain.
5. Define acute and chronic pain.
6. Of the 10 pain therapies, which have you tried? What works best for you? Which would you like to try the next time you have acute pain? Chronic pain? Which therapy would you *never* try and why?

ANSWERS

1. Answers will vary.
2. Pain can be a warning that something is wrong in normal body functioning. It warns of inflammation, tissue damage, infection, bodily injury, or trauma somewhere in the body.
3. The gate control theory of pain: Pain is the result of the summation of the action of both neurotransmitters and neuromodulators at each neural receptor site from the site of injury to the cortex. At each neuron synapse, if the amount of neurotransmitter exceeds the amount of neuromodulator, then the impulse continues to the next synapse where similar interactions are in operation.
4. McGuire describes a short, simple tool for assessing pain:
   - ■ *P* = *place* (patient points with one finger to the pain's location).
   - ■ *A* = *amount* (patient rates pain on scale from 0, no pain, to 10, the worst pain possible).
   - ■ *I* = *interaction* (patient describes what makes the pain worse).
   - ■ *N* = *neutralizers* (patient describes what makes the pain less).
5. Acute pain is recent in onset, usually lasting less than 6 months. Increase in heart rate, blood pressure, and muscle tension, but decrease in salivary flow and gut motility. Chronic pain is continuous or intermittent and lasts longer than 6 months. Generally serves no useful purpose. Associated with decrease in sleep, libido, and appetite.
6. Answers will vary.

GLOSSARY

ACETYLCHOLINE: A neurotransmitter substance that transfers nerve impulses across synapses and neuromuscular junctions.

CORDOTOMY: Surgical division of one or more of the lateral nerve pathways emerging from the spinal cord in order to relieve pain.

ENDORPHIN: One of a group of naturally occurring substances produced by the central nervous system that reduce the perception of pain.

HISTAMINE: A substance present in all body tissues, released by injured cells as part of the body's inflammation process. It functions to dilate capillaries, lower blood pressure, increase gastric secretions, and constrict bronchial smooth muscle.

HYPOPHYSECTOMY: Removal of the pituitary gland.

NARCOTIC: A drug that in moderate doses depresses the central nervous system, relieving pain and producing sleep, but that in excessive doses produces unconsciousness, stupor, coma, and possibly death.

NEUROTOMY: Division or dissection of a nerve.

NEUROTRANSMITTER: A substance produced and released by one neuron that travels across a synapse, exciting or inhibiting the next neuron in the neural pathway.

SYNAPSE: The narrow gap between two neurons in a neural pathway, where the termination (axon) of one neuron comes in close proximity with the beginning (dendrite) or cell body of another neuron.

TRIGGER POINT: Any place on the body that when stimulated causes a sudden pain in a specific area.

Chapter 16
Holistic Health

LEARNING OBJECTIVES

Upon successful completion of this chapter, you will
- Define holistic health care.
- Discuss personal responsibility in relation to holistic health.
- Identify at least two external and two internal environmental factors which influence our health and well-being.
- List at least four influences of personal lifestyle on holistic health.
- Describe the effects of unexpressed negative emotions on our bodies.
- Identify at least seven constructive outlets for negative emotions.
- Define stress and distress.
- List the four basic food groups important to good nutrition.
- Identify at least three dietary goals for the United States.
- Discuss the importance of laughter and play in holistic health.
- List at least five "playful/fun" activities.
- Compare and contrast conditional and unconditional love.
- Discuss the effects of a personal faith on a holistic lifestyle.

HOLISTIC HEALTH AND
HOLISTIC MEDICINE DEFINED

Holistic health is many things: It is a philosophy of life that relates to the whole rather than its parts. It is an attitude. It is an approach to life. Holistic health focuses on enabling good health to emerge in an individual. It encourages the individual to recognize the stresses of life and their impact on one's well-being.

Holistic medicine is a system of care that considers the needs of the whole person. Rather than focusing only on malfunctioning body parts, it also explores the broader dimensions of the patient's life—physical, nutritional, environmental, emotional, and spiritual. Holistic medicine does not espouse one method over another to foster the healing process, but rather encompasses all safe methods of diagnosis and treatment—including medication and surgery when appropriate. Holism in medicine can be traced, in part, to Hippocrates, who emphasized the environmental causes and treatment of illness and the importance of emotional factors and nutrition. Both holistic health and holistic medicine emphasize personal responsibility and encourage the cooperation and participation of patient and practitioner to achieve that goal.

PERSONAL RESPONSIBILITY

The body is not indestructible, and from birth, we need to be taught self-care and responsibility. Often, however, it is not until we see someone become disabled, or die, that a greater appreciation for the body is sensed. From the moment of birth, the road to death begins. And during the period of life, choices continually are made about the body's well-being. Early in life, we are taught and we observe from those close to us either to respect or to ignore our bodies.

If we accept ourselves, feel self-worth, and have been taught well, we ought to listen to our body's signals and seek necessary attention. There is little or nothing even the most influential medical practitioner can do for us when our body breaks down if we do not want help or are unwilling to ask for it.

ENVIRONMENTAL FACTORS

Personal health and well-being are greatly influenced by environment, both internal and external. *Internal environmental factors* include genetic traits, familial tendencies, and physical and psychological characteristics inherent in each person. *External environmental factors* may be more easily defined. They include the air we breathe, the water we drink, the food we eat, and the surroundings in which we live and work.

Unfortunately, environmental factors are not easily controlled, changed, or altered. None of us has any influence on personal genetic makeup; some may choose to influence the genetic makeup of their offspring, however. Familial tendencies are almost as difficult to influence as genetics. For those raised with the same family into which they were born, their lifestyle will reflect much the same patterns as those of their parents.

Physical and psychological characteristics can be altered more easily than either genetic and familial tendencies, but deliberate, consistent, and continuous efforts must be instituted before change occurs. A choice may be made to alter the shape of the nose and a conscious effort can be made to modify a "type A" behavior, but even when such choices are deliberate, they may not greatly influence health.

Is there more influence on external than internal environment? A conscious effort may be made to refrain from smoking, but can one leave a job working in a coal mine all day? The air is cleaner in Seattle than in New York City, but can one move? Food may be purer with no preservatives or additives, but is food poisoning risked? Should the government control the spraying of fruits and vegetables with pesticides, or should persons take their chances in the market? Is nuclear energy safe? How are decisions made?

In the final analysis, one must recognize the influences both internal and external environment have on health. It is important, however, to understand that these factors also greatly affect the body's disorders and diseases.

INFLUENCE OF LIFESTYLE
ON HEALTH AND DISEASE

Lifestyle is the consistent, integrated way of life of an individual as typified by mannerisms, attitudes, and possessions. From the time one is born, choices are made which influence lifestyle. Influences in life come from the following: (1) modeling of family members and peers, (2) education and knowledge, (3) personal attitudes, (4) degree of self-confidence, (5) individual responsibilities, (6) where we are in life, and (7) life's opportunities. All these factors have a strong influence on lifestyle.

From the preceding factors, it becomes obvious that there is a great deal of control in determining a lifestyle. The choices one makes will influence health, positively and negatively. For example, parents who model optimal health will influence their children toward a healthy lifestyle. Increased information and knowledge on cholesterol blood levels encourage proper dietary intake. If a person has a positive attitude and self-confidence, that individual is better equipped to cope with illness. Appropriate personal responsibility mandates that a person acts safely in a potentially dangerous situation. Conversely, choosing to smoke, intentionally avoiding exercise, refusing to fasten a seatbelt, or disregarding prescribed treatment all have a potentially negative impact on health.

MANAGING NEGATIVE EMOTIONS

The human being is an emotional creature. Feelings of joy, sorrow, anger, jealousy, love, resentment, fear, and hate are part of existence. How persons deal with their emotions has much to do with their physical health.

For simplicity, categorize emotions as positive or negative. Fear is a negative emotion, for instance, if it keeps people from functioning as normal human beings; it is a positive emotion if it cautions people to be safe. In this way, emotions are categorized as positive or negative and good or bad in terms of how they cause people to respond in the world.

A sense of joy may warm the body, cleanse the spirit, relax muscles, lighten air passages, and generally make people feel "good all over." Anger or resentment may cause the fist to clench, breathing to accelerate, the heart to pound, the head to ache, and muscles to tighten. Norman Cousins, in his introduction to *You Can Fight for Your Life,* by Lawrence LeShan, states that when we feel despair, panic, depression, fear, and frustration, the healing resources of the human brain are not fully engaged.[1]

However, when we have a great will to live and expect the best in life, the brain has a greater ability to produce chemicals such as encephalens and endorphins which have a very positive enhancement of our bodies. Some may recognize the physical signals of the body. All too often, however, people have "buried" somewhere in their inner consciousness the negative impact emotions may have.

Buried emotions later may exhibit themselves during an illness. Even then, illness may not be attributed to a negative emotion long since unexpressed. The kind of disease that results from unexpressed negative emotion is what is called *psychosomatic illness.* The symptoms of the disease are very real, but if the cause could be carefully traced, you would find one or more unexpressed negative emotions.

It is therefore important to realize that negative emotions that are not dealt with in a wholesome manner probably will express themselves physically in the body. People must learn how to express negative feelings without destroying themselves or others if they wish to live a healthy lifestyle. Refer to Table 16–1 for suggestions on how to express negative feelings in a positive manner.

TABLE 16–1. Some Positive Ways of Working Out Negative Emotions

1. Chop wood.
2. Scrub and wax a floor.
3. Run a mile—or several.
4. Ride a bike.
5. Beat up a pillow.
6. Relax in a hot tub.
7. See a counselor.
8. Wash the car.
9. Knead bread.
10. Lift weights.
11. Cry, weep.
12. Accept yourself.
13. Read a funny book or go to a funny movie. Laugh!
14. Roll up the car windows, scream a little or a lot.
15. Make certain there is someone who loves you unconditionally.

The next time anger or emotions have a negative effect, check the body to see which part is most affected. If you can feel a headache coming on, can feel the fire in your "gut," or feel your heart pounding, remember that you may be needing an emotional release.

STRESS AND DISTRESS

It is generally believed that biological organisms require a certain amount of stress in order to maintain their well-being. Stress is always present. "Good" stress enables the body to meet the challenges of everyday activity. For example, stress keeps one alert when driving in heavy traffic or helps one respond to needs of family members in crises. Without a correct balance of stress, people would be unable to respond to any stimuli.

Distress, however, tends to be a negative influence. When stress occurs in quantities that the system cannot handle, it may produce pathologic changes. These stressors can be either a person or a condition, e.g., children, spouse, boss, other people, the weather, traffic, noise, money, school, environment, retirement, divorce, death, disease—any change that occurs in one's life. The amount of distress experienced depends on how individuals respond to these stressors.

Again, there is the freedom of choice. The recognition of stressors in life and their subsequent management constitute one of the keys to a healthy lifestyle. It has been shown that good nutrition, proper exercise, and a quality support system help alleviate distress.

THE VALUE OF GOOD NUTRITION

How many times have you heard, "You are what you eat"? We understand the logic of advice such as "Beware of saturated fats," "Avoid refined sugar," and "Low salt, no salt, is the best salt." Why does eating often get out of control? Perhaps it comes from the philosophy that it is best to clean all the food from the plate. It may occur, also, because food is used as a reliever of emotions and physical pain and as a reward for "being good."

A popular and excellent guide to an adequate daily diet is the basic four food groups:
- Milk, cheese, ice cream, and yogurt: $2\frac{1}{2}$ to 4 cups
- Meats, poultry, seafood, eggs, legumes, nuts, peanut butter: $2\frac{1}{2}$ to 3 oz, servings
- Vegetables and fruits: 4 servings
- Cereals and breads: 4 servings

Improper nutrition may result in body disorders and/or diseases. Bowel cancer is more common among groups of people who consume high amounts of animal fat and little fiber. There also is evidence that breast cancer may be linked to a high-fat and low-fiber dietary pattern and that where there is high meat consumption, cancer mortality rates are correspondingly high.

The *Dietary Goals for the United States* furthre suggest the following changes in food selection and preparation:

■ Increase consumption of fruits and vegetables and whole grains.

■ Decrease consumption of meat and increase consumption of poultry and fish.

■ Decrease consumption of food high in fat and partially substitute polyunsaturated fat for saturated fat.

■ Substitute nonfat milk for whole milk.

■ Decrease consumption of butterfat, eggs, and other high-cholesterol sources.

■ Decrease consumption of sugar and foods high in sugar content.

■ Decrease consumption of salt and foods high in salt content.[2]

Obviously, the list could go on and on! It is important, however, to realize that individuals have the power to improve their lifestyle by eating properly each and every day. Good nutrition can make a difference—if not to prolong life, at least to enable one to face life's stresses with greater ease.

LAUGHTER AND PLAY

Laughter has been described as "internal jogging." People cannot experience despair and joy at the same time. Therefore, it is important for individuals to allow, even plan for, laughter and play in their lives.

There are several examples of the use of laughter and play in today's health care. Dr. O. Carl Simonton, noted radiation oncologist, tells of his work with teaching cancer patients how to juggle. On his first visit with patients, he gives them a set of juggling bags and one or two simple instructions. He juggles for them and tells them to practice every day and that they will do some juggling together each time they meet. Simonton reports that this activity (1) enables him and his patients to develop a relationship outside of doctor-patient, (2) encourages a lot of laughing together, and (3) gives the patient something other than an illness to think about.

David Bresler, Ph.D., director of the Bresler Center for Allied Therapeutics in Los Angeles, uses long, slender, balloons blown up and shaped into all kinds of animal forms to help children cope with chronic pain. This activity takes their minds off the pain and may stimulate the release of endorphins in the body.

A hospital chaplain whose avocation is that of a clown often visits hospital patients with clown paint on his face. Sometimes it is easier for patients to express their pain or grief in the "make-believe" vernacular. It also brings laughter and joy where there is pain and sorrow.

Norman Cousins reports in *Anatomy of an Illness*[3] about the validity of laughter in healing his illness. He watched old Marx Brothers movies several times a day, laughing to near tears. Following this time of laughter, however, he always was able to function without pain medication.

It seems obvious that play and laughter ought to be a more important and deliberate part of people's daily lives. All too frequently people forget to play as they become adults.

Some ways to interject laughter into life include

■ Become a collector of cartoons.
■ Be a good jokester.
■ Allow humor to get back at the "bad things" in life.
■ Learn to smile, then chuckle, then laugh, then really roar with a deep belly laugh.
■ Read humorous items.
■ Watch a TV program well known for its humor.
■ Laugh at yourself—then share it!

Play time in our lives may require more concentrated effort. Make a list of 40 playful or fun things which cost less than $5 each. Do something on this list every day. Your authors, who work hard at incorporating laughter and play, will share a few of their favorites:

■ Find a beach, take off your shoes, and let the sand squiggle through your toes.
■ Lay down in a snow drift and make an angel.
■ Have a marshmallow or water balloon fight.
■ Finger paint.
■ Throw a Frisbee for a dog—several times.
■ Play in the water while everyone thinks you are watering the lawn.
■ Be creative on April Fool's Day.
■ Take a bubble bath and blow bubbles.
■ Deliver May Day baskets and *run*.
■ Plan a treasure hunt for the neighborhood.
■ Dance.
■ Go to the zoo.
■ Sing crazy rhymes.
■ Fly a kite or model airplane.
■ Play volleyball, Ping Pong, etc.—for fun.
■ Go to a playground—swing, slide, and merry-go-round.
■ If you see a road and wonder where it goes, take it.
■ Feed ducks at a lake.
■ Ride an elephant or camel.
■ Play "Hide and Seek."

Planned play every day may be hard work at first, but it is essential for a healthful lifestyle. The important principles of humor and play are practice, practice, practice, practice.

LOVE, FRIENDSHIP, RELIGION

We learn in most psychology classes that we must love ourselves before we can love another. But what is love? Leo Buscaglia, in his book, *Love,* defines *love* as "a learned, emotional reaction. If one wishes to know love, one must live love, in action."[4] Love is spontaneous. If we love someone, we need to share that love *now*. Love must be given unconditionally. If we expect something in return for love, we are in error. We love because we feel it and want to share it. And we never "run out of" love.

Friendship is one part of love. Each of us needs at least one friend-mentor with whom we can share anything at any time. Our friend must love us as we are and not expect anything from us.

In both friendship and love, we must be willing to assume responsibility for ourselves and be able to take risks. Only then can personal growth occur. Read the following:

Risking

To laugh is to risk appearing unconcerned.
To weep is to risk appearing sentimental.
To express your independence is to risk losing your friends.
To trust others is to risk being taken advantage of.
To make a decision is to risk making a mistake.
To admit a mistake is to risk losing the respect of others.
To reach out to another is to risk involvement.
To show feeling is to risk exposing your true self.
To place your ideas, your dreams before the crowd is to risk their loss.
To love is to risk not being loved in return.
To live is to risk dying.
To hope is to risk despair.
To try at all is to risk failure.[5]

Not every person embraces religion or senses a strong spiritual influence in their lives. But at one time or another, all of us have witnessed its influence in the life of someone.

Some call it worship. Others refer to it as prayer. For your neighbor, it may be meditation. Yoga has been very helpful for many; for still others, it is a mental discipline. The experience is a devotion, a setting aside, an adoration, a refreshing, or an enlightening. It may include service, witnessing, sharing, and a sense of community and/or belonging. Whatever it is, it is a very personal experience.

Practitioners of holistic health recognize the worth of such experiences in a person's life. Religion or a faith in something or someone greater and more powerful than ourselves can make the most desolate of times a little less frustrating.

REFERENCES

1. LeShan, L., *You Can Fight for Your Life,* M. Evans and Company, Inc., New York, 1977, p. xv.
2. Select Committee on Nutrition and Human Needs, *Dietary Goals for the United States,* U.S. Government Printing Office, Washington, D.C., February, 1977, p. 3.

3. Cousins, N., *Anatomy of an Illness,* W. W. Norton, New York, 1979.

4. Buscaglia, L., *Love,* Ballatine Books, New York, 1982, p. 91.

5. Allen C., *Victory in the Valleys of Life,* Fleming H. Revell Company, New Jersey, 1981, p. 114.

REVIEW QUESTIONS

Fill in the Blanks

1. Internal environmental factors which influence health and well-being include
   a.
   b.
   c.
   d.
2. External environmental factors which influence health and well-being include
   a.
   b.
   c.
   d.
3. Personal lifestyle may be influenced by
   a.
   b.
   c.
   d.
   e.
   f.
4. Emotions may be categorized as _____ or _____ .
5. The kind of disease that results from unexpressed negative emotion is called _____ .

Short Answer

1. List at least four constructive outlets for expression of negative feelings beneficial to you.
2. Describe situations which cause stress to have a positive or a negative impact on our lives.
3. Determine a day's eating plan to allow for four servings of fruits and vegetables.

Discussion Questions/Personal Reflection

1. Identify a negative emotion you have difficulty expressing. Discuss with a friend what the consequences of such activity may be.
2. Share a cartoon, joke, or funny story with a classmate.

ANSWERS

Fill in the Blanks

1. a. Genetic traits
   b. Familial tendencies

    c. Inherent physical characteristics
    d. Inherent psychological characteristics
2. a. Air
    b. Water
    c. Food
    d. Surroundings
3. a. Education and knowledge
    b. Attitudes
    c. Individual responsibilities
    d. Modeling of family/peers
    e. Self-confidence
    f. Position in life
    g. Life's opportunities
4. negative; positive
5. psychosomatic illness

Short Answer

1. Chop wood, ride a bike, knead bread, run a mile, etc.
2. Positive—stress keeps us alert in traffic
   Negative—insufficient money to pay heat bill
3. Varies: 6 oz orange juice in morning; 1 apple at noon; mixed vegetables for dinner; fresh strawberries for dessert

Discussion Questions/Personal Reflection

Answers will vary.

Appendix 1

Diagnostic Procedures

A

Alkaline Phosphatase: A venipuncture is performed to measure serum levels of alkaline phosphatase, an enzyme that influences bone calcification and lipid and metabolite transportation. Used in assessing bone and liver function.

Amniocentesis: Surgical puncture of the amniotic sac, which surrounds the fetus in utero, to remove amniotic fluid; can detect over 100 genetic disorders and evaluate adverse uterine environment.

Angiography: Often called *arteriography.* It is x-ray visualization of blood vessels with or without the injection of a radiopaque material. Common types include cerebral, coronary, renal, pulmonary, and abdominal angiography.

Antibodies to Epstein-Barr (EB) Virus: The EB virus is found in patients with mononucleosis. The cells are cultured and the EB virus antibodies are diagnostic.

Anti-DNA Antibodies: Measures anti-native DNA antibody levels in a serum sample obtained by venipuncture.

Antinuclear Antibody (ANA): A test diagnostic of SLE where peripheral blood smears are taken and a fluorescein-tagged anti-human gamma globulin is used. If the LE factor is present, the specimen will fluoresce.

Aortography: X-ray of the aorta after injection of an opaque medium into a vessel to assess possible aneurysm, arteriosclerosis, or congenital anomalies.

Arterial Blood Gases (ABGs): A percutaneous arterial puncture is made to assess the gas exchanges of oxygen and carbon dioxide in the lungs by measuring the partial pressures of oxygen and carbon dioxide.

Arteriogram: See *Angiography.* X-ray of arteries after the injection of a radiopaque material into the bloodstream.

Audiogram: A record made by a delicate instrument, the audiometer, of the threshold of hearing.

Auscultation and Percussion (A&P): *Auscultation* is listening to the sounds within the body, usually using a stethoscope. *Percussion* is using the fingertips to tap the body lightly to determine size, position, and consistency of body structures and fluids.

348

B

BCG Vaccine: Bacille Calmette-Guérin, a form of tuberculosis vaccine that offers some protection to tuberculin-negative persons. Its use is recommended only where exposure to tuberculosis is great and the usual tuberculosis control measures are not possible.

Barium Enema: X-ray of the lower gastrointestinal tract where barium is the contrast medium, given as an enema.

Barium Swallow: X-ray of the upper gastrointestinal tract where barium is the contrast medium, given by mouth.

Blood Serum for Hormones: Radioimmunoassay (see *Radioimmunoassay*) and competitive protein binding are two testing methods commonly used to measure serum hormone levels; blood samples will be carefully drawn so as to correspond with or avoid times of peak secretions for the particular hormones being tested.

Bone Marrow Biopsy: Bone marrow fluid and cells can be removed through aspiration or needle biopsy of bone tissue; examination will give important data about blood disorders.

Bronchography: X-ray of the lung after the instillation of an opaque iodine medium through a catheter into the trachea and bronchi. Bronchoscopy is more frequently used.

Bronchoscopy: Visualization of the trachea and bronchi through a metal or fiberoptic scope with a light; also used for removal of foreign bodies and biopsy.

Burdzinski's Sign: When the neck of the patient is bent, involuntary flexure movements of the ankle, knee, and hip are produced; seen in meningitis.

C

Cardiac Catheterization: A catheter is passed into the right (veins to inferior vena cava) or left (arteries to the aorta) side of the heart; can determine blood pressure and blood flow in the heart and permits collection of samples.

Cardiac Enzymes: See *CPK, LDH,* and *SGOT.*

Carcinoembryonic Antigen (CEA): Blood tests used to monitor the effectiveness of cancer therapy, since serum CEA levels will fall within about 1 month if treatment is successful.

Catheterization of Ejaculatory Ducts: A catheter is passed into the ejaculatory ducts to determine blockage or disease.

Cerebral Angiography: See *Angiography.* X-ray visualization of blood vessels of the brain after injection of radiopaque material into the arterial bloodstream; a less hazardous procedure more commonly used is the CT scan.

Chemistry Screens: Tests performed on blood to determine values of any number of factors, such as calcium, phosphorus, creatinine, uric acid, cholesterol, total protein, alkaline phosphatase, glucose, blood urea nitrogen, sodium, etc.

Cholecystogram: Used to detect biliary tract disease. A series of x-rays of the gallbladder is taken after the ingestion of contrast medium.

Cocciodin Skin Test: A delayed hypersensitivity skin test used to detect an acute self-limiting disease of the respiratory organs—coccidioidomycosis.

Colonoscopy: Visual examination of the lower bowel with a colonscope. Biopsy and surgical excision can be accomplished through the scope.

Complete Blood Count (CBC): A venipuncture usually is performed to give a complete picture of all the blood's formed elements. A CBC usually includes hemoglobin, hematocrit, red and white blood counts, and a differential white cell count.

Complete Neurologic Examination: A series of tests and procedures to assess functioning of cranial nerves, motor and sensory systems, and superficial and deep tendon reflexes.

Convergence Testing: Part of an eye examination to determine the movement of the eyes toward fixation of the same near point.

Coomb's Test, Direct: A venipuncture is done to detect the pressure of protein antibodies on the surface of red blood cells; helpful in diagnosing erythroblastosis fetalis.

CPK, Creatinine Phosphokinase: A venipuncture is performed to measure CPK, an enzyme that speeds up the creatine-creatinine metabolism in muscle cells and brain tissue. Its purpose is to detect acute myocardial infarction or reinfarction and evaluate chest pain and skeletal muscle disorders.

CSF Analysis: Cerebrospinal fluid is commonly obtained by lumbar puncture between the third and fifth lumbar vertebrae. Its purpose is to measure CSF pressure and diagnose viral or bacterial meningitis, brain tumor and hemorrhages, and chronic central nervous system infections.

CT Scan, Computerized Tomography: Noninvasive x-ray technique more sensitive than conventional x-ray; a scanner and detector circle the patient sending an array of focused x-rays through the body; allows a specialist to distinguish tumors, abscesses, hemorrhages, and white and gray brain tissue.

Cystometry: The study of urinary bladder efficiency using an instrument which measures the bladder's pressure and capacity. A catheter is passed into the bladder; then saline, water, or air is instilled with the patient reporting any sensations or the need to void. Pressure and volume are recorded.

Cystoscopy: The urinary bladder is distended with water or air with the patient sedated. Examination of the bladder with a fiberoptic scope is done to obtain biopsies of growth and to remove polyps.

D

Dilation and Curettage (D&C): Involves widening of the cervical opening and scraping with a curet to remove the uterine lining.

Doppler Ultrasonography: Noninvasive test evaluates blood flow in the major veins and arteries of arms, legs, and extracranial cerebrovascular system; a hand-held transducer directs high-frequency sound waves to the area being tested.

E

Echocardiography: Noninvasive diagnostic test using ultrasound to visualize internal cardiac structures. A special transducer is placed on the patient's chest, and it directs ultrahigh-frequency sound waves toward cardiac structures which reflect these waves. The echoes are converted to electrical impulses and shown on an oscilloscope.

Echoencephalography: Involves the reflection of ultrasound waves from structures within the skull; less commonly used since CT scanning.

Ejaculatory or Semen Analysis: Uses semen specimen to evaluate the volume of seminal fluid, sperm count, and sperm motility; also used to detect semen on a rape victim, identify the blood group of an alleged rapist, or to prove sterility in a paternity suit.

Electrocardiography (ECG): The recording of electric currents emanating from the heart muscle. Electrodes are placed on the patient to obtain the reading.

Electroencephalography (EEG): Process of recording the electric currents developed in the brain by placing electrodes on the skull.

Electrolyte Analysis: See *Serum Calcium, Phosphorus, Total Protein, or Serum Electrolytes* and *Chemistry Screens.*

Electromyography (EMG): Recording the changes in electrical potential of muscle using surface needle electrodes, insertion of needle electrodes into muscle, or stimulation of the muscle nerve.

Endoscopic Retrograde Cholangiopancreatography (ERCP): A radiographic examination of the pancreatic ducts and hepatobiliary tree after injection of a contrast medium into the duodenal papilla. It is used to diagnose pancreatic disease.

Endoscopy: Visual inspection of any cavity of the body by means of an endoscope.

ESR, Erythrocyte Sedimentation Rate: A blood specimen is obtained by venipuncture to measure the time required for erythrocytes in whole blood to settle to the bottom of a vertical tube; may be one of the earliest disease indicators.

Exfoliative Cytology: Microscopic examination of desquamated cells or cells that have shred or scaled off the surface epithelium. The cells are obtained from sputum, lesions, secretions, urine, aspirations, smears, or washings.

F

Fluorescein Stain: A dye used to reveal corneal lesions and to test circulation in the retinas and extremities. A sterile fluorescein strip is moistened and touched to the eyelid, and the dye film spreads to the entire eye. A special slit-lamp (see *Slit-Lamp Examination*) is used to detect areas of concentrated dye.

Fluoroscopy: Examination of deep structures by using x-rays. Immediate projection of x-ray images can be visualized.

G

Gastric Analysis: Requires aspiration of gastric contents for culture to detect gastric pathogens; a nasogastric tube will be used to collect the washings.

Gastroscopy: Inspection of the stomach interior using a gastroscope.

Gram's Stain: A staining procedure in which microorganisms are stained with crystal violet, followed by iodine solution, decolorized with alcohol, and counterstained with safranin. The retention of either the violet or pink color serves as a means to identify and classify bacteria.

H

Hemoglobin: A venipuncture or finger stick is done to measure the amount of hemoglobin found in whole blood; is used to measure the severity of anemia or polycythemia.

Hematocrit: Used to measure the percentage of packed red cells in a whole blood sample obtained by finger stick or venipuncture.

Hydroxy-25: See *Hydroxyproline.*

Hydroxyproline: Indicates if hydroxyproline has increased due to bone diseases, especially bone resorption; a 24-hour urine catch is required; circulating hydroxyproline can be checked by a blood sample, too.

Hysterosalpingography: X-ray of the uterus and uterine tubes after the introduction of an opaque material through the cervix.

Histoplasmin Skin Test: A form of delayed hypersensitivity skin testing to detect a systemic fungal respiratory disease due to *Histoplasma capsulatum.*

I

Intravenous Pyelogram: Contrast medium is injected intravenously, and x-rays are taken as the medium is cleared from the blood by glomerular filtration. The renal calyces, renal pelvis, ureters, and urinary bladder are all visible on film.

K

Kernig's Sign: In a sitting position or when lying with the thigh flexed upon the abdomen, the leg cannot be completely extended; a sign of meningitis.

L

Laparoscopy: A small incision is made in the abdominal wall to visualize the interior of the abdomen using a laparoscope. It is used to examine the ovaries or fallopian tubes and as a gynecologic sterilization technique.

Laryngoscopy: Visual examination of the interior of the larynx using a laryngoscope.

LDH, Lactate Dehydrogenase: A venipuncture is done to test for the LDH enzyme, which helps to differentiate myocardial infarction, pulmonary infarction, anemias, and hepatic disease; supports CPK test results; monitors patient response to some forms of chemotherapy.

Lumbar Puncture: See *CSF Analysis.*

Lupus Erythematosus (LE) Test: A blood sample is mixed with laboratory-treated antigens. If the sample contains ANA, it will react with the antigen causing swelling and rupture. Phagocytes from the serum engulf the foreign particles and form LE cells, which are then detected by microscopic examination.

Lymphangiography: X-ray of the lympatic vessels following injection of oil-based contrast medium into a lymphatic vessel in each foot.

M

Magnetic Resonance Imaging (MRI):   An imaging procedure which relies on magnets and computers to produce images of different areas of the body. An individual is surrounded by a magnetic field which causes hydrogen atoms to line up in a certain fashion. A signal is released when the atoms move back to their original places and is processed by the computer. Ionizing radiation is not required.

Mammogram: X-ray of the mammory gland or breast.

Microscopic Urine: A urine sample is centrifuged; then the cells, casts, and crystals are viewed to detect infection, obstruction, inflammation, trauma, or tumors.

Myelography: X-ray of the spinal cord after the injection of a contrast medium; used to identify and study spinal lesions caused by trauma and disease.

O

Ophthalmoscopy: Allows magnified examination of inner structures of the eye; an ophthalmoscope is used which has a light source and a special viewing device.

Opticokinetic Drum Test: Used to determine and measure eye movements; patient looks at a rapidly rotating, vertically striped drum.

Ortolani's Sign: A procedure to evaluate the stability of the hip joints in newborns and infants. With the infant on his or her back, the joints are manipulated, and if a clicking or popping sensation (Ortolani's sign) is felt or heard, the joint is unstable.

Otologic Examination: An ear examination, which may include the use of an otoscope, a tuning fork, and an audiometer.

Otoscopy: Direct visualization of the external auditory canal and the typanic membrane through an otoscope.

P

Papanicolaou (Pap) Test: Diagnostic test for early detection of cancer cells by a simple smear method usually taken from the cervix through a vaginal speculum.

Patch Test: A skin test for identifying allergens to confirm allergic contact sensitization. The suspected substance is applied to an adhesive patch that is placed on the patient's skin. Another patch with nothing on it acts as a control.

Pelvic Examination: Includes inspection of the vulva, vagina, and cervix for abnormalities. A bimanual palpation of the uterus, fallopian tubes, and ovaries occurs also. A Pap smear often is done at the same time.

Pen-Light Examination: Performed with a lighted instrument to check pupil reactivity.

Pericardiocentesis: Surgical puncture of the pericardium to remove purulent pericardial effusion.

pH Studies: Potential of hydrogen. Determines the acidity or akalinity level of gastrointestinal secretions. A pH electrode is used which is swallowed by the patient. Studies also can be done on blood and urine.

Phlebography: X-ray of the veins after the injection of a radiopaque contrast medium.

PKU, Phenylketonuria Test: A heel stick on an infant is done to collect three drops of blood for screening which determines elevated serum phenylalanine; performed about 4 days after milk feeding has begun. Also called the *Gutherie screening test.*

Pneumoencephalography: X-ray of the head after injection of air into the subarachnoid space which permits visualization of cerebral cortex and ventricles. A less hazardous procedure more commonly used is the CT scan.

PPD Tuberculin Test: Purified protein derivative (PPD) involves an intradermal injection of tuberculin antigen which causes a delayed reaction in patients with active or dormant tuberculosis.

Proctoscopy: Visual examination of the rectum using a proctoscope.

Pulmonary Artery Catheterization (PAC): Permits evaluation of ventilation function through spirometer measurements; performed on patients with pulmonary dysfunction.

R

Radioimmunoassay: A technique in radiology used to determine the concentration of an antigen, antibody, or other protein in the serum. See *Blood Serum for Hormones.*

Radioisotope Studies: Radioisotopes are used as tracers or indicators by being added to the stable compound under observation so that the course of the latter in the body can be detected, followed, and tagged.

Rectal Examination: A digital examination to detect polyps, early cancer, lesions, inflammatory conditions, and hemorrhoids. It also can show how far the uterus is displaced in the female; reveals the texture of the male prostate.

Rectal Manometry: Measures rectal sphincter function and peristaltic contractions.

Reticulocyte Count: A venipuncture is performed to determine the number of immature erythrocytes in the blood; important in diagnosing certain blood disorders, especially anemia.

Refraction: Defines any vision or refractive error and determines any correction required with glasses or contact lenses.

Renal Function Test: See *Urine Concentration and Dilution Tests.*

Retrograde Pyelogram: Contrast medium is introduced through a urinary catheter into the ureters and calyces of the kidney pelves while being observed on x-ray.

Rheumatoid Factors: Diagnostic blood test for immune-related diseases, e.g., rheumatoid arthritis.

Rinne Test: Hearing test to evaluate air and bone conduction. A tuning fork is placed on the mastoid process.

S

Scintiscan: Produces a map of scintillations when a radioactive substance is introduced into the body. The intensity of the record indicates the differential accumulation of the substance in the various body parts.

Serum B_{12}: A venipuncture is done for a quantitative analysis of serum vitamin B_{12} levels. Usually done concurrently with a serum folic acid, since the two are common causes of megaloblastic anemia. Also see *Shilling's Test.*

Serum Bilirubin: Measures serum levels of bilirubin; helps evaluate liver function, jaundice, biliary obstruction, and hemolytic anemia.

Serum Calcium, Phosphorus, Total Protein, or Serum Electrolytes: This series of tests performed on a blood sample will determine levels of calcium, phosphorus, and protein in the blood. See *Chemistry Screen.*

Serum Creatinine: Creatinine in blood serum provides a sensitive measure of renal damage. Creatinine levels are directly related to the glomerular filtration rate. See *Chemistry Screen.*

Serum Ferritin: Serum ferritin levels are related to the amount of available iron stored in the body. This test screens for iron deficiency and overload, measures iron storage, and can distinguish between iron deficiency and chronic inflammation.

Serum Folate: See *Serum Folic Acid.*

Serum Folic Acid: This test on a blood sample records the levels of folic acid; helps determine megaloblastic anemia and folate stores in pregnancy.

Serum Human Chorionic Gonadotropin (hCG): The production of hCG begins very quickly after the fertilized ovum is implanted into the uterine wall; the blood test reveals the presence of hCG if pregnancy has occurred.

Serum Gonadotropin: See *Serum Human Chorionic Gonadotropin.*

Serum Iron: A blood sample will estimate iron storage in the blood and help distinguish between iron deficiency anemia and anemia of chronic disease.

Serum Protein Electrophoresis: Measures serum albumin and globulins in an electric field by separating the proteins in size, shape, and electric charge at pH 8.6; helps to diagnose hepatic disease, protein deficiency, blood and renal disorders, and gastrointestinal and neoplastic diseases.

Serum Pregnancy Test: See *Serum Human Chorionic Gonadotropin.*

SGOT, Serum Glutamic-Oxaloacetic Transaminase: A venipuncture is performed to measure this cardiac enzyme. SGOT is essential to energy production; used to detect recent myocardial infarction, to differentiate acute hepatic disease, and to monitor patients with cardiac and hepatic disease.

SGPT, Serum Glutamic-Pyruvic Transaminase: A venipuncture is performed to measure this hepatic enzyme. SGPT is an enzyme necessary for tissue energy production. SGPT in the blood may indicate acute hepatic disease such as hepatitis and distinguish myocardial and hepatic tissue damage.

Shilling Test: Vitamin B_{12} is tagged with radioactive cobalt and administered orally. Gastrointestinal absorption is measured by determining the radioactivity of urine samples collected for the next 24 hours. Measures deficiencies of the vitamin; aids in diagnosis of megaloblastic anemia and central nervous system disorders of peripheral and spinal myelinated nerves.

Sigmoidoscopy: Visual inspection of the sigmoid flexure of the large intestine using a sigmoidoscope.

Skin, Intradermal/Scratch, Test: A small quantity of solution containing a suspected allergen is put on a lightly scratched area of the skin, or an intradermal injection may be used. If a wheal forms within 15 minutes, allergy is indicated.

Slit-Lamp Examination: Allows an ophthalmologist to visualize the anterior portion of the eye. The slit lamp is an instrument with a special lighting system and a binocular microscope.

Snellen Eye Test: A visual screening using a standardized chart with varied-sized block letters arranged in rows of decreasing sizes. Large E chart or one with animals and familiar objects may be used for children.

Sputum Culture: An examination of the material raised from the lungs and bronchi during deep coughing; is important in the management of lung disease.

Stool Culture: Examination of the feces will be performed to determine pathogens that cause gastrointestinal disease; a chemical test may be done on the stool specimen to detect occult blood, too.

Stool Occult Blood: A chemical test performed on a stool specimen to detect occult or hidden blood.

Synovial Fluid analysis: A sterile needle is inserted into a joint space to obtain a fluid specimen; aids in arthritis diagnosis, relieving pain and distension, and administering local drug therapy.

T

Thermography: A test which detects and records heat present in a body part; used to study blood flow to limbs and detect cancer of the breast.

Thoracentesis: Surgical puncture of the pleural space to remove fluid for analysis or treatment.

Thyroid Function Tests: Tests for evidence of thyroid function, including physical examination; some tests include determination of thyroid hormones.

Tonometry: Measurement of tension or pressure, especially of the eye for detection of glaucoma.

Transaminase: See *SGOT* and *SGPT.*

Trendelenburg's Test: The leg is raised above the heart level until veins are empty and then it is lowered quickly. If vein distension occurs immediately, valve incompetence is indicated.

Tzanck Smear Test: The examination of tissue from the floor of a lesion to discover the type of cell present as a means of diagnosing the disease.

U

Upper Gastrointestinal Endoscopy: Allows visualization of the upper gastrointestinal tract to diagnose inflammatory, ulcerative, and infectious disease, neoplasms, and other lesions.

Urate Crystals in Joint Fluid, or Tophi: Synovial joint fluid is examined under the microscope. If the joints are acutely inflamed, urate crystals are found.

Urine Calcium and Phosphates: Measures the urine levels of calcium and phosphates, which are essential for formation and resorption of bone; requires a 24-hour urine specimen.

Urine Catch, 24-Hour: Urine is collected over a 24-hour period to measure quantity and physical and chemical characteristics.

Urine Concentration and Dilution Test: Measures the levels of creatinine in urine and is used to help assess glomerular filtration and to check the accuracy of 24-hour urine collection based on relative contrast levels of creatinine excretion.

Urine Culture: A clean-voided midstream sample is collected for evaluation of urinary tract infections; specimen will be studied under a microscope and a colony count made to determine the presence of infection.

V

Vaginal Smears: With a cotton-tipped applicator or wooden spatula, vaginal secretions are collected for microscopic examination.

VDRL, Venereal Disease Research Laboratory Test: This test is widely used to screen for primary and secondary syphilis. A serum sample usually is used, but a specimen of cerebral spinal fluid may be used, also.

Ventriculography: X-ray of the head following removal of cerebral spinal fluid from cerebral ventricles and replacement with air or contrast medium; x-ray of heart ventricles after injection of contrast medium.

Visual Acuity Test: Part of an eye examination; evaluates the patient's ability to distinguish the form and detail of an object.

W

WBC, White Blood Count: Test made on whole blood to report the number of leukocytes in a cubic millimeter. The WBC may rise or fall in disease and is diagnostically useful only when interpreted in light of the patient's clinical status.

Wood's Light: An ultraviolet light used to diagnose certain scalp and skin diseases. The light causes hairs infected with a fungus to become brilliantly fluorescent.

X

X-Ray of Kidneys, Ureters, and Bladder (KUB): Provides x-rays of the kidneys, ureters, and bladder, which supply data about the urinary tract, kidney structure, size, and position.

Appendix 2
Associations Related to Diseases of the Human Body

Alzheimer's Disease and Related Disorders
360 N. Michigan Ave., Suite 601
Chicago, IL 60601

American Academy of Allergy
611 E. Wells St.
Milwaukee, WI 53202

American Allergy Association
P.O. Box 7273
Menlo Park, CA 94025

American Anorexia Nervosa Association
133 Cedar Lane
Teaneck, NJ 07666

American Cancer Society
777 Third Avenue
New York, NY 10017

American Celiac Society
45 Gifford Avenue
Jersey City, NJ 07304

American Council of the Blind
1211 Connecticut Avenue NW, Suite 506
Washington, DC 20036

American Diabetes Association
Two Park Avenue
New York, NY 10016

American Digestive Disease Society
420 Lexington Ave., Suite 1644
New York, NY 10017

American Geriatrics Society
Ten Columbus Circle
New York, NY 10019

American Heart Association
7320 Greenville Avenue
Dallas, TX 75231

American Liver Foundation
30 Sunrise Terrace
Cedar Grove, NY 07009

American Lung Association
1740 Broadway
New York, NY 10019

American Lupus Society, The
23751 Madison Street
Torrance, CA 90505

American Rheumatism Association
Arthritis Foundation
3400 Peachtree Rd., NE
Atlanta, GA 30326

Amyotrophic Lateral Sclerosis Society of America
15300 Ventura Blvd., Suite 315
Sherman Oaks, CA 91403

Asthma and Allergy Foundation of America
1707 N St., NW
Washington, DC 20036

Biofeedback Society of America
c/o Francine Butler, Ph.D.
4301 Owens Street
Wheat Ridge, CO 80033

Center for Sickle Cell Disease
2121 Georgia Avenue Northwest
Washington, DC 20059

Children's Liver Foundation
28 Highland Avenue
Maplewood, NY 07040

Coalition for Health and the Environment
806 15th Street NW, Suite 450
Washington, DC 20005

Epilepsy Foundation of America
4351 Garden City Drive
Landover, MD 20781

Gluten Intolerance Group
26604 Dover Ct.
Kent, WA 98031

Herpes Resource Center
Box 100
Palo Alto, CA 94302

Human Growth Foundation
4930 W. 77th, Suite 150
Edina, MN 55435

International Society of Endocrinology
9650 Rockville Pike
Bethesda, MD 20014

Juvenile Diabetes Foundation
23 E. 26th Street
New York, NY 10010

Lupus Foundation of America
11673 Holly Springs Drive
St. Louis, MO 63141

March of Dimes Birth Defects Foundation
1275 Mamoroneck Avenue
White Plains, NY 10605

Muscular Dystrophy Association
810 Seventh Avenue
New York, NY 10019

Myasthenia Gravis Foundation
15 E. 26th Street
New York, NY 10010

National Anorexic Aid Society
P.O. Box 29461
Columbus, OH 43229

National Association for Sickle Cell Disease
3460 Wilshire Blvd., Suite 1012
Los Angeles, CA 90010

National Ataxia Foundation
6681 Country Club Drive
Minneapolis, MN 55427

National Foundation for Ileitis and Colitis
295 Madison Avenue
New York, NY 10017

National Genetics Foundation
555 W. 57th Street
New York, NY 10019

National Geriatrics Society
212 W. Wisconsin Ave., 3rd Fl.
Milwaukee, WI 53203

National Hospice Organization
1311A Dolly Madison Blvd.
McLean, VA 22101

National Migraine Foundation
5252 N. Western Avenue
Chicago, IL 60625

National Multiple Sclerosis Society
205 E. 42nd Street
New York, NY 10017

National Psoriasis Foundation
6415 SW Canyon Ct., Suite 200
Portland, OR 97221

National Reye's Syndrome Foundation
426 N. Lewis
Bryan, OH 43506

National Scoliosis Foundation
48 Stone Road
Belmont, MA 02178

National Spinal Cord Injury Foundation
369 Elliot Street
Newton Upper Falls, MA 02164

National Sudden Infant Death Syndrome Foundation
Two Metro Plaza, Suite 205
8240 Professional Pl.
Landover, MD 20785

United Ostomy Association
2001 W. Beverly Blvd.
Los Angeles, CA 90057

United Parkinson Foundation
220 S. State Street
Chicago, IL 60606

United Scleroderma Foundation
P.O. Box 724
Watsonville, CA 95076

A more complete list with a description of each organization can be found in the *Encyclopedia of Associations,* Vol. 1, Sections 8–17, 1983, National Organizations of the United States, by Gale Research Company, Book Tower, Detroit, Michigan 48226.

Index

A page number in **boldface** indicates a main discussion of the topic. A "*t*" or an "*f*" following a page number indicates a table or figure, respectively.

RANDOM
HOUSE
LARGE
PRINT

SHE
SAID

SHE SAID

BREAKING THE SEXUAL HARASSMENT STORY

THAT HELPED IGNITE A MOVEMENT

Jodi Kantor and Megan Twohey

RANDOM HOUSE
LARGE PRINT

Published in the United States of America by Random House Large Print in association with Penguin Press, an imprint of Penguin Random House LLC, New York.

The Library of Congress has established a Cataloging-in-Publication record for this title.

ISBN: 978-0-593-15232-4

www.penguinrandomhouse.com/large-print-format-books

FIRST LARGE PRINT EDITION

Printed in the United States of America

10 9 8 7 6 5 4 3 2 1

This Large Print edition published in accord with the standards of the N.A.V.H.

TO OUR DAUGHTERS:

MIRA, TALIA, AND VIOLET

CONTENTS

SHE
SAID

In 2017, when we began our investigation of Harvey Weinstein for the **New York Times,** women held more power than ever before. The number of jobs once held almost exclusively by men—police officer, soldier, airline pilot—had narrowed almost to a vanishing point. Women led nations including Germany and the United Kingdom, and companies such as General Motors and PepsiCo. In one year of work, it was possible for a thirtysomething-year-old woman to make more money than all of her female ancestors had made in their combined lifetimes.

But all too often, women were sexually harassed with impunity. Female scientists and waitresses, cheerleaders, executives, and factory workers had to smile past gropes, leers, or unwelcome advances to get the next tip, paycheck, or raise. Sexual harassment was against the law—but it was also routine in some jobs. Women who spoke up were frequently dismissed or denigrated. Victims were often hidden and isolated from one another. Their best option, many people agreed, was to accept money as some form of reparation, in exchange for silence.

The perpetrators, meanwhile, frequently sailed to ever-higher levels of success and praise. Harassers were often accepted, or even cheered, as mischievous bad boys. Serious consequences were rare. Megan wrote some of the original articles in which women alleged that Donald J. Trump preyed on them—and then she covered his triumph in the 2016 election.

After we broke the story of Weinstein's alleged sexual harassment and abuse on October 5, 2017, we watched with astonishment as a dam wall broke. Millions of women around the world told their own stories of mistreatment. Large numbers of men suddenly had to answer for their predatory behavior, a moment of accountability without precedent. Journalism had helped inspire a paradigm shift. Our work was only one driver of that change, which had been building for years, thanks to the efforts of pioneering feminists and legal scholars; Anita Hill; Tarana Burke, the activist who founded the #MeToo movement; and many others, including our fellow journalists.

But seeing our own hard-won investigative discoveries help realign attitudes left us asking, Why this story? As one of our editors pointed out, Harvey Weinstein wasn't even that famous. In a world in which so much feels stuck, how does this sort of seismic social change occur?

We embarked on this book to answer those questions. Nothing about the change was inevitable or foretold. In these pages, we describe the motivations and wrenching, risky decisions of the first brave sources to break the silence surrounding Weinstein. Laura Madden, a former assistant to Weinstein and a stay-at-home mother in Wales, spoke out just as she was reeling from divorce and about to undergo post-cancer breast surgery. Ashley Judd put her career on the line, spurred by a little-known period in her life when she stepped away from Hollywood to immerse herself in big-picture thinking about gender equality. Zelda Perkins, a London producer whose complaints against Weinstein had been suppressed by an agreement she had signed two decades before, spoke to us despite potential legal and financial retribution. A longtime Weinstein employee, increasingly troubled by what he knew, played a key, and previously undisclosed, role in helping us to finally unmask his boss. We intend the title, **She Said,** as a complicated one: We write about those who did speak out, along with other women who chose not to, and the nuances of how and when and why.

This is also a story about investigative journalism, beginning with the first uncertain days of our reporting, when we knew very little and almost no one would speak to us. We describe how we coaxed out secrets, pinned down information, and pursued the truth about a powerful man even as he used under-handed tactics to try to sabotage our work. We have also, for the first time, reconstructed our final show-down with the producer—his last stand—in the offices of the **New York Times** right before publica-tion, as he realized he was cornered.

Our Weinstein reporting took place at a time of accusations of "fake news," as the very notion of a national consensus on truth seemed to be fracturing. But the impact of the Weinstein revelations was so great in part because we and other journalists were able to establish a clear and overwhelming body of evidence of wrongdoing. In these pages, we explain how we have documented a pattern of behavior based on first-person accounts, financial and legal records, company memos, and other revealing mate-rials. In the wake of our work, there was little public debate about what Weinstein had done to women; it was about what should be done in response. But Weinstein has continued to deny all allegations of non-consensual sex, and has repeatedly asserted that our reporting is incorrect. "What you have here are allegations and accusations, but you do not have ab-solute facts," a spokesman said when we asked for a response to the revelations presented here.

This book toggles between what we learned dur-ing the course of our original work on Weinstein in 2017 and the substantial amount of informa-tion we've gathered since. Much of the new report-ing we present about Weinstein helps illustrate how the legal system and corporate culture has served to silence victims and still inhibits change. Businesses are co-opted into protecting predators. Some advocates for women profit from a settlement system that covers up misdeeds. Many people who glimpse the problem—like Bob Weinstein, Harvey's brother and business partner, who granted extensive interviews for this book—do little to try and stop it.

As we write this, in May 2019, Weinstein awaits a criminal trial for alleged rape and other sexual abuse and faces a volley of civil suits, in which actresses, former employees, and others are seeking to hold him financially accountable. No matter the outcome of those cases, we hope this book will serve as a lasting record of Weinstein's legacy: his exploitation of the workplace to manipulate, pressure, and terrorize women.

In the months after we broke the Weinstein story, as the #MeToo movement exploded, so did new debates about topics ranging from date rape to child sexual abuse to gender discrimination and even to awkward encounters at parties. This made the public conversation feel rich and searching, but also confusing: Were the goals to eliminate sexual harassment, reform the criminal justice system, smash the patriarchy, or flirt without giving offense? Had the reckoning gone too far, with innocent men tarnished with less-than-convincing proof, or not far enough, with a frustrating lack of systemic change?

Nearly a year to the day after our Weinstein story was published, Dr. Christine Blasey Ford, a psychology professor from California, appeared before a U.S. Senate committee and accused Judge Brett Kavanaugh, then nominated to the Supreme Court, of sexually assaulting her while drunk in high school. He furiously denied the allegation. Some saw Ford as the ultimate hero of the #MeToo movement. Others saw her as a symbol of overreach—a living justification for the mounting backlash.

We saw her as the protagonist of one of the most complex and revealing "she said" stories yet, especially once we began to learn how much about her path to that Senate testimony was not publicly understood. Jodi watched from the hearing room, observed some of her legal team as they worked, and met her the next morning. In December, Megan conducted the first post-hearing interview of Ford, over a breakfast in Palo Alto. In the following months, she had dozens of hours of additional interviews with Ford about how she came to raise her voice and what the consequences were. We also spoke with others who shaped and witnessed her experience. We tell the story of Ford's journey to Washington and how an overwhelming array of viewpoints, institutions, political forces, and fears all came to bear on her.

Many people wonder how Ford has fared since her testimony. The final chapter of this book consists of a unique group interview, in which we brought together some of the women we reported on, including Ford, across these different stories. But something larger is at stake in Ford's odyssey too: that continued question of what drives and impedes progress. The #MeToo movement is an example of social change in our time but is also a test of it: In this fractured environment, will all of us be able to forge a new set of mutually fair rules and protections?

This book recounts two astounding years in the life of women in the United States and beyond. That history belongs to all of us who lived it: Unlike some journalistic investigations that deal with locked-away government or corporate secrets, this one is about experiences many of us recognize from our own lives, workplaces, families, and schools. But we wrote this book to bring you as close as we could to ground zero.

To relate those events as directly and authentically as possible, we have incorporated transcripts of interviews, emails, and other primary documents. There are notes from the first conversations we had with movie stars about Weinstein, a searching letter that Bob Weinstein wrote to his brother, excerpts from Ford's texts, and many other firsthand materials. Some of what we share was originally off the record, but through additional reporting, including returning to the parties involved, we were able to include it here. We were able to depict conversations and events that we did not witness firsthand through records and interviews. All told, this book is based on three years of reporting and hundreds of interviews conducted from London to Palo Alto; the endnotes give a detailed accounting of which information we learned from which sources and records.

Finally, this book is a chronicle of the partnership we developed as we worked to understand these events. To avoid confusion, we write about ourselves in the third person. (In a first-person account of our reporting, which was collaborative but often involved us following separate threads, "I" could be either Jodi or Megan.) So before we slip into that way of telling the story, we want to say, in our own voices: Thank you for joining our partnership for the duration of these pages, for puzzling through these events and clues as we have, for witnessing what we witnessed, and hearing what we heard.

CHAPTER ONE

THE FIRST PHONE CALL

The **New York Times** investigation into Harvey Weinstein began with the most promising source refusing even to get on the phone.

"Here's the thing, I have been treated quite shabbily by your paper at times and I believe the root of it is sexism," the actress Rose McGowan wrote on May 11, 2017, responding to an email from Jodi asking to talk. McGowan listed her criticisms: a speech she had made at a political dinner was covered in the Style section instead of the news pages. An earlier conversation she'd had with a **Times** reporter about Weinstein had been uncomfortable.

"The NYT needs to look at itself for sexism issues," she responded. "I'm not that inclined to help."

Months earlier, McGowan had accused an unnamed producer—rumored to be Weinstein—of having raped her. "Because it's been an open secret in Hollywood/Media & they shamed me while adulating my rapist," she had tweeted, adding the hashtag #WhyWomenDontReport. Now she was said to be writing a memoir intended to expose the entertainment industry's mistreatment of women.

Unlike almost anyone else in Hollywood, McGowan had a history of risking her own career prospects to call out sexism, once tweeting out the insulting clothing requirements on a casting notice for an Adam Sandler movie: "tank that shows off cleavage (push up bras encouraged)." In general, her tone on social media was tough, confrontational: "It is okay to be angry. Don't be afraid of it," she had tweeted a month earlier, later adding: "dismantle the system." If McGowan, as much an activist as an actress, would not have one off-the-record conversation, who would?

Harvey Weinstein was not the man of the moment. In recent years, his moviemaking magic had faltered. But his name was synonymous with power, specifically the power to make and boost careers. First he had invented himself, going from a modest upbringing in Queens, New York, to concert promotion to film distribution and production, and he seemed to know how to make everything around him bigger—films, parties, and most of all, people. Over and over, he had propelled young actors to stardom: Gwyneth Paltrow, Matt Damon, Michelle Williams, and Jennifer Lawrence. He could turn tiny independent movies like **Sex, Lies, and Videotape** or **The Crying Game** into phenomena. He had pioneered the modern Oscar campaign, winning five Best Picture statues for himself and armloads for others. His record of raising money for Hillary Clinton, and flanking her at countless fund-raisers, was almost two decades long. When Malia Obama had sought an internship in film, she worked for "Harvey"—first name only, used even by many strangers. By 2017, even though his movies were less successful than they used to be, his reputation remained outsized.

Rumors had long circulated about his treatment of women. People had joked about them publicly: "Congratulations, you five ladies no longer have to pretend to be attracted to Harvey Weinstein," the comedian Seth MacFarlane said at the Oscar nomination announcements in 2013. But many people had dismissed the behavior as philandering, and nothing had ever been publicly documented. Other journalists had tried and failed in the past. A 2015 investigation by the City of New York Police Department (NYPD) into a groping accusation against Weinstein had ended without any criminal charges. "At some pt, all the women who've been afraid to speak out abt Harvey Weinstein are gonna have to hold hands and jump," Jennifer Senior, a journalist, had tweeted back then. Two years had passed. Nothing had happened. Jodi had heard that two more reporters, a writer at **New York Magazine** and NBC's Ronan Farrow, had tried, but no stories had appeared.

Were the whispers about Weinstein's interactions

with women wrong? Had McGowan's tweet referred to someone else? In public, Weinstein boasted
of feminist credentials. He had just given a large
donation to help endow a professorship in Gloria
Steinem's name. His company had distributed
The Hunting Ground, a documentary and rallying
cry about campus sexual assault. He had even participated in the historic women's marches of January
2017, joining the pink pussyhat throngs in Park City,
Utah, during the Sundance Film Festival.

The point of the **Times** investigations department,
tucked away from the hum of the rest of the newsroom, was to dig for what had never been reported,
bringing to account people and institutions whose
transgressions had been deliberately concealed. The
first step was often careful outreach. So how to reply
to McGowan so as to motivate her to pick up the
phone?

Her email had openings. First, she had written
back. Lots of people never did. She had put thought
into her note and cared enough to offer a critique.
Maybe she was testing Jodi, jabbing at the **Times** to
see if the reporter would defend it.

But Jodi wasn't looking to have an argument about
her own workplace of fourteen years. Flattering
McGowan ("I really admire the bravery of your
tweets . . .") also was not the way to go. That would
sap what little authority Jodi had in the interaction.
And there was nothing to be said about the investigation to which McGowan would be contributing:

If she asked how many other women Jodi had spoken to, the answer would be none.

The note would need to be phrased just so, with no mention of Weinstein's name: McGowan had a history of posting private communications on Twitter, like the Adam Sandler casting notice. She was someone who wanted to blow things open, but that impulse could backfire in this situation. ("Hey, world, check out this email from a **Times** reporter.") The subject matter made the response even trickier. McGowan had said she was an assault victim. Pressuring her would not be right.

In 2013, Jodi had started investigating women's experiences at corporations and other institutions. The gender debate in the United States already seemed saturated with feeling: opinion columns, memoirs, expressions of outrage or sisterhood on social media. It needed more exposure of hidden facts. Especially about the workplace. Workers, from the most elite to the lowliest, were often afraid to question their employers. Reporters were not. In doing those stories, Jodi had found that gender was not just a topic, but a kind of investigative entry point. Because women were still outsiders at many organizations, documenting what they experienced meant seeing how power functioned.

She wrote back to Rose McGowan, calling on those experiences:

Here's my own track record on these issues: Amazon, Starbucks, and Harvard Business School have all changed their policies in response to gender-related problems I exposed. When I wrote about the class gap in breastfeeding—white collar women can pump on the job, lower paid women cannot—readers responded by creating the first-ever mobile lactation suites, now available in 200+ locations across the country.

If you'd rather not speak, I understand, and best of luck with your book publication.

Thank you, Jodi

McGowan wrote back within a few hours. She could talk any time before Wednesday.

The call seemed like it could be tricky: McGowan appeared tough, with a buzz cut and that call-to-arms Twitter feed. But the voice on the phone belonged to someone impassioned and game, who had a story and was searching for the right way to tell it. Her tweets about being raped had just been hints, with few details. Generally, the rule in interviews was that they were on the record—meaning the material could be published—unless otherwise discussed.

But any woman with an assault complaint against Weinstein would probably be reluctant to have even an initial conversation. So Jodi agreed that the call would be kept private until they decided otherwise, and McGowan started in.

In 1997, she had been young and newly triumphant, on a heady trip to the Sundance Film Festival, where she alternated between premieres and parties and a TV camera crew followed her around. She had only been in four or five films, like the teen-horror flick **Scream,** but she was becoming one of the ingenues of the moment, with multiple new movies at the festival alone. "I was the belle of Sundance," she said. Independent films were at the center of the culture, the festival was the place to be, and Harvey Weinstein was sovereign: That was where the producer-distributor had bought small films like **Clerks** and **Reservoir Dogs,** which he had turned into cultural touchstones. In her telling, McGowan didn't remember which year this was; many actresses chronicled the past not according to date but instead to which movie of theirs was filming or being released at the time. McGowan recalled the screening where she had sat right near Weinstein: The movie was called **Going All the Way,** she said with an incredulous laugh.

Afterward, he had asked for a meeting with her, which made sense: The top producer wanted to get together with the rising star. She went to see him at the Stein Eriksen Lodge Deer Valley, in Park

City, where they met in his room. Nothing happened except the usual talk about films and roles, she said.

But on the way out, Weinstein pulled her into a room with a hot tub, stripped her on the edge, and forced his face between her legs, according to McGowan. She said she remembered feeling like she was leaving her body, floating up to the ceiling and observing the scene from above. "I was just feeling massive shock, I was going into survival mode," she said. To get away, McGowan said, she faked an orgasm and mentally gave herself step-by-step instructions: "Turn the door handle." "Walk out of this meeting."

Within a few days, she said, Weinstein had left a message on her home phone in Los Angeles with a creepy offer: Other big female stars were his special friends, and she could join his club as well. Shocked and distraught, McGowan had complained to her managers, hired a lawyer, and ended up with a $100,000 settlement from Weinstein—essentially, a payment to make the matter go away, without any admission of wrongdoing on his part—which she said she had donated to a rape crisis center.

Did she have her records from the settlement? "They never gave me a copy," she said.

The problem was worse than Weinstein, she said. Hollywood was an organized system for abusing women. It lured them with promises of fame, turned them into highly profitable products, treated their bodies as property, required them to look perfect, and then discarded them. On the call, her indictments came fast, one after another:

"Weinstein—it's not just him, it's an entire machine, supply chain."

"No oversight, no fear."

"Each studio does the victim shaming and payouts."

"Almost everyone has an NDA."

"If white men could have a playground, this would be it."

"The women here are just as guilty."

"Don't step out of line; you can be replaced."

McGowan's words were arresting. It wasn't new to say that Hollywood took advantage of women, forced them into conformity, and dumped them when they aged or rebelled. But hearing a direct account of exploitation from a familiar face, in full disturbing detail, and with one of the most renowned producers in Hollywood as the perpetrator, was entirely different: sharper, more specific, sickening.

The call ended with an agreement to talk again soon. The actress was an unusual character, but the sometimes outrageous things she had done or said or whom she had dated didn't matter for these purposes. The question was how her account would stand up to the rigors of the journalistic process, and, if it got that far, the inevitable challenge by Weinstein, and then public scrutiny. Before the **Times** would even consider publishing McGowan's allegations, they would need to be buttressed, and, finally, taken to Weinstein. He would have to be given an opportunity to respond.

The paper had a duty to be fair, especially given the gravity of the charges. In 2014, **Rolling Stone** magazine described what it called a horrific group sexual assault at the University of Virginia without anything close to sufficient evidence. The ensuing controversy set off a series of lawsuits, almost ruined the magazine's reputation, gave ammunition to those who said women fabricated rape stories, and set back the cause of fighting campus sexual assault. The **Washington Post** reported that police had called the story "a complete crock," the **Columbia Journalism Review** called it "a mess," and the article won an "Error of the Year" award.

On first inspection, McGowan's account seemed vulnerable to challenge by Weinstein. He would easily be able to say that he remembered things differently, that she had appeared to enjoy herself. He would have the perfect evidence: her faked orgasm. The old answering machine tape was potentially significant, showing that Weinstein was using his power as a producer to compel sexual favors. But unless McGowan had the tape from two decades ago, it was just a memory of a long-ago message, also easy to deny.

As a sole account, McGowan's story had a high likelihood of becoming a classic "he said, she said" dispute. McGowan would tell a terrible story.

Weinstein would deny it. With no witnesses, people would take sides, Team Rose versus Team Harvey.

But McGowan said she had gotten a settlement. Finding any record of it would be difficult, but there had been lawyers, a signed agreement, money that changed hands, the donation to the rape crisis center. The agreement had to be documented somewhere. It wouldn't prove what had happened in the hotel room, but it could add support by showing that Weinstein had paid McGowan a significant sum at the time to settle a dispute.

Jodi brought everything she had learned to her longtime editor at the **Times,** Rebecca Corbett, who was an expert in complex investigations. They discussed whether McGowan's account could be backed up, and the important question: Did other women have similar stories about him?

Finding that out would require huge effort. Weinstein had produced or distributed hundreds of movies over the decades. With his brother, Bob, he had co-owned and run two companies: Miramax and The Weinstein Company (TWC), his current endeavor. That meant there were a lot of potential sources, a better situation than when critical information was held by just a few people. But there were an overwhelming number of people to contact, actresses and former employees scattered across several continents, most of whom would probably be reluctant to talk.

In mid-June Corbett suggested that Jodi contact

a colleague, Megan Twohey, who was relatively new at the paper. Megan was on maternity leave, but she had a real touch with this kind of work, the editor said. Jodi didn't know what help she would be, but she sent off an email anyway.

When Megan got Jodi's email, she was caring for her newborn child and recovering from the most bruising reporting stretch of her career. She had arrived at the **Times** in February 2016 to cover politics, investigating the presidential candidates. Megan had said yes to the job with some hesitation: Politics had never been her assignment or interest.

But within weeks of her arrival, Dean Baquet, the executive editor of the paper, had tapped Megan for a specific line of inquiry that drew on her reporting expertise: Had Donald J. Trump's behavior toward women ever crossed legal or ethical lines? For more than a decade, Megan had been uncovering sex crimes and sexual misconduct. In Chicago, she had revealed how police and prosecutors in the area were shelving rape kits, robbing victims of the chance for justice, and how sex-abusing doctors had continued to practice. Later, she had exposed a black market for adopted children that had delivered some of them to sexual predators.

Trump had long fashioned himself a playboy, or at least a caricature of one. He was on his third wife and had entered the presidential race with a trail of

Howard Stern interviews in which he bragged about his sexual exploits and engaged in crude commentary about women, including his own daughter Ivanka.

Baquet saw some red flags beneath the bravado. If Donald Trump had simply been promiscuous, that was not a story—the paper didn't peer into people's sex lives, even those of presidential candidates, without a reason. But some of Trump's comments had been made in the workplace, a possible sign of sexual harassment. On **The Celebrity Apprentice,** a show that he helped produce and starred in, Trump had told a contestant, "That must be a pretty picture, you dropping to your knees." Decades earlier, Trump's first wife, Ivana Trump, had reportedly accused him of marital rape, then minimized the allegation. Baquet had already enlisted another reporter, Michael Barbaro, to investigate Trump's treatment of women, and he wanted him and Megan to answer the question of whether Trump was just crude in his behavior toward women or if the problem was more extensive.

Initially, the reporting was slow: Most of Trump's former employees were bound by nondisclosure agreements, his history of being vindictive toward those who crossed him had left a chilling effect, and so many lawsuits had been filed against him over the years that it was hard to know which to examine.

By May 2016, however, Megan and Barbaro were prepared to write an article, based on hundreds of records and more than fifty interviews with people who had worked with or for Trump, dated him, or socialized with him. Trump was a powerful man who had engaged in contradictory behavior toward women. He could be gracious and encouraging to women he worked with, and he had promoted several to the top positions in his company. But he also had a habit of unending commentary about women's bodies and unsettling workplace conduct.

Most significantly, Megan had pieced together multiple allegations of sexual aggression beyond the Ivana rape allegation. A former Miss Utah had explained in detail how, in 1997, Trump had forcibly kissed her on her mouth twice, at a gala after the Miss USA pageant and later at a meeting at his office to discuss a possible modeling career. In two old lawsuits, a former Trump beauty pageant business partner claimed that Trump had groped her under the table during a work dinner at the Plaza Hotel and had taken her into a room at another work gathering and forcibly "kissed, fondled, and restrained" her from leaving.

Caution was essential. If a single allegation in a story turned out to be shaky, it could undermine the entire article. When a former pageant contestant told Megan that Trump had groped her at his Palm Beach mansion, prompting her to flee to her room and place a panicked call to her father, a colleague tracked the man down in another country. "Got the father," the colleague reported back in an email. "In short—he has no memory of this having happened with Trump." That didn't mean the woman had been lying. But it did mean that they couldn't use her allegation in the story.

The article—in which many women's accounts were told in their own words—was published at dawn (ET) on Saturday, May 14, 2016, and it quickly exploded, eventually becoming the most-read **Times** political article thus far that year. That Trump, known for viciously attacking critical stories about him, said nothing about the article all weekend was seen as a sign of its strength. Before publication, Megan and Barbaro had conducted a lengthy interview of the candidate and woven in his responses, including his denials of any misconduct and his insistence that he had always treated women with respect.

On Monday morning, they were in the green room of the **CBS This Morning** news show, preparing to be interviewed about the article, when Gayle King walked in and pointed to the TV: "Did you see, Rowanne Brewer Lane just went on **Fox and Friends** to dispute your story?"

Brewer Lane was the first person quoted in the article. A former model who had met Trump at a pool party at Mar-a-Lago in 1990, she had described in an interview how Trump had focused in on her, led her into a room, encouraged her to put on a swimsuit, and then showed her off to the guests. Brewer Lane wasn't disputing her quotes about the interaction. She disagreed with the way it was characterized: as "a debasing face-to-face encounter between Trump and a young woman he hardly knew."

The account made up a handful of paragraphs in a five-thousand-word story, one that had pointed out that Brewer Lane went on to date Trump. But her public criticism provided Trump with a toehold to attack the entire article. He immediately seized on her comments and started punching back in a series of tweets:

> The @nytimes is so dishonest. Their hit piece cover story on me yesterday was just blown up by Rowanne Brewer, who said it was a lie!

> With the coming forward today of the woman central to the failing @nytimes hit piece on me, we have exposed the article as a fraud!

Soon his supporters were coming out swinging too, taking direct shots at Megan and Barbaro on social media, in emails, in angry phone calls. The article had carefully documented the serious allegations of sexual misconduct against Trump. But because of criticism of a far less grave anecdote, Megan and Barbaro were on the defensive.

The staff of Bill O'Reilly, the bombastic king of right-wing news, called Megan over and over, asking, "Are you a feminist?," as if that would discredit her. Suspicious of their motivations, she refused their interview requests, then watched as the host took to the airwaves to tell millions of viewers not to trust her work. "The problem is, Megan Twohey is a feminist, or so it seems," he said. His argument was absurd—as the **Washington Post** asked, should a chauvinist report the story?—but he used the full force of his influence to blunt the impact of the findings and to try to discredit her.

Those public attacks were unlike anything Megan had ever experienced. She was grateful when June 2016 arrived, and a previously scheduled commitment, her own wedding, took her out of the newsroom.

But did other women have allegations of forcible kissing, groping, or worse? When Megan returned from her honeymoon, she kept reporting on Trump.

Several months later, on Friday, October 7, Megan was on the phone with a source when colleagues started rising from their seats and flocking to TVs throughout the newsroom. The **Washington Post** had obtained a snippet of an audiotape from the gossip show **Access Hollywood** from 2005, in which Trump bragged about his aggression toward women.

I'm automatically attracted to beautiful— I just start kissing them. . . . I don't even wait. And when you're a star, they let you

**do it. You can do anything . . . Grab 'em
by the pussy. You can do anything.**

His words were like nothing ever publicly heard
from a presidential candidate. This sounded like
confirmation of the behavior that Megan had spent
months piecing together.

Trump apologized for his words, then doubled
down on his denials. The comments on the **Access
Hollywood** tape were just locker room talk, he insisted. Two days later, during an October 9 presidential debate, he denied that he had ever kissed women
without their permission or grabbed intimate parts
of their bodies. Yes, he had boasted about it. But had
he ever actually done those things? "No, I have not,"
the candidate said.

Within a week, Megan and Barbaro had a new
article almost ready, with two other women saying
that Trump's words on the audio recording matched
their experiences. Both Jessica Leeds, a seventy-four-
year-old former stockbroker and great-grandmother
who lived in a tidy one-bedroom on the Upper East
Side of Manhattan, and Rachel Crooks, a thirty-
three-year-old PhD candidate in higher education
administration from Green Springs, Ohio, had written emails to the **Times** outlining their allegations.

Leeds had been traveling as a sales representative
for a newsprint company in the early 1980s when she
had lucked into a first-class upgrade on a flight from
Dallas to New York City. In the next seat happened

to be Donald Trump, tall, blond, and chatty. Forty-five minutes after takeoff, Leeds alleged, he leaned over, grabbed her breasts, and tried to put his hand up her skirt.

"He was all over me, hands everywhere," she wrote in her email, explaining that she had fled to a seat in coach.

Crooks was the daughter of a nurse and a mechanic who didn't talk politics but identified as Republican. In high school, she had been all-state in basketball, track, and volleyball and voted Most Likely to Succeed. In 2005, she had wanted to experience New York for herself. She and her boyfriend rented a cheap apartment on the outskirts of Brooklyn, sleeping on an air mattress until they had enough money for a futon. To make rent, she took a secretarial job at a real-estate development firm on the twenty-fourth floor of Trump Tower that worked on deals with The Trump Organization. **The Apprentice** had gone on the air the year before, the most popular new show of the season.

One day that winter, when she saw Donald Trump waiting for an elevator outside her office, she rose from her desk to introduce herself, offering him a business-like handshake. He didn't let go, she said. He kissed her on the cheeks. Then he went for her lips and pressed hard. The whole thing lasted only a minute or two. She was twenty-two. Before that, the only man who had ever kissed her was the boyfriend she lived with.

"I was angry that Mr. Trump had viewed me as so

insignificant that he could impose himself on me in such a way," she wrote.

Crooks was describing a forced kiss almost exactly like those allegedly planted on the former Miss Utah. Leeds was describing groping similar to the kind endured by the former beauty pageant business partner. And it all matched the behavior that Trump had been recorded boasting about. On the phone, both Leeds and Crooks had told Megan they were prepared to go on the record. Neither woman was inclined to draw attention to herself. But they wanted the world to know that Trump was lying.

Mindful of the stakes, Megan and Barbaro checked and double-checked with friends and family members in whom the women had confided. They scrubbed the two women's backgrounds to make sure there were no ties to Hillary Clinton's campaign. Megan even asked Crooks to send her an old picture of her at her desk in Trump Tower, to confirm that she worked there. The due diligence could have seemed insulting to the women. But it was to protect them, and the **Times.**

The final step was to run the allegations by Trump's team. As the sun went down, Megan sat at her dining table glued to her email, expecting a perfunctory denial from a Trump spokesperson. Instead her cell phone rang.

Trump was on the line.

Megan had barely begun her questions before he started lashing out. Jessica Leeds and Rachel Crooks were lying. He had no idea who they were. If he had done those things to them, why didn't they complain to the police?

Megan explained that the women did not claim to have known him but only to have had chance encounters with him. She reminded him of the allegations by the former Miss Utah and of his onetime beauty pageant business partner.

Seething, Trump switched aim. The **New York Times** had concocted the women's accounts. If it published the story, he would sue.

Megan pressed forward, determined to keep him talking. What about the recently leaked **Access Hollywood** tape? She asked him again if he had ever done the things he had bragged about.

"I don't do it," he insisted, his voice rising. "I don't do it. It was locker-room talk."

He began to erupt at Megan. "You are disgusting!" Trump shouted. "You are a disgusting human being."

When the line went dead, Megan relaxed. As brutal as the conversation had been, she had provided Trump with adequate opportunity to respond to the allegations. They could move forward with publishing the article, complete with his comments.

Minutes later, Trump stepped onstage in Florida for a campaign rally, and he set to work directing his crowd's thundering energy and anger toward journalists.

"The corrupt media is teamed up against you, the American people," he said. "And I'll tell you what, it's libelous, it's slanderous, it's horrible, and it's really unfair. But we're going to beat the system."

It was less than four weeks until Election Day. The Republican Speaker of the House said he was sickened by the **Access Hollywood** tape. Senator John McCain withdrew his endorsement. Governor Mike Pence, the vice-presidential nominee, said that he was praying for the Trump family. Some Republicans were saying he should drop out of the race.

Other women stepped forward to level accusations against Trump. One had been out with friends at a nightclub. Another was a former contestant on **The Apprentice.** A third was a reporter assigned to write a valentine of a story on Trump's first wedding anniversary with Melania, his third wife. Some of their stories were essentially the same as those Megan had reported. Trump had allegedly grabbed, groped, or fondled them, pushed them up against walls and thrust his hips or genitals at them. Who could ignore or dismiss the pattern of predatory behavior now?

But journalists were not able to vet all of the allegations. An explosive civil lawsuit alleged that he had raped a thirteen-year-old girl two decades before, at a party hosted by a well-known financier named Jeffrey Epstein who was later investigated for running an underage-sex ring for powerful men and convicted of soliciting a prostitute. But the alleged victim of Trump, referred to only as Jane Doe, had never been identified or made available to reporters, even confidentially. Without a woman whose existence could be confirmed and whose story could be vetted, Megan had refused to cover the case and discouraged her colleagues from touching it either.

Other claims drew attention but did not feel newsworthy. Megan watched as a woman tearfully recounted in a televised press conference an incident that sounded like Trump had accidentally brushed his hand against her breast and heckled her as she waited for a ride.

As the carefully reported allegations of Crooks and Leeds swirled together with the other accusations, Trump moved from firm denials to sweeping attacks. His accusers were liars. Out for fame. Working for Hillary Clinton. Too ugly and unappealing to have drawn his attention. He would sue them.

His supporters listened to his cues and once again sprang into action. Fox Business anchor Lou Dobbs shared with his nearly one million Twitter followers a link to a post from a conservative news site that listed Jessica Leeds's phone number and address, along with the false claim that she worked for the Clinton Foundation.

Leeds did not scare easily; Rachel Crooks, on the other hand, was extremely rattled. She couldn't go outside because of the reporters who swarmed her lawn in Ohio. She couldn't go online either, because of the Trump trolls and their barrage of messages:

You're so ugly. You're getting paid off. Someone should put a gun to your head and do this country a favor. A stranger posted a message on Facebook identifying herself as a family friend and claimed to know that Crooks was lying about Trump. The post became the top hit for any search of Crooks's name. Another man that Crooks had never heard of accused her of stealing from a company she had never worked for.

With every attack, Megan felt worse. She had encouraged the two women to go on the record, telling them it was a public service to share vital information about a presidential candidate. She was the one who had painted intimate details of their lives onto a giant wall, big enough for the whole country to read. Now they were under siege. Crooks, her voice shaking over the phone, had asked what the **Times** would do if Trump followed through with his threat to sue her. The answer was very little. Thousands of people were quoted in the **Times** every week: As with other publications, the paper could not assume legal responsibility for them.

Megan was being attacked too. Threats from Trump supporters arrived through both her phone and computer. She alerted **Times** security after repeatedly receiving anonymous messages from a man who said he was going to rape and murder her and dump her body in the Hudson River. She was pregnant, more visibly so each day, and worried strangers would start tweeting threats about the baby or do even worse.

Trump himself was threatening to sue. His lawyer sent a letter to Baquet, which the Trump team then made public, instructing him to retract Leeds's and Crooks's accounts. "Failure to do so will leave my client with no option but to pursue all available actions and remedies," he wrote.

David McCraw, vice president and assistant general counsel of the **New York Times,** beloved in the newsroom for his unflappability and protection of journalists, replied with equal force.

"It would have been a disservice not just to our readers but to democracy itself to silence their voices," the lawyer wrote.

He all but dared Trump to sue the **Times.** "If he believes that American citizens had no right to hear what these women had to say and that the law of this country forces us and those who would dare criticize him to stand silent or be punished, we welcome an opportunity to have a court set him straight."

It was a rousing defense, not just of journalism but of the rights of women to make allegations against powerful men. When the **Times** published the letter on its website, it went immediately viral.

But inside the newsroom, Megan was afraid Trump would follow through with a lawsuit against her, Barbaro, and the paper, as McCraw suspected he would if he wasn't elected. Trump would ultimately lose in court, but it would be a long, arduous legal process. Megan had begun preserving all of her notes, emails, and text messages, in case of future legal discovery.

On November 7, three and a half weeks later, Megan flew to Illinois to observe what many people thought would be the election of the first female president of the United States. For the sake of symbolism, Megan's editors had asked her to help capture the moment at polling places in Park Ridge, a suburb of Chicago and Hillary Clinton's hometown.

Megan wasn't advocating for Clinton, or for any other candidate. That's not what reporters did. A few weeks before, in an article that had drawn fire from the Democratic nominee's supporters, Megan had highlighted the role that Hillary Clinton had played in battling women who alleged sexual impropriety and worse by Bill Clinton. Her allies insisted the role was minimal, but Megan found evidence that she had signed off on hiring a private detective to dig up dirt to smear the women.

As she stood talking to voters, she knew they would make their decisions based on many factors, beyond the sexual misconduct allegations against Trump. But Megan did expect to encounter concern about them. Using hashtags like #WhyWomenDontReport, in the weeks leading up to the election, a chorus of women had begun speaking up online about other men who had done similar things to them. Rose McGowan, with her tweets about the studio head who had violated her, was among them.

But in interview after interview at the polling place, it became clear that very few of the suburban white women appeared to care much about Trump's alleged trespasses or his own words on the **Access Hollywood** tape. That night Megan hardly needed to look at the television: She already knew Trump had been elected.

That April following the election, Megan and Jodi each watched, with astonishment, a series of developments that would lead directly to the beginning of the Weinstein investigation. Bill O'Reilly, the right-wing television host at the peak of his power, lost his position at the Fox News Network after the **Times** exposed how he and the company had covered up repeated allegations of sexual harassment. The article, by Emily Steel and Michael Schmidt, had taken eight months to report, and it proved that O'Reilly had racked up settlements with at least five women who had accused him of verbal abuse, lewd remarks, and unwanted come-ons. O'Reilly and Fox News had handed over what then looked like a total of $13 million to silence the women: an enormous secret payout from one of America's top critics of feminism.

In that story, only a single woman had spoken on the record about her allegations: Wendy Walsh, a former guest who lost a lucrative offer to be an O'Reilly contributor after she declined an invitation back to his hotel suite. Most of the women in the story were barred from speaking because they had settled with O'Reilly or the network. They had accepted large sums of money in exchange for agreeing never to talk about what had happened.

But Steel and Schmidt had realized something important: Transactions that complex can never be truly secret. The agreements involved lawyers, negotiations, and money, and others inevitably found out too—colleagues, agents, family members, and friends. Together the payments formed a legal and financial trail that told the story of the allegations against O'Reilly. The settlements didn't prevent the story; they **were** the story, a tale of cover-up that illuminated the alleged wrongdoing. This was a new way of reporting on sexual harassment.

Within days, advertisers like Mercedes-Benz and Allstate dropped O'Reilly's show. Most important, other women at Fox started lodging complaints about the host's behavior. On April 19, not even three weeks after the publication of the **Times** story, he was fired. Both he and Roger Ailes, the Republican power broker and architect of the network, had lost their jobs, not due to claims of mistreating women—Fox had known about many of those—but rather because of public exposure of those claims. That it had happened a second time made the story more astounding: It was like a momentary reversal in the physics of power.

Times editors quickly took the measure of the moment. Women seemed increasingly fed up. Just as had been the case after Trump's "grab-'em-by-the-pussy" comments, women vented their frustration at the revelations about O'Reilly. Convincing women to go on the record on matters like these was never simple, but this could be a rare window of opportunity for candor.

The O'Reilly story offered a playbook. Almost no one ever came forward completely on their own. But if patterns of bad behavior could be revealed, there might be a way to tell more of these stories. The editors put together a team of reporters to look at a range of industries: Silicon Valley and the tech industry, a utopian field, supposedly unbound by old rules, which nonetheless excluded women. Academia also seemed ripe for investigation because of the power that professors held over graduate students who wanted careers in the same fields. The journalists also planned to focus on low-income workers who had low visibility, overwhelming economic pressure, and less recourse than women higher on the economic ladder.

A few days after O'Reilly was fired, Rebecca Corbett asked Jodi to pursue the answers to two questions. The first was, Were there other powerful men in American life covering up abusive behavior toward women? Jodi had quietly made some calls for advice, and Shaunna Thomas, a feminist activist, had suggested that Jodi look to Hollywood, Rose McGowan's upcoming book, and Harvey Weinstein. But Corbett also gave Jodi a second assignment: to go beyond individual wrongdoers and pin down the elements, the system, that kept sexual harassment so pervasive and hard to address. How common were these settlements, which seemed to pop up in every story, and how had they masked the problem?

When Jodi phoned for advice, Megan still did not know what stories she would pursue once she returned from leave. But they discussed what had motivated women like Jessica Leeds and Rachel Crooks to come forward and how the O'Reilly article had become proof that the **Times** knew how to execute a project this delicate without a hitch. They analyzed what to say in the very first seconds of a phone call with a stranger who might be a victim, and Megan suggested a few new approaches, including one she had used when getting rape victims in Chicago to share their experiences: "I can't change what happened to you in the past, but together we may be able to use your experience to help protect other people."

That sentence clicked like nothing else had. It did not overpromise or suck up. It suggested compelling reasons to risk talking about a painful, messy subject. It was what Jodi had been trying to say to McGowan in that initial email: We mean business.

The pitch was about helping other people. This was always the truest, best reason to talk to a journalist, and one of the only potent answers to "I don't want the attention" or "I don't need the stress."

After that phone call, Jodi had a question for Corbett: How soon would Megan be back from maternity leave?

CHAPTER TWO

HOLLYWOOD SECRETS

Megan's advice was valuable, but as the Weinstein investigation continued in June 2017, the daunting question was how to even get top actresses on the phone. The vocation of these women demanded they keep up appearances, and they lived in a way intended to limit public scrutiny. The typical procedure to reach these stars was to call their publicists. But that was out of the question, as was contacting agents and managers. Those people were paid to build and maintain barriers and were often loyal to power brokers like Weinstein. Besides, the questions were private, too awkward to share with paid intermediaries. Jodi's only hope was to connect directly with actresses. But she wasn't sure she knew a single one: It was a world in which she had virtually no sources or connections.

Jodi clicked through red carpet photos from the recent Cannes Film Festival in France. As usual, there were few shots of men. Nicole Kidman, Jessica Chastain, Salma Hayek, Charlize Theron, and Marion Cotillard posed for the cameras; Uma Thurman stood in a glittering gold skirt at a charity event annually championed by Weinstein, a black-tie party and auction for the American Foundation for AIDS Research, or amfAR. Was it possible that any of them had been Weinstein victims? What did they know about the experiences of others? The women looked flawless, serene, and hopelessly out of reach.

She began seeking private email addresses and phone numbers for women who had appeared in Weinstein's films—especially Ashley Judd, who had given an interview to **Variety** in 2015, in which she had described being sexually harassed by a producer. Some of the searches for contact information practically turned into full investigations themselves: calls to relatives who were listed in public phone records; searches for go-betweens who might make introductions.

The few times Jodi got actresses on the phone, the conversations were mostly short and unproductive. Then came a tip from a well-connected friend: call the actress Judith Godrèche. She's a household name in France and has said privately that Weinstein victimized her. Plus she's outspoken by nature. Jodi emailed Godrèche. No reply. She tried again and got a note back. "I am so sorry, my lawyer doesn't want me to be involved," Godrèche wrote. A frustrating response, but also a clue: involved in **what**?

Contacting Weinstein's former employees was a little more fruitful. They were certainly more reachable, on LinkedIn or at their office numbers or homes. Their responses fell into conflicting categories. Many sounded unsurprised to hear from a reporter but still refused to speak. Others were willing to provide bits and pieces: old suspicions that had lingered across the years; guidance on which Hollywood stars to try to reach.

Some of the former employees gave lectures: Harvey Weinstein's sex life was his private business. The "casting couch," or the practice of actresses submitting to producers and directors in exchange for roles, was as old as Hollywood itself, an unpleasant but permanent part of the business, they said. (As if to underscore their point, there was an actual casting couch sculpture in Los Angeles, near the famous old Chinese theaters where movie premieres were often held.) Several used the same phrase to describe how Weinstein had treated actresses: "Oh, he may have chased her around a couch," they said of this or that woman as if they were describing a pantomime. Those former employees spoke to Jodi as if she were a naïve idealist. Weinstein's treatment of women had been an open secret for years, they said. Jodi would never get the story, and even if she did, no one would care.

On Friday, June 30, Jodi walked into a tiny West Hollywood restaurant to meet with the actress Marisa Tomei. A former Miramax employee had said

Weinstein harassed Tomei, upsetting her so much that she had cried at work. Jodi had tracked down Tomei through a playwright, and now she was sitting at the other end of the restaurant table.

The tip was wrong. Tomei wasn't a Weinstein victim. But she had decades' worth of frustration with the way women were treated in her business. She had headlined films and television shows from **A Different World** (1987) to **My Cousin Vinny** (1992) to **Empire** (2015). She had struggled with seemingly hopeless pay disparities, and repeatedly found herself reduced to an accessory in scenes revolving around male characters. Often, acting just meant reacting to whatever the men were doing, she said.

Tomei shared a theory: Actresses and the public were stuck in a cycle of mutual misperception. From very young ages, girls were taught to admire and model themselves on the fantasy women onscreen. That made many of them want to become actresses themselves. The lucky ones who made it could never really describe the harassment or the punishing physical standards; that would be self-sabotage. So the cycle continued, with the next generation of girls growing up with Hollywood dreams and little understanding that the industry could mistreat them too.

Tomei was giddy at the thought of an exposé. She had almost never discussed her theory, even with other actresses. Sharing her impressions about a business that was all about appearances would make her too vulnerable, she said. For solidarity, she hung on to a clip from a 2013 **Vogue** magazine profile in which Claire Danes discussed what she had learned from Meryl Streep and Jodie Foster. "You have to ask for money because there's always more money and they won't give it to you because you're a girl!" Danes had said.

"Can you imagine me finding this little part of a paragraph in an article that I actually had to cut out in order to feel connected?" Tomei later asked Jodi. "To feel like it isn't just me."

Slowly, Jodi began to reach a few other well-known actresses, through a mutual friend here, an unusually helpful manager there. Some of their email addresses were pseudonyms, often comical ones, and once they were on the phone, they swore Jodi to secrecy. But they were direct. Hollywood was plagued by rampant sexual abuse, most of them said. Daryl Hannah, her voice familiar from years of hit movies but filled with anxiety, said that she had been victimized by Weinstein but felt too fearful to go into any detail. Another actress, an Oscar winner, said she had wanted to see him stopped for years, but hadn't really known how to help, because the fellow actresses who had confided in her about their encounters wanted their privacy protected. This woman had tracked the failed reporting efforts years earlier at the **New Yorker** and the stalled **New York Magazine** article and wondered why every story in the works seemed to disappear.

The conversations with these actresses would not be made public, but they were telling, contradicting the lectures about how Weinstein was a non-story. Tomei and the others had global success, important roles, awards. They were insiders, but on this topic, they felt they had little ability to spur change, and they wanted the **Times** investigation to succeed.

When Jodi reached out to a few other women they had suggested, nothing came of it: Everyone said no. Soon even some of the actresses who had been helpful stopped responding to Jodi's emails and texts.

The same week she met with Tomei, Jodi received a promising email. Lisa Bloom, a celebrity feminist lawyer and the daughter of famed women's rights attorney Gloria Allred, wanted to talk. She had represented women in some of the most important and high-profile male misconduct cases, including the ones against Bill O'Reilly and Bill Cosby. Jodi figured that Bloom had clients with allegations against Weinstein, had caught wind of the **Times** project, and was getting in touch to help.

Jodi forwarded the email to her colleague Emily Steel, one of the reporters who had broken the story about Bill O'Reilly's settlements. Steel was about a decade younger than Jodi, petite, with a high voice, and Jodi had quickly learned to listen to everything she said. As soon as she got the email, Steel called with a warning. Bloom was in business with Weinstein, she said. The information was public. Bloom had posted a gushing tweet a few months before: "BIG ANNOUNCEMENT: My book SUSPICION NATION is being made into a miniseries, produced by Harvey Weinstein and Jay Z!"

Jodi realized the person behind the email wasn't Bloom. Harvey Weinstein knew what the **Times** was working on and he was going on the offensive.

There had been no obligation for Jodi to give Weinstein notice of the investigation—it wasn't even clear that there would be a story yet—and the duty to ask him for an interview or responses would come later. But now that he knew, it would make the reporting even more difficult. Any investigation into serious wrongdoing was a contest with its subject to control information, to get to sources—a race to expose on the reporters' end, a race to hide on the other.

She would have liked a little more running room, but there was nothing to do but to keep reporting. Jodi arranged a call with Bloom and kept it short, saying little.

Nicholas Kristof, the **Times** opinion columnist, made getting in touch with Ashley Judd simple. He had written the foreword for her autobiography. Days after he made an introduction, Jodi was on FaceTime with Judd, who had already figured out the reason for the call. And unlike Tomei, she had a personal story to tell about Weinstein.

In 1996, when Judd was in her late twenties, becoming a star in films including **Heat** and **A Time to Kill,** she had met Weinstein at a Los Angeles event. The producer had asked to get together, and Judd had assumed they would have a business conversation. They planned to meet at the Beverly Hills Hotel—at the Polo Lounge restaurant there, Judd presumed. She suspected nothing. Her father was on the trip, and she had introduced the two older men at the event. "My own dad didn't see it coming," Judd said.

When she arrived at the hotel, she was directed to meet Weinstein in a suite, where he had a bottle of champagne on ice. She took only a few sips. They made small talk, and "I got myself out of there as fast as I could," she remembered, a little suspicious about what he wanted.

Days later, he issued another invitation, this time to a breakfast meeting at the Peninsula Hotel in Beverly Hills. A conversation so early in the morning would surely be safe, Judd reasoned.

She arrived at the hotel exhausted. She had been up all night filming her first big thriller, **Kiss the Girls,** with Morgan Freeman, and had come straight from the set. When the reception staff told her that she would be meeting with the producer in his suite, instead of the restaurant, she was annoyed: She needed sleep and room service would likely take forever to arrive. She figured she would order cereal to save time.

When she arrived at the room, she recalled to Jodi, Weinstein was in a bathrobe, which was not what she expected. He wanted to give her a massage. She refused. He countered by suggesting a shoulder rub. She rejected that too. Next he steered her toward a closet, asking her to help pick out his clothing for the day. Then toward the bathroom. Two decades later, she could still picture the layout of the hotel room, she said.

Weinstein's requests turned even more overtly sexual, she said. She refused each one, but he kept going. "I said no, a lot of ways, a lot of times, and he always came back at me with some slimy ask," she said. His movements were almost like military commands, she told Jodi, with a chop-chop quality, first you go here, and then you go there. Finally, he raised the possibility of her watching him take a shower, as if that was some sort of compromise.

She recalled feeling trapped in the room and fearful of hurting her film prospects. "There's a lot on the line, the cachet that came with Miramax," she said.

She needed an exit strategy, a way of getting away from Weinstein. "I'll make you a deal, Harvey," she recalled saying. "When I win an Academy Award in a Miramax movie, I'll give you a blow job," she said, before exiting.

Judd said she had been in a no-win situation: To rebuff the producer was to risk career consequences.

So she had quickly come up with a joke that wouldn't offend him while finding a way to leave safely.

At the time, Judd mentally classified it as a creepy incident. Soon after, she described what happened to her mother, the singer Naomi Judd; her father; her agent; and later on, other confidantes. Judd had sounded serene during the call, and maybe that was why: She had not suppressed her story, so there was little confessional rawness to her telling.

A few years later, she took a Miramax role, in the film **Frida,** at the request of Salma Hayek, the star who was playing the Mexican artist Frida Kahlo. (Judd was cautious about Weinstein but wanted to help Hayek.) During filming in Mexico, they spent a day off at a resort, relaxing with their costar Valeria Golino. The three women were sitting together at an outdoor table when Weinstein walked by. He warmly greeted the others, and barely acknowledged Judd, she recalled.

After he left, she told the other two women what had happened in the Los Angeles hotel room. That's his thing, they said. He was always making those kinds of requests. He had done similar things to them too.

Judd asked the others why the women weren't banding together to stand up to Weinstein. "I didn't understand how any of us could be so scared of him," Judd said. But **Frida** was Hayek's labor of love, it was being made by Weinstein, and he had the power to halt production at any moment.

During the hour-long call with Judd, the investigation shifted a little. Judd had described a group of actresses who, years earlier, had identified Weinstein's troubling behavior. He was a powerful boss who used the pretext of business meetings to try to pressure women into sexual interactions, she said, and no one did anything about it.

Loneliness had defined Ashley Judd's upbringing. Born in 1968 with the name Ashley Ciminella, her parents had split early. Her mother was then an amateur musician who practiced harmonies at home but worked as a waitress and then a secretary to pay the bills, and Ashley attended thirteen schools in four states before graduating from high school, each time losing friends. She yearned for playmates and company so badly that she invented a cast of fairies to keep her company. By third grade, "I made myself meals like Chef Boyardee pizza from a box and baked my own chocolate-chip cookies from scratch and walked myself to the school bus, even on the first day of school, although I wasn't entirely sure where I was supposed to go," she said in her memoir, **All That Is Bitter and Sweet.** The refrain of her childhood, she wrote, was "Where is everybody?"

Growing up, she was molested several times, she wrote. In grade school, an old man offered her a quarter for a pinball machine if she would sit in his lap. "I was shocked when he suddenly cinched his arms around me, squeezing me and smothering my mouth with his, jabbing his tongue deep into my mouth," she wrote. She told the adults who were supposed to be looking after her, but they didn't believe her. One summer in high school, when she worked as a model in Japan, she was sexually assaulted by her boss and raped by an acquaintance, she said.

But at the University of Kentucky, she found female companionship in a sorority and gender studies courses. The lighted pathways and call boxes on campus struck her as a sign of unfairness, she said later. Why did women have to confine themselves in order to stay safe? Driven by a sense that things could be better, she discovered a taste for activism, leading a student walkout to protest a trustee's use of a racial epithet. She thought of becoming a Christian missionary, and she applied and was accepted to the Peace Corps, which she intended to join after graduation.

But she became an actor instead—she wanted to try it while she was young and could take chances—and then a star. Still, in her free time, she used her celebrity for advocacy work, visiting poor villages, slums, and clinics all over the world to draw attention to AIDS, violence against women, and maternal health and family planning. In 2006, she and Salma Hayek visited HIV clinics and brothels in Guatemala, where they met with prostitutes who explained that they needed money and could earn two dollars per client, ten or twelve times a day. Despite the problems Judd had seen in Hollywood, she kept her two lives, in entertainment and public health causes, separate.

In 2009, at the age of forty-one, she enrolled in a midcareer master's program at Harvard's Kennedy School. (Secretary-General Ban Ki-moon of the United Nations had completed the same program—and so had Bill O'Reilly.) Privately, she was thinking of going into politics. The state of Tennessee had then never had a female governor or U.S. senator.

At Harvard, she felt more at home than she had in show business, and she wasn't sure she would return to acting at all. "I found my people," she said. Her favorite course, called Gender Violence, Law and Social Justice, was taught by a law school professor named Diane Rosenfeld. Judd bonded with the second- and third-year law students, asking to form a study group, baking biscuits for them, and speaking easily in class, but rarely about Hollywood.

In the course, Rosenfeld argued that the legal system had been constructed to protect men more than women. In contrast, she introduced students to research on the egalitarian behavior of bonobo apes, who over the course of evolution have eliminated male sexual coercion in their communities. If a male does get aggressive toward a female bonobo, she lets out a special cry, Rosenfeld explained. The other females come to her aid, descending from the trees and fending off the attacker.

For Judd, the class was a revelation, and, in some

sense, a return. Rosenfeld was taking things Judd had known and seen her whole life—from her childhood, in Hollywood, on the trips to the brothels and clinics abroad—and giving her the intellectual framework and theory to understand them in new ways. "She metabolized everything in my class with her whole being," Rosenfeld said. Judd showed up to everything, the professor noticed: visiting lectures, receptions, a research presentation on GPS monitoring for high-risk domestic violence offenders.

She channeled her thoughts into a final paper that called for women to recognize their common experiences and take on sexual coercion. "I propose a model based on female-female alliances," she wrote on the first page. She wanted women to follow the example of the bonobos, becoming less separate and secretive, joining together to chase away overly aggressive men.

It would be hard to convince women that things could change, she wrote in her research paper, which won a Dean's Scholar Award. "Bias is built into the very structures of our formal institutions, economy, and daily life," she said. But "something is waiting on the other side."

What was needed, she wrote, was a "bold step of trust that breaks isolation."

Still, in June 2017, Judd was not sure if she wanted to accuse Weinstein publicly. She had already tried to call out his behavior once. In 2015, she had given

that account to **Variety** magazine, without naming
Weinstein, Hayek, or Golino, hoping it would spark
something, maybe a surge of others coming together.

Nothing much happened. The ensuing burst of
attention was directed at Judd, not Weinstein, and it
was brief and sensationalized. Judd had to scale back
publicity for a film, **Big Stone Gap,** to avoid getting
too many questions about the incident. To come forward again might repeat that experience.

This was a cautionary tale. Judd's account in
Variety had been gutsy, but it was a lone account
without a perpetrator's name or any supporting information. Impact in journalism came from
specificity—names, dates, proof, and patterns. Jodi
didn't want Judd to decline to participate in what
might be a much stronger story because a weaker one
had gone nowhere.

Judd was also wary because just a few months
before, she had paid a price for speaking out. Over
the years, she'd had a lucrative contract as a spokesperson for Copper Fit, a line of socks, compression
sleeves, and braces. In commercials, she cheerfully
recited lines like: "I love my hardwood floors, but
they can be hard on my feet. That's why I love my
Copper Fit Gripper socks." Her relationship with the
company was amiable, and she sometimes socialized
with the chief executive.

In the weeks before the Women's March in
January 2017, she had sent him a protest poem
about female rage, written by then nineteen-year-old

Nina Donovan of Franklin, Tennessee, which Judd had discovered and planned to read from the main march stage. "I'm a nasty woman," it began. "I'm not as nasty as a man who looks like he bathes in Cheeto dust." The poem wasn't vulgar, but it was confrontational: "We are here to be nasty like bloodstained bedsheets," Ms. Donovan wrote, making the point that menstruation was part of life. Copper Fit raised no objections. But a few weeks after the march, Judd was fired. Customers were complaining about the poem, the company said.

So Judd had reason to be cautious. But on the call, Jodi had used a word she had been waiting to hear: "pattern." An important factor for her, Judd said, would be how many other stories the reporters were able to track down and whether other actresses were going on the record. True to her Harvard paper, she wanted to be one of many women standing up to Weinstein in unison.

The call ended with a plan: Judd was going to reach out to Salma Hayek. For additional advice, Jodi also spoke to Jill Kargman, lately the writer, producer, and star of the television show **Odd Mom Out,** and a contact who had provided guidance in unfamiliar worlds before. Kargman urged Jodi to talk to Jenni Konner, Lena Dunham's producing partner on the television show **Girls.** Konner, in turn, wanted Jodi to speak to Dunham too. Jodi hesitated. From the outside, Dunham seemed like the opposite of a secret keeper. She tweeted constantly and turned even intimate parts of her life into material.

The calls were worth the gamble. Konner and Dunham had heard stories about Weinstein's alleged predatory behavior and had wanted to expose him in **Lenny Letter,** their online newsletter, but they didn't have the investigative or legal resources. Dunham, who had served as a surrogate for Hillary Clinton during the 2016 campaign, told Jodi she had told Clinton's aides to stop relying on Weinstein as a fundraiser, but her warnings went nowhere. (Later, Tina Brown, the magazine editor who herself had briefly partnered with Weinstein in the late '90s on **Talk** magazine, told Jodi she had delivered a similar warning to the 2008 Clinton campaign. After the revelations became public, Clinton and her team expressed shock and denied the extent of Dunham's warning.)

Konner and Dunham became a two-woman celebrity switchboard, sending Jodi some of the direct contact information she needed, working quickly and discreetly. Another entertainment executive with a feminist bent did the same.

The response rate from the actresses was still low. But by the end of June, Konner had news: Gwyneth Paltrow wanted to talk.

At the outset, Paltrow had barely been on Jodi's list of people to contact. She had been Weinstein's golden girl, one of his top stars, and twenty years later, the memories of her acting career were still tied to him. They had been photographed together many times, a laughing father-daughter pair. In 1999, when Paltrow won the Oscar for Best Actress for her role in **Shakespeare in Love,** Weinstein stood next to her, radiating pride: He had made the movie, molded the star. Back then, Paltrow's nickname had been First Lady of Miramax. She seemed unlikely to help the **Times.** She was hardly a rebel like McGowan or an activist like Judd. She had become a health-and-beauty entrepreneur, and for some people, a love-to-hate figure.

But once their phone call was scheduled, for the final weekend of June 2017, Paltrow cut a different figure: She was a dead-center source who might know more than anyone yet. On the telephone, Paltrow was polite and sounded a little jittery. After the ritual reassurances—yes, this was off the record; yes, Jodi understood the delicacy of the situation—Paltrow shared the unknown side of the story of her relationship with Weinstein.

They had met by an elevator at the Toronto Film Festival in 1994 or '95, when she was around twenty-two, Paltrow recalled. At that point, she barely had a career. Her parents, the actress Blythe Danner and Bruce Paltrow, a director and producer, were successful, and she had gotten encouraging reviews in a film called **Flesh and Bone,** but she was still auditioning for more parts.

Right there at the elevator, Weinstein gave her his vote of confidence. I saw you in that movie; you have to come work for us, she remembered him saying. You're really talented. "I just remember feeling legitimized by his opinion," she said.

Before too long, he offered her two films. If she would do a comedy called **The Pallbearer,** Weinstein said, she could also have the lead in his upcoming adaptation of Jane Austen's **Emma**—a dream job, a star-making role.

Paltrow joined the downtown Miramax fold, which at that time struck her as warm and creative. "I felt like I was home," she said. She was dating Brad Pitt, who was far more famous than she at the time, and flying between New York and Los Angeles. On one of those trips, before shooting started for **Emma,** she got a fax from her representatives at Creative Artists Agency, telling her to meet Weinstein at the Peninsula Hotel in Beverly Hills.

That was the same hotel as in Judd's story. What Paltrow said next also felt familiar. The meeting seemed routine, held in a suite for privacy. "I bounced up there, I'm sort of like a golden retriever, all happy to see Harvey," she said. They talked business. But Weinstein closed by placing his hands on her and asking to go into the bedroom and exchange massages. Paltrow could barely process what was happening, she said. She had thought of Weinstein as an uncle. The thought that he was interested in her sexually shocked her and made her feel queasy.

He asked a second time to move into the bedroom, she said.

She excused herself, but "not so he would feel he had done something wrong," she said. As soon as she left, she told Brad Pitt what had happened, then a few friends, family members, and her agent.

The next part of Paltrow's story diverged from Judd's and made it potentially more consequential. Weeks later, when Paltrow and Pitt attended the same theater premiere as Weinstein, Pitt confronted the producer and told him to keep his hands to himself. At the time, Paltrow felt relieved: Her boyfriend was her protector.

But when she returned to New York, Weinstein called and threatened her, berating her for telling Pitt what had happened. "He said some version of I'm going to ruin your career," she said. She remembered standing in her old apartment on Prince Street in SoHo, fearful she would lose the two roles, especially the starring one in **Emma.** "I was nothing, I was a kid, I was signed up. I was petrified, I thought he was going to fire me," she said.

She tried to put the relationship back on professional footing, explaining to Weinstein that telling her boyfriend had been natural, but that she wanted to put the episode behind them and move forward. "I always wanted peace, I never wanted any problem," she said. For a time, their relationship was restored. "In this funny way, I was like, well, that's behind us," she said. The more successful her partnership with Weinstein became, the less she felt she could say about the ugly episode at the start of their collaboration. "I had this incredible career there, so I could never in a way traverse back over what happened," she said. "I was expected to keep the secret."

The ethos of Hollywood, she said, was to swallow complaints and to put up with exactly that kind of behavior. She didn't think about the encounter as part of something larger or more systemic. During her years with Miramax, she heard the occasional disturbing rumor about Weinstein, but never with specifics attached. Weinstein was abusive in other ways that made the moment in the bedroom seem mild in comparison. He threw things. His tirades were beyond anything Paltrow or others had seen from a grown man. The Miramax employees she knew lived in fear of his volatility. "It's the H-bomb, the H-bomb is coming," they would warn before he approached.

After two Miramax movies starring Paltrow tanked—**Bounce** in 2000 and **View from the Top** in 2003—Weinstein's treatment of her changed, she said. "I wasn't the golden girl with the Midas touch," she said. "My worth had diminished in his eyes." By the time Paltrow was pregnant with her first child, she quietly distanced herself from the producer.

That remained the case until 2016, when Miriam Weinstein, the producer's mother and a beloved figure at Miramax, passed away, and Paltrow wrote Weinstein a brief condolence email. To her shock, he read it aloud at the funeral and called her soon afterward—to thank her, Paltrow figured.

But after the niceties, he began to pressure her again. **New York** magazine was working on an exposé of his treatment of women. They have nothing, Weinstein told Paltrow. He wanted her to promise that she wouldn't talk about the incident at the Peninsula all those years before. "I just really want to protect the people who did say yes," he said, meaning women who had succumbed to his overtures. Paltrow declined the magazine's interview request, but she avoided saying whether she would ever speak.

The story needed to come out, she said to Jodi. For a long time, she had assumed she would never disclose what had happened. But twenty years later, everything looked different, and that's why she was on the phone now.

Paltrow made it clear that she was a long way from going on the record. She was not having a good public relations moment, to put it mildly. At the time, her e-commerce business and lifestyle brand, Goop, was selling a sixty-six-dollar jade egg meant to be inserted into the vagina to "help cultivate sexual energy, clear chi pathways in the body, intensify femininity, and invigorate our life force," as the site put it. The eggs had generated months of derisive laughter and accusations that Paltrow was blithely selling products with dubious or no health benefits. "Organically sourced, fair trade urine pH sticks coming soon to GOOP for seventy-seven dollars I presume?" wrote

Dr. Jen Gunter, an ob-gyn who made cutting critiques of the product and other practices Goop had championed.

On Instagram, Paltrow looked as untroubled as ever. Privately, she was feeling crushed and unsure if she could handle any more controversy. She was certain that any story involving her, Weinstein, and sex was likely to be sensationalized, turned into the trashy celebrity scandal of the week. "I didn't know if I was going to be dragged through the mud," she said. "That's usually what happens to women if you look, historically." More than a hundred people were working for her, paying mortgages and raising children, and wading into more controversy could hurt them too. "I can't wreck the business," as she put it.

But Paltrow decided that she would use her Hollywood network to help Jodi identify and enlist other Weinstein victims so the women could share the burden of speaking up together. (Jodi couldn't mention Judd to her or vice versa.) Paltrow listed a half dozen other famous names she wanted to call, asking for pointers on the protocols of investigative journalism. Jodi suggested others. Paltrow was on vacation with her children in Europe, and her social media feeds showed wine glasses, a picnic, and an Italian lake. Privately, she also was texting old costars and acquaintances for so-and-so's contact information, asking other women if they would speak.

On July 5, Megan returned to the **Times,** undecided about what to cover. On that first day, Rebecca Corbett spelled out Megan's options. The first was to return to Donald Trump. In the final months of her pregnancy, Megan had started scrutinizing Trump's company and ties to Russia, turning up his pursuit of a Trump Tower Moscow during the presidential race and other questionable dealings. The second was to join the investigation of Harvey Weinstein. Jodi was still eager for Megan to join her. Was she interested?

Megan took a day to deliberate, seeking the advice of a few trusted colleagues. Those who covered Trump were unequivocal: He was the story of a lifetime. Much more important than a sleazy Hollywood producer accused of preying on young actresses. Passing up the chance to report on the president would be a huge mistake. But Megan wasn't so sure; she had watched hard-hitting articles about Trump pile up without much impact.

However, the Weinstein investigation was a question mark. The McGowan accusation was grave, but some of the material Jodi had gathered didn't seem that awful compared to the sex crimes Megan had reported in Chicago. How much demonstrable harm was really involved in the massage stories? She had a hard time conceiving of famous actresses as a category of victims. A prime mission of journalism was to give voice to the voiceless, to those who were often ignored. Movie stars, with their fame and fortune, were far from that.

Did the casting couch even meet the legal definition of sexual harassment? The women were not technically employees of Weinstein, and for some of them, there were no specific roles on the line. How much could this investigation really prove?

But, Jodi insisted, if the accounts were accurate, Weinstein personified the way powerful men could abuse their status to establish dominance over women. When he had invited these women to meetings, they had responded because they wanted to work, because they had ambition, creativity, and hopes and dreams. In return, he put them in no-win positions: Submit to sexual demands or risk repercussions. That was sexual harassment, whether or not it met the legal definition.

In perhaps the most famous harassment allegation of all time, Anita Hill had accused Clarence Thomas of asking her out on dates and making pornographic comments at work. While the status of a future Supreme Court justice and a Hollywood producer were different, the claims against Weinstein also appeared to have a predatory edge. And that his accusers were famous women was part of the point: It proved this was a universal problem.

Megan pulled up a seat at Jodi's cubicle and got to work.

Now both reporters were reaching out to some of the most prominent women in the world. Angelina

Jolie had a Weinstein story, they heard from a former Miramax employee. Jodi cadged her email address from the helpful Hollywood executive, sent the star a carefully worded note, spoke to an adviser, and waited to see if she might participate. They also wrote to Uma Thurman: She did not reply, the reporters discovered later, because someone had told her they were not trustworthy. Despite repeated notes, Salma Hayek never responded either.

Ambra Battilana Gutierrez, an Italian model who had allegedly been groped by Weinstein during a meeting at his office in 2015—the incident investigated by the NYPD—appeared to have been the only woman who had reported the producer to law enforcement. In the end, the district attorney's office had declined to prosecute Weinstein, but working with undercover detectives, Battilana had apparently recorded the producer discussing what had happened.

Megan wasn't hearing back from the model, and the New York Police Department was refusing to provide her with a copy of the incident report under a long-standing policy that prohibited the release of such records. So she called around to attorneys and others who might have knowledge of the case. While reporting on DNA evidence in Chicago, Megan had interviewed Linda Fairstein, renowned in the field of sex crimes prosecution. Now Megan reached out to Fairstein again, hoping she might have valuable insight into the same sex crimes division where she had once worked, the one that had declined to press charges. But as soon as she heard the reason for the call, Fairstein's tone turned cool. Ambra Battilana Gutierrez's allegations had been unfounded, she insisted. There was no criminal conduct there. And there wasn't anything irregular about how the case was handled. "I don't think there's a road to go down," she told Megan.

In mid-July, the reporters met in person for the first time with Rose McGowan—over dinner at Jodi's apartment, for privacy. McGowan was anything but relaxed. Her eyes darted around the room. She had no interest in small talk. But she gamely answered question after question, especially about the aftermath of the hotel room encounter and who else might remember it or provide evidence. Jodi and Megan asked her to try to obtain a copy of her settlement agreement, explaining that one of the law firms must have retained a copy.

After the interview with McGowan, the reporters mentioned one particularly confusing question to Matt Purdy, a top editor at the paper who had overseen the O'Reilly story, pulled together the broader sexual harassment team and was keeping a close eye on the investigation. Beyond McGowan, some secondary sources were also suggesting that Weinstein had repeatedly committed criminal offenses: assault, rape. Should the reporters concentrate on finding those claims, prioritizing the most serious kinds of potential violations? Not necessarily, Purdy said: Concentrate first on what you can prove, even if what you can prove are lesser offenses. Get the women's allegations of sexual harassment on the record, the documents, and especially the settlements paid to victims. No one had ever nailed the Weinstein story, so the most important thing was to do it cleanly. Purdy wasn't ignoring the possibility of more severe transgressions; he was saying that if the reporters could break the story, everything was likely to tumble out.

On Saturday, July 15, Jodi checked her phone to find a series of panicked text messages and missed calls from Paltrow. Harvey Weinstein was standing in the living room of Paltrow's Hamptons home. She was hiding in her upstairs bathroom to avoid him.

His timing was the surprise, not his presence. Paltrow had heard from him a week or two before. He had caught wind of a party she was throwing, for potential investors in a musical she was backing, and he asked to come. She felt that he was clearly sending a message—I'm watching you. Paltrow had asked Jodi what to do.

Jodi had not wanted to get in the middle of the action. But they had talked through options. Paltrow could tell him not to come, but that might hint she was talking to a reporter. Maybe it was better to

include him. On the other hand, what if he confronted her and demanded an answer about whether
she was speaking to the **Times**?

Paltrow had decided it was best to say yes and to
hope he got lost in the crowd. But he had shown up
early, probably trying to speak to her alone, throwing Paltrow off balance. Jodi was anxious too, especially when she saw the accumulation of texts
from Paltrow.

From many miles away, Jodi willed Paltrow to
stay the course. After the party, Paltrow called: The
party had unfolded without incident. She had kept
her assistant close. She sounded undeterred—maybe
even a little fascinated by what was unfolding.

On the first Friday in August, Jodi and Megan
met Paltrow for the first time at her home in the
Hamptons. The hope was to encourage her to go on
the record. On a back deck, surrounded by bench
swings and lush hedges, the interview began. In person, Paltrow was earthy and funny. She asked Megan
empathetic questions about new motherhood before retelling her Weinstein story, and she nodded
gamely when Megan carefully pushed for elabora-
tion and told her that the reporters would seek to
contact Brad Pitt for confirmation of her account.
That was standard procedure, Megan told the star:
To corroborate the accounts of alleged victims, they
would reach out to people they had told at the time,

checking to make sure they remembered the stories the same way.

Asking Paltrow to go on the record was delicate. She was still dealing with the furor over the jade egg. Jodi and Megan understood the criticism but didn't want it to prevent Paltrow from participating in what might be a more consequential story. Also, for all of Paltrow's outreach, she had not managed to convince other actresses to speak about Weinstein problems. One declined because she was friendly with the producer's wife. Others hadn't gotten back to Paltrow.

In the middle of the interview, Paltrow picked up a call from a famous friend, walked out onto the lawn to ask if she had ever been victimized by Weinstein, then returned to explain that the woman had said nothing ever happened. Paltrow summarized her own thinking: She wanted to go on the record, but she didn't want the story to be about her. The more women who spoke in the article, the better. "I want to make sure that I'm not in any way at the focal point," she said.

In the car on the way back from the Hamptons, Jodi and Megan were encouraged. Paltrow hadn't said yes, but they had connected in person. Then the reporters realized that they might be able to catch someone who had not answered their inquiries: a former Miramax executive who lived nearby. So they took a detour and pulled up to the woman's summer cottage. She came to the door and greeted them with a smile. But as soon as she understood why they were there, she slammed the door in their faces, leaving them alone on the front porch.

Rebecca Corbett immediately wanted to hear every detail about the Hamptons trip. As an editor, she fully inhabited stories, worrying them forward, living through her reporters while also maintaining a critical eye. Weinstein, who liked to boast of his coziness with media power players, had likely never heard of Corbett. She was sixtysomething, skeptical, scrupulous, and allergic to flashiness or exaggeration, the cohead of the **Times** investigation department but so low profile that she barely surfaced in Google search results. Her ambition was journalistic, not personal.

But she was revered in newspaper circles because of one quality she did share with Weinstein: She had exerted outsized influence by championing other people's work. At the **Baltimore Sun,** she had mentored a twenty-two-year-old reporter named David Simon, pushed him to stop writing short news items about rowhouse fires and murders and pursue more ambitious ones about the sociology of crime and class, and edited him until the day he left the **Sun** to create shows like **The Wire.** (In the final season, the character of the city editor, one of the show's few heroes, was a man, but he was based in part on Corbett.) A few years after September 11, 2001, when two **Times** reporters discovered that the National Security Agency was secretly spying on American citizens without warrants, Corbett kept the investigation alive despite internal debate and intense pressure from the White House not to publish, producing one of the biggest scoops of the Bush years.

Like Jodi and Megan, she had come of age in male-dominated newsrooms, raising a daughter in the middle of story sprints. When she was appointed to the **Times** masthead in 2013, it became 50 percent female for the first time, but the milestone went mostly unremarked. Later, people would say that two women had broken the Weinstein story, but it had really been three.

As Corbett tracked the growing body of hotel room stories, she had one chief concern. "What is your strategy for getting these women on the record?" she asked every few days. Jodi and Megan had a sort-of answer: If we find enough of them, we can urge everyone to go public at once, for safety in numbers.

That was too risky an approach for Corbett. The sources were extremely reluctant, for understandable reasons. There was something inherently unfair in this kind of reporting: Why was it their burden to publicly tell uncomfortable stories when they had never done anything wrong? Corbett was worried that Jodi and Megan could end up with a shocking pile of off-the-record hotel room stories but no article. Even if the reporters did manage to persuade one or two women, that could lead to the old "he said, she said" problem.

The journalists were realizing the Weinstein story would have to be broken with evidence: on the record accounts, ideally, but also the overwhelming force of written, legal, and financial proof.

CHAPTER THREE

HOW TO SILENCE A VICTIM

In mid-July, with Jodi focused on Hollywood, Megan turned to a basic investigative question: Were there any public records of abusive behavior by Weinstein?

After all, there were laws to protect victims of sexual harassment, and at least in theory, government agencies enforcing them. If Weinstein had been a serial harasser, some of his victims might have filed complaints with the federal Equal Employment Opportunity Commission (EEOC) or the corresponding state agencies in New York and Los Angeles, the cities where Weinstein had run his companies.

The federal and New York agencies had nothing. But Grace Ashford, a savvy young researcher on her first month at the **Times,** obtained a report from California's Department of Fair Employment and Housing, which showed several workplace complaints for Miramax. The information was shrouded in the ultraobscure language of state bureaucracy: addresses, dates, and numerical codes denoting the nature of the allegation and how it was resolved, but nothing about who the people were or what had happened to them.

On September 12, 2001, the agency had received a complaint of sexual harassment against Miramax. Strangely, it had been closed the same day.

The report noted "complainant elected court action," which normally meant the agency had signed off on the merits of the complaint and steered it into the civil legal system. But there was nothing further, nor was there any record of a court case in California's docket. How could a complaint filed with the government disappear within hours?

Megan kept calling the agency to ask, but it was like ringing a house where no one was home. When she finally reached someone by email, the government official told her the complaint against Miramax and any other related records had been destroyed under an agency policy that prevented the retention of documents after three years. Another policy prohibited the official from providing the name of the person who had filed the allegation.

This was maddening. After some additional prodding, Megan secured the name of the government investigator who had been assigned the case at the time that it was filed. The woman was retired. No one at the agency knew where she lived. Through social media sites and address searches, Megan found her living east of Los Angeles and finally got her on the phone.

The interview was brief. The former investigator had reviewed hundreds of complaints during her time with the California agency. She didn't recall this one.

"What's Miramax?" she asked.

On the afternoon of July 14, the **Times** team that had convened to work on harassment stories after the O'Reilly scoop—including Rebecca Corbett, Matt Purdy, Emily Steel, and others—filed into the empty Page One conference room for an update. The room had no ornamentation, no pictures of presidents or historic events. But twice a day, top editors gathered to debate which stories would lead the print and digital editions of the paper. Reporters almost never attended those meetings, so being there lent this session a heightened quality.

The new harassment stories were promising. Two weeks before, Katie Benner, who covered Silicon Valley, had published a detailed exposé of harassment in the tech industry, about female entrepreneurs who had sought investment from male venture capitalists and instead were subjected to inappropriate texts, gropes, and come-ons ("I was getting confused figuring out whether to hire you or hit on you"). For a long time, women in the male-dominated industry had mostly stayed silent about the problem, viewing discussion as risky and taboo.

Now more of them were speaking out together. Earlier that year, Uber had been turned upside down when Susan Fowler, a former engineer for the company, had written a blog post describing the harassment and retaliation she had experienced there. In Benner's article, more than two dozen women had come forward. Many had gone on the record or named the investors. In photographic portraits, which had run with the story, the women looked composed and strong: innovators starting companies and expecting fair treatment.

The story had impact. One of the men and one of the firms had apologized. The women were praised by peers and readers for sharing their experiences. Benner's in-box swelled with new accounts and tips.

That meant the success of the O'Reilly story was no longer a one-off. Megan and Jodi had texted Benner's article, and the supportive reactions, to their Weinstein sources, as if to say yes, this is tricky, but our team knows how to do it.

The meeting opened with quick updates: Jodi and Megan were making slow but real progress on Weinstein. Emily Steel was hearing alarming accounts of violations at **Vice.** Catrin Einhorn was immersed in conversations with restaurant, retail, hotel, and construction workers. Susan Chira was focusing on formerly male blue-collar workplaces, like shipyards and coal mines.

In each industry, harassment had its own particular sociology. In restaurants, liquor was omnipresent at the workplace, eroding judgment and loosening inhibitions, and managers were often loath to confront customers who got out of line. Silicon Valley was filled with young men who got rich overnight and felt accountable to no one. In shipyards, construction sites, and other traditionally male workplaces, men sometimes tried to drive out women by putting them in physical danger. Chira had heard of one woman who had been left deep in a mine without any communication device, and another had been stranded atop a wind turbine.

The journalists had come to the project knowing the basics about sexual harassment. Since the 1960s, a body of law had emerged to protect people from unwanted advances in the workplace. Sexual harassment was not a criminal offense, unless it involved rape or assault, but it was a violation of federal civil rights laws. Everyone in the room knew the stories of Clarence Thomas and Bill Clinton. But now as the reporters combined what they were learning across industries, they were coming to a deeper realization: Some of the weapons intended to fight sexual harassment were actually enabling it.

Emily Steel had the first lead, from her work on Fox and O'Reilly. It was common knowledge that many sexual harassment cases settled out of court, and she and Michael S. Schmidt had already revealed that O'Reilly and Fox had relied on settlements that imposed confidentiality clauses—essentially paying victims to keep quiet. But the specific terms of the agreements were crying out for further investigation.

From what Steel was learning, the language of the deals made them look less like aboveboard legal transactions and more like cover-ups. The agreements included one restrictive clause after another. The women were obliged to turn over all their evidence—audio recordings, diaries, emails, backup files, any other shred of proof—to O'Reilly and his lawyers. They and in one case their attorneys were prohibited from helping any other women who might have similar claims against the host. If they received subpoenas compelling them to talk, they were required to notify O'Reilly and his team, who could fight their being called to testify.

The lawyer for one of the women agreed to switch sides, to "provide legal advice to O'Reilly regarding sexual harassment matters," according to the language of the agreement. Another of the alleged victims promised never to make disparaging statements about O'Reilly or Fox News, "written or oral, direct or indirect," and not to respond—ever—to any journalists who might contact her about the matter. As part of the deal, she confirmed that she had not filed a complaint with any of the government agencies responsible for fighting sexual harassment, including the EEOC.

In return, one alleged victim received about $9 million, and another got $3.25 million. If either woman violated any of these clauses, she could lose the money. Whatever O'Reilly had or hadn't done to the women was thus dropped down a deep well, never to be recovered. Cash for silence; that was the deal.

That summer, as Steel continued to look into O'Reilly, she also had broader questions: Were these clauses even legal? Were women across the country signing documents like these every day, often unbeknownst to almost anyone? And were sexual harassment lawyers actually tackling the problem they purported to fight or pumping out settlements for profit?

Steel had suggested to editors that the paper delve into those questions, so this was part of the assignment Corbett had given Jodi. In between trying to reach movie stars, she had been calling attorneys and legal experts across the country, from small town employment lawyers to scholars, and now she shared her findings.

The kinds of clauses that Steel described were not aberrations, the lawyers said. This was standard practice for dealing with sexual harassment, and often one of the only ways of dealing with it at all.

Women signed these agreements for good reason, the attorneys had emphasized. They needed the money, craved privacy, didn't see better options, or just wanted to move on. They could avoid being branded tattletales, liars, flirts, or habitual litigators. This was a way to get paid and get on with their lives. The alternative, taking this kind of lawsuit to court, was punishing. Federal sexual harassment laws were weak, leaving out vast categories of people—freelancers, employees at workplaces with fewer than fifteen employees. The federal statute of limitations for filing a complaint could be as short as 180 days, and federal damages were capped at $300,000—not necessarily enough to cover lost earnings or attract a good lawyer. No wonder many viewed settlements as surer propositions.

The deals worked out for the lawyers too, especially financially. They generally worked on contingency, getting paid only if the client did, taking at least one-third of the client's award as a fee. Losing in court could mean getting nothing. So sexual harassment settlements had swelled into a cottage industry. Some attorneys fought back against egregious provisions, but others rubber-stamped them or capitulated in order to win bigger awards.

Even the EEOC, the government agency that was supposed to enforce sexual harassment laws, often kept its settlements confidential. The agency had very little enforcement authority, and, under its founding mandate, was required to settle whenever possible, often disclosing little. "We know internally who the companies are that have the most charges," Chai Feldblum, then the commissioner of the EEOC, had told Jodi. But the agency was prohibited from making that information public. Before taking a job, a woman could not check with the EEOC to see what kind of record the prospective employer had on harassment. No wonder Megan hadn't gotten anywhere with the old Miramax complaints to the California agency. Such agencies would gather crucial information with taxpayer dollars and then, for the most part, were required to lock it away where almost no one could see it.

Jodi cut to the point: The United States had a system for muting sexual harassment claims, which often enabled the harassers instead of stopping them. Women routinely signed away the right to talk about their own experiences. Harassers often continued onward, finding fresh ground on which to commit the same offenses. The settlements and confidentiality agreements were almost never examined in law school classrooms or open court. This was why the public had never really understood that this was happening. Even those in the room with long histories of covering gender issues had never fully registered what was going on.

Leaving the meeting, Jodi and Megan realized how much needed to be investigated. Would the public be interested in these obscure legal instruments or their ramifications? There was some reason to be optimistic: After the publication of Benner's story, Benner heard from activists and legislators in California who wanted to change the state's rules on the legality of secret settlements for sexual abuse.

But if Harvey Weinstein had entered into settlements with women besides Rose McGowan, and if those claims had been hushed up by lawyers, could those women even be found?

In 2005, the Weinstein brothers had relinquished control of Miramax, their first movie company. But many of its former employees remained connected, bound by having together worked through terrible and wonderful moments, sometimes almost simultaneously. For many, working there had been an education, a crucible, a privilege, and a trauma. You could influence the world's moviegoing taste, negotiate a deal on a yacht in Cannes, and lose every shred of your dignity to the boss's lashings all in the same day. When former Miramaxers held informal reunions in New York and Los Angeles, they jokingly referred to the gatherings as "Mir-anon" meetings, as if they were in permanent recovery together.

Every day that July, Megan and Jodi continued to work that old Mir-anon circuit, one member passing them to the next. The former employees who supposedly knew the most did not return calls; many of the people rumored to have assisted the most with Weinstein's abuses had no interest in seeing their complicity in his misdeeds exposed. But the reporters asked other ex-employees for tips: Had anyone heard anything over the years about women accepting settlements?

On the last weekend of July, two weeks after the

all-hands-on-deck meeting in the Page One conference room, Megan drove north, away from New
York City, through the winding roads of a lush suburb. She was pursuing the mystery of an assistant in
Miramax's early years who had abruptly quit.

Megan knew her name. Starting at Miramax, she
had impressed others as smart and serious and been
quickly promoted. But then, in 1990, she had disappeared, leaving behind only running shoes tucked
neatly under her desk. In phone interviews, several
former Miramax employees had recalled hearing
that Weinstein had done something to her. But no
one knew the details.

The most promising clue came from Kathy
DeClesis, who had served as an assistant to Bob
Weinstein at the time. She said a lawyer for the
woman's father had sent a letter to the office shortly
after her disappearance. The specific language es-
caped her, but DeClesis had the impression that the
letter had threatened legal action. Her recollection
was more than Megan and Jodi had gotten from anyone else. What had the young woman complained
about, how had the matter been resolved, and what
had happened to her?

The former assistant had left little online trace of
who she was or where she had been living the past
twenty-seven years. She wasn't on LinkedIn. She
wasn't on Facebook. But Ashford, the researcher at
the **Times,** eventually found her on a far-flung corner

of the internet, listed in an employee directory in another city. The photo showed no hint of Hollywood or celebrity. Just a regular fortysomething-year-old woman with shoulder-length hair and a face free of makeup.

Contacting the former assistant was even harder than identifying her had been. Megan left several messages with the front desk of the woman's workplace, explaining that she was a reporter from the **Times** wanting to speak with her, but never heard back. Even talking to the receptionists was tricky, because she wanted to avoid making the woman's colleagues aware of the sensitive nature of her questions. Megan briefly considered flying to the city where she lived but didn't want to scare off the woman.

But there had also been a local address for her mother, in that New York suburb. Megan decided to drive there and explain in person why she wanted to learn about the former assistant's experience. If the mother wasn't home, Megan would leave a handwritten letter with her explanation taped to the door. She arrived at the address to find a grand modern house.

Megan had been knocking on doors uninvited as part of her reporting for more than a decade, but it never got easier. It was often necessary in order to get reluctant sources to talk. Over the years plenty of people had welcomed her into their homes, persuaded by the initiative Megan had shown tracking them down. But she had also encountered people who felt violated by her mere presence. As she rapped on the large wooden door, Megan couldn't help but feel like she was intruding into someone's private life.

The person who appeared in the entrance was not the mother but the woman from the picture on the website. Megan was face-to-face with the former assistant.

A young girl was standing by the woman's side, peering out the doorway. Megan introduced herself as a reporter with the **Times,** and a flash of recognition—or perhaps fear—crossed the woman's face. "I can't believe you found me," she said. She and her daughters were back in New York for summer vacation, she explained. Megan had caught them in the middle of a visit with family friends. Reluctant to say too much in front of the other people in the house, Megan asked if the woman would be willing to join her on the front steps for a minute. She agreed.

As they sat side by side, Megan explained that she and Jodi were hard at work on an investigation of Harvey Weinstein. Their reporting had turned up what appeared to be a pattern of predatory behavior. They had reason to believe that Weinstein may have hurt her when she worked at Miramax. Megan wouldn't have gone to such trouble to find her if it wasn't important.

As she spoke, the corners of the woman's mouth turned up ever so slightly. It wasn't a smile, but it was some hint of recognition. "I've been waiting for this knock on my door for twenty-seven years," she said. "All I can say is that I had a business dispute with Miramax, the dispute was resolved amicably, and we've agreed not to discuss it."

Megan paused, turning over the lines in her head. Technically, the woman was saying nothing. But there was meaning to her nondisclosure, as if she were working in the blank spaces between the words. She seemed like she might be saying: **Something bad did in fact happen to me years ago, but I must feed you this carefully crafted line.**

This was exactly how a woman who had signed a settlement would answer. There are times in journalism when the right thing to do is turn and walk away, to leave a source alone. But this was not one of them. Megan was determined to keep the woman talking, if only about unrelated things. How old were her daughters? Megan's own daughter was only four months old. The woman was close in age to Megan, with so many similar reference points. The conversation was easy.

After another half hour of chatting, Megan made her pitch. She asked the former assistant to consider contributing to the **Times** investigation. Megan appreciated how risky it was to break a settlement, but, she said, there were ways to bring settlements to light while protecting sources. Her colleagues had done it with payoffs made by Bill O'Reilly. The woman nodded along. She didn't say no. She didn't say yes. Instead she agreed to give Megan something always coveted by journalists: her cell phone number.

But on her drive back to Brooklyn, Megan got a phone call that punctured her optimism. The woman said she had just spoken to her lawyer. He had instructed her not to talk to the **Times.** Megan maintained a positive tone even as her heart sank. She told the woman that her attorney's advice was predictable, but she didn't have to make a final decision yet. All Megan asked was that they stay in touch and continue to discuss options. Reluctantly, the woman agreed.

As she drove, Megan's suspicions were growing. The rumors about the producer had involved actresses, but now she and Jodi were glimpsing an entirely new category of possible victims: employees of Weinstein's companies. The woman who had stood next to Megan in the kitchen—perhaps the Patient Zero of the Weinstein investigation—wasn't famous at all. And she had been young and vulnerable when she worked at Miramax. Could the producer have abused women more systemically than she or Jodi had ever contemplated? How many women had he victimized since, and would things have been different if the former assistant had been able to speak freely?

On that final weekend of July, Megan still didn't know exactly what had happened to the woman twenty-seven years earlier. But she wanted desperately to keep their conversation going, and so two days after the house visit, she sent the former assistant a text:

I know I must have thrown you a
curveball into your trip home. But
please know it's only because this
story is so important. There's a real
opportunity to make a difference.
My hope is that we can continue to
be in touch—that I can keep you
abreast of what's happening on
our end. I suspect you've had some
more conversations about this—
with family and perhaps others.
Seems to me the most important
conversation of all is the one you
have with yourself.

She also sent a link to the **New York Times** article on O'Reilly's history of settlements. Even as she typed, Megan suspected she might never hear from the woman again.

A few nights later, Megan took another drive, to the home of John Schmidt, a former Miramax executive who had served as the company's chief financial officer in 1990, the year the young assistant had disappeared. Megan figured that Schmidt, who still worked in the film business, would be aware of any settlement the woman might have signed, but he had been dodging her phone calls. So she was staking out his house in Riverdale, a leafy Bronx neighborhood, slouching down every time the local private security patrol drove by, waiting for the living room lights to flick on to indicate that someone was inside. Soon she was face-to-face with Schmidt, apologizing for showing up unannounced at dinnertime, feeling awkward because his wife was also there, listening to her every word.

These settlements were insidious, making victims feel they couldn't speak, potentially saddling them with substantial financial damages if they did, Megan explained to Schmidt. If other people were aware of the payoffs, they were uniquely positioned to provide crucial help. Megan wasn't asking Schmidt to go on the record. She just wanted his perspective on what might have happened all those years ago.

But Schmidt wasn't prepared to speak with her, at least not yet. He told Megan he needed to think about it and escorted her to the door. The reporter understood that people often needed time to come around, but it was frustrating. Some former Weinstein employees appeared aware of problems, and they still wouldn't talk.

One Friday evening that same July, Jodi spoke on the phone with a Hollywood executive named Matt Brodlie who had worked at Miramax many years ago. He listened with unusual care, and she got the feeling that he was assessing her. Shortly afterward, he called her back to give a name and number. He had a close friend from Miramax who had been holding something inside for years, he said. She was both wary and bursting to talk. Her name was Amy Israel and she was also a respected entertainment executive.

"I want to have a long career, I don't want to be marked by this," Israel said as soon as she got on the phone. "I do not want to be quoted, period, end of story." But a memory had troubled her for almost twenty years and she wanted to share it.

In the autumn of 1998, she had attended the Venice Film Festival with Weinstein, scouting for new films to buy. During a meeting in Weinstein's hotel suite, she saw that something appeared visibly wrong with two female assistants, Zelda Perkins, a fixture of the London office, and Rowena Chiu, a more recent hire.

"The two of them were sitting there trembling," Israel recalled. "They were literally vibrating with fear." Weinstein seemed fine, talking about films as usual. Something had just happened involving the two women, Israel had intuited. Weinstein was refusing to acknowledge it.

Israel knew about Weinstein's offenses from firsthand experience. He had praised her, trusted her with significant responsibility at a young age, and harassed her, she said. One year at the Toronto Film Festival, when she arrived at his hotel to pick him up for a gala screening, a male assistant summoned her up to the boss's hotel room. She had complied, thinking the assistant would be in the room as well. Instead she found a nearly naked Weinstein, wearing only a tiny towel, entreating her for a massage. She blurted out that she needed to call her mother and pretended to dial her on the spot, she said.

A year or two later, after being promoted to the head of her department, she was screening a film for Weinstein in New York when he asked her, out of nowhere: "Why don't you take off your shirt and do some cartwheels?"

"Go fuck yourself, you fat fuck," she shot back, and he turned to a game of tic-tac-toe. (Weinstein denied her account.)

But all these years later, she feared that what had happened in Venice was worse. She knew only bits of the aftermath. Zelda Perkins had left the company and signed some sort of contract that prevented her from speaking about what happened—a settlement, Jodi thought. Israel also recommended she call another former employee of the London office, a woman named Laura Madden: She might have something to say too.

Israel was also asking a bigger question: What had all of them, the whole former Miramax crowd, tolerated? That was what she really wanted to know, and the reason she was on the phone with a reporter. Back in the day, Israel had taken small steps to protect colleagues, like forbidding female subordinates from being alone with Weinstein. Doing more had felt impossible—she had only suspicions about what had happened in Venice, and there were few realistic avenues for complaint. When she had reported her own hotel room encounter with Weinstein to one of her supervisors, she was told that another colleague had been victimized too, but no action was taken.

She and her peers focused on their work. "He counted on my shame to keep me silent," she said. Ever since the news of Bill Cosby's crimes had broken, she had been waiting for mention of Weinstein, willing that story to emerge too.

"Why are we not speaking out?" Israel said on the phone. "Why are people still not talking twenty years later?"

Three weeks later, on Wednesday, August 2, Jodi was in London, sitting across a restaurant table from Zelda Perkins in South Kensington, hearing her account of what had taken place in 1998.

Perkins had the no-nonsense manner of a good producer. She was mostly a theater person, a longtime hand to one of the top stage and screen producers in town, working on prestige plays and occasionally television series like **The Crown.** She spent time in a cottage in the countryside where she tended to a flock of sheep and returned to London frequently for work. Because she was legally prohibited from talking about it, only a small number of people knew the full story of her career.

This meeting was the most Perkins had opened up to any of the journalists who had contacted her over the years about the Weinstein rumors. (The others had all been men, she said pointedly.) With her voice low, she plunged back into the story she had started to tell on the phone, when Jodi had first contacted her.

In 1995, Perkins had ended up working for Weinstein when he was near the peak of his powers. She was only twenty-two years old and had gotten the job through a chance encounter. "I didn't know who he was, and I didn't have a driving ambition to work in the movie industry," she said. "I wasn't sophisticated enough to understand that I had landed myself an incredibly rarefied position."

Weinstein had harassed Perkins from practically the first day, she said. "He was pathologically addicted to conquering women," she said. "That was what got him out of bed in the morning." She wasn't speaking figuratively. Each morning, Perkins, or whichever assistant from the London office was on the early shift, had to rouse the partially or fully nude Weinstein out of bed in his hotel room, and turn on his shower, as if he could not rotate the handle himself. Sometimes Weinstein tried to pull Perkins into bed with him, she recalled. There was no one to complain to about this behavior, no human resources operation in the tiny London office, no pretense of policies or rules.

Perkins never succumbed to Weinstein's come-ons.

She was small but tough and she had come to the job prepared. Another female colleague had instructed her to sit in armchairs, not sofas, in his presence, so he couldn't sidle up easily, and to wear her winter parka for protection even if she was warm. "I always managed to say no," she said.

While the hazards of working for Weinstein were beyond anything she had ever seen, so were the perks. On trips to Paris and Rome, "he would just hand out the cash, which was your blood money," she said. "You'd come back from trips with him with a weird comedown of guilt and relief that you'd survived." Each trip felt like a bungee jump, she said, exhilarating but close to the void. Sometimes, he would close the trips on a benevolent note, saying to Perkins: Take the company jet, keep the suite at the Ritz for the weekend, invite your boyfriend to come, have fun. "We all took the gifts," she said.

In 1998, Perkins hired another assistant, Rowena Chiu, an aspiring producer so creative and driven that as the president of the Oxford University Drama Society, she had staged a Brecht play in the round and Euripides in the original Greek. Perkins warned her to be careful around the producer. That September, the two women flew to Italy for the Venice Film Festival and the standard Weinstein festival routine: screenings, a stay in a top hotel, and meetings with colleagues from New York, including Amy Israel.

But before the meeting that Israel had remembered, Chiu had come to Perkins for help. When

Chiu confided the disturbing details of what Weinstein had done to her the night before, Perkins teared up, said it was unconscionable, and had set off in pursuit of him.

But she couldn't share the details of what Chiu had told her, Perkins said at lunch. Those were for Chiu to describe or keep forever private.

Much later, Chiu told Jodi that part of the story herself. On the Venice trip, it had been her job to tend to Weinstein in the evenings, putting her alone with him in a hotel room for long hours at night. He made advances on her from the beginning, she said, but on the second or third night of the festival, according to Chiu, his behavior worsened. They were supposed to be going through a stack of scripts, and as they paged through, he flattered her, telling her she had real insight and a feel for the business.

That night she had worn two pairs of tights as protection. But as she tried to work, he interrupted with an escalating series of sexual requests, for massages, a bath. She tried to appease him by taking off one set of tights and letting him massage her, she said. When his hands wandered further, she protested that she wanted to get back to the scripts, that she had a boyfriend. He responded by making grandiose promises of career help for him as well.

"I didn't directly say no, I didn't want to be that confrontational," she said. "He was much bigger than me, and as long as he was being pleasant, I wanted to be pleasant too."

This continued for four hours, she said: She would push back to work, and then he would resume pressuring and touching her, saying that they could have oral sex, that he had never had sex with a Chinese girl before. Weinstein removed her second layer of tights. But when he asked her to remove her underwear, she refused.

"It's exhausting, he tries to whittle you down little by little," Chiu said. "I was on high alert; I was worried about being raped." He managed to get her on the bed—he was holding her down, she said, not forcefully, like it was a game. He parted her legs, and told her that with one single thrust, it would all be over. Before anything further happened, she rolled over, wriggled away, and dutifully continued on her shift, leaving the hotel room around 2:00 a.m., when the work was finally done.

Later, Weinstein denied the whole story. "There is not a bit of truth," he said through a representative, "and any reporting retelling this narrative is just continuing the falsehood."

In London, Perkins continued with her story: She had found Weinstein at a business lunch on the hotel terrace. In front of all the other guests at the table, she commanded him to follow her. He was almost docile, she remembered, trailing her down the hallway as if she were the boss and he the assistant. When she confronted him, he swore on the life of his wife and children he had done nothing wrong, Perkins remembered.

She was twenty-four years old by then, the older of the two women and the employee of longer standing. Chiu, her assistant, had her account of the incident, but Perkins knew about her boss's record of misbehavior. Chiu and Perkins banded together and resigned. "I had to protect her," Perkins said. "She couldn't have done anything on her own; it would have just been her word against his. I was her shield."

Perkins consulted with a more senior figure, Donna Gigliotti, a producer who would go on to win accolades for **Shakespeare in Love,** and, many years later, **Hidden Figures.** She was far better connected than Perkins, the relatively rare female producer with the clout and experience to get major movies made. Gigliotti urged Perkins to get a lawyer, recommending one in New York, participating on a call with her, and offering other forms of quiet support. At the time, Perkins was grateful; now, years later, she questioned whether Gigliotti could have done more. (Later, Gigliotti emphasized that she tried to help Perkins find a lawyer who would take the lead.)

She and Chiu, a part-time law student at the time, found an attorney in London, from the firm Simons Muirhead & Burton, and assumed that the next stop would be criminal proceedings.

The lawyers told the two women otherwise. They

had no physical evidence. They had not called the police in Venice. They were two twentysomethings going up against Weinstein and potentially Disney, which now owned Miramax. Instead they were told that their best course of action was a settlement— maybe a year's salary, around 20,000 pounds. This is how such cases were typically handled, they were informed. Perkins and Chiu protested that they did not want any money: It had to be donated to charity, which they hoped would create a public flag. That wasn't how things worked, they were told. Weinstein's attorneys weren't likely to even enter a negotiation without a financial request.

Indignant, Perkins named an even higher figure and then attempted to craft a settlement that would go some way to stopping Weinstein's behavior. She demanded that Weinstein attend therapy and that she be present for his first session. Miramax would finally have a sexual harassment policy, with training and a group of three people to evaluate complaints, one of whom had to be an attorney. If anyone made a similar allegation in the next two years, with a settlement of at least 35,000 pounds or six months' salary, the matter would be reported to Disney or Weinstein would be dismissed.

Weinstein's lawyers fought back. A London law firm, Allen & Overy, represented him and a Miramax attorney named Steve Hutensky, who generally handled deals and contracts with actors, directors, and writers, disappeared from the New

York office and materialized in London to work with them. (Hutensky later said that this was the only sexual assault claim against Weinstein of which he was aware, and that the producer insisted to him that the encounter was consensual, and that he was settling the matter to protect his marriage.) One negotiating session lasted until five in the morning. In the end, each woman would receive 125,000 pounds, but both had to agree to extraordinary restrictions.

As Perkins and Jodi ate lunch and talked in London, written proof of those restrictions was sitting in Perkins's bag. Though Jodi and Megan knew about Rose McGowan's settlement, and suspected that one had been struck with the former assistant Megan had met, the reporters had never actually laid eyes on any of the Weinstein settlement papers. In investigative journalism, knowing about incriminating documents was good; seeing them was excellent; and having copies was best. In the days before Jodi's trip, Megan had given her pep talks and sent her encouragement by emoji: You'll see the papers. I know you will.

Now Perkins hesitated before drawing the battered sheets with the distinctive old Miramax logo out of her bag. She began to read aloud. She was not permitted to speak to anybody about her time working at Miramax. Any "medical professional" she consulted about what happened would need to sign a confidentiality agreement. She could not be truthful with her own accountant about the money she received. In the agreement, she had to list everyone she had already told about the events in Venice—not by name, Perkins had fought off that part. Instead there was an odd, anonymous list of parties who knew: She told three employees and her boyfriend that she left Miramax "because of an act," and for moral reasons; she told her two closest friends the precise nature of what happened, and so on.

The roll call of restrictions went on. She was not to speak to "any other media now or hereafter existing" about what happened. (**God bless Perkins,** Jodi thought, sitting here with a reporter almost twenty years later.) "In the event there is disclosure by the parties," Perkins continued, she would be required to provide "such reasonable assistance as it may request in taking such steps as are prudent to deal with the foregoing to prevent any further disclosure or as the case may be to mitigate such effect." In other words, Perkins was required to help conceal the truth even if it somehow got out.

These restrictions were insults to common sense. Though the settlement shaped Perkins's life, she wasn't even allowed to hold on to a complete copy of the paperwork. Instead she was allowed limited visitation rights—if she wanted to see it, she could view a copy at her lawyer's office. The papers that Perkins had brought to lunch were bits and pieces, cadged together. When she had asked her lawyer how she could possibly abide by an agreement she couldn't consult, she had given her these excerpts. Worst of all, after intense pressure from the Weinstein lawyers, Perkins and Chiu, who had a matching agreement, had assented to confidentiality clauses that implied that the two of them could never discuss the matter again.

The date on the documents was October 23, 1998. The mess in Venice had taken just weeks to erase. Chiu sent Perkins a thank-you gift, a Filofax planner, then disappeared from her view.

Afterward, Perkins felt "broken and disillusioned." Her search for a new job was uncomfortable because she couldn't explain to prospective employers why she had left a top company so abruptly. Her career in film was over, she realized. She went to Guatemala to train horses. She had fought hard in the settlement negotiations for the right to attend therapy with Weinstein and had chosen a therapist for him, but she had trouble making the sessions happen and gave up.

The 1999 Academy Awards, which took place five months after the papers were signed, belonged to **Shakespeare in Love.** The film won seven Oscars, more than any other movie that year. Gwyneth Paltrow won Best Actress. Weinstein and Donna Gigliotti took home Best Picture. (Later, she briefly returned to working with him: in 2010, Gigliotti was Weinstein's president of production.) Perkins's name was in the end credits for the film.

Over the nearly two decades since, Perkins's perspective had expanded. She was no longer driven, she said, by wanting to get Harvey Weinstein. Perkins wanted to publicly question the fairness of the entire settlement system, to prevent other women from being pressured to sign away their rights.

"For me, the bigger trauma was what had happened with lawyers," she said later. "I wanted Harvey to be exposed, but what broke my heart is what happened when I went to the lawyers."

Perkins was tempted to defy her stifling confidentiality agreement and speak out, and Jodi was impressed by her courage. So many other women would barely get on the phone, and here Perkins was thinking of exposing herself to serious financial and legal risk. Before traveling to London, Jodi had phoned a top employment lawyer there for an assessment of how much a woman with a settlement would risk if she broke the agreement and spoke out. The attorney was unequivocal. "They'll sue her, ask for the money back," he said. In all of his years practicing law, he said, no client had ever breached a confidentiality agreement. "They're paying for silence," he finished. Perkins decided, like everyone else, that she wanted company: If Jodi and Megan could get other women to break their settlement agreements, she would too.

A safer, if less satisfying, way to proceed was to document the basic facts of her settlement by speaking with others. Amy Israel knew a chunk of what happened, and she wasn't the only one. But that still left another problem. Chiu, the alleged victim, was not responding to emails or phone messages. She did not want to be found.

The week before the London trip, Jodi had gotten on an airplane to the Bay Area, rented a car, and driven up to Chiu's house in Silicon Valley. Like Megan a few weeks before, she had a note on nice stationery and a mental script.

A man stood in the driveway, fiddling with a car. Jodi introduced herself and asked if Rowena Chiu was home.

No, she was out of the country, he said. But he was her husband, and he was certain that his wife didn't want to speak to any journalists. Could she please leave?

Jodi nodded in assent. Before she went, she asked the husband if they could just speak for a few moments, off the record, right there in the driveway. She wanted to explain why she had come all the way from New York.

He didn't say his name, but she already knew it: Andrew Cheung. She tried to read his face. It must have been strange to be cleaning out the car in the driveway one moment, then finding a reporter there the next.

Cheung nodded tentatively. As soon as Jodi laid out the broad strokes, he started asking questions. You're not the only journalist who has been contacting my wife, he said. Why are all of these reporters trying to reach her?

Surely, he knew the answer, Jodi wondered. It seemed impossible that multiple reporters were approaching his wife and he had no idea why. He was probably testing Jodi to see how much she knew and was employing the same script that Megan had heard from the former assistant in the New York suburbs, not even acknowledging that anything happened.

How to respond? She could not lie. She had shown up in this man's driveway asking to speak. If she wanted this couple to be forthcoming with her, she had to be transparent with them too. But at that point, she did not yet know the specifics of the allegations, and if he really had no idea about whatever had happened in Venice, Jodi should not be the one to inform him.

Jodi gently shared that she thought his wife might have been victimized by Harvey Weinstein, making clear that she could be wrong. When she mentioned a settlement, Cheung laughed and gestured at the ordinary-looking house behind him. "Do I look like a man whose wife got a settlement?" he asked.

He really doesn't know, Jodi realized with dread. This woman had never told her own husband. All these years later, the confidentiality clauses had left all three of them in bizarre positions: a woman barred from sharing her own experiences with her spouse. A husband standing incredulously in his own driveway, learning his wife's secrets from a stranger. He promised to relay a message to her but said he was sure that she wanted to be left alone. If Weinstein had victimized so many women, he asked, can't you just do your article and leave her out?

Before she drove away, hoping she hadn't just made things worse, Jodi answered his question. "If everyone takes that stance, the story will never be written," she said.

After she left, Cheung asked his wife, who was then staying with her parents in her native United Kingdom, about Jodi's visit, but Chiu brushed it away, and Cheung didn't want to inquire further. He knew she had worked at Miramax, but because he had no idea about the alleged assault or the settlement, he was also ignorant of one of the most telling details of her employment: Nine months after the Venice film festival, she had returned to the company.

She hadn't wanted to. But like Perkins, she found interviewing for other film jobs in London hopeless under the unexplainable circumstances. As part of the agreement, Miramax had already given her a reference letter, so she asked Hutensky, the company lawyer, for job leads at other organizations.

The message she got back was: **Harvey really values you and would like you back.**

Chiu caved and returned to Miramax in the summer of 1999, to a job based in Hong Kong, scouting for Asian films that could be made into Hollywood productions. She had no contact with Weinstein, save for one conference call, with Hutensky on the line to supervise, and wondered what other employees knew—but of course she couldn't tell them.

"I did my best to make a fresh start. It was a whole new country," she said. "I tried to see it as, 'I'm building my own empire and I'm far from New York and the abuse of Miramax headquarters.'" At the start, she threw herself into finding Asian films but found that Miramax was not serious about the material. She slowly began to suspect that the job was a concoction designed to keep her under Weinstein's control.

"It was a deal with the devil," she said. She fell into a depression and attempted suicide twice before finally leaving Miramax for good and moving back to London, where she studied for an MBA and began to create a new life for herself.

By the time Jodi showed up in her driveway, she had a résumé full of accomplishment and adventure in the world of business and economics, and four children, including an infant. Chiu told her husband to ignore Jodi's visit. Journalists had turned up from time to time, she assured him, but they never wrote anything, and she didn't think they ever would.

Twenty-four hours after the lunch in London with Zelda Perkins, on Thursday, August 3, Jodi was sitting at a picnic table opposite the other woman Amy Israel had recommended: Laura Madden.

When Jodi had asked if she could come see her, Madden had hesitantly said yes. She lived in Wales, but that week she would be on vacation in Cornwall, in the far southwest of England, and she could only spare an hour or so. Jodi went anyway. The flights from London were sold out, so she took a five-hour train ride. In the final hour, the train broke down, so she took a bus. She absolutely had to see Madden, because her story, which she had already started to share haltingly over the phone, brought together so much of what the reporters had already heard.

In 1992, Madden had been just twenty-one or twenty-two, a girl from rural Ireland with little life experience, who had grown up feeling isolated on an estate her family had owned for generations. There was no great fortune left—her parents kept the place going as a hotel—but her family struck locals as too posh, too British. As a child, her pleasures were books and roaming the family property, which held farms and gardens. Madden did not attend university, and aside from a few months of language study in Spain, she had never really been away from home.

When a film began shooting nearby, she got a job wrangling extras and caught the movie bug. That crew told her to look for work on **Into the West,** a film starring Gabriel Byrne and Ellen Barkin. She was hired, and that was how she found herself dispatched to Weinstein's hotel room in Dublin one day, excited for the chance to answer calls and run errands for the producer, whom she had never met. When she arrived, champagne and sandwiches were waiting. Weinstein complimented Madden, telling her everyone on the production had noticed her talent and hard work.

"He told me that I was guaranteed a permanent job in the Miramax London office, to start immediately," Madden wrote in an email to Jodi later. "I was delighted, as this was literally my dream job."

Weinstein, wearing a bathrobe, told Madden that he was worn out from travel and wanted a massage from her. She resisted. He pushed, telling her that everyone did it, that it wasn't a romantic request, he just needed to relax, she remembered. "I felt completely caught in a situation that I intuitively felt to be wrong but wasn't sure whether I was the problem and it was completely normal," Madden wrote.

When he took off the bathrobe and Madden placed her hands on him, she froze. He suggested that he massage her first, to put her at ease. She took her top off, as he had instructed, then her bra, and he put his hands all over her, she recounted. She felt disgusted and scared she would lose the job in the London office.

It was only months later, after the story had broken, that Madden shared the worst details of her account. Soon her pants were off too. Weinstein stood over her, naked and masturbating. "I was lying on the bed and felt terrified and compromised and out of my depth," she wrote. She asked him to leave her alone. But he kept making sexual requests, the same kind Judd had described—can we do this, can we do that. Weinstein suggested a shower and Madden was so numb she gave in. As the water poured around them, he continued masturbating and Madden cried so hard that the producer eventually seemed annoyed and backed off, she said. That was when she locked herself in the bathroom, still sobbing. She thought she could still hear him masturbating on the other side of the door.

Omitting those details, Madden described how she hurried back into the room to recover her clothes and belongings and ran away. (Later, Weinstein denied her account in its entirety.)

The most painful part was that she had felt so enthusiastic at the start of the assignment, tingling at her opportunity and luck. "The overwhelming feeling I can still remember was shame and disappointment that something so full of promise had become reduced to this," she said. "All the optimism I felt for my future was robbed by him. Any hope that I had been offered a job through my own merit was gone."

Afterward, a female colleague she'd enlisted for support phoned Weinstein to confront him about his behavior and he readily apologized. "I was to take the job and never feel compromised," Madden said. The producer swore that it would never happen again.

Madden did take the London job, and she spent six years working in production for the man who had abused her, she said. It had seemed safe in part because he was based in the States. The work was what she had wanted, after all. Her father, at first livid at the mistreatment, eventually backed the decision.

But Madden was never happy at Miramax. When

the producer visited London, she never knew which version of him she would see: the charming or the dangerous one. She had plenty more uncomfortable moments in hotel rooms with Weinstein, she said, even if none were as bad. She spent the whole of her employment feeling "compromised"—her word—by what had happened at the start. "I carried the weight of feeling responsible for the assault and that I should have outright turned him down and never taken the job," she wrote later.

Madden's story was a kind of distillation, bringing together the elements of what Jodi and Megan were starting to call The Pattern: Weinstein's hallmark moves, so similar from account to account. Each of these stories was upsetting unto itself, but even more telling, more chilling, was their uncanny repetition. Actresses and former film company employees, women who did not know one another, who lived in different countries, were telling the reporters variations on the same story, using some of the same words, describing such similar scenes. Eager young women, new recruits to Miramax, hoping to connect with the producer. Hotel suites. Waiting bottles of champagne. Weinstein in a bathrobe. They had been so young, so overpowered. They had all wanted what young Laura Madden had wanted: their own equivalent of that job in the London office, the chance to work, participate, and succeed.

———

As she and Madden talked, Jodi did not mention the lunch with Perkins the day before, nor had she mentioned Madden to Perkins. She couldn't: The conversations were confidential. Though the two women had worked alongside one another in the London office, they had never shared their painful stories with each other. Both women were isolated; no one could see the whole picture. It was tempting to daydream about bringing all of the alleged Weinstein victims together somehow, to show them that they had each been part of something larger. But that would be perilous, even with their permission, for the reporters as well as the women. One source could not know who the others were. Anxiety was contagious, the reporters knew. One woman could talk the rest out of participating. One leak could compromise everything.

Earlier, on the phone, Madden had said she would never be able to tell the story publicly. Now, as they sat on the beach, Jodi registered a clearer impression of her. There was something quietly impressive about Madden: She was careful about what she did and didn't remember, and judicious in her descriptions, with an eye for nuance and detail. After Miramax she had gone on to experience deep happiness from motherhood. But now she was at a profound point of struggle. Her marriage had just ended. She was figuring out how to be a single mother to her four children, ages eleven to sixteen. She had recently had breast cancer, had lost one breast, and would need a second mastectomy in addition to full reconstructive surgery in coming months. She'd never worked full-time since leaving Miramax, only briefly running a small catering business, and was just trying to finish a landscape design course, but her confidence was low. She didn't say this to Jodi at the time, but between the loss of her marriage and her breasts, she felt like her whole womanhood was in question, and she wondered if she would ever feel attractive or wanted again. As they talked on the beach, Jodi realized that even the vacation was trying for Madden. She wasn't used to spending summers on her own.

Besides, her feeling of having been somehow at fault had never lifted. (That was why she had told Jodi only an abbreviated version of the story.) She could never speak out, she had told Jodi, because she was too afraid of being judged for not running away.

But she was speaking privately to Jodi because of a call she had gotten prior to any of their conversations, from an ex-assistant of Weinstein's named Pamela Lubell, to whom she had not spoken in almost two decades. Lubell had effused about how lucky they had all been to work for Miramax, how kind Weinstein had been. Then she asked if Madden had gotten calls from any journalists—"cockroach journalists," she had said. Lubell had wanted assurances that Madden wouldn't speak to them. Madden had refused to make any promises, so Lubell continued to call and push. "If you ever have a project you want to make, you can bring it to me; I can bring it to Harvey," she remembered Lubell saying. Madden was certain that Weinstein had put her old colleague up to the calls. She was direct with Lubell. Yes, Weinstein had harassed her. No, she could not provide any assurance that she wouldn't speak. In fact, she was outraged by the attempt to silence her. That's why she had taken Jodi's first call.

On the beach, Jodi asked Madden to just imagine going on the record with her story. She sketched out the growing scale of the allegations, without using names; told Madden that her story would mean a great deal to others; and promised to go over everything before publication and do whatever she could to make the experience as dignified as possible. If Weinstein retaliated in any way, that would only seal the case against him, she added.

Madden said, cautiously, that she would think about it. She wanted the story to work. Now that Jodi understood the level of personal difficulty Madden was facing, she worried the timing was just wrong for the former assistant. But privately, Madden was thinking the opposite: "Everything felt like it was imploding," she said. "An added bit of implosion didn't seem like such a bad thing." She was craving something proactive, something positive.

And in her own mind, Madden was formulating an even more potent argument to herself. She realized that she was free. She no longer worked in Hollywood. Even more important, she had neither

received money to stay silent nor signed a nondisclosure agreement. She began to wonder if she had a
responsibility to speak because others could not.

Back in New York, Megan was making one final effort to track down the mysterious 2001 complaint
against Miramax filed at the California Department
of Fair Employment and Housing. She needed help
from someone who knew the territory, who would
understand why Megan didn't want to give up. She
sent an email to Gloria Allred.

Megan had become acquainted with the feminist attorney in October 2016 while reporting on
Trump's treatment of women. After the release of
the **Access Hollywood** tape, Allred represented several women who had come forward with allegations
against Trump. She had put on tightly controlled
press conferences, comforting her clients when they
teared up in front of the cameras. When Trump
lashed out at his accusers, Allred fought back.

Some journalists and critics saw her as a shameless
self-promoter. But after having read Allred's autobiography, spoken with her at length, and interviewed
some of her former clients and coworkers, Megan
took her very seriously. She knew that as a young,
single parent, Allred had struggled to collect child
support, been raped at gunpoint at age twenty-five,
and gotten an illegal abortion, which almost killed
her. Allred's drive to help protect other women and

give voice to victims appeared to be the product of her own suffering.

One thing made Megan cautious about seeking help from Allred on the Weinstein investigation: the strange outreach from Lisa Bloom, Allred's daughter. So when she spoke to Allred, she didn't mention Weinstein's name, only that she needed advice on how to obtain an old sexual harassment complaint from a government agency in her state. Allred was muted, with little advice to give. Megan didn't realize, and would never have suspected, that Allred's firm was sitting on separate records about Weinstein, ones that had never come to the attention of the government or the public.

While the attorney cultivated a reputation for giving female victims a voice, some of her work and revenue was in negotiating secret settlements that silenced them and buried allegations of sexual harassment and assault. In 2011, she and a partner had negotiated a settlement with Bill O'Reilly—one of those so breathtakingly restrictive that it had alarmed Emily Steel. In late 2016, when the public was first starting to learn about abuse of elite gymnasts by former team doctor Larry Nassar, Allred was working on a settlement that muzzled Olympic-medal-winning gymnast McKayla Moroney, one of the top names in the sport.

Megan only learned months later that in 2004, Allred's firm had also negotiated a settlement with Weinstein. His alleged victim—the firm's client—was

Ashley Matthau (then Anderson), who had worked as a backup dancer in **Dirty Dancing 2: Havana Nights,** a movie produced that year by Miramax. Matthau was twenty-three years old at the time but felt much younger. She had spent her teenage years in the sheltered world of dance, traveling with the American Ballet Theater. Afterward, she had been swept into a world of music videos, Playboy Mansion parties, and other settings where she was expected to look good and say little.

But what happened during the shooting of the film had triggered a deep anger in Matthau, she said. During a visit to the **Dirty Dancing** set in Puerto Rico, Weinstein had insisted Matthau come to his hotel room for a private meeting to discuss future projects. Once they were alone, she said, he had pushed her onto the bed, fondled her breasts and masturbated on top of her. "I kept telling him, 'Stop, I'm engaged,'" Matthau later told Megan. "But he kept saying: 'It's just a little cuddling. It's not a problem. It's not like we're having sex.'" The next day, Weinstein had kept promising her more work, as if they were doing a business deal. "I didn't want him to get away with it. I wanted to stand up for myself."

At the urging of her fiancé, Matthau had turned to Gloria Allred. The fiancé had seen the lawyer on television and thought she could help. Allred steered Matthau to her partner, John West, who encouraged Matthau to enter a private out-of-court settlement. Fearful of going up against Weinstein, and all his power, in public, Matthau had quickly agreed to accept $125,000 in exchange for a legally binding promise to never speak of the allegations again, she said. "I remember John not negotiating that much because he thought I was an emotional wreck and couldn't handle it," Matthau explained. "He suggested I just take the money and move on and try to heal." The firm's cut was 40 percent, she said.

West and Allred refused to comment on the firm's representation of Matthau. But in a separate interview, Allred made the same case for confidential settlements that the reporters had already heard: They were better for clients, many of whom wanted privacy and feared being shunned by employers; going to court was risky and could take years. "Nobody has forced anyone to sign an NDA," she told Megan. "Nobody is holding a gun to their head."

Allred also acknowledged the harsh truth about confidentiality clauses: They served perpetrators of sexual misconduct too. "A client will say, 'I want to be compensated, this is a significant amount you've been able to achieve for me, I'm very happy with that, but why should I have to keep secret?'" Allred said. "That's because that powerful figure wants peace, wants to end it, and wants to move on in the same way that you want to move on."

By 2017, a group of consumer lawyers in California, Allred's home state, had come to see danger in that line of thinking. They thought victims of sexual harassment deserved financial compensation, but settlements shouldn't be used to cover up—and thus perpetuate—predatory behavior. "If there's a serial perpetrator out there, you can't keep these secrets repeatedly because the actions will continue," Nancy Peverini, a lobbyist for the consumer lawyer group, later told Megan.

That January, Connie Leyva, a state legislator, had considered sponsoring legislation, requested by those lawyers, that would transform settlements for sexual harassment in California by banning confidentiality clauses and ensuring that future victims could speak out and name the perpetrators. This was the push that Katie Benner had mentioned to her **Times** colleagues in the Page One conference room.

Then Allred stepped in. On a tense phone call with lobbyists and an aide from Leyva's office, Allred was adamant: Sexual harassers would never make payments to victims without getting silence in return. If the legislation was proposed, she would travel to the state capitol to oppose it.

No bill to protect victims could possibly survive public attack from Gloria Allred, the consumer lawyers knew. She could deploy the many fans who thought of her as the ultimate advocate. Not surprisingly, Connie Leyva backed away from sponsoring the bill. With Allred's threat, an effort to reform the system and protect victims' voices died before it was ever introduced.

CHAPTER FOUR

"POSITIVE REPUTATION MANAGEMENT"

On July 12, Dean Baquet, the executive editor of the **Times,** gathered Jodi, Megan, Corbett, and Matt Purdy in his office. He wanted to hear about the progress of the Weinstein story. But he also had instructions.

Within the newsroom, Baquet's corner office was a place apart, roomier and quieter, containing mementos from a lifetime in the newspaper business. Baquet had grown up in New Orleans, in an apartment behind his parents' Creole restaurant, which was so modest that a cigar box had served as the original cash register. He was the first black editor of the **Times,** but he rarely opened up to his staff about his personal experience of race. Instead, he liked to talk about holding the powerful to account, when to be aggressive or restrained in dealing with them.

That day, Baquet wanted to communicate one thing in particular: Watch out. In 2014, when an early version of Weinstein's troubled theatrical production **Finding Neverland** opened in Cambridge, Massachusetts, Weinstein had tried to get the paper not to review it, knowing that one bad notice could doom the show. He had complained to Baquet and Arthur Sulzberger, then the publisher, making a not-so-subtle reference to the money he spent on advertising in the paper and citing a tradition of New York publications not reviewing out-of-town tryouts. But one of the culture editors had persuaded Baquet that the rule was outdated: **Finding Neverland** was a big budget production, and in the online era, the show was no secret. When Weinstein heard that answer, he told Baquet to expect a call from none other than Meryl Streep.

The call from the famed actress never came, but Baquet was contacted by David Boies, one of the most distinguished lawyers in the country. Boies had tried the government's antitrust case in the 1990s against Microsoft, represented Al Gore in the 2000 presidential recount, and helped convince the Supreme Court to overturn California's ban on gay marriage. He had been serving as counsel for the producer since 2001. But when he dialed Baquet in 2014 to argue against reviewing the **Finding Neverland** tryout, Boies had opened by saying: "I'm not calling as Harvey's lawyer, I'm calling as Harvey's friend." The attorney was being disingenuous about his relationship with Weinstein, Baquet felt, and he had found Boies's chummy,

I-just-want-to-straighten-things-out-for-you tone condescending. Baquet refused to change his stance.

The following year, **Finding Neverland** was about to make its Broadway debut, and the **Times** was preparing a story on the production. Weinstein yelled at an editor in the **Times** Culture department to omit any mention of a glaring development: He had just come under police investigation in New York, for the groping complaint from Ambra Battilana Gutierrez. The producer insisted that the accusation was false, and he argued that the **Times** should ignore it, even though it had already gotten widespread coverage in the paper and elsewhere.

Baquet told his staff to keep the reference, and he instructed Weinstein never to speak to his journalists that way again. "You and I are going to have a pretty rough talk soon about how you talk to my editors," Baquet had written in an email to Weinstein in March 2015. "And it will be very rough, trust me."

An investigation of the producer's treatment of women had far higher stakes than any theater coverage, and Baquet predicted that Weinstein would do just about anything to try and stop it. The editor didn't make a big deal of it, but both Weinstein and Boies had already begun calling him and the publisher, requesting off-the-record conversations.

Baquet wanted Jodi and Megan to follow two rules as they went forward. First, expect Weinstein to turn to increasingly desperate practices: employing investigators to trail them or their sources, digging into their pasts. He leveled his gaze at the reporters. "Assume you're being followed," he told them. "Talk like every call is being taped." Second, Baquet did not want the reporters to speak with Weinstein off the record. That would take discipline. What reporter wouldn't want to engage with a subject directly? But Jodi and Megan needed to be strategic, Baquet said. To allow Weinstein to talk in confidence could mean letting him lie with impunity. If he had something to say, he had to say it out loud, on the record.

But in the first week of August, Megan began to question Baquet's rules of engagement after Jodi got an unexpected phone call. It was from Lanny Davis, a Clinton-era Washington lawyer, who ran a lucrative business working as a crisis counselor, often representing unsavory characters, including African leaders who had been investigated by the paper. He had just been hired by Weinstein and wanted to chat off the record. Jodi told him that all communication had to be on the record, but when he resisted, she took the request to Megan and Corbett. As Jodi waited, Davis kept asking her more questions: Could they meet—immediately? Could David Boies join them? "He is a close friend of the client," Davis emailed, repeating the line that had annoyed Baquet years before.

Jodi and Corbett had dealt with Lanny Davis before. He was old school and outwardly cordial, though he had also been known to yell at reporters he thought were treating him or his clients unfairly.

Despite everything Baquet had said, Megan pushed to meet with Davis. She understood the boss's argument, but in her experience, if you engaged with people who had things to hide, they often hung themselves by accident. Besides, she was curious. How had Weinstein supposedly killed previous investigations by journalists? If the producer was up to something, she wanted to know, sooner rather than later.

Megan proposed that she and Jodi talk with Davis on background, meaning they could further report and write about what he said, as long as they didn't attribute any of it to him by name. A couple days later, Corbett said that Jodi and Megan could move forward with the meeting with Davis. But she and Baquet stipulated that the session couldn't serve as a substitute for an on-the-record conversation with Weinstein. Boies was not welcome. And while the reporters had to be straightforward, they would reveal nothing of the actresses and former employees who had begun to quietly tell their troubling stories.

As soon as Jodi called Davis to iron out the details, the loquacious PR man started spilling information about his client. "He's obviously going through very rocky times," Davis said of Weinstein. "And he's not always that rational."

———

On August 3, Davis pulled up a seat at a long table in a **Times** conference room, chatting about baseball, being one of Hillary Clinton's closest friends, and his years at Yale Law School. Corbett had joined Jodi and Megan for the meeting, a mark of the seriousness of the moment. Megan took out her iPhone and, with Davis's permission, began audio recording their conversation. As often happened, the click of that button ended the small talk.

"The reason I'm here is not to try to kill anything or not to try to spin or misdirect," Davis said. He had several other goals in mind.

The first was to defend. He mentioned the veiled rape claim Rose McGowan had made against Weinstein on Twitter the year before. His team knew she might include the allegation in the memoir she was writing. If Jodi and Megan were intending to report the charge, Davis wanted a chance to respond to the accusation.

That was easy. Of course, the **Times** would ask Weinstein to address any allegations.

The second was to probe: "I don't expect you to name sources, especially in a story like this one—but if it's possible for you to let me know overall what your story is about, it would help me basically do my job, which is to answer your questions and make sure they're true," Davis said.

Another simple one. Jodi and Megan told Davis they were looking into problematic behavior toward women by Weinstein and left it at that.

His third goal was to pitch. While Weinstein adamantly denied any allegation of rape or assault, he was aware of a growing number of complaints about his treatment of women, Davis explained. Weinstein had started to see his previous behavior in a different light. Powerful men of an older generation were changing their understanding of the meaning of the word **consensual,** Davis said—and "why women don't feel it's consensual even if a man convinces himself it is."

Where was Davis going with this? It wasn't easy to say. They saw that day, and in the following weeks, that he was a challenging professional communicator. He delivered statements that lacked precise meaning. He parceled out some useful information about his high-profile clients, but some of his claims proved wrong.

"I believe that there is a story to be told here about the evolution of men, and in particular Harvey Weinstein on this subject," Davis said.

His words grew even more elliptical: "So the bigger story may well be here that what has been out there for a long time about Harvey and lots of people in Hollywood who are men, powerful men, there may be something that when you're done with your article that is speaking much more broadly to men reaching a different awareness of this issue."

Just what did Davis seem to be tentatively offering? Was Weinstein willing to give Megan and Jodi an interview, in which he would discuss his own questionable behavior toward women?

Davis had just started talking to Weinstein about this possibility, he said, noting that his client had to "deal with his wife and children before anything else." But he thought the producer might be willing to have this discussion with the reporters. "I've been at least a little bit encouraged" that it could happen, he said.

This was only the first meeting with Weinstein's team, and his side seemed to already be acknowledging misconduct. That was a hint that the full extent of the findings could be far worse. If Weinstein was already really willing to talk about wrongs he had committed, the interview could be monumental, and the investigation much easier than any of them had anticipated. But the idea of Weinstein coming into the newsroom and opening up about sexual transgressions was implausible. Almost no one ever admitted to these things without being confronted with evidence.

The journalists told Davis that of course they'd be open to hearing anything the producer had to say—on the record. They left it at that: If Davis was trying to dangle some sort of trade, a halt to their investigation in exchange for an interview, they weren't engaging.

Instead, Megan changed the subject back to Rose McGowan. Davis was adamant that her rape accusation was false, and that a main reason she should not be trusted was the absence of any "contemporaneous outcry" at the time of the alleged attack. "Did she tell anybody right away? Did she show signs of distress?" he asked.

But McGowan had told Megan and Jodi that she had indeed appeared upset immediately after her encounter with Weinstein in a hotel room in 1997. She had told her manager, and then a lawyer, who had helped her obtain the $100,000 payment from Weinstein. McGowan had not yet gone on the record with the reporters, and they were still searching for corroboration that she had gotten a settlement. Maybe by pressing Davis on his characterization of events, Megan could back him into a corner and confirm that a settlement had been paid.

Megan leaned in: Was Davis **sure** McGowan hadn't shown any signs of distress at the time? Was last year's tweet the **first** time Weinstein had learned of any concerns that the actress had about an encounter with him?

Davis's narrative shifted. "Concerns?" he said. "Yes, there—he was aware that there were concerns, but not that she was accusing him of rape. So I'm making a bright line on the word **rape.** Anything below that line, he was aware of feeling, concerns . . ."

Corbett asked, "Of what kind?"

"And if the concerns were not about rape," Jodi asked, "then what were they about?"

Davis had intended to tell the journalists what Weinstein **hadn't** done to McGowan. Now he had to explain what the producer **had** done. "The only way I can answer, Jodi, based on what I now know, is a sense of being exploited because of that disparate power relationship. Taken advantage of, exploited, a wide range of verbs that post facto, or even in the middle of an incident, women are made to feel in an unequal position."

"There's mental coercion that isn't physical coercion," Davis said, adding that Lisa Bloom had been working with Weinstein to help him recognize the difference. "I know that he's mentioned that Lisa has looked at this, looked at him, looked at his past conduct, and has helped him understand that."

Lisa Bloom! The attorney who had emailed Jodi a few weeks before. What else was there to know about her relationship with the producer? But instead of asking that question they needed to press Davis on what Weinstein knew about McGowan and when.

If Weinstein had in fact been made aware of McGowan's concerns at the time, how did he respond?

"I believe he had dealings legally with her about them," Davis said.

"How would you characterize those legal dealings?" Megan asked. They were that close to confirmation of a settlement.

"I think he became aware that she did not regard what happened as okay with her," Davis said. "I'm not talking about rape; I'm talking about the effect that he had on Rose McGowan. She says that it was a severe effect. That rather than fighting . . ."

"Rather than fighting—then what?" Megan asked.

"I think that he has agreed to settlements rather than litigating what he might have litigated," Davis said. As Weinstein saw it, Davis explained, "It's better to settle even if you haven't done anything wrong."

Yes! They had been interacting with Weinstein's side for only minutes, and Davis was already confirming the settlement Weinstein had paid to McGowan and hinting at a larger pattern of payoffs.

Were there other cases of "questionable intimate relations with women in which Weinstein settled?" Megan asked. The reporters didn't say so, but so far they were aware of McGowan, Perkins, and Chiu, and they believed one might have been paid to the assistant who had fled the New York office. Megan had also come to suspect that Ambra Battilana Gutierrez, who made the police complaint in 2015, had been paid off. Did Davis know the truth?

Now Davis was squirming. "So I was trying to be careful because I'm not sure what my legal position is on admitting that there have been settlements and that the settlements involved sexual personal behavior. So let's say for now, even on a background basis, that I need to find out what my limits are legally, even if on background I am confirming settlements. I need to just find out where I stand. But the answer is, yes, there have been, but I just need to find out how I can better define that for you."

Before he departed, Megan wanted to ask one more thing. Baquet's warnings about private detectives, intimidation, and threats lingered in her mind. She asked the lawyer: Aside from hiring Davis, what else had Weinstein done in response to the interviews she and Jodi were conducting? Had he tried to interfere with the reporting in any way?

"Listen, the guy can be a jerk," Davis said. "Depends on the mood he's in and how much food he's eaten."

But, no, he insisted, the producer had no intentions of getting in the way of their reporting. Davis said he had asked Weinstein that question directly during their first meeting: "Do you have any plans to engage people to go on the attack for anyone who's cooperating with the **New York Times**? I need to know."

Davis said Weinstein's answer was unequivocal: "No" and "I don't intend to do that."

Davis left the conference room promising to pursue the potential interview with Weinstein. The journalists were still skeptical but felt encouraged. Perhaps Weinstein recognized that he couldn't halt the **Times** investigation. Just as important, Davis was recorded saying Weinstein wouldn't even try.

But the producer had been ahead of the investigation from the start. His efforts to conceal his alleged offenses had begun all the way back in October 2016, when McGowan had first tweeted, **New York** magazine had tried to pursue the story, and Weinstein had told Paltrow not to speak. He had spent hundreds of thousands of dollars to identify people who might talk, to cover his tracks, and even to have obtained passages from McGowan's memoir as she was drafting it. By the time of Davis's meeting at the **Times,** he had been combating Jodi and Megan's work in ways that went far beyond labeling them "cockroach journalists."

The astounding thing was how much help he had.

On July 10, two days before the meeting in Baquet's office and about a month before the conversation with Lanny Davis, David Boies was preparing to board a private helicopter in East Hampton following a family birthday celebration. Weinstein rang his phone—again. The producer had been calling the lawyer frequently, according to Weinstein's assistants. Cloaked in the secrecy of attorney-client privilege, the two men were plotting how to fight any **Times** story.

Weinstein was calling to share a fresh idea, Boies later recalled. The producer explained that he considered Arthur Sulzberger Jr., the **Times** publisher, to be a friend. Weinstein's companies had been a major advertiser over the years. The two men had shared business lunches and long moved in similar circles. Now Weinstein could use that relationship to lean on Sulzberger Jr. to kill the story, he suggested.

The producer and the lawyer, who had been working together for sixteen years, had contrasting styles. Weinstein was bold but erratic, brutish, and sometimes unsophisticated; Boies was polished and persuasive. The lawyer curbed some of the producer's worst instincts but enabled others to protect a man he knew had been repeatedly accused of predatory behavior.

The son of teachers from Illinois, Boies had grown up with undiagnosed dyslexia that stunted his learning. Yet he had gone on to earn a law degree from Yale and slay corporate giants. Boies was daring. He had been an enthusiastic card player since youth, had been expelled from the first law school he attended for having an affair with a professor's wife (he later married her), and had offended previous law partners with his renegade ways.

He also liked to be at the center of popular culture. When Boies left one law firm to start his own—to avoid a conflict of interest that would have prevented him from representing a new client, New York Yankees owner George Steinbrenner—he quickly attracted other celebrities, including Calvin Klein, Don Imus, and Garry Shandling.

Among those seeking his services were the editors of Miramax Books, a new publishing imprint that Weinstein and his brother, Bob, had launched. It was 2001, and Boies had just lost **Bush v. Gore,** a defeat of immeasurable consequence that the attorney had somehow used to win over legions of new fans. The editors wanted Boies to write a memoir, but the famous lawyer wasn't returning their calls.

Then, one day, Weinstein himself phoned, asking for a lunch date, Boies later recalled in a series of interviews with Megan.

Soon, Boies was meeting the Weinstein brothers at Tribeca Grill. The lawyer was clear: He didn't have time to write a book, and he wasn't that self-reflective. Weinstein wouldn't let it go. Boies said Weinstein made the task sound easy: All he had to do was write down the story of some of his cases. By the end of the meal, Boies had agreed.

The next year came and went without him writing a single word. One afternoon his wife looked up from the computer. "Sweetheart, you didn't tell me that you'd finished your book," she said. "What book?" Boies replied. "Well, the book for Harvey," she replied. "I just looked it up and it says it will be published this fall." Boies felt completely boxed in. If he didn't follow through, he would look like he had failed. He wrote every day until the book was on his editor's desk. From the start of the relationship, Weinstein seemed to know just how to conscript him, and Boies did not say no.

Weinstein got more than the book. He had secured new legal representation, and within months of their first lunch in 2001, the lawyer was privately helping the producer fight off a potential article about Rowena Chiu's allegation of sexual assault.

In 2002, the **New Yorker** writer Ken Auletta had heard from a source about the settlements that

Weinstein had paid to Zelda Perkins and Chiu—
the same ones Jodi and Megan were now piecing
together. Auletta had been unable to get Perkins
and Chiu to speak with him, but he was still hoping to write about the payoffs and the incident that
prompted them.

Auletta, David Remnick, the magazine's editor,
another editor, and its lawyer met with Weinstein,
his brother, Bob, and David Boies to discuss the
matter. At first, Boies appeared to be playing referee. When Weinstein insisted he would file an
injunction against the magazine, Boies patted
Weinstein's arm, saying that there was something
called the First Amendment that he couldn't get
around. But then Boies turned his attention to the
journalists, saying that running the story would be a
grave mistake.

Boies later told Megan that he had believed
Weinstein's claim that his encounter with Chiu
had been a consensual, extramarital dalliance. He had
thought it was plausible that women were lying in
order to milk Weinstein for money, a point he emphasized in the meeting at the **New Yorker.** In a follow-up session with the **New Yorker** journalists the
next day, Bob Weinstein handed over copies of personal checks that he had written to pay off the two
women on behalf of his brother: proof, he claimed,
that no company money had been used for Weinstein's
personal affairs. Without an on-the-record allegation

of assault, or any proof of misuse of company funds, Auletta said he and his editors agreed he could not write about the settlements.

By then, Boies had become counsel to the Weinstein brothers, and he was increasingly enmeshed in their work. The brothers were battling Disney. When the parent company refused to distribute Michael Moore's **Fahrenheit 9/11,** Boies helped the brothers regain control of the film and take it to Lionsgate Films. When the Weinsteins decided to leave Disney altogether and form The Weinstein Company in 2005, Boies helped secure contracts that specified the brothers could be fired only if convicted of a felony.

Weinstein and Boies attended film openings, charity events, and political fund-raisers together, two celebrities among celebrities. Boies admired that "Harvey's always selling something," and in Weinstein he had a valuable link to the film world. His daughter, Mary Regency, was an aspiring actress. Boies invested in the industry himself, forming a production company, the Boies/Schiller Film Group, in 2012, with one of his law partner's sons. Over the years, Boies and the group did business with The Weinstein Company, and Weinstein provided his lawyer invaluable favors, including discussing a role for Boies's daughter, who had appeared in a minor role in a little-seen, hardly reviewed 2011 film called **Son of Morning.**

Dear David,

I hope you're doing well. Thank you
for sending me SON OF MORNING.
I watched it with my team—Mary is
wonderful in the film. The movie is a
tough one—I don't think it is commercial
or the right fit for me—but Mary shines
through in it.
    If you can get me all of her scenes
and previous work. I'll have my team
put together a great promo reel for her
and get it to the right casting agents.
I'll also put her in touch with my people
internally to get her a small role in
my upcoming production I DON'T
KNOW HOW SHE DOES IT with Sarah
Jessica Parker. Anything I can do
to help.

All my best,
Harvey

That part never materialized, but the next year,
Mary Regency got a part in his film **Silver Linings
Playbook.** In October 2011, Jon Gordon, a former Weinstein assistant who was helping produce
the film, sent an email to Weinstein about the actress, asking for instructions on behalf of David O.
Russell, the director:

David read and wants David Boies' daughter, Regency, to play Dr. Patel's secretary.
    DAVID O. DID NOT OFFER HER THE PART YET AS HE WANTED TO KNOW IF YOU WANTED/NEEDED TO DO SOMETHING FIRST WITH DAVID BOIES.

Did these film entanglements with Weinstein explain why Boies had worked to conceal mounting allegations of sexual misconduct against the producer? "Well, it could, you know?" Boies said. "If I'm Harvey's lawyer, I'm going to try to keep things under wraps. That's my job, right?"

Boies said that with or without entanglements, "I am very dedicated to my clients."

In the following years, the lawyer continued learning of other accusers. Time and again, he came to Weinstein's defense, and helped him to conceal, spin, and silence. He chose to believe Weinstein's claims that he was guilty only of philandering. "I thought, like a lot of people in Hollywood surrounded by very attractive women who want to make him like them, he ended up in multiple affairs," Boies said.

Even years later, after the scale of Weinstein's alleged offenses were revealed, Boies saw no problem with the lengths he had gone to protect him.

"When I look back I don't have any regret that I represented him the way I did," he said.

O n a summer evening in 2017, when Weinstein raised the prospect of leaning on Sulzberger, Boies swatted away the idea as a waste of time. Exerting pressure like that might have worked elsewhere, but it would prove worthless at the **Times.**

Instead, Boies was focused on a stealthier way to try to block a **Times** story, just a variation of something Weinstein was already doing.

The producer had long relied on private detectives to protect his reputation. Those companies were basically professional watchers: They observed journalists, wrote reports, sometimes even picked through reporters' garbage. According to the unwritten rules of journalist-subject interactions, using private detectives was a shady practice, but not a surprising or illegal one. As Baquet had said, it was something Jodi and Megan should expect.

But nine months earlier, Weinstein had begun a secret relationship with an Israeli firm of a whole different order: "The black cube group from israel contacted me thru ehud Barack," Weinstein had written in an email to Boies on Oct. 16, 2016, later obtained by Megan. "They r strategists and say your firm have used them." Black Cube did far more than watch other people. It manipulated them as well, even using an actor who adopted a fake identity in order to dupe unsuspecting targets. Others were former military intelligence experts. At the time of the email, two of its operatives had just been arrested on hacking charges in Romania. Boies's law firm, Boies, Schiller & Flexner, had in fact used Black Cube before, and soon the law firm was executing an agreement between Weinstein and the Israeli company. Under the terms of a contract struck that October, Weinstein agreed to pay the professional manipulators $100,000 a month to shield his behavior from scrutiny.

Soon the relationship was in full swing.

Seth Freedman, a British freelance journalist, fed Black Cube information that he was collecting from women whom Weinstein feared would go public with damaging information about him. Freedman told the women he was a reporter who had worked for the **Guardian,** sometimes claiming he was writing about life in Hollywood, other times the film industry. Katherine Kendall, an actress, and other women who fielded phone calls from Freedman, said they spoke freely, never suspecting he was doing anything aside from straightforward journalism.

Black Cube went to work on Benjamin Wallace, the writer investigating Weinstein's treatment of women for **New York** magazine. Freedman had contacted him offering information of interest but never delivering. Wallace had also been approached by a female Black Cube agent posing as a potential source. When they met, Wallace didn't say much to the woman, who called herself Anna, suspecting she might be working for Weinstein. Eventually, he and his editors decided to suspend the investigation. No one was talking, Wallace later explained; the Weinstein story felt like a dead end.

By May 2017, the same agent was targeting McGowan. This time, the woman called herself Diana Filip, and said she was the head of sustainable and responsible investments for the wealth-management firm Reuben Capital Partners in London. She spoke with a German accent, used a UK cell phone number, and offered McGowan $60,000 for a speaking event. Over the next months, they met at least three times in whichever city was convenient to McGowan, conversing for hours about women's issues and the woman's stated desire to invest in McGowan's production company. McGowan read her a passage of her memoir.

"She presented as someone who really cared about women," McGowan later told Megan.

Now, in July 2017, Boies helped renegotiate Weinstein's contract with Black Cube with the goal of solving two problems. The first was Jodi and Megan's reporting. The second was that Weinstein and Black Cube were in a billing dispute. The Israeli firm expected a bonus for procuring information about McGowan's memoir, but Weinstein refused to pay, arguing that the pages mostly reiterated her tweet, Boies said.

Under the contract that Boies helped revise, Black Cube's mission became much more explicit: to halt Jodi and Megan's investigation.

Black Cube would "provide intelligence which will help the Client's efforts to completely stop the publication of a new negative article in a leading NY newspaper," along with gathering more information from McGowan's book. The agent "Anna," aka Diana Filip, the woman who had approached McGowan and Wallace, would be on the case full time. So would a so-called freelance journalist. The contract also promised continued "avatar operators" to create fake identities on social media, linguists, and "operations experts" to concentrate on "social engineering," all of whom would be advised by former heads of the Israeli intelligence services. If Black Cube was able to stop publication of the article, it would earn a $300,000 bonus. Boies signed the new contract on July 11, weeks before Lanny Davis met with Jodi, Megan, and Corbett at the **Times.**

In genially dangling the prospect of an interview to the journalists, Davis had never mentioned that at his first meeting with Weinstein a Black Cube agent had been present. He only told Megan that much later, saying that he had not known exactly what the agent was doing for his client.

The same week as the meeting with Davis, Jodi received a series of emails and texts from the same Diana Filip. Jodi had never heard of her, but she said she was from an organization called Reuben Capital Partners in London and that she was staging a series of events devoted to advancing women in the workplace and wanted her to contribute. Jodi had already brushed off the requests, but in an email the woman was persistent:

Hi Jodi,

Thanks for clarifying.

We are planning a series of round table discussions about gender inequality and discrimination in the workplace. Our aim is to get policymakers, different industries executives, journalists and other stakeholders to discuss these issues from different perspectives.

Some prominent individuals have already expressed their willingness to take part in this initiative, and we are now in the process of finalising the schedule and agenda.

At some point along the way I would love to get your input (in any way possible, even if not as a speaker), given your work in the field.

I want these events to have real impact and value and be much more than just empty talk, so I want to make sure that all the right questions are asked. As you can probably tell, I am very passionate about this project—in fact, this is very much my own initiative.

I understand the difficulties in you

having a direct role, but, nevertheless, I would love to have a quick chat with you and hear your thoughts.

Thanks so much for your time,
Diana.

Something about the email seemed slightly off—Jodi couldn't say exactly what. She sent the message to the paper's online security expert, who said the URL looked fine. The website, showing a smiling picture of a woman in a business suit, was a call for gender equality in the corporate sphere. "Women earn less, get promoted less, and are under-appreciated in the workplace," the site said. "This initiative will not only focus on combating all forms of discrimination against women in the workplace, but also work towards promoting the inclusion of women in business—actively and at all levels." By the standards of corporate feminism, the language was tougher than usual, calling for "progressive ac-tivism" and "full transparency" from companies.

Instead of beckoning to Jodi, this warned her off. Her job was to gather information and uncover secrets, not participate in activism. And because **Times** ethics rules prohibited journalists from ac-cepting corporate speaking gigs, to protect the paper against attempts at buying influence, she couldn't have accepted the money. Nor did she have time for nice-to-meet-you coffee dates.

A few days later, Filip emailed again. Jodi wrote back tersely to convey her lack of interest: "I am tied up, but good luck w your project."

Later Ronan Farrow would uncover some of Black Cube's work for Weinstein. Boies said he believed the best way for Weinstein to beat back critical stories about his treatment of women was to provide facts that reinforced his defense, and that he thought Black Cube would gather that information. He said he was unaware of the underhanded tactics the firm used against journalists and regretted not paying closer attention. Remarkably, Boies's firm had helped execute a contract to undermine the **Times** investigation even as it was representing the newspaper in legal cases. Boies insisted this did not constitute a conflict of interest, but the paper fired his firm, calling its actions "reprehensible."

But in the summer of 2017, Jodi never guessed that the rah-rah feminist messages she was getting were from an actor-agent hired to sabotage their investigation and undercut victims' stories. Nor did she suspect they were connected in any way to Boies. At Baquet's instructions, she and Megan had rejected the attorney's requests to meet with him. He seemed like a distant suit relegated to the sidelines.

Just as Megan and Jodi were sizing up Weinstein's team, Emily Steel sent over a glowing, newly published profile of Gloria Allred and Lisa Bloom in

W magazine. "Gloria Allred and Lisa Bloom Are the Defenders of Women in 2017," read the headline.

The article described Allred's daughter as her heir and equal, the two standing together at the forefront of civil rights issues, especially "the sexual harassment and assault of women by powerful men." The lawyers posed against the beachscape of Allred's Malibu home, looking more like sisters than parent and child.

As with her mother, Bloom's métier was public attention. Over the course of her career, she had appeared as a legal analyst on many networks and even hosted her own show on **Court TV.** She had her own Los Angeles firm, and she appeared to more or less replicate her mother's model: She cultivated high-profile clients and then often scored big settlements for them in private.

Her public relations skills were on display in the **W** profile. Bloom boasted about the confidential settlement she had just reached: "Women who were sexually harassed became millionaires," she said. For the interview, Bloom had shown up wearing a "Notorious R.B.G." T-shirt, as if to claim a link with the most supreme feminist lawyer of all, Ruth Bader Ginsburg.

So why had Bloom signed on to work with a rumored sexual predator? Was it related to the movie deal, the one Bloom had tweeted about triumphantly a few months before? What motivated her, and how did she operate?

Megan told Jodi and Steel that she had first become suspicious of Bloom in 2016 when the lawyer got involved in the lawsuit alleging that Donald J. Trump had raped a thirteen-year-old girl at a party hosted by Jeffrey Epstein in the 1990s, the one that Megan had refused to cover because it had been impossible to vet the anonymous victim's claims. One week before Election Day, with debate raging about the **Access Hollywood** tape, and the mounting allegations against Trump, Bloom had announced that she was representing the Jane Doe victim. Megan had never spoken to Bloom, but she quickly sent her an email.

> I've long viewed this as a dubious case and have doubted the existence of a real plaintiff/victim.
> Have you met with the actual plaintiff and concluded this is legitimate?
> I'd really value your perspective.

Megan never got a response. Instead, she watched as Bloom convened a press conference at her office in Los Angeles, where Jane Doe was to make her first public appearance.

The only person who stepped in front of the cameras that day was Bloom. She announced that the victim, who she said was there at her office, had gotten death threats and was too terrified to go public. Perhaps that was true; maybe Bloom's client had in fact been raped by Trump and was genuinely fearful to speak out. But to Megan the whole thing looked like an elaborate effort to draw media attention to unsubstantiated allegations against the presidential candidate.

Later, Bloom acknowledged that she solicited money from a pro-Clinton political advocacy organization, saying that she needed the money to vet Jane Doe's claim, and that after the lawsuit was dropped, she had accepted $700,000 from pro-Clinton donors for security, relocation, and a possible "safe house" for other potential Trump accusers. When the other women chose not to come forward, Bloom reportedly gave back $500,000 of the donations, but kept the other $200,000, later telling the **Times** that she needed "some funds to pay for her out-of-pocket expenses." When the financial arrangements were later revealed, Republicans accused Bloom of offering money to women to make up lies about Trump. Others saw it as the lawyer manipulating shaky Trump accusations for her own financial gain.

Bloom said later that she had spent months vetting Jane Doe and that, in the end, the woman was too afraid to go public, so she had instructed her team to drop the case and not discuss it further. She said she did not take any fees for her work with Trump accusers.

Around the same time, some of Bloom's own clients came to criticize her. In 2016, Steel had quietly begun interviewing Tamara Holder, a politically progressive lawyer and former Fox contributor, who had filed a complaint with the network, alleging that she had been sexually assaulted. According to legal documents that Steel had seen, Holder claimed that in February 2015, when she was working as host of a show called **Sports Court,** a Fox executive named Francisco Cortes had trapped her in his office and tried to force her to perform oral sex.

As Steel was conducting her reporting, Bloom helped Holder secure a settlement worth more than $2.5 million. Holder said she had not understood the terms of the agreement, which were especially ironclad. If the **Times** or the **Wall Street Journal** published articles about her experience, Holder would lose much of the money. "I never signed this with the understanding that if Steel"—or a **Wall Street Journal** reporter—"wrote a story, I would lose the 2nd payment," she later wrote to Bloom.

Holder was outraged. As she saw it, Bloom had pressured her to accept an agreement without disclosing the extent to which it placed Holder at financial risk. Even worse, she feared she had lost the option to go public with her story, something she had made clear to Bloom was more valuable to her than any payout. When she voiced her concerns shortly after the settlement was struck, she said, Bloom fired her as a client, walking away with $1 million.

"She did not care about me," Holder later told Megan. "She cared about the money."

Bloom denied ever pressuring her to settle, said she goes over settlement agreements line by line with her clients, and that it's standard for representation to end once a settlement is complete. Bloom also pointed out that Holder, herself, is an experienced civil rights attorney.

On Saturday night, August 26, Megan unexpectedly heard a story about Lisa Bloom that began to illustrate the work she was doing for Weinstein.

Megan was meeting someone who she hoped would explain an unusual financial transaction involving **Finding Neverland,** the Weinstein Broadway production that Baquet had mentioned, and amfAR, the AIDS charity for which he helped throw splashy gala auctions in Cannes. As the show struggled to get off the ground, Weinstein had arranged for $600,000 raised at a 2015 amfAR auction to flow into the pockets of the **Finding Neverland** investors, without disclosing that to the charity. Some of the charity's leaders felt duped and feared that something illegal had happened.

Megan was meeting Tom Ajamie, a lawyer who had been hired by amfAR's board to look into the matter. He told Megan how investigating Weinstein was like nothing he had ever been through. The producer had blocked his review of the financial transaction at every turn. David Boies had muzzled members of the board with NDAs. Meanwhile, the more Ajamie asked around about Weinstein, the more he heard about allegations of sexual harassment and abuse.

Ajamie was so troubled by the claims that he raised them with Bloom when he met her for a drink in Los Angeles in October 2016. Ajamie had met Bloom once before, was impressed by her feminist credentials, and hoped to forge more of a professional relationship. If she was willing to go after powerful men like Donald Trump, surely she wouldn't be afraid to take on Harvey Weinstein, he reasoned. Maybe she was already working with some of his victims?

Bloom told Ajamie that she had never heard any complaints about Weinstein's treatment of women and asked him to keep her posted, he said. But several months later, things got weird. Bloom accepted Ajamie's offer to stay with him and some friends at a condo he rented in Park City, Utah, during the January 2017 Sundance Film Festival. After attending a party hosted by Weinstein and Jay-Z, Bloom had returned saying that Weinstein wanted to meet with Ajamie. Reluctantly, he allowed Bloom to bring him to Weinstein's suite at the Main and SKY hotel for breakfast. One minute, Weinstein was lashing out at Ajamie for digging into his past. Moments later, he was pleading that they work out a deal of some kind. All Ajamie had to do was sign an

NDA drawn up by Boies agreeing to keep anything he had learned about Weinstein secret. "Let's just be friends," Ajamie recalled Weinstein telling him. "We can do business together."

Ajamie rejected any deal in exchange for his silence, and he left the room convinced that the $600,000 amfAR transaction was the least of what the producer had to hide.

Afterward, he recalled, as he and Bloom were leaving, she turned to him. During the meeting, Bloom had presented herself as a neutral party and mostly kept quiet. Now she had some advice.

"You know, I think you really should reconsider your position toward him," she said.

"What do you mean?" Ajamie asked.

"He can really help your career," she replied.

By the time of the Park City trip, Bloom had already been working with the producer for six weeks, at a rate of $895 per hour.

Much later, Bloom said that representing Weinstein in 2017 was a "colossal mistake" which she "deeply regretted." "I was naïve to believe he had only used inappropriate language with women, and to think that I could get to the root of the problem in a different way, by encouraging him to apologize, which he did when the story broke," she wrote in an email to Jodi and Megan. "Clearly my approach did not go over at all and I should have known better.

Should I have assumed that it could have been a lot worse than what I knew at the time? Yes. That's on me."

But contrary to what she wrote in that email, when Bloom was retained by Weinstein in December 2016, she appeared to know a lot about what she was getting into—and proposed a role for herself that was far darker than just encouraging him to apologize. She laid out that vision in a memo, later obtained by Megan, that she sent to Weinstein, along with private investigators named Jack Palladino and Sara Ness:

> Harvey,
>
> It was a treat to speak with you today, though yes, we'd all prefer better circumstances. I've spent the rest of the day reading Jack and Sara's thorough reports about Rose, who truly comes across as a disturbed pathological liar, and also your former assistant . . . who seems to be less of a concern. I also read through a lot of Rose's Twitter feed, to get a sense of her, and watched her short film, Dawn. (I'm no film critic, but I found it dreadful, but telling as to who Rose is: boy meets girl. Girl trusts boy. Boy murders girl. All men suck. The end.)
>
> I feel equipped to help you against the Roses of the world, because I have represented so

many of them. They start out as impressive, bold women, but the more one presses for evidence, the weaknesses and lies are revealed. She doesn't seem to have much going on these days except her rapidly escalating identity as a feminist warrior, which seems to be entirely based on her online rants. For her to keep her "RoseArmy" following she must continue ramping up the outrageousness of her diatribes.

Clearly she must be stopped in her ridiculous, defamatory attacks on you. She is dangerous. You are right to be concerned.

Options after my initial read, which I can flesh out on our next call:

1. Initiating friendly contact with her through me or other good intermediary, and after establishing a relationship work out a "win-win." Key question: what does she want? To direct, it appears?

2. Counterops online campaign to push back and call her out as a pathological liar. A few well placed articles now will go a long way if things blow up for us down the line. We can place an article re her becoming increasingly unglued, so that when someone Googles her this is what pops up and she is discredited. We have all the facts based

on publicly available information. This can begin simultaneous with #1.

3. Cease and desist letter from me, warning her of the violation of agreement with you and putting her on notice of causes of action for CA claims of false light, invasion of privacy, defamation etc. Risk: she posts the letter online, generating heat and backlash. (Sara: I need to see the agreement, please.)

4. You and I come out publicly in a pre-emptive interview where you talk about evolving on women's issues, prompted by death of your mother, Trump pussy grab tape, and maybe, nasty unfounded hurtful rumors about you. This will be headline grabbing if you express genuine contrition for anyone who you hurt, while emphasizing it was always adult consensual behavior. You thought that was enough at the time but now realize it's more nuanced, that a power imbalance means something, etc. You reached out to me to help understand rapidly evolving social mores around sexual misconduct because you are a good and decent person (as evidenced by your life's work making films on important social issues and extremely generous philanthropy). Example: Charlie Sheen, as women were set to come out against him re

HIV status, did a Today Show interview recently where he came out with it himself, receiving massive praise. I represented a few of the women and their stories were largely drowned out by his interview and the love he got for it. It is so key from a reputation management standpoint to be the first to tell the story. I strongly recommend this. If you agree, I'd like to come out and meet with you to go over the story in some detail, so this is done for maximum effectiveness. You should be the hero of the story, not the villain. This is very doable.

5. Start the Weinstein Foundation, focusing on gender equality in film, etc. Or establish the Weinstein Standards, which seek to have one-third of films directed by women, or written by women, or passing the Bechdel test (two named female characters talk to each other about something besides a man), whatever. Announce you will immediately raise standards re gender parity in very specific ways on all films under your control. Announce partnership with Geena Davis' group that works for gender equality in film, for example by mandating that half of all extras in crowd scenes will be female. You get the idea. These details can be worked out, but the point is you decide to

be a leader and raise the bar in a concrete, headline-grabbing way.

6. Positive reputation management. I Googled your name, and a few obnoxious articles pop up. I work with the leading reputation management company that can backlink to the positive articles to make a "firewall" which prevents negative pieces from ranking well on Google. Your first page of Google is key as 95% never go beyond the first Google page. Let's improve this. Easy to do. This should happen simultaneously with other option.

A reminder: would you please connect me with David Boies so that I can get retained?

Also, given that your emails with the Clinton campaign were hacked recently, I recommend you set up a secure new email account for emails with this team. We shouldn't be emailing on these sensitive matters to your company email as your IT people and others may have access.

Thanks and really honored to be brought into this team.

Talk tomorrow?

Best,
Lisa Bloom

Weinstein paid her an initial retainer of $50,000. The billing records that followed provided her own private accounting of what she did to help Weinstein.

She collaborated with the Black Cube agent "Anna," aka Diana Filip. She huddled with Weinstein and Boies. She helped orchestrate the collection of information on Rose McGowan, Ambra Battilana Gutierrez, Ashley Judd, and other women who might accuse Weinstein. Bloom worked hand in hand with Sara Ness, the private investigator who was compiling dossiers on journalists investigating Weinstein, tracking their social media accounts for clues on who their sources were. Just as Baquet had predicted: Weinstein and his team were watching the reporters, using their every click on social media to try to figure out with whom they were talking.

"Based on social media activity and comments made by HW, so far the following names appear to be among the more relevant/important potential sources for Kantor and Farrow," Ness said in the dossier, which Jodi and Megan only saw months later. It went on for pages, listing who they followed on Twitter and when they had started following them. Several of Jodi and Megan's most important sources were on the list.

Some assessments turned out to be off-kilter. "It is difficult to predict whether McGowan would grant either Farrow or Kantor an interview," the investigator wrote, after Jodi and Megan had already been in conversation with McGowan for weeks. "It seems unlikely Judd would want to go on the record and rehash the 2015 **Variety** article," she noted. And Weinstein, "does not believe Paltrow is a threat."

But other notes were scarily on point. Several of the women were described as potential "adverse sources," including the assistant who had fled Miramax in 1990, the one Megan had found at her mother's home.

"Adverse sources" sounded a lot like another word: adversaries. With the help of a large team, Weinstein was waging war.

CHAPTER FIVE

A COMPANY'S COMPLICITY

Throughout August and into September 2017, Jodi and Megan had a growing problem: For all they had learned about Weinstein's alleged mistreatment of women, there was little that could be said in print.

One night, Rebecca Corbett took the reporters to a quiet Midtown Manhattan bar and asked for an update. Jodi and Megan listed what they knew, so far. The stars who had told them Weinstein stories. The former employees. The settlements.

Corbett knew exactly what material they had. She was making a point. How many women were on the record? How many settlements had been confirmed? Of the women with firsthand accounts of abuse, only Laura Madden had said yes to going on the record, and her answer was not final. Their evidence of the payoffs was incomplete.

"You do not have a publishable story," Corbett said.

Persuading former Weinstein employees to speak was not getting any easier, particularly when it came to the innermost circle of executives who had served with the producer over the years. Talking was not in their self-interest. Why would they want the world to know that they had risen in their careers by enabling a man who seemed to be a predator? The best shot was to convince them that the **Times** investigation was a way to mitigate past wrongs, a safe way to address behavior that had, perhaps, eaten away at them.

At the end of a not particularly revelatory conversation with one executive, Jodi heard something intriguing. The subject was one of Weinstein's top lieutenants, Irwin Reiter, The Weinstein Company's executive vice president for accounting and financial reporting. Former colleagues had described him as the company's institutional memory: He had done the books for the brothers since 1989. He had also been described as a loyalist, gruff, and unlikely to be concerned about his boss's treatment of women. But this executive also said something no one else had mentioned. "Irwin Reiter **hates** Harvey Weinstein," the source said.

Jodi had been holding on to Reiter's phone number, waiting to call until she had some insight into him. Now that moment had come. When she rang him, he said he didn't want to speak—but before he hung up, he gave her his private email address. Jodi tapped out a note.

Friday, Sep. 15, 2017, 4:46 PM
To: Irwin Reiter
From: Jodi Kantor

Dear Irwin,

Thanks for the email address. We're documenting allegations that have to do with a pattern of mistreatment of women over the years. Our reporting is turning up evidence of numerous settlements. I've been told that this is something you may have been concerned about over time. Helping us get this story right could provide an opportunity to do something about the situation, without anyone else knowing. I'd value the chance to have a confidential conversation with you, and run our information by you to see if it's right.
    My sister lives near you, and I was planning on being in New Jersey soon. Can I buy you a cup of coffee, just so you can suss this out more?

Friday, Sep. 15, 2017, 8:27 PM
To: Jodi Kantor
From: Irwin Reiter

Your background is impressive. In 2017,
things being what they are, I have a
healthy respect for reporters. Have
a great weekend.

Jodi immediately forwarded Irwin's note.

Friday, Sep. 15, 2017, 8:37 PM
To: Megan Twohey
From: Jodi Kantor

What's my line?

Friday, Sep. 15, 2017, 9:11 PM
To: Irwin Reiter
From: Jodi Kantor

Thank you, that means a lot to me.
Carefully documenting the truth
seems more important than ever. I can
swing by your place around 11 a.m.
on Monday to introduce myself. (The
phone book says 3 Hebron Drive in
East Windsor.) Let me know if there's a
better day or time.

Friday, Sep. 15, 2017, 9:46 PM
To: Jodi Kantor
From: Irwin Reiter

> You're a great reporter but you really
> stink at addresses. I've never in my life
> lived in New Jersey. I'm thinking about all
> of this. I will let you know on Monday
> what I've decided.

To keep the dialogue over email going, Jodi made small talk, with Megan invisibly reading his responses and advising on Jodi's replies.

Soon Reiter sent instructions: Meet me at 9:30 p.m. at the bar behind the restaurant Little Park in Tribeca. He set rules for the meeting: He would ask the questions; he reserved the right to leave after five minutes; he would pay the check. That was fine, but Jodi was surprised at his choice of location. Tribeca was Weinstein's world. When he had moved the Miramax offices there decades ago, the company's rise had helped transform the formerly gritty neighborhood to a place of wealth, prestige, and power, home to multimillion-dollar lofts, expensive restaurants, and a famous film festival. Little Park, pricey and stylish, seemed like the kind of spot the movie producer might frequent. His office at The Weinstein Company, cofounded with his brother in 2005, was six blocks away. But she didn't question the choice. If Reiter wanted to meet under Weinstein's nose, that's what they would do.

On Monday night, September 18, Jodi walked into the bustling restaurant, glancing around: Even if Weinstein wasn't there, she wanted to make sure she didn't know anyone, lest an acquaintance come over and interrupt. She continued to an almost hidden space in the back that was sparsely populated: a dim bar that looked like a clubby living room, ideal for private conversations, with plenty of room between one cluster of couches and wing chairs and the next. Where was Reiter? And was he a spy, positioned to find out what the reporter knew?

But the short, fiftysomething man in an armchair in the back seemed too nervous to be a plant, glancing over his shoulders and making dark jokes about evading the goons he was sure Weinstein was employing. He had an avuncular manner, with a bridge-and-tunnel cadence to his speech.

A few minutes into the conversation, Reiter was still jumpy, but he didn't ask Jodi many questions, and he didn't seem inclined to leave, so she ventured a few of her own: She wanted to know if he had any of the financial details of some of the long-ago settlements. As she probed him about the past, he looked a little puzzled, or maybe even disappointed. Finally he asked: Why are you asking about ancient history when Weinstein had committed so many more recent offenses against his own employees?

Recent offenses.

Jodi and Megan didn't know about many of those; aside from the 2015 police investigation of Weinstein's behavior, they only had a few unconfirmed tips. When Jodi asked Reiter to say more, he tensed, then started speaking elliptically. He mentioned a young development executive who read scripts and another who had worked at The Weinstein Company while in business school. He used initials: EN, LO, and a scramble of others. He was unwilling to offer more. What he really cared about, he said, was stopping Weinstein from what he had been doing in recent years to young women who worked at the company.

For the next two weeks, Jodi and Reiter met every few nights, always late, almost always at the bar behind Little Park. Jodi and Megan told no one beyond the editors. In emails and texts to one another, the journalists just referred to him as "the source" or "Jodi's guy." The accountant swore that each meeting would be the last. His job was on the line. He spoke in a nervous rush, willing to reveal some things but not others, sometimes refusing to attach names, zigzagging between episodes that sounded central and others that seemed irrelevant or hard to prove. He did not claim to understand everything that had happened at the company, and he wasn't telling the story in order.

In between those interviews, Jodi and Megan worked to decipher, track down, and back up what he was saying, by speaking with other former employees, obtaining records, and contacting the women Reiter alluded to. They were focused on the fundamentals: What had Weinstein done to these young women and what evidence could they find?

But it was also dawning on them that Reiter was providing glimpses of a story that would take much longer to report. During two harrowing years inside The Weinstein Company, 2014 and 2015, the producer's danger to women had become much more visible within the company's top ranks, with problems surfacing with disturbing regularity.

Harvey Weinstein had long conscripted some of the people and practices of his illustrious companies—from lawyers to assistants, contracts to work expenses—to further his predation or hide it. Some employees knew little or nothing as they worked on movie marketing posters and release dates. But over that two-year period, Reiter, the company's most active board member, and Weinstein's own brother and business partner all became increasingly aware and worried about allegations of sexual harassment and abuse against Weinstein. One by one, they all failed to address the problem, and the producer showed a remarkable ability to create his own reality, to make a series of problems simply disappear.

How could a company become so deeply complicit in abuse?

For a long time, Reiter looked away from his boss's treatment of women. He had started at Miramax on July 15, 1989, thirty years old, a Brooklyn College–trained accountant awed by the daring films Weinstein was releasing, so different from the movies shown at most multiplexes. The next year, he noticed the sudden, mysterious departure of the assistant from the tiny New York office—the same woman Megan later approached at her mother's house. He was told that Weinstein had acted inappropriately with her, she had negotiated some sort of settlement, and that was that.

Almost a decade later, Reiter heard Zelda Perkins had a problem in the London office and knew a company lawyer was dispatched to England to help dispose of it. And like many colleagues, Reiter heard rumors of "affairs" between the producer and actresses but felt unsure about who was taking advantage of whom: Weren't actresses known for doing anything for a part? Besides, he was the back-office numbers guy, paid to do the books, without the authority to question Weinstein. He didn't inquire further.

Until 2014, when he became more alarmed. Over the summer, Reiter picked up some worrisome office chatter about Weinstein's behavior toward women. That October, women of all different backgrounds and ages were publicly accusing Bill Cosby of sexual assault. As the news broke, Cosby's TV projects and tour dates evaporated. When he did perform, protestors and hecklers began expressing disgust.

In light of the Cosby news, Reiter felt he had to

intervene. He wasn't yet grappling with whether women had been hurt or how. He was anxious about the state of The Weinstein Company, which projected an image of success—it made prestige hits like **The King's Speech,** and the television show **Project Runway**—but was more precarious than outsiders knew, with many failed projects and hundreds of millions of dollars in losses. A sex abuse scandal could send it on a path to destruction.

In November 2014, he composed an accusatory email to Weinstein, naming some of the women he had heard about through the office grapevine. "Stop doing bad shit," he wrote to his boss, according to a draft of the email. He didn't care about what Weinstein was doing with the women "unless and until it costs the company. Has it?" he asked. The next day, Weinstein confronted Reiter, admitting nothing. Afterward, the producer turned cold to him and began referring to him as "the sex police" around the office. (Weinstein denied this.)

Weeks later, in December 2014, just as the company was supposed to go dark for the holidays, Reiter arrived at work one morning to find some other executives astir with concern. A twenty-five-year-old woman named Emily Nestor, a graduate student, had taken a temporary job as a receptionist in the Los Angeles office, filling in during the holiday period. By her second day of work, Weinstein had badgered her into breakfast at the Peninsula Hotel in Beverly Hills and had offered to exchange sex for mentorship, boasting of all the actresses who had supposedly accepted and gone on to fame and fortune. Nestor kept saying no. He kept offering. When she finally extricated herself and returned to the office, she told other employees about what had happened, and they alerted their counterparts in New York.

Reiter was worried: The company was facing what sounded like an episode of sexual harassment. Nestor didn't want to file a complaint with human resources. So Reiter and several other executives persuaded the employees in Los Angeles who had heard her account firsthand to write everything down. One record noted how long it had taken her to fend off Weinstein: "She said he was very persistent and focused though she kept saying no for over an hour."

In early 2015, Reiter sat in a midtown restaurant arguing with his daughter Shari, who was twenty-six, about the same age as Nestor, a psychology student, and a firm feminist. When her father told her what was happening in his workplace, even passing his phone across the dinner table to show her and a law student friend some of the emails and documents, she was appalled. Shari urged her father to act, both recalled later, and she told him he had to find a way to stop Harvey Weinstein's behavior.

Reiter wanted to. He was no longer just afraid for the company: He was starting to fear for the safety of female employees and was troubled by the idea of the boss hurting women in his own employ. But he

didn't see what could be done. The company's outside counsel had advised the executives that because
Nestor did not want to file an official complaint,
sharing her account with the company's board might
not make sense. Pushing further felt futile. Besides,
he added to his daughter, they both knew what happened in these situations: Victims often ended up
being blamed, as if they had done something wrong.

Shari pressed forward anyway. The conversation
grew heated enough to attract glances from other
diners, she remembered later. He had power, she
told her father. He could help create an environment
conducive to women coming forward, and he was
obligated to do more.

That winter, Reiter heard concerns from another young female employee. Sandeep Rehal was
Weinstein's personal assistant, twenty-eight years
old, working in her first professional job beyond
an hourly retail gig. She began to confide in him
and a few other executives about duties she found
uncomfortable. Weinstein had ordered her to rent
him a furnished apartment, using his corporate
credit card to stock it with women's lingerie, flowers,
and two bathrobes. She had to maintain a roster of
women, which she referred to by a phrase Reiter had
heard around the office before: "Friends of Harvey."
Managing their comings and goings had somehow
become part of her job.

Rehal had been too ashamed and scared to tell
the male executives about her worst experiences,

she said later. How she had to procure and organize Weinstein's personal supply of an erectile dysfunction drug called Caverject, administered through injection into the penis. How she had to keep a supply of those shots at her desk, hand them off to him in brown paper bags, and sometimes run the drugs to hotels and elsewhere, just before his meetings with women. And how, after she spent a week finding a new supplier of the drug, and paid for it with his company card, Weinstein gave Rehal a $500 bonus, paid for by the company, according to an email she saw him send to human resources. He had implied there would be consequences if she told anyone about these duties, mentioning her student loans and where her younger sister attended school, and saying he could have her kicked out. Staying silent would come with rewards, he suggested. "You are at Harvey Weinstein University, and I decide if you graduate," he told her, she said. Soon Rehal left the company, and Reiter did not hear from her again.

But the accountant began grousing more to colleagues about another issue Rehal had raised—use of company expenses. Weinstein charged massive amounts to his company card, relying on a loose system to classify which personal expenses he would reimburse. On top of his generous salary—$2.5 million in 2015—he sometimes demanded the film company pick up questionable bills, including a $24,000 tip for yacht staff—which he eventually reimbursed—and a private jet stop in Europe to pick up a model. (Weinstein denied that he ever misused company funds.)

After Weinstein requested payments for a new round of women in movie production roles without clear jobs or tasks, Reiter wrote to Tom Prince, the head of physical production at The Weinstein Company:

Tuesday, Feb. 10, 2015
To: Tom Prince
From: Irwin Reiter

How many??????????
How many are enough????
How many are too much???

To: Tom Prince
From: Irwin Reiter

There is no thinking about it . . . it will happen . . . how old is Cosby? How long was he harboring his sexual sickness? Its gonna happen I hope humously not post . . .

To: Irwin Reiter
From: Tom Prince

It truly is mind boggling

In between Jodi's late-night discussions with Reiter, the reporters continued to scramble to confirm what the accountant was saying. Emily Nestor did not wish to comment publicly about what had happened. But soon Megan was on the phone with another young assistant, whose initials Reiter had provided, who had left The Weinstein Company in the summer of 2015. The woman's voice was shaky. But slowly, she started to explain that she had left the company "for moral reasons." Because she had signed a nondisclosure agreement, she was afraid to tell Megan everything she had experienced. Weinstein had preyed on her, bombarding her with solicitations for sex and massages that she repeatedly refused. She hadn't wanted to miss the opportunity to be part of such a highly regarded company, so she had worked her way into a new position that provided more distance from him.

When Weinstein demanded that she resume working for him directly, she complained to a top executive about assignations she was forced to arrange for Weinstein, hoping the executive would help keep her out of the boss's reach, she said. Instead, Weinstein himself called her, pressuring her to deny her allegation, submit a letter saying she had a "positive experience" with the company, and exit.

At the same time, Jodi was having eerily similar conversations with a former assistant named Michelle Franklin, who had worked in the London office in

2012. She was also very anxious about speaking and wanted to talk only off the record. Weinstein had never pressured Franklin for sex. But like the young assistant to whom Megan had spoken, she said she had to arrange hotel room encounters for "Friends of Harvey"—the same term Reiter and others had used. Like Rehal, she was charged with procuring penile injection drugs from the pharmacy, and while tidying his hotel rooms, had even picked up the discarded syringes off hotel room floors. (Weinstein denied their accounts.).

One day, as she had walked a young woman to Mr. Weinstein's hotel room, Franklin confronted him. "It's not my job, and I don't want to do it," she remembered saying. "Your opinion doesn't count," she said he responded. Soon afterward, she was fired.

On the afternoon of September 19, Megan got her own firsthand experience in Weinstein's ability to exert pressure, conscript others, and shamelessly pretend that problems did not exist.

For two weeks, she had been piecing together more details of how the $600,000 raised at the 2015 AIDS charity auction had instead, through a series of complicated transactions, landed in the account of investors in Weinstein's **Finding Neverland** production. Jodi and the editors were worried that she was pursuing a distraction from the larger target of how Weinstein treated women.

But Megan couldn't let go. She had confirmed that the New York Attorney General's office was investigating. She had obtained internal records showing that people inside amfAR had expressed grave concerns. In an email, the chief financial officer had written, "Nothing about this deal feels right to me." Legal experts were telling Megan the arrangement might amount to fraud. Even if he hadn't broken the law, Weinstein appeared to have siphoned off more than half a million for AIDS research to reimburse his own investors.

The story, Megan believed, would show how Weinstein could bend an institution to his will. The producer had maintained a cozy relationship with amfAR for years, helping the organization throw its star-studded fund-raiser in Cannes, France—the one with the splashy red-carpet photos Jodi had studied months earlier. David Boies had helped Weinstein silence amfAR's board when it sought an outside investigation. In a recent interview, Boies had walked Megan in a verbal circle for nearly two hours, with Lanny Davis and Charlie Prince, a Weinstein Company attorney, reinforcing the there's-nothing-to-see-here defense.

Now, Weinstein himself had arrived at the fourth floor of the **Times** building, determined to face off against Megan and beat back the story.

The interview had been approved by Corbett and Baquet under two conditions: first that it was on the record, and second that it focused solely on the financial transaction, not the allegations about mis-treatment of women. Megan was eager to push for answers but also to size up the man she and Jodi had been reporting on for months. Corbett would participate in the meeting to help keep it on track.

The producer wore rumpled clothes and walked with a slight limp. He growled hello, his voice low and nasal with an old-school New York accent.

Behind him trailed a posse. Megan wasn't sur-prised to see Davis and Prince. Another attorney, Jason Lilien, who had apparently just been hired by Weinstein, introduced himself as former head of the Charities Bureau for the New York State Office of the Attorney General. "I know this sounds self-serving, but I quite literally wrote the law in New York on these areas," he told Megan.

The presence of two other members of the contin-gent was baffling. Megan shook hands with Roberta Kaplan, the litigator who had successfully argued **United States v. Windsor,** the landmark Supreme Court case that had paved the way to federal gay marriage. Then Megan recognized a tall, striking middle-aged woman with dark hair and a strangely familiar face. She was Karen Duffy, aka "Duff," an MTV video jockey of her youth. Why had they cho-sen to be by Weinstein's side in a matter that they surely knew nothing about?

Corbett wanted to set the expectations clearly: The meeting was to stay tightly focused on the amfAR transaction.

But Weinstein, it became clear, intended to produce his own narrative. About his awakening to the heartbreak of AIDS, his extensive philanthropic giving, and his concern for the suffering of others. The visitors now seated around the conference room were his supporting players.

At first Weinstein's tone was friendly, if condescending. He began with a tutorial of how the world of charitable fund-raising **really** worked. If the journalists dug deeper, he explained, they would see that creative transactions like the one involving amfAR were extremely common. Everyone did them. You had to run charities like a business if you wanted to do good in the world, he said, pointing out that other money that he helped raise at the auction did go to amfAR.

"And legal schmegal," he said, spreading a smile around the room. "Our idea was to get people help."

It was time to discuss how much he had done to battle AIDS. He recalled first seeing the ravages of the disease close-up when the Broadway director Michael Bennett, of **A Chorus Line** fame, became ill decades ago.

"One day I get a phone call from his person saying that Michael's got pneumonia. And I . . ." Weinstein paused, as if to steady himself. "Okay, all right. I'm gonna get through this," he said.

Soon Weinstein was reading from an actual script, a written statement from a former vice president of amfAR who could not attend the meeting. Using the third person, he described his own compassion and generosity:

"Harvey came forward and said: 'Do you need help'?" Weinstein said. "We did, and he literally took over the auction, badgering people."

He appeared to choke up and struggle to get the words out.

"I'm not acting," the producer said.

He started again, stopped, as if he was overcome by emotion, and then slid the script over the table to Duffy, who read the rest. With tears in her eyes, she said that Weinstein had helped save her life when she was diagnosed with a rare disease. Now, she said, it was important "to represent the people who really can't talk right now," AIDS victims who had benefited directly from Weinstein's generosity.

Megan let them finish, then launched into more questions. Shouldn't people bidding on items at a charitable auction know where their money was going? Was it appropriate for charitable contributions to ultimately flow back to Weinstein and other **Finding Neverland** investors?

With each round, Weinstein became visibly annoyed.

Did Megan and Corbett know their own employer was taking money from outside nonprofits to subsidize investigative journalism? "Who gets the write-off? How are they doing it?" he snapped. He quickly swung from attacking the paper to expressing his devotion. "I love the **New York Times**," he said.

"My famous story is 1977, I'm in this snowstorm in Buffalo, New York, as a student, you know, a guy goes out, it's my friend Gary, 'What are you gonna get at the store?' He says, 'I'm gonna get Twinkies.' The other guy is gonna get milk, the girl says 'I want Cheerios,' whatever. And my famous—and this is a longtime quote, you can probably look it up. I said: "Just get me the last copy of the **New York Times**."

If there was anything untoward about the $600,000 transaction, he insisted, Megan should be pressing the lawyers who were responsible for it. And if the bidders of the auction hadn't figured out that their money was serving his business deal, well, that was their problem. "You don't want to make a donation to that, don't," he said.

Kaplan said that she served on the board of another AIDS charity and suggested that if the **Times** followed through with this story, it could hurt AIDS patients around the world. She did not appear to understand the underlying financial transaction that she had come, in effect, to defend.

Megan asked: Would Weinstein do this type of financial arrangement again?

"Not with you around," the producer joked.

"I think we need to wind this up," Corbett said.

But Weinstein had one last point: He wasn't just fighting for good; he was battling villains. The charity board members who had reported him to the attorney general just wanted to take over the organization to serve their own dark interests.

The Weinstein Company attorney tried to cut in, but Weinstein swatted him away.

"I'd rather go down with the truth," Weinstein told the journalists. "That's what I grew up with. I grew up with the truth."

Megan thanked the group for their time. For all of the theatrics, she was still going to write her story about the $600,000 transaction. She watched the producer leave, trailed by his supporters, and was struck by the display of this man forcing his way through the world, expecting everyone to fall in line.

When Jodi saw the group filtering out, she went down to the lobby. She had made a point of introducing herself to Weinstein before the meeting started, and as he left, she wanted to see him once more, to remind him of Lanny Davis's suggestion of a possible interview.

The producer was standing outside the security turnstiles, amid the usual mix of office workers and tourists snapping pictures of the **Times** sign. When she approached him, he leaned in to Jodi with such intensity that she had to remind herself not to show any signs of intimidation. She told him that while that day's meeting had been about amfAR, she and Megan hoped to interview him later about his treatment of women.

Weinstein started mocking that investigation to his retinue, describing the findings even though the reporters had never shared them. "Luring them to hotel rooms," he said dismissively.

Let's sit down and talk about it **now,** he suddenly proposed. "I'll tell you everything. We'll be transparent and there will be no article," he said. "Go ahead, let's do it."

Jodi declined. She and Megan would reach out when they were ready, she said.

He stepped in closer, and Jodi let out a nervous laugh. He hadn't done the terrible things that women were accusing him of, he said. He wasn't that bad.

He smiled sardonically, then said: "I'm worse."

The tactics Weinstein used during the in-person interview over the amfAR transactions were a guide to how he operated. Later, they helped Megan decipher what had happened at his company in March 2015, when the next and most perilous complaint landed, from Ambra Battilana Gutierrez, the Italian model. Emily Nestor and Sandeep Rehal had just left, but this allegation caused far more tumult than the others, because for the first time ever, a woman made an accusation against Weinstein in full public view. After going to Weinstein's office for a work meeting, Gutierrez went to the New York Police department and accused the producer of groping her. The news made headlines. And for the company, the timing could not have been worse: It was poised to sell its TV division to ITV, a British broadcaster, for over $400 million, a deal that would have served as a potential lifeline. Reiter, who said he had been promised a million-dollar bonus from the sale, was appalled—this was just what he had feared, a public mess.

The police helped Gutierrez secretly record Weinstein discussing the incident and later said they had been eager to see him charged with sexual abuse.

But the district attorney's office soon announced through a spokesperson that it would not prosecute, saying only that "after analyzing the available evidence, including multiple interviews with both parties, a criminal charge is not supported." Gutierrez left New York without giving interviews or otherwise publicly discussing her complaint against Weinstein, making Reiter and others wonder what had happened behind the scenes.

What almost no one knew at the time was that Weinstein had conducted an elaborate campaign to make the model's allegation disappear.

The criminal lawyer, Elkan Abramowitz, a former partner of District Attorney Cy Vance, was the public face of Weinstein's legal team.

Privately, Linda Fairstein, the famed former Manhattan sex crimes prosecutor, provided help too. She was in touch with Weinstein's office about the case and helped connect Weinstein's legal team and the lead prosecutor. (During the summer of 2017, when she had insisted to Megan that the model's allegation was unfounded, Fairstein had not disclosed her ties to the case. Fairstein said later that it was Megan's fault for not asking and that there was nothing unusual about her actions.)

Weinstein's private investigators went to work collecting records from two Italian court cases involving Gutierrez. In 2011, she had testified for the prosecution at the trial of Silvio Berlusconi, the former Italian prime minister who was charged with patronizing an underage prostitute. Gutierrez had described a sex party with teenage girls at Berlusconi's house, in which she said she had refused to participate in lewd acts. On the stand, the defense had pressed her about a sexual assault allegation she had made years earlier against a man in his seventies. Prosecutors had declined to pursue that case when Gutierrez refused to cooperate. During her cross-examination, she denied the original facts that she had provided in a sworn affidavit.

The court records weren't proof that Gutierrez was lying about Weinstein. They weren't even proof that she had lied about the older man. But New York prosecutors would later acknowledge they worried about how credible she would come off in a trial given the history that Weinstein had highlighted on her.

Boies and Abramowitz shared the documents from Italy with Ken Auletta, the **New Yorker** writer. Auletta had been contemplating writing about the case. But the lawyers convinced him Gutierrez was not trustworthy, Auletta later explained.

Rudolph Giuliani, the former New York mayor, had fielded one of Weinstein's first phone calls following the police complaint and steered him to Daniel S. Connolly, a partner in his firm.

After prosecutors declined to press charges, Weinstein paid Gutierrez a seven-figure settlement in exchange for her silence, with Connolly's representation. As part of the agreement, he also secured Gutierrez's copy of the audio recording she had made of him at the direction of the police.

To the company's leadership and others, Weinstein insisted the entire episode was an elaborate effort to blackmail him, but never revealed that he had paid Gutierrez a hefty financial settlement.

"She's a shakedown artist, she's done this—she did this to some older guy in Italy, and she went to Berlusconi's bunga-bunga parties," Lance Maerov, a member of the board, recalled Weinstein telling him. "And, if you don't believe me, I'll have Rudy Giuliani sit down with you."

In a final stroke, Weinstein drew on the power and resources of his own company to help seal his secret deal to silence his accuser.

On Saturday evening, April 18, 2015, the producer summoned two prominent female executives to Giuliani's firm. Gutierrez was present, along with her lawyer. At the producer's instruction, the two women walked the model through steps she could take to break into acting and boost her public profile, people who attended the meeting later recalled.

This was part of the deal both sides had struck: Weinstein would quietly arrange for career assistance for Gutierrez. For the model, it was a way of picking herself up and moving on. For the producer, it was a familiar form of leverage: If you stay quiet, my people and I will help you succeed.

That evening, Weinstein wrote the two executives an email of thanks, which Megan later obtained.

> I appreciate you participating in the meeting at Giuliani's offices today at 6:00 pm. I want to assure you that any financial cost to you will be paid for by me. You are totally indemnified by me and I appreciate everything you're doing. . . . there will be a $10,000 bonus for each of you, and my heartfelt appreciation.
>
> All my best,
> Harvey

No one had more incentive to hold Weinstein accountable for his behavior than Bob Weinstein, his brother and long-term business partner.

The brothers had risen in the movie business by relying on a bond that dated back to the childhood bedroom they shared growing up in a modest apartment in Queens. From the age of ten or twelve,

Weinstein had been a voracious reader, tracker of talent, and celebrity maven, noting who was on the late-night shows, in the gossip columns and the hot nightclubs. "Do you know Sinatra's in town tonight?" he would ask around the dinner table, the rest of the family incredulous at what the young kid knew. Bob was more inclined toward numbers, later remembering how the family had to stretch when its rent was raised from $86 to $92 a month.

When they launched Miramax, Weinstein commandeered the prestige movies, while Bob ran the financial modeling and built a lucrative business in horror movies and other mass-market franchises. In those early days of the company, the brothers often stayed on the phone with each other all evening, from nine or ten until one or two in the morning. Some people found Bob difficult to work with in his own right. He was socially awkward and volatile: kind one moment, lashing out the next. In his older brother, Bob found inspiration, creativity, and drive, comparing their relationship to a marriage, to the "ultimate friendship," to one long, rolling conversation, he said in a series of interviews with Megan.

But The Weinstein Company, founded in 2005, never reached Miramax's cultural or financial heights, and the brothers soon fought about money, Bob's more disciplined approach versus Weinstein's insatiable appetite to buy and greenlight films, rack up massive expenses, then buy and do more. Bob watched with concern as his brother grew obsessed with personal fame, eventually turning himself into a single name: Harvey.

He had also seen evidence of the threat his brother posed to women. Bob had participated in discussions about the confidential settlement that was paid to the young assistant who fled Miramax in 1990, two people familiar with the agreement would later tell Megan, though he denied any knowledge. When Harvey Weinstein needed money to pay off Zelda Perkins and her colleague, Bob wrote the checks. (He later said his brother told him the money was to cover up extramarital activity.)

But Bob regarded his brother's sexual behavior as just one more form of excess, he told Megan. In his eyes, his brother was "crazy, out of control—out of control with money, out of control with buying, out of control with your anger, out of control with your philandering."

One day in 2010 or 2011, the brothers were arguing about finances in a little antechamber near Weinstein's office. As Bob rose to leave, Weinstein punched him in the face. Several other executives were right there: Reiter, the assistant general counsel, the chief operating officer, and comptroller. Everyone watched as blood gushed down Bob's face. No one, not even Bob, did anything to hold his brother accountable for the violence.

By that time, even though they shared responsibility for their company, their employees, and the huge sums that had been invested in their business, Bob had decided that he was not his brother's keeper.

From then onward, Bob distanced himself from his brother. They technically co-ran the company, and the world still saw them as a team, but they communicated less and less. The bosses had already been working out of separate buildings. Now the distance took on more meaning.

Bob periodically considered splitting the company in two. He would sneak off to discuss the plan, code-named "splitco," with bankers, but the financial challenges were overwhelming, he said. Whenever Bob raised the suggestion, his brother would reply: "Sure we can split the company. I'll get everything, and you'll get nothing." Ultimately, Bob was unwilling to walk away. "I wasn't ready to give it up," he said. "Not so easy to start over."

His attitude was also colored by a private experience he rarely discussed at the office but that had come to define the way he thought about his brother.

During Bob's divorce from his first wife in the early '90s, he began to drink himself to sleep every night, he told Megan. Only with the help of Alcoholics Anonymous and Al-Anon had he been able to recover from alcohol addiction, and now he saw almost all human behavior through the insights he had gained while fighting substance abuse. He believed the bedrock 12-step principles: No one can change anyone else. People have to want to change.

Bob convinced himself that his brother's problem

was sex addiction, and that no one could stop Harvey Weinstein other than Harvey Weinstein. It was a convenient, and arguably disastrous, moral choice, by which Bob justified his failure to do more. He stayed in business with his brother but excused himself from intervening in his brother's actions. He refused to take responsibility or even help employees who came to him upset about his brother's belittling language or lacerating tactics.

"People would come into my office and say, 'Your brother's screaming and yelling at me,'" he said. "I said, 'Quit. You're talented.'"

That was what passed for his management credo. "Send a note to HR," he would sometimes say to his employees, even though the human resources operation at the company was weak and offered little recourse. "Write a letter."

But in the weeks after the public accusation from Gutierrez, Bob finally felt compelled to act. The deal to sell the television division was now dead, a major business blow. He feared that without intervention, his brother could do something else even more destructive to the company. Thanks to an accident of timing, he thought he had just the right opening: The contracts for the Weinstein brothers and other top executives were expiring at the end of 2015. Bob would seize the chance to ensure his brother underwent in-depth professional treatment for his sexual behavior.

That summer, Bob sent David Boies an email

containing a letter for his brother. In the email, later obtained by Megan, he explained that his hope was that Weinstein and Boies would come back to him with a "responsible plan of action."

Dear Harvey,

First let me acknowledge how pleased I am that you have begun, taking the first steps with Dr. Evans and Dr. Carnes towards addressing problems that have plagued you for many years. That is a huge start toward facing these issues sincerely and with the seriousness that they deserve for the first time.

From my own experience I want you to see in writing how your past actions have affected me. I only speak for me personally and no one else.

Over the past 15 to twenty years I have been personally involved with the repercussions of your behavior. The reason I state that is for u to truly see how long this has been going on and how it has only gotten worse over time.

There have been instances of behavior that I and David Boies have had to assist u with in getting out of trouble. I am referring to a situation in England. In that case and every and I mean every time u have always minimized your behavior, or misbehavior, and always denigrated the other parties involved in some way as to deflect the fact of your own misdeeds. This always made me, sad and angry that u could or would not acknowledge your own part.

Over the years I can if I wanted to list at least one hundred times, I am not exaggerating, that's five times a year, over twenty employees have come to my office complaining that they have been verbally and emotionally abused by you. They have reported to me that you have called them stupid, incompetent, idiots, etc. you were not speaking about their work, but about them personally. You denigrated these people as human beings.

I would defend you to them, saying you didn't mean it, or it would blow over, but I knew and they knew this was the way that you treated employees and it would continue. And it did and it only got worse. On many occasions I would tell these people if they could to find the courage to quit. These people had families to provide for and that was not an easy choice for them.

For my part I started to feel sad and

angry. I looked at you, as someone who had completely lost his way and did not value people as separate human beings. That u did not care about their basic right to have dignity.

I knew in my heart you were a typical bully, acting out of your own insecurities on those that were weaker than you.

I also began to look at myself and my relation to you. I saw my own weaknesses and co dependency on you and realized, I too did not have the courage to face you down. And I too continued at my own will to suffer abuse. I have begun to seriously address this problem in my own recovery. I am not waiting for your recovery to guide my decisions anymore. It is a hard and slow process, but I am getting better.

For the record you have physically assaulted me in your office and lied about it and minimized it as recently as a few weeks ago in Your therapists office, when I brought it up, u said u had told me you were sorry!! You said it with no sincerity or one ounce of real care.

See I said I'm sorry, so let's move on. I feel hate and sadness for you when you display that behavior.

Lastly would u ever hit your children

as u have me, would u ever call your children idiots, stupid, incompetent etc. or would u tell a movie star or financial equal or chief that. I highly doubt it.

There are other behaviors that I will not describe that u are aware of that need to be addressed.

You recently told me that anger was your real issue as if to minimize the other one. That is classic addict behavior. Creating a smokescreen to give up one behavior so that u can hold on to another "misbehavior."

You have hurt many people with this behavior as well. You have picked on people and used your power over them. You have brought shame to the family and to your company through your misbehavior.

Your reaction was once more to blame the victims, or to minimize the misbehavior in various ways. If u think nothing is wrong with your misbehavior so in this area then announce it to your wife and family. You told me in Bart Mandels office that u were ashamed of this behavior and didn't want anyone to know.

So slowly I have watched you get worse over the years to the point where

from my point of view there is no more
person or brother Harvey, that I can
recognize, but merely an empty soul
acting out in any way he can to fill up
that space and hurt that will not go away.

The reason I can say everything about
without any judgement is because I have
gone done this road as well, brother. I
speak from experience. I have suffered,
I have acted out and in the end I was
completely lost and defeated. And after
admitting complete defeat, that I realized
I needed help.

I asked for it and received it.

Once I got that help I was told that I
get better only if I continued to work at
this my whole life, and that if I expected
an easy fix or I could quit treatment after
a while that I would surely fall back on
my bad behavior. I have never had to
experience that.

So what do I want to happen. First is
that I want you to understand that this
letter and following request only comes
out of love and caring for my brother.

What I am asking is for u to outline the
exact nature of the treatment that u will
be engaging in with Dr. Evans and Dr.
Carnes etc. how many times a week you
will see each of them and for how many

years you are committing to your on
going treatment.

I would like to know if u are going to
commit to a group therapy plan. How
many times a week or month are u going
to do it and for how long a duration

I would like to have one talk or session
with each of these Doctors to explain my
experience with u.

I would like u to give me, David Boeis
and Bert Fields your word that u will
follow thru with your agreed upon plan.
The three of us know fully that we have
no power to make you keep your word,
we just want it for ourselves and for
you as a record to indicate that u once
gave it.

What I will not do, is share this letter
or commitment with any member of our
mutual families. I will not share this with
any business relation past or present. It
is between the three of us.

For my own self of self, I am advising
you that should you ever strike me
again or verbally abuse or denigrate
me that I will take the proper action to
protect myself and my family and my
interests. This is not a threat. It is merely
stating that I will exercise my right as a
human being.

As regard to other misbehaviors that do not affect our company I have no intention or care to police u or call u out in any way. That's not my job.

Please discuss the above with David Boies and thru him let me know what you decide. You probably won't realize this now, but this is all for your benefit.

More than anything I look forward to the return of that person that was just Harvey. I knew him when and I can assure you he was quite a great guy, all by himself.

Love Brother, Bob

At the same time, another company leader separately felt motivated to act.

The Weinstein brothers had packed the company's board with allies. Almost all of them were male—only one woman, the AIDS pioneer Dr. Mathilde Krim, had ever served, and she was not an entertainment or business specialist. Most of the seats were taken by wealthy executives from the finance and entertainment industries who took a hands-off approach.

But Lance Maerov, who had been appointed to one of the three independent seats in 2013, was different: He was supposed to be a watchdog. Maerov's employer, the advertising giant WPP, Goldman Sachs, and other major investors wanted him to make sure the brothers didn't rip off the shareholders. "Just make sure to keep these guys honest," Maerov told Megan later. "That's what my mandate was."

At first he had given little thought to Weinstein's treatment of women. He had heard rumors about the producer putting "friends" in his films, and Weinstein seemed to always have a young woman on his arm at movie screenings and other events, but Maerov believed it was extramarital cheating, nothing more. His focus was ferreting out financial misconduct and trying to address the broader toxicity at the company. "You would walk out of a board meeting and it felt like the most dysfunctional Thanksgiving dinner you've ever sat at," he said of the verbal brawls that erupted between the Weinstein brothers.

But when the groping accusation made headlines, Maerov, like Bob, feared that Weinstein might be engaged in a pattern of sexual behavior that could pose a liability to the company, and wanted to use the contract renewal to force the issue. He and Bob weren't acting in tandem; Bob saw Maerov as a threat to his own power. But Maerov was one of the board members in charge of renewing the contracts. In the process, he could take the routine step of examining Weinstein's personnel file— which would give Maerov a chance to see if it held anything questionable.

Weinstein refused to let Maerov see the file, with David Boies backing him up. Boies countered that he would review the file himself and report to the board about any potential legal problems for the company.

Maerov found the proposal ludicrous and was growing distrustful of Boies. Sometimes Boies said he worked for the company, other times for Weinstein, creating what felt like a conflict of interest when it came to potentially damaging information that Weinstein might want to hide from the board.

On the morning of July 1, 2015, Maerov received a secret peek inside the file anyway, thanks to someone who was trying to aid his efforts: Irwin Reiter. The accountant and two other executives sat him down for breakfast at the Four Seasons Hotel in Beverly Hills, and began to outline complaints of verbal abuse that had been made against Weinstein over the years. Then Reiter slipped Maerov several pieces of paper, Maerov later recalled. It was the memo outlining what Weinstein had done to Emily Nestor. Reiter and the other executives, who were taking a risk, were afraid to let the board member leave with it, so Maerov flipped through the pages at the table, finally seeing some of the information he had sought—and evidence of the exact type of behavior that Maerov suspected.

Maerov, Reiter, and Bob Weinstein all felt the situation could not stand. But four months later, in October 2015, Harvey Weinstein signed a brand-new contract that secured his power for years to come.

With David Boies's assistance, Weinstein had mis-
led, placated, and otherwise outmaneuvered Maerov,
Reiter, and his own brother.

For Maerov, attempting to scrutinize Weinstein
was like nothing that he had experienced in decades
of corporate life. Weinstein and Boies worked in
concert, alternating the producer's brute pressure
with the attorney's artful persuasion. At a movie premiere during the summer of contract negotiations,
Weinstein threatened to punch Maerov, according
to the latter. When Maerov complained, Boies responded in a tersely worded letter, calling the claims
"exaggerated," "a bit hysterical," and proof "that anyone who feels as you do about Harvey should not be
in a position of trying to negotiate with him." Boies
threw Maerov what looked like a bone on the personnel file: Rodgin Cohen, one of the most prominent corporate lawyers in the country, reviewed the
file and reported back that nothing in it "could result in liability to the company." (What Maerov only
learned afterward was that Cohen's son was a junior
employee of The Weinstein Company, seeking to get
his start in the film business.)

Maerov also brushed aside key information. When
Boies acknowledged to him that Weinstein had paid
settlements to women over the years, emphasizing
that no company money had been used, Maerov
didn't press for details. He also chose to disregard the
memo about Emily Nestor he had seen. He would
later downplay its significance, telling Megan that

it looked like a bad Xerox copy, or a scan of a scan, and that he had noted that it had come from the woman's colleagues, not Nestor herself.

He considered the matter taken care of, because in the contract negotiations, Weinstein had agreed to a concession. The company would put a new code of conduct in place. If it ever had to pay settlements as a result of Weinstein's misconduct, Weinstein would be required to cover the costs and be hit with a further series of financial penalties—$250,000 for the first settlement, $500,000 for the second, and so on, up to a million dollars, a whole fee structure for potential future allegations. The contract specified that Weinstein could also be terminated for misconduct. It almost read as if the company expected Weinstein to keep accumulating allegations and that the resultant financial penalties could take care of the problem.

Maerov's main concern was liability: He was trying to make sure that if anything went wrong, the company wouldn't suffer. That was different than trying to guarantee that women would not be harassed or hurt. Once Maerov felt assured that the organization was legally protected, and with some additional financial controls in place, he decided he had done enough.

Irwin Reiter didn't know what more to do. He had plotted with Bob Weinstein on ways to separate his brother from the company only to watch Bob lose his nerve. He had slipped documents to a board member to no avail. He was only working three days a week, and that summer, the company tried to bring him back full time, at double his salary, for a total of $650,000 a year. He refused. He was more deeply worried than ever: "There is almost no deal I wouldn't sign if HW wasn't my boss and there is no deal I would sign if he is," he wrote to a board member in the summer of 2015. But he remained at the company, working at essentially the same job he had held since he was thirty years old.

Bob Weinstein, who held the most responsibility, walked away satisfied, because his brother finally gave him what he wanted: a promise to stick with intensive therapy for sex addiction. Originally, Bob had wanted the requirement that his brother get treatment to be solidified in writing, like the code of conduct, and the series of escalating penalties. Boies talked him out of it, saying that Maerov would use the information to try to gain greater control over the company. Instead, Bob accepted a private promise, one that was impossible to enforce.

"There were many emails where he'd swear that he would do it, and he's going, and he always delayed it, which has led me to go, addict, addict, addict, addict, addict," Bob said.

"You start to hear this, you get worn down— you get worn down. They come at you hard with their lying, just nonstop. I got worn out. I said, 'I surrender,' see?"

———

Late on the evening of September 28, 2017, five days after Megan's article about the amfAR mess was published, Jodi again met Reiter at the bar behind Little Park. As the employees at The Weinstein Company had read and discussed the article, Reiter had texted Jodi, narrating the reaction from inside the company. He had not been involved in the questionable transactions with the AIDS charity, since Weinstein's theater business was separate. But he and other employees were riveted by the article, he said: They were finally watching someone hold his boss to account. (Weinstein continued to deny wrongdoing, but later, the authorities took action: Federal investigators in Manhattan opened a criminal inquiry into the transactions but have made no public comment about where their examination stands. The New York Attorney General's office wrote a letter to amfAR, saying the transactions raised several concerns, including whether they "resulted in benefits to private interests," and told the charity to strengthen its corporate governance.)

Reiter had already been so helpful, and back at the paper, the editors were already urging Jodi and Megan to start composing a first article about Weinstein. But the reporters wanted more—in particular, more documentation of what had happened at The Weinstein Company during those tumultuous two years, which could be published without anyone fingering the source. Reiter had mentioned a memo written by a well-respected junior executive named Lauren O'Connor, who he said had departed over Weinstein's treatment of women.

Without giving too much away, Jodi wanted to show Reiter that his mounting outrage since 2014 had been justified. A few minutes into the conversation, Jodi reached into her bag, drew out a printout she had prepared a few hours before, and passed it to Reiter. For all his knowledge about what happened inside the company, he knew very little about what had transpired between Weinstein and actresses in hotel rooms. Jodi explained that this was an account she had heard from a well-known actress. The text was just one paragraph, with no names other than Weinstein's, no location or time. It described how the woman had arrived, unsuspecting, to a meeting at a hotel with Weinstein, and to her surprise, been shown upstairs instead. When she got there, he was waiting in a bathrobe and asked for a massage. He tried to pressure her into sex by saying he could help her career. She fled.

As Jodi had guessed, Reiter appeared aghast. She told him that this actress was far from alone, that she and Megan had heard variations on this same narrative again and again, which closely matched the accounts by employees that had already been disturbing him. She and Megan didn't know how many women had these kinds of stories about Weinstein, she said, but based on what they were hearing, the number might be very high.

Jodi asked him again for the O'Connor memo. He had already read her a few quotes, which she had jotted down, but she wanted to understand the document better. Could he pull it up again on his phone? He started to read the memo aloud, then paused.

"I'm going to pay a visit to the little boys' room," he said. He threw Jodi his phone, open to the email with the memo, rose from the table, and left her alone.

After all of his indignation, his fruitless attempts to intervene, and the moments when he had thrown up his hands, the accountant was finally doing something irrevocable to stop his boss.

The first time Reiter had seen the memo had felt like a case of déjà vu. In November 2015, shortly after Weinstein's new contract had been signed, he had arrived at work to find colleagues huddled in an office, once again examining a complaint about Weinstein. This one was from a woman they knew and trusted: O'Connor was an up-and-comer at the company, respected for her taste and work ethic. Unlike Nestor, she had filed a long, detailed complaint, and it went far beyond one incident. Weinstein had said offensive things to her, but she was writing a much larger indictment, a portrait of how he treated women and how that behavior corrupted the company.

Reiter and the others informed Bob Weinstein, who read the document and agreed that the board needed to know about these accusations. Instead of forwarding the document—too risky—Bob dictated a memo inviting the board members to come to the office to read it in person, waiting half an hour before informing his brother what he had done.

After months of frustration, Reiter felt new hope. The next day at the office, he watched with satisfaction as Maerov sat at a table, looking over the memo. Maerov took photos of the first and last pages, noting all the witnesses and other details that O'Connor had included. "It felt very credible," Maerov said later.

But after that, O'Connor's complaint evaporated, just like the Gutierrez accusation. Reiter couldn't explain it. He figured that Bob Weinstein had lost his nerve yet again. He assumed that David Boies had stepped in to cover his client's misdeeds once more. Soon O'Connor was on her way out the door with little explanation.

Except the allegations had not disappeared: Reiter had seen the memo, and so had several other colleagues. Right after he read it, he stashed away a copy for himself. Nearly two years later, Jodi was sitting blocks away from The Weinstein Company offices with the document in her lap and her source on a very deliberate trip to the bathroom. **He's telling me, without telling me, to copy the memo,** Jodi thought.

She worked quickly, not pausing to read the

document, willing her fingers not to make a mistake. After a few clicks, the full memo was in her possession.

When Reiter returned to the table, his phone was waiting on his chair, and Jodi thanked him but didn't overdo it.

As soon as he left, a few minutes later, she headed for the bathroom to send the screenshots to Megan and Corbett. She didn't want sole electronic possession for one more second than necessary. In the subject line of the email, Jodi just wrote **Memo.**

Lauren O'Connor had sent the document on Tuesday, November 3, 2015, with an innocuous subject line ("For your records") and introduction: "As requested, I took some time to catalog and summarize . . ." Then she cut to the heart of the matter.

> There is a toxic environment for women at this company. I have wanted nothing more than to work hard and succeed here. My reward for my dedication and hard work has been to experience repeated harassment and abuse from the head of this company. I have also been witness to and heard about other verbal and physical assaults Harvey has inflicted on other employees. I am a 28 year old woman trying to make a living and a career. Harvey Weinstein is a 64 year old, world famous man and this is his company. The balance of power is me: 0, Harvey Weinstein: 10.

I am a professional and have tried to be professional. I am not treated that way however. Instead, I am sexualized and diminished.

I am young and just starting out in my career, and have been and remain fearful about speaking up. But remaining silent and continuing to be subject to his outrageous behavior is causing me great distress.

The rest of the memo was a detailed portrait of Weinstein's behavior, including an assistant's confession to O'Connor that she had to give him a compulsory massage:

She told me Harvey made her give him a massage while he was naked. I asked what happened, and she relayed that she was in the other room of the suite, setting up his electronics and when she went into the bedroom, he was on the bed naked and asked her to give him a massage. She told me she offered to have the hotel call a masseuse, to which he told her not to be silly—she could just do it. She said she didn't want to and didn't feel comfortable. My colleague told me she was badgered by Harvey until she agreed to give him a massage. It was horrible to see her so upset. I would have liked to report this but she asked me to keep it confidential as she feared the repercussions of complaining.

During the Gutierrez scandal, O'Connor wrote, she had to sit and wait outside Weinstein's sex therapy office. When a female "personal guest" of Weinstein's had to wait in a hotel lobby for an hour for a room, he blew his top at O'Connor, telling her she'd be better off marrying some "fat rich Jewish fuck" and "fucking making babies." On another trip, he acknowledged to her that he was a "bad boy" but tried to shush her with muddled logic: "We don't talk about it—can I trust you? I mean, I'm a bad boy but what's important is that I'm honest about it."

When O'Connor complained about Weinstein's verbal abuse toward her to a Weinstein Company human resources executive, "the response was basically—let us know if he hits you or crosses a line physically," she wrote.

Her most fundamental complaint was that her job had been turned upside down by Weinstein's upsetting sexual behavior. She had joined The Weinstein Company to turn books into enthralling films, so how had she ended up entangled in her boss's questionable sexual activities?

On other trips with Harvey, I was instructed by him to meet with aspiring actresses after they have had a "personal" appointment in Harvey's hotel room. Harvey instructed me to greet them when they came down to the hotel lobby and facilitate introductions for them to managers, and agents, as well as assisting in

casting them in Weinstein Company projects. Notably, only female executives are put in these positions with actresses with whom Harvey has a "personal friendship," which to my understanding means he has either had or wants to have sexual relations with them. Female Weinstein employees are essentially used to facilitate his sexual conquests of vulnerable women who hope he will get them work.

I am a literary scout and production executive. I was hired to find books The Weinstein Company could make into films, and my role expanded to handle production. Clearly, managing Harvey's past and present sexual conquests was never something I imagined being part of my job responsibilities.

Late that night, when Jodi, Megan, and Corbett read the memo in full, the moral stakes of the investigation suddenly transformed and expanded. What had once been a historical corrective suddenly seemed a far more urgent pursuit. No one had ever stopped this man. If the reporters failed to publish their findings, he might go on to hurt someone else.

CHAPTER SIX

"WHO ELSE IS ON THE RECORD?"

Friday, September 29, 2017

By morning, Corbett had already shared the memo with Baquet and Purdy. The secret document, from inside the company, which confirmed and elaborated on the pattern the reporters had been piecing together for months, was invaluable. They were looking at the situation from the outside. O'Connor had seen it from the inside. Her memo was like a key turning in a lock.

Corbett, Purdy, and Baquet gave the same instruction: **Write!**

But the team debated what to write. Baquet and Purdy, with the O'Reilly article fresh on their minds, were pushing for a narrower story, documenting the settlement trail, which they hoped to get into the paper as quickly as possible. They wanted to lay down a marker, because in recent days, Jodi and

Megan had begun to hear footsteps from Ronan Farrow, who was contacting their sources and had apparently taken his findings to the **New Yorker.** The **Times** team had little sense of his material or how close he was to publication.

Jodi, Megan, and Corbett shared the desire to break the story, but they also knew the material better than Baquet and Purdy. They believed the first article had to be broader and capture the power of what they had heard and documented. The sickening repetition of the hotel room stories. The apparent targeting of women who were new on the job. The terrible bargain of sex for work, and the long-standing silence of those who knew. Corbett pushed the reporters to write the story that the three women were beginning to see in their heads as fast as possible, while trying to hold back Baquet and Purdy.

That story would need names, dates, legal and financial information, on-the-record interviews, and documents. Jodi and Megan pushed aside the half-verified accounts and rumors they were still chasing and made a list of the material that could potentially be solidified enough to be included in a first article, with allegations of harassment and assault marked in black and settlements in red:

1990—Assistant at Miramax, New York.
    Settlement.
1992—Laura Madden, Ireland.

1994 or 95—Gwyneth Paltrow, Los Angeles.

1996—Ashley Judd, Los Angeles.

1997—Rose McGowan, Park City, Utah.
Settlement.

1998—Zelda Perkins and Rowena Chiu,
Venice, Italy. Settlement.

2014—Emily Nestor, Los Angeles.

2015—Ambra Battilana Gutierrez, New
York. Settlement.

2015—Lauren O'Connor, New
York. Settlement?

2015—Assistant in NY leaves for
"moral reasons."

A few days before, Lanny Davis had finally given Megan an answer, on background, about how many payoffs Weinstein had made to women: eight to twelve settlements. Megan paused, somewhat shocked that Weinstein's team would reveal such damning information.

Do you think that's **normal** for men to make so many payoffs? she had asked Davis. "I do," he had replied, in a matter-of-fact tone.

But they still needed a second source to corroborate those figures. They also needed to contact everyone who might go on the record, including former Miramax and Weinstein Company employees who could attest to the findings. Everyone the reporters planned on mentioning—like Steve Hutensky, the

Miramax in-house lawyer who helped negotiate the Perkins and Chiu settlements—would have to be offered a chance to comment. Now was also the time for them to let O'Connor know that they had a copy of her memo.

The draft would be a work in progress, nearly every line requiring negotiation, fact checking, adjustment, or deletion.

By Friday afternoon, Corbett, Jodi, and Megan were on a conference call with O'Connor and her attorney, Nicole Page.

Page did most of the talking. O'Connor didn't speak, but it was clear she was distressed that the **Times** had her memo and planned to publish part of it. She had never wanted to go public. She had tried to move on after the debacle of the Weinstein job, with a fresh start at a new company.

She was afraid that Weinstein would retaliate, and Page asked the journalists to reconsider using the memo, or at least to omit O'Connor's name, describing the stress the article would place on her. The journalists exchanged worried glances. The last thing they wanted to do was cause O'Connor trouble. She was young, not yet thirty. And she had spoken up for others who she believed had been victimized, becoming one of the rare figures in the entire Weinstein saga who had dared to raise questions formally about his conduct.

But newsworthy documents are rarely withheld from readers in newspaper reporting. O'Connor wasn't a source who had confided to the reporters with a promise of anonymity; she was the author of a critical indictment of Weinstein that had been circulated at the highest levels of his company and then covered up. Many publications omit the names of sexual assault victims at their request because of the uniquely private nature of that crime. But O'Connor's situation was different: Although she described verbally abusive treatment from Weinstein, the power of her memo came from her role as a witness, documenting sexual misconduct by Weinstein toward other women.

Corbett assumed control of the call, tucking strands of her neat silver bob behind her ear as she spoke. Her style was always to hear people out as neutrally as possible, and like Baquet, Corbett usually left reporters to deal with sources. But now she spoke for the institution in a way the reporters could not. The paper had to publish the memo, she said gently but firmly. No, not the whole thing. Yes, they could point out that O'Connor had declined to comment, to try to make clear that she was not the source of the memo, and to spare her from retaliation. Yes, the paper intended to name her as the author of the memo to establish its credibility. Corbett added that if Page or O'Connor wanted to make a further case for leaving her name out, they should.

Page did not respond, and her client remained silent. Page said later that the paper's decision sounded set in stone. The attorney ended the conversation saying she appreciated what the journalists were trying to do.

Megan had suspected the reason why O'Connor had not talked during the phone discussion, and with a few more calls she confirmed it: O'Connor had accepted a settlement too. She was legally prohibited from speaking.

Much later, Megan learned the backstory. Right after O'Connor had sent the memo, she was told not to come into the office. Within days, Page was negotiating a settlement with Boies and a Weinstein Company attorney. Boies said he helped craft a cover story for O'Connor: She would stay at the company a few more weeks to finish projects, working in locations that allowed her to avoid any contact with Weinstein. But her career there was over. In an interview with Megan, O'Connor later explained that the company's response to her complaint was: "How can we quickly make this go away?"

Six days after she had sent the memo, the exit agreement had been finalized, Boies said. As required, O'Connor had written a letter to Weinstein thanking him for the opportunity to learn about the entertainment industry, as well as this follow-up note to HR:

Monday, Nov. 09, 2015, 3:23 PM
From: O'Connor, Lauren
Subject: For your records

Because this matter has been resolved
and no further action is required, I
withdraw my complaint. Lauren

Jodi and Megan agreed the next move was to
contact Lance Maerov, The Weinstein Company
board member. In that first story, they wanted to be
able to demonstrate what they had started to learn
from Reiter about the company's complicity.

Maerov answered the call to his cell phone as he
was walking into his Park Avenue office building
with a cup of coffee. Megan introduced herself and
explained that the **Times** was preparing to publish a
story about allegations against Weinstein stretching
back decades. She read an excerpt from the O'Connor
memo, then asked: "What did you do about it?" The
cup slipped from Maerov's hands, spilling scalding
coffee. **How the fuck does she have those records?**
he later recalled thinking.

Only hours afterward, Megan was meeting
Maerov in Bryant Park in Midtown Manhattan.
Maerov, with his carefully parted hair and expensive
scarf, looked every bit the polished businessman.

Maerov explained that, yes, he had been concerned

about Weinstein's treatment of women, especially after the NYPD investigation. He told Megan about how Weinstein had called it attempted extortion and the board had approved a code of conduct designed to curb misbehavior. When the board was notified later that year about the O'Connor memo, he said, he wanted an outside lawyer to investigate. But within a day or two, Boies had informed him that the matter was resolved. "Boies told me the complaint was withdrawn," Maerov told Megan. So Maerov had let it go.

Megan nodded as he talked, pressing for more details. She suspected he wasn't telling her everything he knew, but what Maerov was saying was already valuable, especially if she could get it on the record. The Weinstein Company board had in fact been aware of claims of sexual misconduct against Weinstein and, aside from a written code of conduct, had basically looked the other way.

Maerov agreed to be quoted, but he told Megan that he had a duty to tell the other board members that the **Times** story was coming and that he had talked to her. She asked him to please keep quiet over the weekend. Once Weinstein found out they were close to publishing their article, he would intensify his efforts to stop it. She and Jodi needed more time. Maerov agreed to give them two days.

Before they parted, Maerov had a question. "Are you sure this isn't just young women who want to sleep with a famous movie producer to try to get ahead?"

Maerov felt some relief as he walked out of the park, he told Megan later. For years, he had mostly failed to hold Weinstein accountable. No matter what surfaced, Weinstein always wiggled out of trouble. "It was like watching one of those crime movies where someone like Al Capone keeps getting away with it; he's constantly one step ahead of the law," Maerov explained. Finally someone was closing in.

But Maerov, as usual, felt duty bound to protect The Weinstein Company. Back at his desk, he immediately broke his promise to Megan. He called Bob Weinstein and David Glasser, the company's president, and relayed everything she had told him.

Saturday, September 30, 2017

By that morning, Weinstein somehow knew the details too and called Maerov, begging him to help kill the story: "Lance, I know we have had our differences over the years, but can you just circle the wagons once on my behalf?" Maerov found the conversation so offensive that he took notes.

When Maerov balked, Weinstein turned to threats, he said. Years earlier, Maerov had dated the model Stephanie Seymour when she was separated from her husband, a financial executive named Peter Brandt. Weinstein told Maerov he had obtained a letter that Maerov had written to Seymour and would use it against him. The letter to Seymour is "disgusting," Weinstein said.

Maerov refused. His job was to safeguard the company, not the producer. And he felt there was nothing improper in the letter, he said later.

The next day, he emailed Weinstein a single sentence: "We need to discuss a plan to protect TWC in the event that Megan Twohey runs her article."

Meanwhile, Jodi and Megan were at their keyboards, writing. Jodi typed:

> Actors and former assistants told the **NY Times** variations on the same story, in some cases without any knowledge that others had experienced the same.
>
> Because he usually worked out of his [London] hotel room, rarely coming into the office, the women were often alone with him and there was little escape.
>
> Along the way, he enforced a strict code of silence, threatening women who complained, locking employees in nondisclosure agreements.

Megan wove in what they knew of the remarkable events that unfolded in 2015. Gutierrez's police report had never been made public, but a source had read every word to a **Times** colleague over the phone. Now Megan drew on that language to describe how at the work meeting, Weinstein had allegedly "grabbed her breasts after asking if they were real and put his hands up her skirt." It had never been reported before that behind the scenes, Weinstein had quietly "made a payment" to silence Gutierrez. When O'Connor's memo hit, "with page after page of detailed allegations," Maerov wanted to investigate, but then Weinstein reached a settlement with O'Connor as well.

By Saturday night, they had something resembling a draft to show Corbett. She created a secret file in the **Times** editing system, which only the reporters and relevant editors could open. Typically, stories were labeled, or "slugged," by topic along with dates of when they would be published, for example, 16TRUMPSPEECH, 07EARTHQUAKE, 21BEYONCE. Corbett slugged this one with the generic label 00INQUIRY, so that even colleagues who happened to scroll past the slug in the editing system could not know what the story was about.

Even as the reporters wrote, they were verifying—and to trying to expand—exactly what they could say about which alleged offenses, with which sourcing. Jodi and Megan had only one interview with an alleged Weinstein victim on the record: Laura Madden, with her account of her first meeting with him in Dublin in 1992. Because Zelda Perkins was still locked into her confidentiality agreement and

Rowena Chiu had not spoken at all, their entire saga shrank down to four short but crucial paragraphs, meant to show that there had been serious allegations and a settlement while still protecting the two women involved.

The assistant from 1990, the one Megan had found at her mother's house, was essential to the story.

In the end, John Schmidt, the former Miramax executive to whom Megan had made an unannounced visit earlier in the summer, confirmed on background that the former assistant had been paid a settlement following a troubling episode with Weinstein. He had agreed to speak with Megan, explaining that he had been impressed by her amfAR article. Megan had not abandoned hope that the woman would go on the record. But when she had reached out to her, this was the response:

Dear Megan,

I'm sorry but please do not try to contact me again, directly or indirectly. I have nothing to say, nor do I give anyone else authority to speak on my behalf. I do not want to be named or cited as an anonymous source in any article and I will take legal action if this happens.

Because her story seemed to involve a sexual assault, Jodi and Megan would not use her name without permission. They decided to simply refer to her as a young woman who left the company abruptly after an encounter with Weinstein, according to several former employees, and who later received a settlement. They quoted her old boss, Kathy DeClesis, who said: "It wasn't a secret to the inner circle."

Later, Megan would learn that the assistant had allegedly been sexually assaulted by Weinstein when she ran an errand at his home, and Schmidt would tell Megan more: that Weinstein had confessed to him shortly after the encounter that he had done "something terrible." "I don't know what got into me. It won't happen again," Schmidt later recalled Weinstein telling him. (Weinstein denied saying this.)

Next, Megan called Rose McGowan, who had appeared determined to expose Weinstein. But McGowan said she was not in a position to go on the record with her allegations against the producer. Weinstein had recently offered McGowan a $1 million payment in exchange for her silence, and her lawyer was encouraging her to take the money, she told Megan. She wasn't planning to accept it. But because of a host of complications, she was going to sit this story out. She said her lawyer had sent a cease-and-desist letter to make sure Ronan Farrow didn't use any of the interview she had done with him. "I'm sorry," McGowan said. "I just can't."

But at Jodi and Megan's urging, McGowan had obtained a copy of the settlement she struck with Weinstein in 1997. Remarkably, the one-page document did not include a confidentiality clause. McGowan was able to share it with the reporters without facing potential legal or financial consequences. McGowan declined to comment for the story, but their article could quote from the document, saying that following an episode in a hotel room during the Sundance Film Festival, Weinstein had paid McGowan $100,000. The payment was "not to be construed as an admission" by Weinstein but intended to "avoid litigation and buy peace."

Most of the former Weinstein employees whom the reporters wanted to quote were scared, fearing retaliation. Jodi and Megan argued that the story would include overwhelming evidence, that even after all these years, it wasn't too late to speak up. Most of them refused. ("I have a **life**!" protested one executive.) Another offered a quote: "Sexual harassment was often rumored, rarely revealed. Sadly, shamefully, very few of us had the courage or wherewithal to confront it."

But a few hours later, his employer, a major corporation, nixed the quote, saying it didn't want to be even tangentially associated with the article.

One of the few who came through was Mark Gill, the former president of Miramax Los Angeles. "From the outside, it seemed golden—the Oscars, the success, the remarkable cultural impact, but behind the scenes, it was a mess, and this was the biggest mess of all," he said, describing the producer's alleged offenses against women. Jodi and Megan counted his line, and a few others, as victories and inserted them into the draft.

At midday on Monday, Jodi texted Ashley Judd, asking if she could speak. Baquet and Purdy were still urging the reporters not to get hung up on the actresses. The crucial task, they said, was to break the story, and after that, they predicted, everything would spill out. It would be fine to get Judd and Paltrow on the record then.

Jodi and Megan disagreed. The Weinstein story had two strands: the producer's apparent menacing of generations of his own employees as well as of actresses who wanted parts. The reporters had the first strand well documented. Without the second— many actresses, even some top stars, said they had been harassed by Weinstein—the story would be incomplete.

Judd texted right back. Yes, she was in a dentist's waiting room and could talk.

For more than three months, Jodi had been laying the groundwork for this moment. Two weeks before, she had met Judd in person while the actress was in town for the United Nations General Assembly. On a terrace high above Manhattan's East Side, Jodi asked her to imagine what going on the record would look like and stressed that she was working to get testimonies from other actresses as well. Judd had listened carefully and said she wasn't sure.

Now the ask felt wrong. The story would be published just before the season premiere of Judd's television series, **Berlin Station,** a scenario that she had wanted to avoid. Worse, all Judd had wanted from the beginning was the company of other actresses. But even after dozens of conversations, those accounts had not materialized. Salma Hayek, Uma Thurman, and Angelina Jolie had not gotten on the phone. Jodi was still coaxing Gwyneth Paltrow, but she was still a question mark. Rosanna Arquette, who had also described a harrowing hotel room encounter to Jodi, did not feel ready to go public. Other actresses, prominent and unknown, had told the reporters Weinstein stories and sworn them to secrecy. The pattern that had protected Weinstein for decades—no actress wanted to be the one to speak up and name Weinstein—still held.

On the phone with Judd, Jodi didn't plead or tell the actress how badly she yearned for her to go on the record. Instead she tried to show Judd how strong the article would be: twenty-five years of allegations, a clear pattern, names and examples, human resources records, legal and financial information, and quotes from male and female employees characterizing the problem.

Even as Jodi spoke, she braced for rejection. Judd didn't show her hand. She promised to take the request seriously and call back soon.

A few hours later, a text from Laura Madden popped up. Jodi had been worrying about losing Madden. The speeded-up time line for the article had created an uncomfortable conflict: Madden's long-dreaded next round of breast surgery, a second mastectomy plus reconstruction, was scheduled for October 10. Jodi couldn't give Madden a firm publication date, and it looked like the operation and publication could collide. That was too much stress for any one person to take—but for the journalists, losing Madden would be a disaster.

But instead Madden was worried about being the only woman from the London office on the record. If so, she was out. She asked Jodi more questions about the article: How many women, how many women from this place, this office, this year?

Everyone wanted company, and understandably so.

Monday, October 2, 2017

Just after noon, the reporters filed into Dean Baquet's office to discuss the final step of the investigation: when to take the findings to Weinstein and how much time to give him to respond. After protecting the sources for so long, it was time to approach Weinstein and his representatives, describe the story, and share every allegation they planned to make public. Every anecdote, every date, every woman's name. (They would not mention Judd or Paltrow, who were maybes to go on the record.) Then Jodi and Megan would incorporate his answers into the article. If he denied the accusations, they would say so. If he apologized, they would print that, in his own words. If he refused to comment, they'd go with that. And if he could refute any of the allegations, those claims would have to be omitted.

Presenting findings was standard journalistic practice, the right way to treat any story subject, even a completely untrustworthy one. But the group could not settle on how much time to give Weinstein to respond. They would need to provide him with a deadline: Here's how long you have until we publish. But once Weinstein knew what the **Times** planned to publish, he could pressure women into recanting, intimidate others into contradicting their accounts, or try to undermine the accusers. He could leak information to another outlet, to blunt the story's impact, or preempt publication by rushing out some sort of statement of contrition. The journalists had to protect the victims—and the article.

Six people, all with some form of authority and some final responsibility for guiding the Weinstein story safely into the paper, sat in Baquet's office. Baquet was the boss, the journalist charged with supervising the entire, encyclopedic newspaper every day. The ultimate calls were always his. But Corbett had guided the project from the beginning, and Baquet relied on her in part because her instincts were a little different. They were in running conversation with Matt Purdy, who amid the tumult of supervising many stories across the newsroom was still keeping close watch on the investigation.

But Jodi and Megan as reporters had their own

form of authority and responsibility. They had gathered the information. They had the relationships with the sources. They were writing the story, their bylines would appear at the top, and they would take a great deal of the blame or credit for whatever happened.

The sixth figure in the room was David McCraw, the **Times** attorney. He was there to keep the paper out of legal trouble, so no one present wanted to reject his advice.

Corbett felt they needed to give Weinstein forty-eight hours, as much for the journalists' sake as his. They would be able to say they had done things right and avoid giving Weinstein an opening to say they'd been unfair.

To Baquet, that seemed like too much. Nobody in the group trusted Weinstein, but he was the most suspicious. His instincts told him that Weinstein was just going to run out the clock. Besides, the team figured that however long they gave Weinstein, he would take more time. This was a negotiation and the journalists had to start on the short side.

But Baquet also wanted the investigation to be irreproachable. At the start of his newspaper career, he had covered the case of Gerald Hatcher, a small-time actor who was accused of posing as a talent scout to lure aspiring actresses as young as fourteen into private meetings about their future movie careers and then raping them. The way Baquet had written those stories still made him cringe all these years later. The man was guilty, Baquet was sure. But he had been too quick to convict him on the page, he thought, writing in a way that was too sensationalized and melodramatic, without enough fair summary of the arguments for the defense. "It was even probably disrespectful to the women," he said later. "I always felt like everyone in the courtroom lost a little respect for me, including the prosecutors." Baquet wanted to expose Weinstein, but correctly.

Everyone, including Jodi and Megan, took turns arguing every side, trying to weigh which risk was greater: compromising an investigation by moving too quickly in the final moments or being too generous to a proven manipulator. When the reporters stepped away to write more, the editors were still deliberating.

By the time darkness started to fall over Times Square, they had made a decision. Megan called Lanny Davis to put him on notice: She and Jodi wanted to speak to Weinstein and his team at 1:00 p.m. the following day to share the allegations.

Suddenly the journalists were as little as a day or two away from launch. All around them, colleagues were taking the small steps that turn a collection of words into a **Times** article. They needed the right picture of Weinstein for the top of the story and the front page, and Beth Flynn, the photo editor, sent a selection. Should he be smiling, not smiling? On a red carpet? With a woman—**which** woman? Was it a problem if his wife, Georgina Chapman, appeared in one of the shots? Come to think of it, should the article mention that he was married, for the second time, and that he had been married when most of the alleged transgressions occurred?

Only one journalist could log in to the story file at a time, so Jodi worked on the article, then Megan, then Rebecca, then Rory Tolan, a second editor taking an especially close look at language. They were trying to find the exact right phrasing and were rewriting based on notes from McCraw, who had offered recommendations to fireproof the story legally.

Shortly after midnight, Megan and Jodi left the office and shared a car back to Brooklyn. For the first time, they allowed themselves to speculate on how readers might react to the story. Megan suspected that the board of Weinstein's company would be forced to act against him, but would the broader world care? Jodi cited Purdy, who in classic skeptical-newspaper-editor fashion had pointed out earlier in the investigation that Harvey Weinstein wasn't **that** famous. Perhaps many people would find sleazy behavior by a Hollywood producer unsurprising.

Tuesday, October 3, 2017

As they prepared for the 1 p.m. call, Corbett received a peculiar message from Lanny Davis:

Dear Rebecca:

This is a very personal note.
   I just learned about the Lauren email late last night and read it for the first time. Will do my best to do what should have been done a long time ago. I am not optimistic re. a statement. I am shooting for 1 pm today since that seems to be the absolute deadline. Correct me if I am wrong.
   In any event, I thank you for your consideration and courtesy— way beyond what is customary or even necessary.

   Lanny

To an outsider, the note might have seemed routine: Sorry, I got some of the documents late; I'm just catching up and will do my best. Translated into the language of journalism and public relations, the note read this way:

Can you believe that Weinstein hired me to deal with your article but never even shared the Lauren O'Connor memo with me? This is embarrassing, and by the way, that memo is powerful. Bear with me, I'm trying to get Weinstein to give you some sort of a statement to print in the story, but this client is challenging.

David Boies would be unavailable to join the call, but he was still trying to intervene on Weinstein's behalf. At 12:19 p.m., Baquet received an email from the attorney, who was pushing for more time for Weinstein to respond in order "to make the article fair and balanced (not in the Fox News sense, but in the **New York Times** sense)." Boies, who reiterated the claim that he was not Weinstein's lawyer in this matter, insinuated the **Times** should follow the lead of other media outlets.

"Three major publishers/broadcasters, including the **Times,** have researched this story over the last several months, and insofar as I can tell considered the same allegations and evidence," Boies wrote, in reference to NBC and the **New Yorker.** "One of the other two has said it has decided not to publish the story; the other has said that before they publish they will take the time to thoroughly review with Harvey the charges against him and give him adequate time to prepare a response. I would hope the **Times** would at least do the same."

"I'm not responding," Baquet told the reporters.

Just before 1:00 p.m., the reporters and Corbett settled in for the call. They had written out almost every word they planned to say. Foremost on their minds were the women whose names they would be mentioning. In the hours beforehand, Jodi and Megan had warned Madden, Perkins, and the others, saying: **We're about to go to Harvey for response, and we need to share every allegation** in the article with him, including yours. I know this sounds scary, but it will protect you and us, because we can say this is a fair process that gives him a chance to respond to the charges. We don't think he or his representatives are likely to contact you. But carry around a notebook just in case, and if you get any calls, write down every word. Any threats or intimidation need to go straight into the article. The only way to combat those tactics is to expose them.

The women had agreed, their final act of trust.

When the call itself began, Weinstein was joined by not just Davis and Bloom but also a new lawyer, Charles Harder.

Harder had made a name attacking publications that criticized his wealthy or famous clients. He had recently helped shut down the gossip website Gawker, suing it into bankruptcy on behalf of Hulk Hogan over a sex tape, in a case secretly bankrolled by the technology investor Peter Thiel. Harder believed that libel laws, which governed who could say what about whom in print, were too loose. The prevailing legal standard had been established in 1964, when the Supreme Court decided in **New York Times v. Sullivan** that a successful libel suit had to prove not only that journalists printed false information but that regarding public figures, they did so with "actual malice," defined as "reckless disregard for the truth." That was a high bar that generally protected journalists—too high a bar, Harder thought.

He had represented Roger Ailes in his efforts to beat back media coverage of Ailes's alleged sexual harassment. After he negotiated a $2.9 million settlement from the **Daily Mail** over its false report in 2016 that Melania Trump had once worked as an escort, President Trump hired him too. **GQ** magazine had recently called Harder "perhaps the greatest threat in the United States to journalists, the First Amendment, and the very notion of a free press."

On the phone, Harder was clipped and courteous, hearing out the reporters as they presented their material and repeating variations on "we'll get back to you."

His client had no such restraint. From the first moment of the call, Weinstein kept interrupting the reporters, intent on figuring out whom they had spoken to, who had betrayed him. Coming through the phone's speaker, his voice was even more of a force than it was in person, low, gravelly, and insistent, and he had a tactic of repeating the same question over and over. As Megan and Jodi went through the allegations, Weinstein tried to seize control with a stream of interjections:

"Who else is on the record?"

"Is there somebody on the record who said that?"

"Why don't you tell me who's on the record and let me respond to that?"

"And this woman's on the record?"

"And do you have somebody on the record who said this?"

He was so busy trying to grill the reporters that he did not seem to absorb the fact that the journalists had not just interviews but also settlement records and other documents, including the O'Connor memo.

Megan raised the crucial question of how many settlements Weinstein had paid out over the years. She had already heard the answer—eight to twelve—from Davis, but she needed a second source, and getting confirmation from Weinstein would be ideal. But when she cited the number Davis had given, Weinstein lashed out at his own adviser. "That's you talking; that's not me talking," he shot at Davis. "If Lanny spoke, he spoke for himself and not on behalf of his client," he said.

Megan tensed. The circle of people who knew about the settlements was tiny. Was that important figure slipping away?

When the journalists finished listing the allegations, Harder asked how much time they could take to respond. "Our expectation is that you can get back to us by the end of the day," Corbett said, as the editors had agreed.

"That's impossible," Harder shot back. "You've giving us three hours to respond to a laundry list of stuff going back to the early 1990s?" He asked for two weeks, which Corbett rejected, then he reduced his request to forty-eight hours. Corbett agreed to get back to him.

Weinstein's voice surged through the speaker again. "If the timing isn't good, then we will cooperate with someone else," he threatened, reading the journalists' fears that he would hang up from the call and go straight to another outlet with a softened, distorted version of the story.

"I'm not a saint," Weinstein said, "but I'm not the sinner you think I am."

He launched into a lecture about journalism.

"Get the facts right," he said. "We'll help you get the facts right. If I wasn't making movies, I would've been a journalist. I read every book on the **New York Times,** every book about journalism, and I read every newspaper and magazine. The journalists that impress me the most are the ones who go out of their way to be fair."

Weinstein went on. "When you were kids you grew up to tell the right story, to tell the truth," he continued. "You weren't about deadlines. You wanted to tell the truth. If you mess up and you don't tell the truth, and you write just to write, how do you look yourself in the eye?"

Finally, after ninety minutes on the phone, it was over. Corbett and the reporters sat in the conference room.

Corbett was thinking about how to shore up some of the allegations to further strengthen the story and that the paper should agree to Harder's request for more time. An expert in Baquet's thinking, after years working with him, she was crafting an argument to share with him about a new deadline.

Megan was mentally reviewing Team Weinstein's

reactions for clues about whether it had information that could refute or weaken the findings. Instead of addressing the grave matters at hand, Weinstein was asking questions that would not help his cause. He was fighting with Davis. He had been trying so hard to turn the tables that it was not clear how much of the information he had even processed.

Jodi was bracing for Weinstein's next move, certain he had a plan to use the information they had provided on the call to try to undermine the article. She felt sure what he would do: leak an item to the gossip pages saying, "The **New York Times** is trying to do a Harvey Weinstein story but barely got one woman on the record."

With one phone call, he could make the article seem like a failure before it was even published.

An hour later, Judd called Jodi.

The actress was as composed as ever. "I'm prepared to be a named source in your investigation," she said. She had thought deeply on the decision, gone for a run in the woods, consulted her lawyers, considered her obligations as a woman and a Christian, and decided this was just the right thing to do, she said.

Standing amid the neat lines of glass wall and gray carpet, Jodi lost it, like a marathoner collapsing at the finish line. She and Megan had spent months living in a state of suspense and responsibility. They would land the story or they would blow it; they would get actresses on the record or they would not. Weeping, Jodi searched for something to say to Judd that was equal to the moment but still professional. The best she could muster was: "This means the world to me as a journalist."

The rest of the team was standing down the hall in a cluster, and Jodi walked toward them, still on the phone with Judd, gesturing to say that she had news. Megan knew what was happening before Jodi could say it.

They celebrated by rewriting the story draft. The lede, or beginning, was Judd's long-ago account from the Peninsula suite, and the first section of the article ended with a quote of Judd's that was also a call to action: "Women have been talking about Harvey amongst ourselves for a long time, and it's simply beyond time to have the conversation publicly." By that evening, they had a new version of the article, with Judd on the record.

Meanwhile, Corbett prevailed: They would give Weinstein until noon the next day, Wednesday, October 4. That became the new target publication date for the article. Internally, the reporters set their clocks and expectations.

At nine o'clock that Tuesday night, the journalists were still at the office, eating takeout and sweating over the story draft. Their hum of anxiety was nothing compared to what was going on at The Weinstein Company, a few miles to the south, where

Weinstein was on an emergency conference call with Boies and the board. Maerov had insisted on the meeting, outraged that Weinstein had hired lawyers and Davis's firm to deal with a story that the board knew nothing about.

Boies did most of the talking. After years of minimizing Weinstein's problems to the board, he was suddenly more forthright. The **Times** story was coming, he told them, and "it's going to be bad" for the company, participants in the call later recalled to Megan. He outlined the conclusions, including the eight to twelve settlements, adding that the number could very well be higher. He didn't think Weinstein in fact remembered how many payoffs he had made to women over the years, he said. Defending Weinstein or terminating him were both extreme and inappropriate, Boies argued. The goal was to find a middle ground and present a unified front. "Guys, if we don't stick together, this is going to be like a circular firing squad," he said.

By 11:38 p.m., Lisa Bloom was advising Weinstein to acknowledge that after all their efforts, they would not succeed in killing the **Times** story. "We can nip at it around the edges—and we should—but it is going to run," she wrote in an email to Weinstein, Harder, Davis, and Boies as she prepared to board a flight from Los Angeles to New York to be by her client's side. Bloom's pitch: Weinstein should acknowledge that he had engaged in the core issue of sexual harassment, express remorse, and promise to do better. "I have often thought of Jesse Jackson, caught saying 'Hymietown,' asking for forgiveness, saying "God isn't finished with me,'" Bloom wrote in the email later obtained by Megan, citing the former presidential candidate's apology for an anti-Semitic remark. "Got my vote in '84."

Bloom, comparing the Weinstein allegations to a single comment by Jackson, proposed a statement to give to the **Times** that emphasized her own role and even her movie project:

"As a women's rights advocate, I have been blunt with Harvey and he has listened to me. I have told him that times have changed, it is 2017, and he needs to evolve to a higher standard. I have found Harvey to be refreshingly candid and receptive to my message. He has acknowledged mistakes he has made. And as we work together on a project bringing my book to the screen, he has always been respectful towards me."

Her message: She was the one who had helped Weinstein see the light. After privately working to help Weinstein foil investigations into his behavior, she wanted to publicly cast herself as the person who forced him to change his ways.

For his own self-protection, Davis had decided to stay in Washington, DC. By then, he could tell that whatever Weinstein did, the producer would not be able to wiggle away from the article's findings. Even Boies was pushing contrition.

But Weinstein was not prepared to give in.

That day, Weinstein had called an IT staff member over to the computer of one of his executive assistants and ordered him to delete a document called "HW friends," according to people who were there. (That was essentially the same term Megan and Jodi's sources had used: "Friends of Harvey.") The document was a list of names and contact information for women categorized by city.

With the help of Bloom, Weinstein also tried to pressure employees into signing written declarations saying they had enjoyed a positive experience at the company.

The next morning, Megan checked in with the young woman who had left the company "for moral reasons." She explained by text message that Weinstein had called her three times that morning, suspecting she was a source.

"I'm scared," she wrote.

CHAPTER SEVEN

"THERE WILL BE A MOVEMENT"

Wednesday, October 4, 2017

The reporters came to work knowing they had to tell Team Weinstein that Judd was on the record but fearing the producer would weaponize the information somehow—use it to delay the response further or, worse, launch some sort of preemptive public smear campaign against Judd in the tabloids. ("Eccentric activist Ashley Judd has been threatening to go public with wild accusations . . .") But it had to be done. At 8:40 a.m., Jodi called Lanny Davis, who took the news stoically.

The phone call with Weinstein and his team the day before had dealt a potential blow to the crucial finding that Weinstein had struck settlements with as many as twelve women over the years. But now that other executives at The Weinstein Company knew the **Times** story was coming, Megan suspected they might be angry that Weinstein had jeopardized the company through his actions. Maybe that anger would translate into an incentive to talk.

Megan called David Glasser, The Weinstein Company president, in California. It wasn't yet dawn in Los Angeles, but Glasser picked up, sounding sleep-deprived and frazzled. Megan told him she was calling because she thought it only fair that other executives be given a chance to respond to the **Times** story.

Sure enough, Glasser acknowledged it had been a rough night. There had been an emergency board meeting by conference call. Boies had spelled out what the **Times** was preparing to publish, Glasser said, adding that he had been shocked by what he heard.

Really? Megan asked. What was most surprising? Did Boies mention the number of settlements Weinstein had paid to women? Yes, Glasser said: eight to twelve. Could she believe it? What's more, Boies had told the board the number might be even higher.

Megan told Glasser she was eager to include his perspective in the **Times** if and when he was ready to go on the record. Meantime, could she use him as a source for the settlement figure if she didn't name him? He agreed. When Megan told Corbett the news, she jumped up from her seat and hugged her.

The journalists kept their eyes on the clock: The noon deadline was approaching. As it passed, Weinstein's team provided little more than a wild phone call, in which they sort of denied some of the allegations, rambled about episodes that weren't even in the article, and again protested that they didn't have enough time.

A few minutes later, Baquet watched as Megan stood outside his office fielding yet another phone call from Davis, who didn't have any answers. For so long, Baquet had refused to speak to Weinstein or any of his representatives. Now he asked Megan to hand him her phone. "Lanny, I'm sick of this shit," Baquet said, his tone harder-edged than usual. "You've got five different lawyers reaching out to us. We're not talking to five different lawyers. Get your people in line and get back to us with your response."

At 1:43 p.m., Team Weinstein's answer landed, in the form of an emailed letter from Charles Harder marked "CONFIDENTIAL / OFF THE RECORD / NOT FOR PUBLICATION." The journalists didn't consider that binding. Keeping material off the record required agreement on their part. But it was a fitting start to the letter, an eighteen-page exercise in intimidation, all of which boiled down to one message: If the journalists proceeded, Weinstein and Harder would sue the **Times.**

The core team reassembled in Baquet's office. David McCraw handed out printed copies so everyone could review what they were facing. "Demand to Cease & Desist and Preserve Documents and Materials," the subject line said. For all those months—and in the previous few days in particular—they had been waiting to see what stance Weinstein would ultimately take: denial or apology. Now they saw the answer on the page:

> All accusations by NYT and its alleged "sources" that my client engaged in sexual harassment, including toward employees and actors, are untrue. My client did not engage in the wrongful conduct that you are accusing him of.
>
> My client would likely incur more than $100 million in damage from your false story. Should you publish it, he would have no alternative but to hold NYT legally responsible for those damages.

Weinstein and Harder had another, more tactical demand:

> Because these accusations will have the effect, as you know, of causing considerable damage, if not total destruction, to the highly successful career and business that my client has built over the past forty years, and because you have been working on this story about him for several months now, and the alleged events go back more than 25 years in time, at the very

least it would be appropriate for NYT to
afford my client and his counsel with a
reasonable amount of time—we request
two weeks—to research these issues
and make an appropriate presentation
of the facts and evidence which **refute**
the many false accusations that NYT is
prepared to publish about my client. A
court of law affords a defendant at least
a year to conduct discovery and present
their case at trial. We are asking you for
two weeks.

Weinstein was going to fight. According to the
letter, he was the real victim, pursued by the **Times.**
The letter, seething with contempt for journalism,
conjured a dark alternative reality in which newspapers that aired incriminating information about
the powerful were violating—not upholding—the
public trust.

The letter took direct aim at Laura Madden, calling her a liar. "The accusation is false," Harder wrote:

We expect to be able to provide you with
documents and witnesses that will refute
this allegation, but it will take us time to
locate documents and witnesses from
25 years ago. You are now on notice of
the truth. Should you publish this false
accusation before my client has had a

> reasonable opportunity to locate and
> present to you further evidence
> (witnesses and documents) of the falsity
> of this allegation, will easily demonstrate
> reckless disregard for the truth.

That phrase was how a plaintiff could win a libel suit: by proving that journalists had heard their information was false and maliciously publishing anyway.

Jodi thought of Madden, somewhere in Wales. If Weinstein had any kind of genuine refutation of her story, she needed to know about it immediately. Or was he just gambling, thinking that this was just one woman with no power and little proof, and that his best bet was just to deny?

The former employees helping the reporters were "disgruntled, have ulterior motives, and seek to supply you with false and defamatory statements," the letter said. "You are on notice that your sources are not reliable; they do not have personal information; and they are seeking to use NYT as a vehicle for their wrongful and tortious efforts to defame and harm my client and his company. The publication of any such false accusations about my client by NYT will be with actual malice and constitute defamation." There was the possibility that Team Weinstein would try to publicly cast the gutsy ex-employees as bitter outcasts, losers.

In the final section, Weinstein and Harder took direct aim at Jodi and Megan:

> Please be advised that you are under a
> legal duty to maintain, preserve, protect,
> and not destroy any and all documents,
> communications, materials and data, in
> digital, electronic and hard copy form,
> that may be relevant to the dispute
> including without limitation all
> documents, materials and data that refer
> or relate to Harvey Weinstein, The
> Weinstein Company and/or any of its
> executives, employees and/or
> contractors (collectively, "TWC").

That meant everything: every text, instant message, voice mail, calendar entry. Harvey Weinstein was saying he was going to force the **Times** to turn over the entire contents of the investigation, everything the reporters were sworn to protect.

The journalists sat in Baquet's office and came to a unified decision: There was no reason to change a single element of the story. Harder's letter was essentially legalistic bullying. The journalists would stay open to whatever evidence Weinstein wanted to present, but to capitulate based on this letter was unthinkable.

McCraw reassured the group that the law would protect them. The world that Harder had conjured up sounded scary, but it didn't actually exist. "When the facts protect us, and the law protects us, it's hard to argue with our legal position," McCraw said later.

At 3:33 p.m., McCraw forwarded the reporters
a copy of the reply he had just sent to Harder, just
three paragraphs long. To the eighteen pages of complaints about journalistic technique, McCraw had a
simple answer: "Any notion that we have dealt unfairly with Mr. Weinstein is simply false, and you
can be sure that any article we do will meet our customary standards for accuracy and fairness."

In the final paragraph, he delivered his real
counterpunch:

> I note your document preservation
> demands. In light of that, please provide
> me with assurances that you have taken
> immediate steps to secure all data and
> records that may be relevant to this
> matter, whether in the possession,
> custody, and control of Mr. Weinstein or
> one of his business entities. In particular,
> I ask that you immediately secure all
> phone, email and text records of Mr.
> Davis, Mr. Weinstein's press
> representative, as well as the personal
> and business phone, email and text
> accounts of Mr. Weinstein; all records
> pertaining to any complaints of improper
> workplace behavior, whether in the
> possession, custody and control of Mr.
> Weinstein or one of his business entities;
> and all records relating to settlements

with employees, whether in the possession, custody and control of Mr. Weinstein or one of his business entities.

Translated from legalese, this meant: Harvey Weinstein, if you want to drag this story into open court, go right ahead. If you try to come after our information, we will demand even more of yours, including every single document related to your treatment of women.

The paper's one concession was to give Weinstein more time. Two weeks was out of the question. But the journalists felt they had to say yes to Harder's earlier request of forty-eight hours, even though it was painful to leave the material hanging with Weinstein for so long. Anything less could give credence to his argument about unfairness. The new and final deadline would be 1 p.m. the following day, Thursday, October 5.

Jodi and Megan were exhausted, but McCraw's response buoyed them. He had invoked generations of journalistic tradition, a court system that still protected the free press, and a country where, despite everything, the First Amendment was still sacrosanct. They also realized that Baquet was savoring each moment of the face-off with Weinstein. The rest of the world could not see Harder's offensive. But standing together against it was thrilling.

———

That afternoon, Jodi felt she had to try one last time to convince Paltrow to go on the record. Hearing from his former top star would be so shocking to readers across the world; even many of the reporters' savviest sources did not expect that Paltrow had a story of being victimized or threatened by Weinstein. Three paragraphs about her could rewrite the history of the Miramax years and give cover to so many of the other women who wanted to come forward. Jodi summoned every last bit of persuasion she had, pushing so hard that she worried the pressure would backfire, and that the star was going to tell her to get lost.

The two had been in near-constant dialogue for a week, in phone calls and texts, and Paltrow seemed to be truly deliberating. She had helped with the project from their first contact. But everyone close to her was telling her to stay quiet. Of course, going on the record sounded crazy to them: They were not on the inside of the investigation. Jodi could tell that some part of Paltrow wanted to ignore them, so in phone calls and texts, she continued to gently push.

But Paltrow couldn't bear the thought of weeks of tabloid headlines about her, Weinstein, and sex. She was still afraid the news would devolve into a lurid celebrity scandal.

She was also facing a private reckoning very different from Judd's, because Weinstein had played a far greater role in her life: "The most important man of my career," as she put it later. She wanted to finally call him out. But publication was coming sooner than she'd expected, and she wanted a little more time to sort it out in her own head.

> Since I feel underequipped to make
> this decision under a barrel, I'm
> going to hold.
>
> I feel sorry to have let you down. I
> really do. I'm so torn.

Paltrow's dissatisfaction with her own decision meant that if she did not join this article, Jodi wanted her to be ready for the next one; she could watch from the wings and then enter. Jodi let up with the texts for a few hours, and then started again.

From the beginning, Jodi and Megan had stuck to Baquet's rule: All communication with Weinstein had to be on the record. But around 3 p.m., Megan was informed by Davis that Weinstein was already on his way to share some sensitive, crucial information off the record.

The reporters were confused. He was on his way **where**? To the **office**? Should they refuse to let him in? They had to make a choice, fast: Weinstein would be on their doorstep in minutes, no doubt looking to smear his accusers without leaving fingerprints.

Megan decided to take the meeting. She wanted to know what he had, and the dirty trick of the impromptu meeting gave her another chance to square off against him in person.

Weinstein stepped into the lobby of the **Times,** with an unshaven face, bags under his eyes, and high-profile legal help by his side: not just Bloom but also Abramowitz, the former prosecutor turned criminal attorney who had represented Weinstein in the Gutierrez case. Bringing up the rear was Linda Fairstein, the former sex crimes prosecutor who had told Megan there was nothing to Gutierrez's allegations.

Megan led the group to one of the newsroom's small glass-walled meeting rooms along a heavily trafficked corridor, which put Weinstein on display for all of their colleagues to see. Office passersby lingered at the sight of the producer and his representatives stuffed in the equivalent of a fishbowl. Megan told Weinstein and company that they had fifteen minutes to talk, not a minute more.

The information the group sought to supply was nasty, dubious, and thin. Abramowitz and Fairstein painted Gutierrez as an opportunist with a sleazy past. From a folder, Bloom pulled out pictures of McGowan and Judd smiling alongside Weinstein, as if polite red-carpet photos were proof that nothing untoward had happened. Weinstein accused both women of being mentally unstable. At one point, Judd had sought in-patient psychological treatment for issues stemming from her childhood, and now the producer used descriptions from her own memoir to paint her as a nut.

Megan betrayed as little reaction as possible. This off-the-record meeting had clearly been an ambush, but it did nothing to undermine the investigation. With the help of a colleague in Italy, Jodi and Megan had done background checks of Gutierrez. They had also examined Judd's history, asking Grace Ashford, the researcher, to plow through her memoir, just to make sure there were no surprises that could be used against her or the paper. The only thing the meeting had done was reveal more of the tactics Weinstein and his allies were prepared to use.

The day got stranger. That afternoon, Jodi and Megan sat down to read about themselves in **Variety** and the **Hollywood Reporter:**

> Is **The New York Times** about to expose damaging information on Harvey Weinstein?
>
> The Weinstein Co. film and television mogul has enlisted an army of attorneys and crisis managers in recent weeks and has unleashed them on the **Times** over a planned story on his personal behavior, multiple sources familiar with the behind-the-scenes battle tell **The Hollywood Reporter.**

The story had few details but did mention the **New Yorker**'s efforts as well. **Variety**'s article was similar, with Weinstein denying that he even knew about an upcoming **Times** story. "I've not been aware of this," Weinstein told **Variety.** "I don't know what you're talking about, honestly."

"The story sounds so good I want to buy the movie rights," he added.

If the reporters had any remaining doubts about Weinstein's integrity, here was a final sign: He had just told another publication a flat-out lie.

The **Variety** and **Hollywood Reporter** stories meant that Jodi and Megan were on public display. The guessing games about who had spoken to them would begin. Sources would get nervous. The project was exposed for everyone to see, including the competition. Right when the reporters needed the tightest possible control, they were losing it.

"This is bad, gang," Baquet wrote in an email.

The reporters' phones and in-boxes began to fill with messages from people who had seen the stories in the Hollywood trade publications. Jodi and Megan barely responded. They were still too deep in the text of the article, reworking the lede again, targeting problem areas, and carrying out McCraw's instructions for further fine tuning.

———

Sometime after midnight, the reporters realized they were too depleted to be effective anymore. They had gone with little sleep for many nights in a row. The conversations with Rebecca and Tolan were sputtering in circles. Jodi and Megan gave up and shared a taxi home. About an hour later, Tolan left too. Corbett refused to pull away from the keyboard. They had fiddled so much with various parts of the article that Corbett wanted to stop to reread the whole story and measure what could still be gained and strengthened on the page.

Even under more routine circumstances, Corbett's reporters worried that she did not take care of herself. She never seemed to stop working—because many of her projects were secret, it was hard to gauge how much she was really fielding—and at times appeared to survive on black tea and dark-chocolate-covered almonds. Her days were frenzied, with consultations every few minutes.

But in the hush of a newsroom finally drained of activity, she was able to edit stories with real concentration. (Being "in the zone," her husband called it, acknowledging that his wife was temporarily inaccessible.) Corbett often stayed at work so long that the ceiling lights sometimes automatically clicked off, leaving her working in darkness until she got up and waved her arms.

That night, she sat and worked away, slowly making the words in the story tighter, clearer, and stronger. Sometime before dawn, she fell asleep at her desk for forty-five minutes. When she woke, she worked some more.

At 7 a.m., she finally stopped and left the building. She couldn't go home: Corbett lived in Baltimore, spending every Tuesday through Friday in a hotel room down the street from the **Times.** She showered and changed her clothing. Soon afterward, she was back at her desk.

Thursday, October 5, 2017

Just as Corbett was returning to her hotel, Jodi received an email from Laura Madden, who was now five days away from her surgery. The previous evening, she had stood in her kitchen in Wales and told her older two daughters, Gracie and Nell, that she had to share something. The teenagers assumed it was about the operation. Instead Madden told them what Weinstein had done to her all those years before and that the incident was about to be recounted in a newspaper article.

They looked at her in shock, trying to picture her as a twenty-year-old victim. "My mom is just my mom," Gracie said. "She's such a gentle person. The idea that people could be reading what happened to her . . ." They confessed to Madden that similar things had recently happened to some of their girl-friends: drunken boys preying on them, the young women unsure what to do. It was Madden's turn to be shocked. She knew these kids but had never dreamed of what they were facing.

In the email, Madden wrote to Jodi:

> I feel obliged to talk about the events that happened to me at Miramax as I realise that I'm in the fortunate position of not being employed in the film business and so my livelihood won't be affected. I'm also not one of those that have been silenced even though individuals under Harvey Weinstein have tried to persuade me to be silent. I do not have a gagging order against me either. I feel I am speaking out on behalf of women who can't because their livelihoods or marriages may be affected. I am the mother of 3 daughters and I do not want them to have to accept this kind of bullying behaviour in any setting as 'normal.' I have been through life changing health issues and know that time is precious and confronting bullies is important. My family are all supportive of my decision.
>
> I am happy to go on record.

Just as remarkably, Jodi and Megan were starting to hear from women they had never contacted who had their own Weinstein stories they wanted to share. For months the reporters had been pursuing women, aching for them to speak. Now they were coming to Jodi and Megan, finding them through the **Variety** and **Hollywood Reporter** articles, like a river suddenly flowing in the opposite direction. The journalists did not have enough time to do the reporting, corroboration, and response to include their accounts in the first article. They would have to wait for the next story. But the journalists took the messages as a silent rejoinder to Harder's letter.

At 10:30 a.m., Jodi gave Paltrow one final try. She was sitting in a makeup chair in Atlanta, shooting an **Avengers** movie. That day she was supposed to pose for a big **Avengers** class photo, with all the characters from the preceding decade. Instead she was feeling sick and barely able to get through her scenes. She even pulled aside Michelle Pfeiffer, her costar, quickly briefing her on the situation for one final round of counsel.

At 11:22 a.m., she sent Jodi a text.

> I'm on set in Atlanta. I feel intense pressure because of the time frame. I can't believe his response to the Hollywood Reporter, I can't believe he is taking this tack. I would have hoped he could have seen his way to contrition. I feel like he's setting himself up for an even steeper fall.
>
> I think it will be best to hold and then do something with you as a follow up.

This made the email that arrived from Davis at 12:04 p.m. especially puzzling. Weinstein's team had fifty-six minutes left on the clock until the **Times**'s deadline. But instead of focusing on the many allegations that would be in the article, Weinstein, through Davis, was pelting the reporters with questions about Paltrow, who he seemed convinced was in the story.

Jodi and Megan were dumbfounded. There was no trace of Paltrow in the story. Why was he focusing on an irrelevant matter? Had he never intended to give any response to the allegations at all? One o'clock came and went. Team Weinstein insisted the statements were almost finished, but by 1:33 p.m., nothing had arrived.

Baquet watched as Megan fielded yet another phone call from Davis, who once again had nothing to offer. Baquet instructed Megan to deliver a message. "Tell Lanny the deadline has passed!"

Suddenly, Weinstein himself was on the phone, asking about Paltrow. "Why shouldn't I just do a fucking interview right now with the **Washington Post** and get this over with, based on your lack of transparency?" he asked. "I will do that interview in the next five minutes unless you come clean. If you don't want to come clean, you'd better write this fast."

Megan and Jodi were back in one of the glass-box conference rooms. Outside, Corbett and Purdy hovered over Tolan's shoulder, reviewing the article.

"You want some sort of list of who we've spoken to for this story?" Jodi asked. "And if we don't disclose it to you, you're threatening us?"

"I'm not threatening you," he said. "If you're using Gwyneth Paltrow, tell me." However scared Paltrow was of going on the record, he seemed much more fearful.

"We're **not** using Gwyneth Paltrow," Megan said. He did not seem to understand: If Paltrow were in the story, they would have told him so and given him time to respond.

He asked twice more, then a third time. "If you're going to lie to me, don't, okay? Just don't. You're going to slaughter me anyhow, that's the idea of it. I get it. And you know what? I respect your journalism and I respect what you're doing. You're dealing with an important subject matter and people like me need to learn and grow. I get that. You'll read that in my statement. I've known when I hear something that's hidden from me, you know what I mean? I am a man who has great resources. Tell me the truth."

He did seem certain that Jodi and Megan had been speaking with Paltrow. Even months later, they never figured out how he knew.

Megan tried again: "Harvey, we have not robbed you of the opportunity to speak to anything that's in our story," she said.

"Are you talking to Gwyneth Paltrow?" Weinstein repeated.

A figure appeared next to Megan. Dean Baquet

was leaning over her shoulder. So many times over the prior few months, Weinstein had wanted to reach him directly, influence him, Important Man to Important Man. Now Weinstein was finally getting the audience he wanted.

"Hey, Harvey? This is Dean Baquet," he started. "Here's the deal. You need to give us your statement now. I'm about to push the button."

Weinstein interrupted. "Hey, Dean, let me tell you something about intimidation." The producer repeated the threat to give the **Washington Post** an interview, to undercut the **Times** story. Baquet had been a journalist for nearly four decades, run two of the country's top newspapers, and gone up against the CIA and foreign dictators. Was he about to explode?

Instead his voice eased, the slight New Orleans lilt returning. "Harvey, call them," he said. "That's fine. You can call the **Post.**" He sounded like he was reassuring a child. "Harvey, I'm not trying to intimidate you, I'm trying to be fair with you."

"You **are** intimidating me, Dean," Weinstein said.

Now Corbett and Purdy were in the room too. "No, Harvey, here's the deal," Baquet said. "We're trying to get your statement to be fair. Please give it to us now because we're about to publish."

"I **want** to give it to you," Weinstein said.

"Thank you," Baquet said, hoping for finality.

"But while you're on the phone this is my career, my life," Weinstein said.

He started asking about Paltrow again.

"She's not in the story," Baquet, Megan, and Jodi said nearly in unison.

"Harvey, I'm about to end this part of the conversation," Baquet said. "So here's what we need to do now, Harvey. We want to give you every word that you want to say. So say it. I also have a newspaper to put out. So give them your statement. I'm going to walk out. Talk to the reporters. Take care. Good luck." And with that, he left.

A minute later, at 1:41 p.m., multiple statements from Weinstein's team began arriving—the final elements the journalists needed to be able to publish.

On the phone, Weinstein was still making speeches ("Even if it costs me at the end of the day, investigations like this are important"), and Bloom was complaining that the paper had "a reckless disregard for the truth" and was going to publish "a hit piece" filled with "false accusations," which would soon be discredited. Corbett and Purdy had slipped out of the room without the reporters noticing.

Megan, who was scanning the statements from the Weinstein side, suddenly saw something important in the text in front of her and interjected. "Lisa, you said that Harvey needs time off to focus on this issue?"

Yes, Weinstein said. He was going to take time off.

"From . . . the company?" Megan asked, wanting to make sure this was what she thought it was.

Yes, Weinstein said, he wanted to spend some time learning.

"Learning and listening to **me,**" Bloom chimed in.

Weinstein was still talking, advising Jodi and Megan that they needed more of a sense of humor, and that he prayed every single day for the **New York Times.**

But Megan and Jodi were looking at one another in wonder. Weinstein was taking a leave of absence from his company. In the parlance of journalism, public relations, and business, that meant one thing: He was conceding wrongdoing. No one took a leave of absence from his own company when he was planning on fighting with full force. Suddenly, the reporters knew he probably wasn't going to sue the paper or even contest the article much.

Megan pushed him for more specifics on his plans, but he promised to call back later. "We have the Chinese newspaper to do the press conference with," Weinstein joked, wisecracking about his threat to take the story to a competing publication.

Megan laughed out loud.

"She laughed!" Weinstein exclaimed. "They laughed for the first time," he said to Bloom. Maybe this was the rough charm others had tried to explain. Or perhaps Weinstein was looking for one moment of dominance and control amid his own ruination.

It didn't matter. Megan and Jodi hung up from the call and fell together, laughing and crying with relief, esprit de corps, and sisterhood.

The reporters came out of the glass conference room ready to go. But Corbett and the other editors were already far ahead of them. They had been editing as the call was taking place, examining the statements of the Weinstein team, lifting out the crucial material to use, and transplanting those lines into the article.

Together, the written statements of Weinstein and his lawyers were baffling. Lisa Bloom's statement denied "many of the accusations as patently false," but she didn't say which. Weinstein's was vaguely contrite ("I realized some time ago that I needed to be a better person . . . My journey now will be to learn about myself and conquer my demons . . . I so respect all women and regret what happened.") In rambling paragraphs, he talked of working against the National Rifle Association and referenced non-existent Jay-Z lyrics.

"I'm making a movie about our President, perhaps we can make it a joint retirement party." It was the most inchoate, least professional statement any of the journalists could remember.

"He wasn't intimidating, really, he was just a screamer," Matt Purdy said. "He had a lot of lawyers. He had a lot of words. He had a big voice. But we had all the facts."

Now the two reporters and three editors lined up behind Tolan, who sat at the keyboard, all of their eyes reviewing the article on his computer screen. The old way of publishing newspaper stories was to send them to presses with giant rolls of paper and vats of ink, and then rumbling trucks, then newsstands and lawns. The new way was to push a single button.

Baquet, jumping out of his skin, thought the story was ready to go. Purdy suggested that the six journalists read through it together one last time.

They started at the top, with the headline:

HARVEY WEINSTEIN PAID OFF SEXUAL HARASSMENT ACCUSERS FOR DECADES

The article started by stacking three separate stories from the Peninsula hotel. The reporters had the reference to at least eight settlements, and the string of allegations they had worked to document, starting with the young assistant in New York in 1990, then Madden in Ireland, the terrible pattern continuing until 2015. "Dozens of Mr. Weinstein's former and current employees, from assistants to top executives, said they knew of inappropriate conduct while they worked for him. Only a handful said they ever confronted him," they had written. The article described the way women who had come forward had been shut down or silenced.

The team read every line in silent unison. When they finished, no one had any fixes or suggestions. At

2:05 p.m., only twenty-four minutes after Weinstein sent his statements, Tolan pushed the button.

Weinstein had not grasped that the article would be published right away. At that moment, he was in his office with Bloom, and other defenders, planning their next move, when an assistant popped his head in. "The story's up," he told them. Employees throughout the office became fixed to their computer screens, taking in the news about their boss.

Back at the **Times,** Jodi's phone rang. "I have Harvey Weinstein for you," an assistant said in a routine singsong.

"There was no sexual harassment in the room with Ashley Judd," Weinstein bellowed as soon as he got on the line. "There was no police report. This is a dead issue."

Jodi and Megan asked him if he planned to retaliate against the women whose names appeared in the story. They wanted that answer on the record.

"The retaliation is going to be about your reporting," he said. His joking tone from an hour before had turned more menacing, and then it switched again. "I'm sorry to the women too," he said. "I'm no saint, we all know." On the phone, as in the statements, he was hopping between denial and remorse and back again. How could the **Times** call his actions harassment, he wanted to know, if the girls had come up to his hotel room?

The final notes he played were of self-pity. "I'm

already dead. I'm already dead," he said. "I'm going
to be a rolling stone."

The thirty-three-hundred-word article triggered an
immediate crisis for The Weinstein Company.
Within hours, the company's board convened an
emergency meeting by conference call to determine
how to respond, according to notes made from
an audio recording of the meeting later obtained
by Megan.

An enraged Bob Weinstein and several other
board members insisted his brother follow through
with a leave of absence and more mental-health treatment while the company investigated his conduct.
But Weinstein pushed back, making it sound like
the statement he provided to the **Times** was more
show than substance. The board was engaging in a
"rush to judgment." In retaliation, he would use his
connections with the Murdochs to launch a negative story about Maerov in the **Wall Street Journal.**
Weinstein refused to submit to an investigation that
would "put me in jail." He would sell the company
before being pushed out. "I will not be railroaded,"
he told the board.

But after so many years of clouded vision and
compromise, Bob Weinstein finally had a clear view
of his brother and what the story meant for him.
"You are finished, Harvey," he told him.

In the following days, most of the directors would

resign without making public comment. But in this private meeting, their views were on display. Richard Koenigsberg, a onetime accountant to the Weinstein brothers, proposed that the company's board walk a "fine line: We don't approve of the behavior, but we can't be held responsible for what Harvey Weinstein did twenty years ago." Tim Sarnoff, of the production and distribution company, thought it would be impossible to disconnect Weinstein from the company Technicolor, and, as a result, the directors "need to protect Harvey." Paul Tudor Jones, an investor, sounded at times downright optimistic, convinced "it will be forgotten."

Even at that late hour, they sounded more concerned with the welfare of the company than the welfare of the women, which had been the problem all along. By focusing so narrowly on liability, they had allowed the problem to grow and ultimately destroy what they had sought to protect.

During that board meeting, Weinstein was already touting a comeback narrative, with the help of Lisa Bloom. They would win the support of women's organizations, forty, fifty, sixty of them.

"There will be a movement," Weinstein asserted.

That evening at 9:07 p.m., Bloom wrote a defiant email to the board, her conciliatory tone from her statement to the **Times** gone.

This is the worst day.
This is the day the **New York Times**

came out with a largely false and
defamatory piece, in a major violation of
journalistic ethics, giving only two days
to respond to dozens of allegations,
and then refusing to include information
about eyewitnesses and documents
negating many of the claims.
  Tomorrow there will be more
and different reporting, highlighting
inaccuracies, including photos of several
of the accusers in very friendly poses
with Harvey after his alleged misconduct.

Bloom was right about more reporting. It wasn't the kind she envisioned.

On the next day, Friday, October 6, Jodi and Megan began hearing from so many women with Weinstein stories that Corbett recruited other colleagues to help call them all back. Tomi-Ann Roberts, a psychology professor, said that in 1984, when she was twenty, Weinstein urged her to audition for a film and invited her to a meeting; when she arrived, he sat nude in a bathtub and told her she needed to disrobe for a shot at the part. Hope Exiner d'Amore, sixty-two, described Weinstein raping her in a hotel room in Buffalo in the 1970s. Cynthia Burr, an actress, said Weinstein forced her to perform oral sex on him during the same period.

Katherine Kendall said that in 1993, Weinstein gave her scripts, invited her to a screening, and then took her home, removed his clothes and pursued her around his living room. Another former actress, Dawn Dunning, said that in 2003, Weinstein appointed himself a mentor to her, arranged a hotel room meeting, laid out contracts for three upcoming films, and told her she could have the parts if she had three-way sex with him and an assistant on the spot. Judith Godrèche, the French actress who had refused to speak earlier, opened up about how he had invited her to a Cannes hotel room to discuss an Oscar campaign, pressed against her and pulled up her sweater.

Jodi and Megan faced a question they never thought they would contemplate: How many Weinstein victims could they actually write about?

After the **Times** article was published, Ronan Farrow was finishing his own powerful, detailed account of Weinstein offenses. Lauren Sivan, a television journalist, told Yashar Ali of the **Huffington Post** that Weinstein blocked her in a restaurant hallway, exposed himself, masturbated, and ejaculated into a potted plant.

Angelina Jolie's representatives arranged a time for her and Jodi to speak. Rosanna Arquette went on the record. And Paltrow was also ready to join the next **Times** article, about Weinstein's casting couch harassment, and how orchestrated it was—"meetings," business discussions, assistants, the promise of stardom as a means of predation.

"This way of treating women ends now," she said

in the new article that Jodi and a colleague were just beginning to write.

Lisa Bloom suffered through an uncomfortable appearance on **Good Morning America,** which appeared even more awkward when Megan later revealed in the paper that she had promised the Weinstein Company board publication of photos of Weinstein's accusers posing with him. By then, Bloom had resigned from Weinstein's team, as had Lanny Davis. Now Megan was pressing forward, determined to learn more about what Weinstein's companies knew about the allegations against him and when.

The only person who did not hear much of the escalating roar of reaction was Ashley Judd. Just before publication, she had left for the Great Smoky Mountains National Park to go camping alone. She had almost no cell reception, had made a vow not to check Twitter, and asked her representatives to deal with whatever inquiries came in. About once a day, when she got a few bars of cell service, she sent Jodi pictures of serene, lush mountain landscapes. Hiking amid the dogwoods and magnolias, she had only hints of how her statements about Weinstein had been received and whether the story had meant something to others as well.

CHAPTER EIGHT

THE BEACHSIDE DILEMMA

The Weinstein story was a solvent for secrecy, pushing women all over the world to speak up about similar experiences. The name **Harvey Weinstein** came to mean an argument for addressing misconduct, lest it go unchecked for decades, an example of how less-severe transgressions could lead to more serious ones. An emerging consensus that speaking up about sexual harassment and abuse was admirable, not shameful or disloyal. A cautionary tale about how that kind of behavior could become a grave risk for employers. Most of all, it marked an emerging agreement that Weinstein-like conduct was unequivocally wrong and should not be tolerated.

The aftermath, starting in October 2017, was like nothing Jodi and Megan had ever imagined. In the weeks after the first article on Weinstein, an overwhelming surge of tips flowed into the **Times** and other news organizations—a messy, unvetted,

alarming record of what women in the U.S. and beyond said they had endured. The investigations became a project across journalism.

The **Times** sexual harassment team expanded,
digging into the stories of restaurant waitstaff, ballet dancers, domestic and factory workers, Google
employees, models, prison guards, and many others.
When Jodi got a tip about the comedy megastar
Louis C.K., she and two colleagues documented five
women's damning accounts of his misbehavior, and
he lost the distribution of his about-to-be-released
film, the backing of his television network, and his
agency, manager, and publicist. The entire process
felt concentrated and accelerated: a trip from tip to
downfall in less than a month.

That autumn, women from every arena of life
posted #MeToo stories on social media, coming forward in new solidarity and of their own volition—
without the months of trust building or persuasion
required in the Weinstein investigation. Late one
night when Megan took a break from working to absorb the declarations on own social media accounts,
the sight of such posts from women she knew made
her weep.

The key to change was a new sense of accountability: As women gained confidence that telling their
stories would lead to action, more of them opened
up. The volume and pain of those stories showed the
scale of the problem and the way it had upended lives
and undermined workplace progress. Businesses and

other institutions investigated and fired their own leaders. Those consequences—the promise that telling the truth could lead to action—persuaded yet more women to speak up.

There were revolts in state legislatures over long-buried allegations. Swarms of protestors in the streets of Stockholm. The resignation of the British minister of defense. The instant professional evaporation of men whose power had seemed fixed: the television hosts Charlie Rose and Matt Lauer and the celebrity chef Mario Batali. Growing consensus that all sorts of previously tolerated practices were wrong: sexual overtures from the boss, corporate mandatory arbitration policies that kept harassment and abuse secret, and even smaller-scale behaviors like bra snapping in school hallways and laughing at movie scenes in which girls were taken advantage of by conquering male heroes. So much was suddenly open to question. The reckoning, and the feeling of rapidly shifting social standards, seemed like a sign that progress was still possible, even at a time of partisan fracture and nonstop conflict.

In its first few months, the post-Weinstein reckoning was mostly transcending partisan politics: Republicans had fallen and Democrats too. The offenses were universal and forced many people into self-examination. It felt like a fresh break from the depressing old formula that had dominated the public conversations around the allegations against Clarence Thomas, Bill Clinton, and Donald Trump, which were characterized by opinion split along partisan lines, and results something more like holy wars than true moral accountings.

However, the conversation was also circling back to President Trump's treatment of women, in an unexpected way. **Times** readers came to Megan wanting to know if he would now be held accountable for the sexual misconduct accusations leveled against him in 2016, and whether additional women would emerge with new ones. There was little evidence of that happening. Instead, she was quietly pursuing a separate path of reporting, which involved attending a porn industry awards show in Los Angeles, in search of a woman named Stormy Daniels. Megan was among the journalists trying to piece together a secret settlement that Trump had paid to Daniels during the presidential race to keep her from going public with her allegation of an affair with him. She marveled that these obscure legal instruments were now at the center of the public conversation; in the case of Trump, they might amount to a criminal violation of campaign finance laws. California was among the states preparing to pass new laws to lift secrecy from sexual harassment settlements.

The Trump and Weinstein stories were converging in other ways too: It was becoming clear that both men had used American Media Inc., the parent company to the **National Enquirer,** to help conceal damaging stories about women. In 2016, American Media Inc. had purchased, then buried, another account of a Trump affair. Around the same time, one of the company's executives had directed a reporter to dig up dirt on Weinstein's accusers.

So much was surfacing so suddenly, and so many people were asking: What had really happened in the past? What had been concealed? Who was responsible?

Seven months after their first piece on Weinstein's alleged misdeeds had been published, Jodi and Megan sat in a Manhattan courtroom. They were waiting for Weinstein, who had spent that morning at a precinct house a few blocks away being booked, fingerprinted, and recorded in a series of mug shots. The producer had already lost his job and reputation. But that day he would begin to face the ultimate accountability. He was on the defendant docket behind other workaday cases. Outside the courthouse, long lines of cameras were waiting, strangely reminiscent of the red carpets he had walked for so long.

With the bars of a holding cell momentarily visible behind him, Weinstein entered the courtroom in a posture of humiliation. His arms were immobilized behind his back with three sets of handcuffs to accommodate his girth, and he was led by two detectives, one of them female. The judge called the proceeding to order, and the female prosecutor called out the counts, her voice ringing out: "Your honor, the defendant is before the court, charged with two

violent B felonies for two separate forcible assaults."
In a terse few minutes, Weinstein was charged with
raping one woman and forcing another to have oral
sex in a criminal sexual act. He surrendered his freedom, in the form of his passport, before posting a
million dollars' bail.

There was no way of predicting the outcome of
the trial. Weinstein could not be tried for sexual
harassment. That was a civil offense, and though
many women had filed lawsuits against him, it was
unclear how those would be resolved. Some of the
most serious criminal allegations against the producer were not represented that day and would
never land in court because they were beyond New
York's statute of limitations. Other alleged victims
had thus far chosen not to cooperate with the authorities, intent on protecting themselves or pessi-
mistic about the prospect of conviction. Jodi and
Megan had not vetted the two women behind the
day's charges; they were among the dozens who
came forward after their story broke, and one woman's name had not even been made public. (Later,
prosecutors dropped a set of charges based on one
of those accusers, then added another set related to
a third alleged victim.) Sex crimes were notoriously
difficult to try, and Weinstein's defense attorney was
promising vindication.

But after nearly fifty years of alleged misdeeds,
prosecutors finally had Weinstein in their sights.
"He's now experiencing all the things he's put

everybody else through," Cynthia Burr, who had accused Weinstein of forcing her into oral sex in the 1970s, told the **Times.** "Humiliation, worthlessness, fear, weakness, aloneness, loss, suffering and embarrassment. And it's only the beginning for him."

In the final moments of his day in court, Weinstein was given a bulky electronic ankle bracelet to monitor his whereabouts. He protested, fighting the inevitable, then gave up: What choice did he have? When he exited the courtroom, Weinstein looked dazed, as if he was still absorbing what had happened.

As spring turned to summer, Jodi and Megan began to focus on a new question: how much was truly changing, and whether it was too much or not nearly enough.

The old rules on sex and power had been partly swept away, but it was not clear what the new ones would or should be. There was little agreement, and rancorous debate, over what behaviors were under scrutiny, how to know what to believe, and what accountability should look like. Years before, Tarana Burke had started the #MeToo movement to promote empathy and healing for victims of sexual violence, but now that label was being used as a catchall for a huge range of complaints, from verbal abuse to uncomfortable dates, many of which lacked the clarity of workplace or criminal violations. Earlier that year, babe.net, an online magazine, published an article accusing the comedian Aziz Ansari of behaving badly in a private romantic situation. But it was hard to tell whether his behavior was just overeager and clueless or worse.

That story was based entirely on one incident, recounted by an anonymous accuser, highlighting another dilemma: Though many publications continued to publish exposés based on in-depth investigation and on-the-record evidence, others were running stories that relied on a single source or unnamed accusers, much lower standards. Once published, some of those stories flushed out additional allegations and more evidence of wrongdoing. But other stories appeared thin and one-sided, raising questions of fairness to those facing accusations. So did allegations leveled on social media without any backup or response from the accused.

"Believe Women" grew into one of the catchphrases of the day. Jodi and Megan were sympathetic to the spirit behind that imperative: They had spent their careers getting women's stories into print. But the obligation of journalists was to scrutinize, verify, check, and question information. (A former editor of Megan's displayed a sign on his desk that read: IF YOUR MOTHER TELLS YOU SHE LOVES YOU, CHECK IT OUT.) The Weinstein story had impact in part because it had achieved something that, in 2018, seemed rare and precious: broad consensus on the facts.

Accountability was easy to insist on, but in some cases, much trickier to assign. Democrats were split over the case of Senator Al Franken of Minnesota, who resigned in January over a variety of incidents that mostly dated from before he took office. Some of the allegations involved unwanted kissing, but others seemed like jokey gestures that stemmed from his comedy background. Many companies, mindful of the lessons of The Weinstein Company's failures to act, started boasting of zero tolerance policies, but for what: An unwelcome hand placed on a back? A stray drunken comment at a holiday party? More and more critics were complaining that men were becoming the victims.

Even Weinstein's then attorney, Benjamin Brafman, seized on the criticism. In June, a month after Weinstein was charged, Brafman gave a radio interview in which he articulated the rising sense of grievance. He argued that the charges against Weinstein were just another way in which the #MeToo movement was becoming a witch hunt, a moral panic. Because of women making exaggerated claims, it was "proving to be so over the top" that it had lost "some of its own credibility," becoming so extreme that officemates now feared telling "an attractive associate that they're wearing a nice outfit." Instead of addressing the strength of the overall complaints against Weinstein, he seemed to be using the most strained #MeToo claims to sow doubt.

As the backlash developed, others argued that the changes hadn't gone nearly far enough. Social attitudes were shifting, and there were dramatic accusatory headlines almost daily, but the fundamentals were still largely the same. Sexual harassment laws largely were outdated and spottily enforced, and aside from some revisions in a few states, they did not appear likely to change anytime soon. Secret settlements were still being paid—in fact, some lawyers said the dollar amounts were higher than ever—allowing predators to remain hidden. Race and class often had an outsized influence on how cases were handled.

Jodi reported on low-income workers, whose experiences suggested little had shifted structurally. Most of the employers she called, from Walmart to Subway, said their long-standing policies were just fine. Many of the workers she spoke to were inspired and angry: They had watched the actors speak up and felt connected to the experiences of those distant celebrity figures. But they felt unclear about whether they had any avenue for addressing the problem.

Kim Lawson, a twenty-five-year-old McDonald's employee in Kansas City, Missouri, told Jodi that she had been harassed in two settings, the first time around 2015 at the run-down studio apartment she shared with her young daughter. Her landlord had repeatedly hit on her, and as she turned him down, he had raised the rent four times, until it was beyond what she could pay. With nowhere to live, Lawson had reluctantly decided to send her toddler, Faith, to reside with her mother, who lived four hours away.

A few months before she became homeless, she

had managed to get a new job at McDonald's. But soon after Lawson had started, she said, she faced similar predatory treatment: One coworker stood far too close to her, so that every time she turned around, she couldn't help but brush against him. She had asked the general manager to admonish him, but he didn't stop. Soon one of the shift supervisors started bothering her too, making comments like "You are a chocolate drop" and "You should leave your boyfriend." She hadn't known what options or recourse she had in the situation with the landlord, and when she and Jodi spoke, it hadn't been clear to Lawson what more she could do about the work problems either. As far as she could tell, McDonald's had no sexual harassment training. (It did, but company officials later acknowledged that it didn't reach many employees.) She didn't know how to reach anyone at the parent company for help, and had feared that doing so would trigger retaliation.

"I have no idea of any number to call," Lawson told Jodi. "I don't know if there's anyone else I could talk to."

Jodi and Megan were hearing these sorts of questions—Who do I contact? What process do I follow?—from numerous women of all backgrounds. The reporters' mobile numbers and email addresses had been passed around, and every day, they were contacted about experiences of harassment, violence, and quiet suffering. On uncomfortable phone calls, women begged Jodi and Megan to investigate their cases; certain that, if they were to write something, it could create some sort of justice.

But there were too many alleged victims of Weinstein, and many other perpetrators, to ever possibly write about. The reporters stumbled trying to explain that the paper was overwhelmed with stories of abuse, that not all could be told, and that even the nation's most powerful publications could not bear the entire weight of the reckoning. Journalists had stepped in when the system failed, but that wasn't a permanent solution.

In a way, those who felt #MeToo had not gone far enough and those who protested that it was going too far were saying some of the same things: There was a lack of process or clear enough rules. The public did not fully agree on the precise meaning of words like **harassment** or **assault,** let alone how businesses or schools should investigate or punish them. Everyone from corporate boards to friends in bars seemed to be struggling to devise their own new guidelines, which made for fascinating conversation but also a kind of overall chaos. It was not clear how the country would ever agree on effective new standards or resolve the ocean of outstanding complaints.

Instead, the feelings of unfairness on both sides just continued to mount.

On a Saturday afternoon in early August, Jodi received an urgent text. The attorney Debra Katz, who specialized in sexual harassment, employment issues, and whistleblowing, wanted to speak immediately. No, it couldn't wait an hour.

In the course of their reporter-source relationship, Jodi had turned to Katz for legal analysis, quoted her in articles, and talked to her about Irwin Reiter, who was now one of her clients. This time when Jodi dialed her number, Katz's voice took on a this-is-complicated tone. She wanted to talk about a new client who might be a potential story. But this was all off the record, she said.

Just a few days before, she had started representing a woman who said she had been attacked by Judge Brett Kavanaugh, Trump's Supreme Court nominee. The two had been in high school at the time in suburban Maryland. According to Katz's client, a drunken Kavanaugh had pushed her into a bedroom during a party with the help of a friend, locked the door, pinned her down, grinded against her, and covered her mouth when she tried to yell. The client said she managed to get away, but that encounter had caused her anguish and anxiety ever since, Katz said.

There was not a lot of corroboration of the alleged assault, Katz said. The woman hadn't told anyone at the time. In recent years, she had discussed the matter with her husband and a few friends—they were still sorting out which. She had also told therapists. Some of the particulars had faded: She didn't know precisely when it happened or some other details.

She had already passed a lie detector test Katz had arranged, and she seemed to be mentally preparing to tell her story more widely.

This was the most worried the lawyer had ever sounded to Jodi. She described her client as a research scientist who was careful and precise, who had no reason to fabricate something. But, she continued, the woman had none of the armor that came from being in public life. She was so earnest about sharing her story and didn't seem to grasp how utterly torn apart she, her family, and her life could be. Weeks before she had spoken with Katz, the woman had written a letter with her account to an elected official. That document could easily be leaked, Katz said. If that happened, the attorney wasn't sure how the country would react.

Katz was calling for two reasons. She wanted to tip off the **Times** to do more digging on Kavanaugh's treatment of women, to see if there was a pattern of misbehavior.

She also raised the prospect of her client telling her story to Jodi and Megan in the **Times,** getting ahead of any possible leak. Her client had sent a tip to the **Washington Post** and spoken with a reporter there, but it wasn't clear if the **Post** was moving on the story.

Jodi suggested the first step was for her to talk to the client, off the record, to hear the story firsthand. Katz agreed and also warned: Don't try to figure out this woman's identity on your own or show up on her doorstep. She's frightened and surprise tactics will backfire.

As soon as Jodi hung up, she texted Corbett and Megan: "Need to talk to you asap. Kavanaugh, assault."

From that very first, nameless sketch, the scenario that Katz had described summoned some of the most complicated and unresolved issues in the #MeToo conversation: The dilemmas of how to deal with painful incidents from the past. The challenges of coming up with fair processes for accusers to complain and the accused to respond. The debates over accountability: If this woman's story was true, should job candidates be judged based on something they did in high school?

Had a novelist tried to conjure a scenario to capture the swirl of strong feelings around #MeToo, it would have been hard to write one more flammable. The lack of corroborating evidence from the time of the alleged assault meant that the facts were probably going to be in dispute. If Katz's client went public with her allegation, some people would regard it as a serious attack, even criminal, but others were likely to dismiss it as drunken horseplay. At the time of the encounter, Kavanaugh had been a teenager at a private party, so this was very different from the workplace complaints at the heart of the Weinstein investigation. Then again, she was describing behavior that could be relevant as he was considered for one of the most influential jobs in the country, in which he would help make far-reaching decisions, including about the lives of women and girls.

If this allegation went public, it could be a return to the experience of Anita Hill's testimony in 1991 at Clarence Thomas's hearings. All of this would play out in Trump's Washington, with the retirement of the court's swing justice, at a time when Democrats were enraged by Republicans who had denied President Obama his final pick, and via a nomination process that had been fully politicized long before Trump's election. A Justice Kavanaugh could rule on abortion, perhaps still the single most divisive issue in an utterly divided country. Because the midterm elections were approaching, the political consequences of this woman coming forward could be profound.

Corbett quietly shared the tip with several editors at the paper. Reporters had already been checking into Kavanaugh's interactions with women, but she asked a small group to focus even further and to prepare for the likelihood that an accusation could surface at any moment.

Her name was Christine Blasey Ford. At the beginning of the summer of 2018, she was an established scientific researcher, an independent thinker, and a mother of two sons, who had not fully tuned in to #MeToo news and debate. She had expected that the next couple months of her life would be filled with controversy, because of a paper she and her colleagues were about to publish about the anti-depressant effects of the drug ketamine.

Washington, DC, figured in her life mainly as a place she had rejected. She had grown up in the same preppy, privileged suburban circles as Kavanaugh. But she had fled that world back in her twenties for California and immersion in the science of the brain. At fifty-one, she was a professor of psychology and a biostatistician at a consortium made up of professors from Palo Alto and Stanford. Twitter was a foreign land to her. She was a casual Democrat who had made a few campaign contributions here and there, including one to Bernie Sanders, but had little affinity for the pinball dynamics of national politics. Like her peers, she wrote her papers in a language of high science that most people would barely understand. Her name had appeared on studies on trauma, depression, and resilience, but her memories of the attack she had described had never been front and center in her life.

She hadn't known much about what happened to Kavanaugh until 2012, when she happened to read on the internet that George W. Bush had attended his wedding. For the first time, she realized how high Kavanaugh had risen in his legal career. It wasn't unusual for people from her high school crowd to ascend to prestigious positions. "That was the moment when I thought, 'I wonder if he'll be nominated to the Supreme Court,'" she later recalled in a series of interviews.

That same year, she and her husband had gone to counseling for help with communication issues, including resolving some fights that lingered from remodeling their Palo Alto house a few years earlier. Ford had insisted that they build a second front door, explaining that she would feel trapped without it, much to her husband's frustration. At the therapist's urging, Ford for the first time told her husband that in high school, she had been trapped in a room and physically restrained by a boy who molested her while another boy watched. This was why she needed multiple exit routes.

"She said she was eventually able to escape before she was raped, but that the experience was very traumatic because she felt like she had no control and was physically dominated," Russell Ford later wrote in a sworn affidavit. "I remember her saying that the attacker's name was Brett Kavanaugh, that he was a successful lawyer who had grown up in Christine's home town, and that he was well-known in the Washington, DC community."

Through counseling, Ford had become more aware of how she had struggled with the fallout from the incident, how confined spaces could trigger severe anxiety in her, and how she often had the urge to flee in the face of conflict. Over the years, she told her story to other therapists, including a PTSD specialist, and several friends.

In the spring of 2016, she and a friend, Keith Koegler, were watching their sons play sports together one day, when Ford turned to him and expressed outrage. Brock Turner, a Stanford student who had been convicted of sexually assaulting an unconscious woman on campus, had just been sentenced to six months in jail and three years' probation, which critics saw as a miscarriage of justice. Ford told Koegler that she had been assaulted as a teenager, by someone who was now a federal judge. "Partly because the kids were running around, partly because her face didn't show an interest in saying more, I didn't push," Koegler said in an interview. "I had no context, no idea who he was."

That autumn, Ford had been appalled by the **Access Hollywood** tape, with Trump's crude comments, but she hadn't followed the stories of the women who made allegations against the presidential candidate. A few months later, she joined in the women's march in San Jose, where other women wore pink hats, in protest of sexual violence, but she felt more invested in a separate march that year, to protest federal cuts to scientific research. She and friends wore gray knitted hats, for the gray matter in the brain. After the Weinstein story she had written "#metoo" on social media and left it at that.

But in June 2018, when Trump's short list for the Supreme Court circulated with Kavanaugh's name included, she emailed her friend Koegler about her unease:

The favorite for SCOTUS is the jerk who assaulted me in high school. He's my age, so he'll be on the court the rest of my life. ☹

Koegler wrote back:

I remember you telling me about him, but I don't remember his name, Do you mind telling me so I can read about him?

"Brett Kavanaugh," Ford replied.

By the time the July Fourth holiday approached, she felt rising panic. President Trump was running a reality-show-style search, and he had promised to make an announcement by the following Monday, July 9.

If Kavanaugh was to be nominated for a lifetime appointment, she felt she had relevant information to provide. Still, she wanted to protect her privacy and did not want to embarrass her family back East by hurting a hometown hero's candidacy. Their fathers were still members of the same small, private golf club, awkwardly enough. She didn't want to shame Kavanaugh publicly. She just wanted to pass on her account of what had happened in high school, and she wanted to do it **before** he became the nominee.

If she intervened early, those in charge could consider the information and perhaps move on to a candidate with no such liability. But who could she tell discreetly, who would handle the information in a trustworthy but effective way?

Ford realized that her perspective was limited, that she didn't know if the behavior she remembered from Kavanaugh was a lone incident or part of a pattern of predation. **Was that an episodic state, or was it part of a personality trait?** she asked herself.

Ford was trying to figure out whether or how to influence a Supreme Court nomination in an unlikely setting. A serious surfer, she and her husband had met through a website that had identified their common interest in riding waves. Their second date had taken place afloat in the waters off the San Mateo coast. Once, a great white shark had risen up beside her in the water. The thrill had been so great that she did not sleep for two days. Ford often used surfing analogies in her classroom and longed for the wide beaches and free-spirit atmosphere of Santa Cruz, her summer escape an hour or so to the south of her Palo Alto home.

Now she and her friends huddled on the sand, gazed out at Pacific vistas, took long swims, watched their kids train in the California State Parks Junior Lifeguard program, and weighed her options for quietly intervening. Ford did not call any lawyers. But she wondered if she should call Kavanaugh directly to tell him to withdraw from consideration for the court post so as to avoid putting his family through the humiliation that would come from her stepping forward. Or she could call Mark Judge, the other man who had been in the room during the assault, and ask him to pass along the message.

"I was just freaking out," she recalled of that time. "What am I going to do?"

She didn't speak extensively with her husband: He was commuting back and forth to Palo Alto for work. Russell Ford was an engineer who built medical devices, and he had the same type of scientific mind as his wife, with the same type of blinders. He was also an optimist by nature. At that point, she said, neither understood that quietly passing on decades-old information could have substantial consequences for their family.

On Friday, July 6, she walked off the Rio del Mar Beach and, from her parked car, called the office of her congressional representative, Anna Eshoo, a Democrat. When a young woman answered, Ford blurted out her message:

Someone on the Supreme Court short list sexually assaulted me in high school. I need to talk to someone in the office. It's urgent; Trump is about to make his selection.

She would hear back as soon as possible, she was told.

Ford picked up her iPhone again. Unsure about when Eshoo's office would respond, she would pursue another route. She clicked on the **Washington Post** anonymous tip line and starting typing:

> 10:26 AM
> Potential Supreme Court nominee with assistance from his friend assaulted me in mid 1980s in Maryland. Have therapy records talking about It. Feel like I shouldn't be quiet but not willing to put family in DC and CA through a lot of stress.

An hour later, she returned to the tip line to clarify:

> 11:47 AM
> Brett Kavanaugh with Mark Judge and a bystander named PJ

"I had thought my phone would ring immediately," Ford said later. But she got no immediate response from the **Post** either.

On July 9, three days later, President Trump announced his nominee: Brett Kavanaugh, distinguished judge, wholesome figure, coach of his daughter's basketball team.

In a text message to friends, she typed out a sad emoji and added:

> Ugh

> Double ugh.

Ford was a rabid football fan—she competed in a fantasy league and had even volunteered to house a Stanford player at her home during summer training—and now she turned to a quarterback analogy to explain what had happened. She had tried to pass the football to her member of Congress and the **Washington Post.** But they had let it drop. The play was over.

The next morning, July 10, Ford returned to the **Post** tip line with the equivalent of a journalism threat: She might go to senators or the **Times** with her story. By late morning, she was on the phone with Emma Brown, a **Post** reporter eager to hear her out.

That same afternoon, her phone rang again. Eshoo's district chief of staff was on the line. The aide had called the day before, asking, "Is it the person who was picked?" Now they agreed Ford would come in to Eshoo's office on Wednesday, July 18.

That was a week away. As she waited, Ford read flattering coverage of Kavanaugh that highlighted his support of women and girls. The **Post** published an opinion piece by a mother who raved about what a terrific girls' basketball coach he was. An old friend from high school told Ford how proud the community was to be producing another justice. (Neil Gorsuch also had attended Georgetown Prep, the same high school as Kavanaugh.) **The math is not in my favor,** Ford recalled thinking.

She could live with him being appointed: "I really consciously divested from the outcome," she said. But the prospect of watching Kavanaugh on the court, while knowing she had not shared her memories, seemed intolerable: "Not saying something is what's upsetting," she said.

So she undertook a mission to gather evidence, driving to her doctor's office in Silicon Valley and requesting copies of the notes from the therapy sessions in which she had recalled being assaulted, the ones she had referenced in her tip to the **Post.**

In the meantime, she told her sons the minimum. "A person who the president wants to hire for an important job did something bad to me when I was your age," she said. "I'm trying to figure out a way to get the information to him. He may find it useful."

"Cool," said her older son, who was the same age she had been at the time of the alleged assault.

On July 18, she met with Karen Chapman, Representative Eshoo's district chief of staff. Ford provided an exhaustive account of everything she recalled, even drawing her a map of the suburban house where she remembered being trapped in the bedroom. Chapman took copious notes and expressed support, but Eshoo wasn't there, so two days later, Ford had to return to the office, relaying her account all over again.

Eshoo promised to be back in touch and issued strict instructions: All of this was to remain confidential. Ford had only told a handful of people other than her husband, including Emma Brown, the **Post** reporter; Keith Koegler; several other friends; and two work mentors. "You can't be talking about this," Eshoo told her. "If it does get around, it will be because you told other people." Eshoo said word traveled fast, and it could impact Ford and how she chose to proceed.

Ford, who still had no idea exactly where this was going, thought the meeting felt like progress: She had gotten her message to someone in a position of authority. "I trust her office," Ford emailed one of her mentors, "and we are consistent in the goal of public service." Following Eshoo's advice, Ford ignored texts from the **Post** reporter.

But during that time, Ford began to get high-pressure texts with messages passed along from strangers. One of her friends had told someone, who had told someone, and soon word of her allegations was traveling around Palo Alto feminist circles. These women, some of them high-powered academics, had come together through the Brock Turner case and the Women's March, and the previous few months of #MeToo activity had strengthened their conviction. Now local activists—one Ford knew, but most she did not—were pushing her to come forward. "This is a crucial time in history," one of her friends stressed in a text.

Ford mostly ignored the outreach. Were it not for Kavanaugh, she would not be paying attention to the nomination process at all, she said, and she was not considering whether or how her actions would affect the #MeToo movement.

But the messages were harbingers: that this situation was going to attract intensely strong feelings from others, that she could lose control of her own story, that other people with various agendas might operate without taking her wishes into account. By ignoring the messages, she was missing important clues.

In the last week of July, Ford was pulled back to the Washington area. Her grandmother had suffered a stroke and was about to die. Ford hated to fly, but she and her sons traveled to stay with her parents at their summer home in Rehoboth Beach, Delaware, for a hot, humid ten days.

Her parents had no idea about her secret—they had never had, she said—and she didn't want to trouble them especially while they were tending to her grandmother. When Eshoo's office called, she stepped out to the porch for privacy. The aide was asking her to write a letter detailing what had happened with Kavanaugh for the Senate Judiciary Committee, which held hearings for Supreme Court nominees. The writing was straightforward: By now, Ford was used to repeating the story. But she debated whom to send it to. The aide told Ford to address the letter to Senator Dianne Feinstein, the top Democrat on the committee, as well as Senator

Charles Grassley, the Republican chair. Ford worried that would raise the chances of her name and story becoming public. So she addressed the letter to Feinstein only, who she assumed would have to abide by constituent confidentiality, based on what Eshoo's office had said.

July 30, 2018

CONFIDENTIAL

SENATOR DIANNE FEINSTEIN

Dear Senator Feinstein:

I am writing with information relevant in evaluating the current nominee of the Supreme Court. As a constituent, I expect that you will maintain this as confidential until we have further opportunity to speak.

Brett Kavanaugh physically and sexually assaulted me during High School in the early 1980's. He conducted these acts with the assistance of his close friend, Mark G. Judge. Both were 1-2 years older than me and students at a local private school. The assault occurred in a suburban Maryland area home at a gathering that included me and 4 others. Kavanaugh physically pushed me into a bedroom as I was headed for a bathroom up a short stairwell from the living room. They locked the door and played loud music, precluding any successful attempts to yell for help. Kavanaugh was on top of me while laughing with Judge, who periodically jumped onto Kavanaugh. They both laughed as Kavanaugh tried to disrobe me in their highly inebriated state. With Kavanaugh's hand over my mouth, I feared he may inadvertently kill me. From across the room, a very drunken Judge said mixed words to kavanaugh ranging from "go for it" to "stop." At one point when Judge jumped onto the bed, the weight on me was substantial. The pile toppled, and the two scrapped with each other. After a few attempts to get away, I was able to take this opportune moment to get up and run across to a hallway bathroom. I locked the bathroom door behind me. Both loudly stumbled down the stairwell, at which point other persons at the house were talking with them. I exited the bathroom, ran outside of the house and went home.

I have not knowingly seen Kavanaugh since the assault. I did see Mark Judge once at the Potomac Village Safeway, where he was extremely uncomfortable seeing me.

I have received medical treatment regarding the assault. On July 6, I notified my local government representative to ask them how to proceed with sharing this information. It is upsetting to discuss sexual assault and its repercussions, yet I feel guilty and compelled as a citizen about the idea of not saying anything.

I am available to speak further should you wish to discuss. I am currently vacationing in the mid-Atlantic until August 7th and will be in California after August 10th.

In Confidence,

Christine Blasey
PALO ALTO, CALIFORNIA

"Got it!" the aide wrote back. "Will hand deliver to her today."

Soon the aide was on the phone with Ford, describing every move of another Eshoo staff member in Washington who was walking a hard copy of the letter to Senator Feinstein's office. "Now he's handing it over," the staff member narrated, as if they were discussing the nation's nuclear codes.

Next Senator Feinstein herself was on the phone. The eighty-five-year-old legislator seemed to be hard of hearing. She was yelling out questions about the precise nature of the incident, and Ford was yelling back, to make sure the senator could understand what she was saying. Senator Feinstein said she would keep the letter confidential and promised to be back in touch.

As she hung up the phone, Ford began to envision the power her letter would take on under the Capitol dome, in a way that she had not on the beach in California. For weeks, Ford's confidantes had been telling her to get a lawyer, to protect and retain control of her own story, but she had resisted. She and her husband had been saving for a down payment for a condo in Hawaii, where they could surf and retire and didn't want to deplete their funds, she said. Now she realized she definitely needed an attorney.

The first Washington firms that she contacted did not want to touch the case, but she found one attorney, Lawrence Robbins, who had argued multiple cases before the Supreme Court and listened carefully. "She did not try to minimize the gaps in her memory," Robbins said. "She was extremely clear about the things she could recall. She provided forms of corroboration, perhaps not bulletproof, but good enough that I thought they should be taken seriously. My impression was that she was believable and deserved to have someone go to bat for her." But he couldn't represent her publicly: His partners feared it could harm their appellate court cases if it looked like the firm had done something adverse to a Supreme Court justice, so any help he gave would have to be behind the scenes.

On Monday, August 6, just after Ford's grandmother passed away, right before she was scheduled to leave the Washington area, she was talking with two new lawyers, this time face to face. Senator

Feinstein's office had flagged a pair of law partners, Debra Katz and Lisa Banks, explaining that these two were among those who worked with these types of allegations. Ford had studied their website and noticed that they had done whistle-blower work. But the most valuable thing about them was that they were available to meet immediately. She said she could squeeze in a quick meeting at a hotel near the Baltimore airport.

Katz and Banks quickly agreed, not sure what to expect. A couple days before, Feinstein's office had reached out to them, with general questions—if you have a very old allegation of sexual assault, what can you do to confirm it?—then followed up with the broad outlines of Ford's account without naming her. Ford, for her part, wasn't sure what to make of the two lawyers or all their detailed, personal questions about her story and background.

She didn't grasp that she was dealing with two of the top gender discrimination lawyers in the country. Debra Katz—Debbie to almost everyone—was Ford's temperamental opposite, a take-charge activist who was steeped in Washington and feminist fights. Katz thought in civil rights terms, and saw the law as a means to progress. She had begun her career as a junior member of the legal team that strategized over how to best argue the first sexual harassment case ever heard by the Supreme Court, **Meritor Savings Bank v. Vinson,** about a bank teller who said that the branch manager had repeatedly assaulted her and told her he would fire her if she did not comply. In 1986, the court ruled in Vinson's favor, nine to zero, establishing the precedent that sexual harassment is a form of discrimination.

Three decades later, Katz was still a diehard lefty but had a closet full of pin-striped suits she wore to negotiate on behalf of employees who felt wronged. Her law partner, Lisa Banks, also her best friend outside the office, had a cooler presence, an impassive glare that could be useful with adversaries, and perseverance that stretched back to childhood, when at age seven someone had shattered her dreams, informing her that she would never be able to play for the Boston Red Sox because she was a girl.

Their office above Dupont Circle was decorated with polished furniture, potted plants—and a painting of Rose McGowan holding Harvey Weinstein's severed head that had been made by a friend of Katz's son. When the attorneys met Ford in Baltimore, they had already been in overdrive for months, trying to make the most of what they saw as a rare window of opportunity post-Weinstein. For most of their careers, progress on harassment and abuse had felt stalled, with the same kinds of cases cropping up repeatedly. They had often won awards for individual women, sometimes very large ones, typically in the form of secret settlements, which they regarded as imperfect but necessary tools.

But the Weinstein case had galvanized their practice, they said later, because their client's complaints were suddenly being taken far more seriously. In the ten months since the Weinstein story, Katz had represented staffers on Capitol Hill whose harassment complaints triggered resignations by a member of the House of Representatives and a high-level congressional staffer. After she and Banks filed a lawsuit against a Washington-area celebrity chef, his partners eventually fled and his empire dissolved. They had met with representatives of Congress and state legislatures, pushing for new laws to better protect victims of sexual harassment. All summer, Katz and Banks had been feeling exhilarated but worried: This moment was so valuable, they felt; change was so overdue. They wanted as much progress as possible, as fast as possible, before too much backlash mounted.

After a few hours with Ford, the attorneys walked out of the conference room with their heads spinning. At first, they just kept muttering to one another: **Oh my God. Oh my God.** They had vetted an untold number of witnesses over the years, and Ford struck both attorneys as very credible, they said. They were also moved by what she called her sense of civic duty. But this woman, with her formidable scientific intellect, also seemed so naïve, a quality that could land her in serious trouble. She seemed unaware of the potential gravity of her own case, but that sense of consequence was part of what drew them to it. Unlike Ford, they had immediately understood the charged nature of the letter she had written to Feinstein. If that letter leaked, she would need protection; if not, she would need counsel on whether and how to pursue the matter further. The lawyers knew they wanted to represent Ford and do it pro bono.

To prepare for what might come, the lawyers set Ford to work on some practical tasks. She soon underwent, and passed, a polygraph test administered by a former FBI agent. She also took on the embarrassing task of calling two of her ex-boyfriends, one from high school and one from right after college. No, I'm not calling to get back together, she told them. I need to know, do you recall if when we were together I ever mentioned being assaulted? Neither did, she said. It became increasingly clear that Ford had told no one about the alleged attack for years.

The lawyers pored over Ford's life history, searching through public records to identify any information that could be used to smear her. Katz called Senator Feinstein's staff and told them that she thought the accusation was credible and suggested that they start searching for evidence of any other assaults Kavanaugh might have committed.

That was when Katz first called Jodi, on Saturday, August 11, asking her to pass the tip to the **Times.** Rebecca Corbett had overseen some of the paper's vetting of prospective Supreme Court candidates over the years and was now doing the same for Kavanaugh. As Corbett pressed the expanding team of reporters to look for any problematic treatment of women, she checked in with Jodi every few days, wanting to know if there was anything more on that Katz client with the allegation.

But Ford declined to speak with Jodi, or to return the latest calls from the **Post.** She was focused on another choice, one that came with a pressing deadline.

Kavanaugh's hearings were scheduled to begin September 4. Three things could happen before then: The letter to Feinstein could leak. Ford could remain silent and likely watch Kavanaugh sail through confirmation. Or she could decide to speak up publicly, which might change the course of the hearings. That's what she, in her heart of hearts, was inclined, if frightened, to do.

Katz and Banks understood why. Ford had a right to tell her story, they believed, and a vital point to make. The violations committed against high school girls, against entire generations of women, mattered, even if those women had maintained long silences or didn't have perfect evidence. The two-part question was what price Ford would pay personally and what impact her coming forward would have—on the nomination, and on the entire raging debate about sex and power.

Other lawyers reinforced the idea that Ford had an important story to tell. In addition to retaining Katz and Banks, she had kept Robbins on as an adviser—and at his referral she took on another adviser named Barry Coburn, a tough criminal defense attorney. Coburn told her he saw a clear distinction between high-school sexual horseplay and what Ford described, "unambiguous attempted rape." "It's not sexual harassment," he later recalled telling her. "It's not a boundary violation. It's not like being insensitive. It's a felony." But Robbins and Coburn understood that this was about more than the underlying incident, and they let Katz and Banks take the lead.

At Katz's request, one more person joined the growing council of professional advisers: Ricki Seidman, a deliberative, discreet veteran of three decades' worth of Democratic judicial fights, who had worked as an aide to Bill Clinton's presidential campaign and served in his administration. Katz had never met Seidman, but she knew that the operative came with deep knowledge and experience of Supreme Court nominations that she and Banks did not have. Seidman had been involved in battles ranging from Robert Bork (who Democrats defeated in 1987) to Sonia Sotomayor (who Democrats confirmed in 2009). She had played a direct role in the only historical proxy for Ford's case: Anita Hill's testimony against Clarence Thomas. In 1991, Seidman had been working for the Senate Labor and Resources Committee as chief investigator, watching the Thomas nomination, when she got a call tipping her off about a professor who said she had been harassed by the nominee. She was the first member of the Senate committee staff to speak with Anita Hill about her experiences, and she had encouraged Hill to engage further with the committee.

Republicans later saw Seidman's history and accused her of harboring a political agenda, of weaponizing Ford to derail a nomination. In fact, that August, Seidman's instinct was that Ford should remain silent.

It was a matter of math. Given Republican control of the Senate, Kavanaugh would likely be confirmed even if Ford spoke up. Her first reaction was that the bar for coming forward was very high, because she didn't think it was going to make a difference in the outcome.

In the decades after Anita Hill's testimony, the adviser had struggled with her role in encouraging the professor to come forward. Hill had prevailed in some ways, catalyzing awareness of sexual harassment. But Seidman thought that any social progress had come at a great personal toll to Hill. She felt the attack apparatus of the Republican Party would almost certainly try to destroy Ford, and the prospect of watching history repeat itself filled her with dread.

Ford's advisers suspected that Kavanaugh had victimized other women, that this had not been an isolated incident—it was just a matter of finding them. **If there were two more women, I would feel better,** Katz thought to herself. **With one more woman, it's risky.** They had zero.

Katz and Banks were trying to stay neutral, sketching out the potential consequences for Ford on each side, knowing that she was the one who would have to live with her decision.

But their worries extended beyond their client's own welfare. In that moment, Katz was also fearful that a national discounting of Ford's story could be detrimental for the entire #MeToo movement. Critics would say it had gone too far, raising violations that were ancient, unprovable, and lacked the more demonstrable harm of workplace sexual harassment or rape. Some men would instinctively side with Kavanaugh, afraid of out-of-the-blue accusations. The wheel of progress could slow, or even spin in the opposite direction, a consequence the lawyers saw as too painful to bear.

The public conversation was still tumultuous. That summer, more men were still being accused, suspended, and fired by the week: the personnel chief of the Federal Office of Emergency Management, a UC Berkeley professor, a Goldman Sachs salesman, two dancers from the New York City Ballet. In August, Ronan Farrow published the first sexual harassment allegations against CBS chairman Les Moonves in the **New Yorker**—but Moonves remained defiantly in place, backed by the company's board. Louis C.K. made his first appearance at a comedy club since the **Times** article, to cheers in the room and jeering outside it. Bill O'Reilly, who had continued writing history books since his ouster from Fox, was about to release his latest book: The previous one had sold nearly half a million copies, his fans ever loyal.

By August 10, Ford was back in Palo Alto, weighing her decision as she was completing a pile of student dissertation evaluations. She barely knew these Washington advisers in whom she had placed her fate; the group's deliberations were taking place by phone or text message. They all said they would support Ford no matter what she decided, but from afar, she could feel their hesitation. **Are they trying to push me forward? Or are they trying to shut me down?** she wondered.

Ford was mulling her own personal concerns. She feared that if she were publicly to point a finger at Kavanaugh, others might point fingers back at her. She had done her fair share of drinking in high school, and early in college, her partying had escalated, and her grades tanked. Shortly after, she had stabilized and succeeded in her studies. In a speech at her old high school in 2014, she had offered herself as an example of how to get a life back on track. She had floundered in statistics in college. Now she taught it. Still she worried that critics would focus only on her younger self's shortcomings and mistakes, she said.

But Ford believed that if she did come under attack, she could withstand it. In 2015, she had been diagnosed with cancer and suffered complications from the treatment. It was the first time Ford had been forced to measure her own mortality, and afterward, she felt she had emerged stronger—with a greater capacity to endure, she said. Her husband had been encouraging her to step forward, to get it over with, predicting the whole thing would die down after a single news cycle.

On August 24, Katz shared an update with Ford: No other allegations of sexual misconduct by the judge had surfaced. If she were going to come forward, she would be a lone accuser. If she did not want Senator Feinstein to share her letter with the rest of the committee, including the Republicans, she needed to say so. To help Ford come to a decision, they agreed on an internal deadline: She would make a call by August 29, seven days before Kavanaugh's hearings were set to begin.

By August 26, Ford was still paralyzed with indecision. Two days later, with no progress, Katz and Banks said they would draft and edit three different letters. Because there was no established process for reporting this kind of story about a nominee, the lawyers were trying to show Ford what various paths could look like. Each version led to a different variation on her future, maybe a different composition of the Supreme Court, even a different version of American history.

In one version, addressed to Senators Grassley and Feinstein, the lawyers used Ford's name and explained that she wanted to meet with them privately to report an allegation of assault against the judge. The second version made the same request, but referred to Ford as Dr. Jane Doe, for a little more protection. The third option, addressed only to Senator Feinstein, used Ford's name but said she was declining to pursue the matter. "She has determined that the personal and professional costs of coming forward before the Judiciary Committee are too great," the letter said. The group agreed that Ford would choose one of the letters by the end of the next day.

The first one struck everyone as too risky: Ford's name would immediately reach the White House. Ford seemed to be leaning toward the second letter, which could allow her to negotiate terms of confidentiality. Together, the women tweaked the language of that letter, and then changed it again, no one fully satisfied.

The more they envisioned delivering the letters, the more the discussion shifted to the question, Then what happens? Ford's lawyers and Seidman told her it would likely be impossible to try to move forward in reporting the claim without having her identity revealed. They predicted she would come under the same type of public attack as Anita Hill had, more than once likening it to the equivalent of stepping in front of a train.

As the self-imposed deadline neared, Seidman flew to California and met Ford for the first time. Once again she warned her from following in Hill's footsteps. Telling the story of the alleged assault still caused Ford pain. She was so unversed in public life, a stranger to scrutiny, not even close to fluent in the flow of the news cycle. Seidman still believed Kavanaugh would be confirmed even if Ford came forward, and the only thing she would accomplish would be turning her life upside down.

At the coffee date with Seidman near the San Francisco International Airport, Ford felt overcome with stress. She didn't know the woman sitting across from her. "I just wanted to leave," she recalled feeling at the time.

Ford spent August 29, the appointed decision day, in academic meetings for hours, consulting with graduate students on their dissertations. As the sun set that evening, Ford was still unable to choose.

"Made edits and having some panic symptoms," she wrote in a text to Katz that evening. "I'll send to you edits soon and we can decide in early a.m. whether to go. Anxiety about leaks and Washington Post."

"Just sent you edits," she wrote again an hour later, "no green light yet."

She didn't have one in the morning either. She was beginning to believe what her team had already told her: that the anonymous letter was pointless, her name was likely to leak, and it was all or nothing. Katz and Banks were twisting too, caught between believing their client was in the right and wondering how many others would feel the same way, unsure which was worse, incineration or silence.

It was Thursday, August 30. The next day marked the start of Labor Day weekend. The following Tuesday morning, Kavanaugh's hearings would begin. In Washington, Katz called Ford.

"This is a life-defining decision, and it's yours," she said.

That afternoon, Ford still wanted a few more

hours to think, to go for a walk, to speak to a friend one last time.

In the end, Ford did not choose any of the letters—none of them felt right to her, she said. That, in effect, became the choice she made.

Katz called Senator Feinstein's office to notify them that Ford did not want to take her account further. On August 31 Feinstein replied by email:

"I am writing now to confirm that my office will continue to honor the request for confidentiality and will not be taking further action unless we hear from you. Assure that I understand and regret the deep impact this incident had on her life."

Katz forwarded the letter to her client. "It felt like a 'goodbye and good luck,'" Ford said.

That night, at Ford's house in Palo Alto, she sent one of her sons to sleep with her husband and climbed into his Ikea bed for refuge. Her mind turned to surfing. She had paddled out into choppy waters and had been prepared to ride a rough wave. Maybe she would have stayed upright until she reached shore. Maybe she'd have gotten blasted. But she had worked hard to get in position, and she had deserved the chance to try. Why were the advisers so worried about the apparent lack of other victims? Wasn't what happened to her enough?

Curled up all alone in her child's bed, she sobbed.

CHAPTER NINE

"I CAN'T GUARANTEE I'LL GO TO DC"

Five days later, on Tuesday, September 4, Christine Blasey Ford sat in the Palo Alto office of a PTSD specialist she had seen on and off for a couple years and asked for advice on putting her brush with the Kavanaugh nomination process behind her.

Across the country in Washington, DC, the hearings on his nomination were starting that day, already at top decibel. Democratic senators were trying to halt the proceedings on the grounds that they had been denied access to documents from Kavanaugh's past, and were failing. Protestors lined the Senate halls, some dressed in red robes and white bonnets, a reference to Margaret Atwood's dystopian feminist novel **The Handmaid's Tale,** interrupted the testimony ("More women are going to be subject to back-alley abortions!") and were arrested by the dozens by the Capitol Police. Republicans, unified behind

Trump's pick, were lashing back, calling Democrats a disorderly mob.

Ford's failure to further report her allegation nagged at her, but she wanted to mentally store away the whole episode. Repeatedly revisiting the upsetting memory that summer had taken an emotional toll, and now she was trying to get back on track, she said. Her sons had returned to school. She was preparing for the first day of work teaching.

The therapist listened but expressed doubt that he could help just yet. As part of his treatment method, he encouraged patients to stop talking about the underlying cause of their PTSD. What she had described made him cautious. "You're not ready to pack this away," she recalled him telling her. He wasn't sure her involvement in the Kavanaugh story was over yet.

A week later, on Monday, September 10, Ford showed up to teach the opening session of her Introduction to Statistics doctoral course. She began with the same pep talk she used every year, promising her students that they would work through the intimidating material together. Three hours later, someone asking questions stopped her as she departed. Not a graduate student. A reporter, from BuzzFeed. The journalist said she knew about the letter as Ford ordered her to leave.

Outsiders were starting to push and pull more

forcefully on Ford's previously private story. Increasing numbers of prominent women and #MeToo activists seemed to know about it, and now journalists were contacting Ford's colleagues and showing up at her home.

Outraged, Debra Katz confronted a leading Palo Alto feminist whom she suspected of trying to out Ford. This is so unprincipled, Katz recalled telling the woman in a heated phone call. My client doesn't want to come forward. In a phone call the previous week, Eshoo's staff had asked whether Ford wanted them to do more, like put her in touch with a second member of the Senate Judiciary Committee. But in the end, Ford reiterated that she had not changed her mind about coming forward. When the journalists came knocking, she refused to talk to them.

On Wednesday, September 12, an article appeared anyway. **The Intercept,** an online publication, revealed that Democrats on the Senate Judiciary Committee were trying to obtain a letter about Kavanaugh that Feinstein had received. According to the story, the letter supposedly described "an incident involving Kavanaugh and a woman while they were in high school" and someone affiliated with Stanford University had authored it. "Kept hidden," the article noted, "the letter is beginning to take on a life of its own."

That made Feinstein look as if she was withholding vital information about a nominee. The following day, the senator announced by press release that she had sent the letter over to law enforcement for review. She was referring the matter to the FBI, which forwarded it to the White House for Kavanaugh's background file, prompting him to issue a denial for an accusation that was still vague. For more than a week, Ford had been reconciling herself with silence. Now it seemed like she was days, maybe hours, from being fully outed.

By then, Ford was determined to regain control over her own account. She had decided that if anyone was going to reveal her identity to the public, it would be her. On Wednesday, she had driven thirty miles outside Palo Alto to one of the Ritz-Carlton restaurants in Half Moon Bay, where Emma Brown, the **Washington Post** reporter who had fielded the anonymous tip that Ford had sent to the paper weeks before, was waiting. In intermittent phone calls and text messages, Ford had stayed in touch with Brown, telling her bits of her story about the high school encounter with Kavanaugh and her initial plan to report it to Congress. Brown had listened attentively, never pushing Ford too hard. The journalist's deference had been a comfort to Ford.

The interview process was more extensive and difficult than Ford had imagined. It began that Wednesday evening, resumed the next morning, and continued by phone in the following days. Ford cringed at the thought of seeing graphic material in the newspaper, especially explicit references to her body. Brown wanted to know whether Kavanaugh had ever penetrated Ford in any way, whether he had raped her. No, Ford explained. She had to provide excerpts of therapy records in which she discussed what had happened. Brown asked to talk to Ford's husband, who confirmed that she had named Kavanaugh as her attacker as early as 2012.

But as she drove back to Palo Alto, Ford felt almost relieved that her hand had been forced. She would finally be out of purgatory. Katz and her other advisers said they thought the article was the right step, to ensure that her allegation was reported correctly. Her husband maintained the same line he had all summer: The sooner she went public, the sooner their lives would go back to normal. She was thinking wishfully as well, telling herself she would be able to cling to some privacy throughout. After she had married, Ford kept her maiden name for professional purposes, in order to maintain a consistent byline on the scientific papers she wrote. Just before the **Post** article was published, she debated using her husband's last name instead, hoping that because Ford was such a common name, it would be more difficult for readers to identify her on the internet. "In my fantasy world, Googling Ford and Blasey are two different things," she said. Instead, she settled on Christine Blasey Ford. Wherever possible, she also removed photos of herself online. But she had not yet succeeded in taking down her LinkedIn profile, which included a photo of her in sunglasses. Ford dropped her sons with friends, booked a hotel for the evening, and hoped for quick, calm passage through the news cycle.

As soon as the **Post** published the story, on Sunday, September 16, Ford's cell phone went into an uninterrupted state of rings and pings. On her LinkedIn page, she had thousands of requests to connect. Her Palo Alto University email account flooded with so many messages, supportive and scathing, that the account crashed.

Around the world, people were absorbing the article paragraph by paragraph:

> Earlier this summer, Christine Blasey Ford wrote a confidential letter to a senior Democratic lawmaker alleging that Supreme Court nominee Brett M. Kavanaugh sexually assaulted her more than three decades ago, when they were high school students in suburban Maryland. Since Wednesday, she has watched as that bare-bones version of her story became public without her name or her consent, drawing a blanket denial from Kavanaugh and roiling a nomination that just days ago seemed all but certain to succeed.
>
> Now, Ford has decided that if her story is going to be told, she wants to be the one to tell it.

Back in Brooklyn, Jodi and Megan read the **Post** article and saw the eruption it was surely going to cause.

Based on the evidence in the story, Ford and Kavanaugh were each going to amass armies of believers. As Katz had indicated earlier, there were blank spaces in Ford's story, extensive ones: holes in the accuser's memory, no corroboration that dated from the time of the alleged event. Kavanaugh's denial, issued the Friday before by the White House, was forceful: "I categorically and unequivocally deny this allegation. I did not do this back in high school or at any time."

But Ford readily admitted the gaps in her memory, which some saw as a mark of a credible victim. She described specific details: the sound of rock music playing at high volume and both boys laughing "maniacally." "Kavanaugh pinned her to a bed on her back and groped her over her clothes, grinding his body against hers and clumsily attempting to pull off her one-piece bathing suit and the clothing she wore over it," Emma Brown had written. "When she tried to scream, she said, he put his hand over her mouth." The reaction to the **Post** story was far more supportive of Ford than her lawyers had anticipated, a testament to the potency of #MeToo. People around the world, already linked and mobilized in support of victims of sexual violence, were rallying to Ford's cause.

She was becoming an instant symbol for women

who had been abused, a figure of great hope for justice—but she also seemed likely to become a focal point for the backlash. Megan—who remembered how Trump had yelled at her on the phone almost two years earlier and knew the ferocity with which he fought these kinds of allegations—wondered if Ford was also about to become his target. In Bob Woodward's **Fear,** Trump was described saying to a friend who had admitted problematic behavior toward women: "You've got to deny, deny, deny and push back on these women." Trump said, "If you admit to anything and any culpability, then you're dead."

Trump might do more than attack Ford: He was likely to take aim at the entire #MeToo movement. The reckoning had already posed a danger to Trump, who still faced multiple allegations of sexual misconduct. Now it threatened his Supreme Court nominee. Just two months before, the president had mocked the phrase #MeToo at a political rally and defended a member of Congress accused of ignoring sexual abuse accusers when he worked as an assistant wrestling coach at Ohio State University. "I don't believe **them** at all. I believe **him,**" the president had said.

Legal thinkers were split. Old sources, prosecutors and defense attorneys, told Megan that if the details of Ford's allegation were true, if the two boys had blocked her in the room and turned up the music, if Kavanaugh had put his hand over her mouth when she tried to scream, then he had committed a serious crime. In the criminal justice system, a single credible victim's testimony had weight: eyewitnesses, DNA, and other types of corroborating evidence were not necessarily required for a conviction.

However, others were stressing why statutes of limitations existed. "I oppose Kavanaugh's nomination, think senators should vote no based on his judicial record, but am uncomfortable with asserting that his behavior as a teen tells us anything about his 'character' now," Rosa Brooks, a Georgetown law professor who had served in two Democratic administrations, tweeted. She pointed out that "after thirty-five years, it is nearly impossible to conduct a full or fair investigation."

That afternoon, Jodi talked to Katz, who was in a new and more advanced state of anxiety. "I'm scared for my client," the lawyer said. "She is going to be annihilated by the White House." She didn't trust the Democrats either. With the midterm elections two months away, she feared they might try to use Ford as a prop or foil.

Before they hung up, Katz had one more detail to add. This is beyond off the record, she said.

"My client can't testify," she said.

It was out of the question, Katz said. It had taken everything Ford had to go ahead with the **Post** piece, and she had assumed that once it was published, little else would be required of her. She feared cameras and flying and didn't want to come back to Washington.

If members of the Senate Judiciary wanted to question her in California, she would oblige. But being grilled by senators, on live television? It just was not going to happen, Katz said.

But the next morning, Monday, September 17, Katz was on morning news shows, assuring the hosts that her client was prepared to testify in front of Congress.

"The answer is yes," Katz told CNN when asked directly.

It was the bluff of Katz's life. Nothing had changed since the day before. Ford was barely aware that her attorney was asserting that on television.

"We had to say she was coming," Katz explained later.

Weeks before, Katz, Banks, and Seidman had urged caution to Ford, mindful of the dangers of exposure. But now they thought that the best course was for her to testify in an open hearing with cameras, convinced that once many Americans saw and heard her for themselves, they would believe her account. Speaking to senators or their staff behind closed doors would only provide them with an opportunity to spin, conceal, or otherwise dismiss Ford's words.

In that moment, they felt their paramount priority was to preserve Ford's options. "If we had been equivocal, we would have looked weak," Katz said. Republicans would have said Ford was not serious enough to show up and articulate her claim. "If you cede that, you're done," Katz said. So they plunged in, deciding to negotiate the form and timing of the testimony, pushing it off as long as possible, buying their client a few more days to warm up to the idea. (And, they thought, possibly for new allegations to surface.) If Ford was unwilling to show up later, fine—better to fold late than to give everything away at the start.

"You need to trust us, to keep your options open," the advisers told Ford. "You will drive this."

Okay, Ford had replied. But I'm never coming, she told her team. The advisers stepped in for Ford, carving a path, hoping she would follow, and becoming yet another escalating force.

By virtue of a Republican Senate, Judiciary Committee chairman Chuck Grassley controlled almost everything about how Kavanaugh's hearings would unfold. Standing just behind him was Senator Mitch McConnell, the Republican majority leader, known for his brass-knuckled tactics, such as blocking former president Barack Obama from filling an empty Supreme Court seat in his final year.

But Grassley and Trump were already promising that they would treat Ford with respect, a sign perhaps of how much had changed over the past year. That summer, the Senate Judiciary Committee had held a hearing in which Grassley and other committee members had come down hard on allegations of sexual harassment within the federal judiciary. The Republicans in power appeared eager to respect Ford.

They also seemed mindful of the potentially damaging optics of a showdown, the all-male members of their side of the Judiciary Committee against a vulnerable woman, just like in the Clarence Thomas hearings. Trump's aides were reportedly stressing to him that it would be a political mistake for him to go into attack mode. "She should not be insulted," presidential counselor Kellyanne Conway told reporters in the White House driveway that Monday morning. "She should not be ignored." With the midterm elections approaching, and Republicans already bleeding female voters, they seemed almost deferential to Ford. In that stance, Ford's team saw a toehold.

Their plan was for Seidman to craft the team's terms behind the scenes, while Katz and Banks negotiated directly with Grassley's staff.

But unbeknownst to television viewers, Katz had a second secret, in addition to a reluctant client, that morning. After the television appearances, she took a car to the hospital, donned a patient's gown, handed her phone over to her wife, and was put under anesthesia. On that day of all days, she was having long-anticipated breast surgery.

Years before, Katz had lived through breast cancer and recovered fully. But like many women, she had an implant that needed to be replaced. She had scheduled the surgery weeks before and her insurance provider would not let her change the date.

She had already sworn to Ford that it wouldn't be

a problem. Jodi and Megan were reminded of Laura Madden's surgery just after the Weinstein story. But this was an even more precarious situation, though, because Katz would be going unconscious when she had so much work to do. Was the lawyer so dead set on this testimony that she was going to negotiate with Grassley while still groggy from anesthesia?

Seidman, meanwhile, was out of town. Her mother had died the week before, and she was in Atlanta, sorting out her family's affairs.

At the law office on Connecticut Avenue, Lisa Banks monitored the situation with rising panic. Grassley's office was already sending messages asking to schedule a call with Katz and her client, and his aides weren't sure why Katz wasn't replying.

"I'm honestly wondering how I ever let her out of my sight," Banks half joked in a text message to Katz's wife. "This is a total shit show. And I'm trying to navigate the country's future by myself here. This would drive a lesser person to drink, or worse. Please tell her everything is fine and delete." She closed with a martini emoji.

As the day went on, #MeToo activists continued to mobilize, with no idea that Ford was unwilling to testify and that her chief public representative was lying on a hospital table.

The following morning, Tuesday, Katz woke up at her family farm in a far corner of Maryland.

Katz had stitches, swelling, and doctor's orders to stay out of the office for at least a few days. But she swore off any medication that might fog her thinking, propped herself up in bed, and flipped open her laptop to review the emails from Senator Grassley's staff and begin negotiating.

As a first step, Ford's team had already requested an FBI investigation of Ford's allegation, in an attempt to have impartial law enforcement officials try to shed light on what had happened that day three decades ago. But the FBI was refusing to get involved, saying it considered Kavanaugh's background check closed. Republicans on the Senate Judiciary Committee were insisting that it had the authority and skill to investigate.

Ford's team was rejecting offers by Grassley's committee to interview Ford in private. So it was now a matter of negotiating the terms of a hearing, in effect making up the rules as they went along. That morning, in an opinion article in the **Times,** Anita Hill worried aloud about that very prospect. Twenty-seven years before, during her own testimony, the committee's members "performed in ways that gave employers permission to mishandle workplace harassment complaints throughout the following decades," she wrote. That the committee, made up of some of the exact same senators, still lacked a specific protocol for evaluating claims of sexual harassment or assault against a nominee suggested that it "has learned little from the Thomas hearing, much less the more recent #MeToo movement," she wrote. Everything about how Ford might deal with the committee was up for grabs: the timing, the format, the question of who else might participate.

Over the following days, the two sides traded carefully worded emails and terse phone calls. Katz and Banks pushed the committee to subpoena Mark Judge, Kavanaugh's old friend, and according to Ford, the other person in the room during the attack. As Ford had described in her letter to Feinstein, she remembered seeing him looking visibly uncomfortable at a neighborhood grocery store afterward, as if he felt bad about what had happened. A recovering alcoholic, Judge had written two memoirs about life at Georgetown Prep that described an extreme party culture of regular blackout drinking. One book, **Wasted: Tales of a GenX Drunk,** mentioned a Bart O'Kavanaugh, presumably a veiled reference to the judge, and a night when he "puked in someone's car" and "passed out on his way back from a party." At the very least, Ford's team thought Judge could substantiate excess drinking by his old friend.

How could the committee ascertain the truth without requiring Judge to testify in person? Katz and Banks asked. Grassley's staff refused, saying they did not take subpoena requests from witnesses as a condition of their testifying. Instead, his staff accepted a written statement from Judge in which he acknowledged being friends with Kavanaugh in high school but said he did not recall any such party and had never seen Kavanaugh act as Ford had described. The staff also accepted a similar written statement from P. J. Smyth, another friend of Kavanaugh's whom Ford recalled being at the party, saying that he had no memory of the gathering, knew Kavanaugh to be a person of "great integrity," and had never seen him engage in any improper conduct toward women.

Republicans had eliminated potential witnesses, reducing the situation to: Do you believe her, or do you believe him?

When it came to their official correspondence, Ford's team tried to curb its outrage. In dealing with an institution like the Senate, the whole world was watching. Ford had requested that her attorneys speak as collegially as possible to the committee. She insisted that coming forward was not a partisan move, and that she would still have spoken up if Kavanaugh had been from her own party. It was not clear if she understood that many others saw her differently: She was working with Democratic lawyers, whom she had learned of from the top Democrat on the Senate Judiciary Committee, and with Seidman, a Democratic operative, making an accusation that might topple a Republican Supreme Court pick. To Mike Davis, who was the Republican staff member leading the committee's negotiations, it appeared as if Ford's team had exploited her allegation for political purposes, and that dragging out the negotiation was part of a coordinated strategy to derail Kavanaugh's nomination, Davis said later.

Back in Palo Alto, stuck in a hotel, Ford was receiving reports from the negotiations but not quite keeping track of all the elements, she later explained. She had been heartened by much of the response to the **Post** article, including from colleagues who were quick to defend her character and former high school classmates who released a letter saying her alleged assault was "all too consistent with stories we heard and lived" at the time. "I can't believe the media—and friends from all times in life—Stanford facility and PAU faculty ready to help," Ford had texted Katz the day the article was published.

But by that Thursday, she still wouldn't even commit to traveling to Washington. When Katz gently pushed her, Ford resisted:

> Ford: I'm feeling way too much
> pressure at moment

Katz was trying to be patient, but she couldn't keep the Judiciary Committee waiting forever.

> Katz: Believe me—i don't want to be
> another pressure. I'm just cognizant
> of the time constraints. We need
> to get an email out to grassley and
> Feinstein soon

Ford: I can't go there ☹ To DC

Katz: That's okay. We can always pull out on the basis that they wouldn't come up with fair rules. This is the right next step

Still, the lawyer needed her client's green light to move forward with the negotiations.

Katz: To clarify—you are okay with us sending the email which we need to do soon. But you want us to be clear that if they don't agree to fair terms that are fair and provide for your security you won't go forward

Ford: I want you to know as you are writing that I can't guarantee I'll go to DC ☹ Can I see final version?

Ford: I'm so scared I can't breathe

Ford was still not acknowledging what was really happening. (This was a pattern: She had written the letter to Feinstein without fully absorbing its potential to leak; she had gone forward with the **Post** story, convincing herself it would cycle out of the news within a week.) She had started, weeks before, by trying to make a small, discreet intervention, and at every stage, things had gotten harder and larger. Now she had a life-altering choice for herself and potentially for the country, and she was trying to avoid it. Katz, Banks, and Seidman were nudging Ford through the process by saying, Leave it to us. They didn't want to operate against their client's wishes, but they were taking the reins, determined to lead Ford forward.

That Thursday night, Ford arrived in a dark French restaurant tucked along a quiet street in San Francisco. Coburn, another one of the Washington attorneys advising her, was in town and was eager to finally meet in person. As she took a seat across from him, Ford pointed to her baseball hat. "This is my disguise," she said trying to force a smile.

Over a long dinner, she made clear why she was so scared to travel to Washington. Her family had been forced to hire twenty-four-hour private security. It was uncertain when it would be safe for them to return home. Ford had already experienced enough disruption and danger.

She pressed Play on her phone at the dinner table. "You lying fucking cunt!" came a voice from her phone. The lawyer told Ford she was right to be frightened by the messages and encouraged her to share them with the FBI. "You've got three months," another voice said. Others repeated similar phrases and sounded like they might have come from the same voice-altering machine, making her think they were somehow coordinated. "Don't be messing with my boy, Brett." "Don't be messing with my boy, Trump."

The next day, Friday, September 21, Katz stopped by her doctor's office to get her stitches removed. In the waiting room, she glanced at the television. The Republicans were losing patience.

CNN was flashing a confidential list of demands that Katz had sent to Grassley's team, apparently leaked by one of the Republican staff members. Trump was now directly casting doubt on Ford's allegation, tweeting: "I have no doubt that, if the attack on Dr. Ford was as bad as she says, charges would have been immediately filed with local Law Enforcement Authorities by either her or her loving parents." At a gathering of Evangelical activists, McConnell was promising that the Senate would "plow right through" and move to confirm Kavanaugh.

That evening, the Republican Judiciary staff announced that the entire committee would vote on Kavanaugh's confirmation the following Monday, September 24. Period. If Ford wanted to appear, she needed to confirm immediately, that Friday night, by 10:00 p.m. The evening news anchors were talking as if the whole thing was already over. "We were about to get steamrolled," Katz said.

Working from their office, Katz and Banks, with cups of coffee in hand, penned a barn-burning public letter to Grassley's staff, accusing them of browbeating a vulnerable woman who was dealing with death threats.

"The imposition of aggressive and artificial deadlines regarding the date and conditions of any hearing has created tremendous and unwarranted anxiety and stress on Dr. Ford," they wrote. "Your cavalier treatment of a sexual assault survivor who has been doing her best to cooperate with the Committee is completely inappropriate."

"The 10 p.m. deadline is arbitrary. Its sole purpose is to bully Dr. Ford and deprive her of the ability to make a considered decision that has life-altering implications for her and her family," they continued. "Our modest request is that she be given an additional day to make her decision." They released the response directly to members of the media, and it was immediately broadcast on TV.

Two hours later, Grassley tweeted out word of his concession, in an odd format that made it look like he was posting a text to the judge:

> Judge Kavanaugh I just granted
> another extension to Dr Ford to
> decide if she wants to proceed w
> the statement she made last week to
> testify to the senate She shld decide
> so we can move on I want to hear
> her. I hope u understand. It's not my
> normal approach to b indecisive

With no road map and no Democratic control of any of the branches of government, Katz, Banks, and Seidman had positioned Ford to testify on their time frame, even though their client had not even signed on to do so. Later, the world would talk about the power of Ford's testimony without understanding the less visible role that the other women had played.

But now they needed to get their client to Washington.

By Saturday, it was clear Ford was never going to give one firm and final yes to testifying in an open hearing. Her ambivalence was paralyzing. So her advisers worked in tandem, coaxing her from one baby step to another.

A sympathetic tech executive had offered his private jet for Ford to travel to Washington. Ford warned her team that any mention of the aircraft would make her more nervous, not less. Katz texted her photos of it anyway, to convey the reality of the situation.

Next, the advisers asked Ford to consider who she would invite to Washington if she decided to move forward. The plane could accommodate some of her friends. Her husband would stay in Palo Alto to care for their sons; both parents were determined not to disrupt the boys' lives any more than necessary. Ford considered who of her friends would be steadiest. One was a mother of triplets and a fourth daughter less than two years apart, who had served as a confidante that summer, starting with the beachside talks in Santa Cruz. She would know how to help Ford keep her cool. So would Keith Koegler, her friend and confidante, who would submit a sworn affidavit to the Senate Judiciary Committee about the time years earlier when Ford had told him about being assaulted by a prominent judge. Two friends, faculty members from the Stanford School of Medicine, would also be useful to have by her side.

By talking through these hypothetical scenarios, Katz, Banks, and the other advisers convinced Ford to go to Washington to talk to the senators. By Sunday, their team and Grassley's staff finally reached consensus: The hearing would take place the following Thursday, September 27.

But that Sunday, September 23, the entire dynamic of the Kavanaugh fight shifted. The material that Ford's team had spent weeks wondering about finally arrived: two additional allegations against the judge, which surfaced almost simultaneously. Suddenly, he was being portrayed in a far darker light, as a repeat offender.

The **New Yorker** published the account of Deborah Ramirez, who alleged that Kavanaugh had exposed himself to her during a drunken party when they were classmates at Yale. She said she had been intoxicated "on the floor, foggy and slurring her words" when Kavanaugh thrust his penis in her face, and she touched it as she was pushing him away. "Brett was laughing," Ramirez was quoted saying. "I can still see his face, and his hips coming forward, like when you pull up your pants."

At practically the same moment, Michael Avenatti, a California plaintiff lawyer who represented Stormy Daniels, the porn star who had accepted a settlement from Trump, tweeted out more ominous-sounding accusations about Kavanaugh from a new client:

> We are aware of significant evidence of multiple house parties in the Washington, D.C. area during the early 1980s, during which Brett Kavanaugh, Mark Judge and others would participate in the targeting of women with alcohol/drugs to allow a "train" of men to subsequently gang rape them.

Avenatti didn't name his client, but published leading questions directed to the judge on Twitter, such as "Did you ever target one or more women for sex or rape at a house party?" He claimed to have multiple witnesses who were prepared to testify.

As Katz, Banks, and Seidman followed the developments, they believed that Ramirez was telling the truth about Kavanaugh exposing himself and that the allegation would help boost Ford's credibility.

But they thought what Avenatti was doing felt like a sideshow, one that could potentially cause harm.

That same Sunday morning, Rebecca Corbett, working at home from Baltimore, had known the **New Yorker** story was coming, the way journalists at competing publications often know these things: through overlapping reporting and common sources. When she learned the **New Yorker** was about to publish, she assumed the magazine had nailed the story, and she had asked her reporters to begin to draft a story that would summarize the magazine's findings. That kind of article, humbling to write, had a name in journalism: a "follow."

But as soon as Corbett, Baquet, and Purdy read the **New Yorker** article that evening, Corbett told her reporters to pause. The magazine had obtained something crucial that the **Times** had not: an interview with Ramirez. Some aspects of the story were similar to Ford's: The **New Yorker** article included no eyewitnesses. (An unnamed classmate said he had heard about the incident, but not seen it.) People Ramirez recalled being at the party denied the incident ever happened or said they didn't remember the party at all.

But Ramirez's account came with other asterisks. The article acknowledged that Ramirez had been reluctant to speak, partly because she had memory gaps from the drinking, and that it had taken her

six days of assessing her recollections to describe
Kavanaugh's role in the alleged incident with cer-
tainty. (Ronan Farrow, a coauthor of the story, later
said that many victims struggle with memory gaps
and that the six days were a sign of her carefulness.)
If Ramirez had named Kavanaugh as the perpetrator
to others, before he was nominated, the **New Yorker**
did not have any examples. Perhaps they had further,
off-the-record support for Ramirez's account, but it
was not in the article.

The standard practice in journalism was for com-
petitors to try to match one another's reporting on a
significant story. If the **Post** had a scoop on Trump's
dealings with Russia, the **Times** would attempt to report on the same material, and vice versa, to inform
their own readers but also for additional confirmation. It was like scientists performing peer reviews:
If separate, even rival, teams were able to execute the
same experiments with the same results, the findings were more trustworthy. In the Weinstein reporting, the **Times** and the **New Yorker** articles had
mostly—if not entirely—matched up, an indication
of the strength of the material.

This was a different scenario. **Times** reporters
had also interviewed dozens of former classmates
and hallmates in recent days and found no one
with firsthand knowledge of the incident. What's
more, the **Times** had learned that Ramirez had
told some of her former Yale classmates that she could
not be certain Kavanaugh was the one who exposed

himself. The **Times** editors were not drawing conclusions about what had happened that night at the party—only that based on the **Times**'s own reporting, the allegation was not well-supported enough to publish as a stand-alone follow story.

Avenatti's tweets presented a separate and much graver set of concerns. He had made veiled allegations of gang rape against the judge without even saying who the accuser was. The lawyer seemed to have his own agenda. In representing Stormy Daniels, Avenatti had dispensed information to the media while cultivating his own presidential ambitions. As that story had played out months before, the brash lawyer had explained to Corbett that he would offer some tips to the **Times** and other news organizations, but his primary strategy was to get on television. "I'll sleep with you, but I'm not going to marry you," he said.

That Sunday, Corbett instructed the **Times** journalists to continue finding out more about the new allegations. But that evening's article about the politics of Ford's upcoming testimony only mentioned the Ramirez allegation in the fourteenth paragraph, and also pointed out the **Times**'s different findings. There was no mention of Avenatti and his unnamed client.

By Monday morning, Republicans were using the weak points in the new allegations to more fiercely defend Kavanaugh. The assumption by Ford's team that additional allegations would bolster their client's story looked like it might be mistaken. Instead, they could detract from Ford's story. A week before, Kellyanne Conway had been arguing that Ford deserved to be heard. Now, in an appearance on **CBS This Morning,** Conway said the allegations against Kavanaugh were "starting to feel like a vast left-wing conspiracy" and implied that the judge was a victim of "pent-up demand" of victims of sexual harassment and assault.

Standing on the Senate floor, McConnell accused Democrats of engaging in a "shameful smear campaign" against the judge. Emboldened, Kavanaugh released a letter saying he wasn't going anywhere.

Mike Davis, the Republican staffer on the Senate Judiciary Committee, said later that the emergence of Avenatti had been especially significant. "He jumped into this thing and turned it into a circus, undermining the credibility of the other accusers," Davis said.

By the morning of Wednesday, September 26, the day before the testimony, Ford was secretly ensconced at the Watergate Hotel, chosen less for its legacy than its location off the grid of downtown Washington.

Ford had flown in the day before, on the borrowed private jet, with prescription Ativan to help her relax, she explained later. As soon as she had disembarked, Conway, of all people, had materialized, apparently waiting to board another plane. Ford had pulled down her baseball cap while friends who had accompanied her from California flanked her protectively, but Conway had given no sign of recognition. That wasn't surprising: Though Ford was at the dead center of the news, the public did not know the sound of her voice or what she looked like. All that had been published was a photo that had been taken decades ago and the shot in sunglasses. At the Watergate, she was protected so tightly that every time she opened her hotel room door, her security guard, positioned in the room next door, opened his in unison. Until the next morning, she would still be mostly a mystery to the country.

As her friends headed out to visit Washington monuments, Ford went to a conference room on a lower floor of the hotel. Katz and Banks were there, dashing back and forth from their law office to the secret prep room. So was Larry Robbins, who had continued to counsel Ford behind the scenes, and Michael Bromwich, a former colleague of Robbins's, who had joined the team the previous Friday and helped with the final round of negotiations with the Judiciary Committee. Seidman was at work across the hall.

The narrow, unassuming room had spotty wi-fi, but someone had stocked each seat at the conference table with Watergate-logo pads, pens, and water bottles. Katz, a junior attorney in her office, and Bromwich had drafted an opening statement, drawing on the details that Ford had provided to them and the **Post,** steering clear of sexually explicit language that she knew made Ford uncomfortable. Ford read the draft and rewrote it almost entirely. "I crossed almost everything out," she said. Not because of factual errors but because it just didn't sound like her. "It wasn't my language. It wasn't in the right order. I had to make it my own." Ford wrote and rewrote, as she did when working on scientific papers, tuning out the lawyers in the room.

Bromwich and Robbins spent an hour walking Ford through some questions they thought she might face during the hearing and offered her general advice on how to handle the testimony chair: You're there to tell the truth; don't worry about the outcome, they explained. If the senators use ambiguous words, don't speculate about their meaning. If they ask a question in three parts, ask them to break down each part one at a time. Bromwich explained that he would sit next to Ford during the hearing. When senators paused, she should look at them, breathe deeply, and not concern herself with what they were saying.

Robbins and Bromwich, both specialists in congressional testimony, knew that the key to performing well in that format was practicing ahead of time, anticipating questions, polishing replies. Everyone practiced for congressional testimony, even for cut-and-dried regulatory matters. Not practicing answers was considered incautious, even a little reckless. The lawyers would need to run Ford through those drills very quickly: Some corporate executives spent weeks, even months, preparing for their own turns in front of Congress, and they only had one day.

Ford took some notes but found it hard to concentrate because the lawyers were talking over each other. When they asked her to practice her responses, she refused. "She was very insistent," Robbins said.

In less than twenty-four hours, Ford would be giving the most sensitive testimony anyone in Washington had heard in a long time. To avoid the impression of an all-male bank of Republican interlocutors, those senators were ceding their question time to an experienced prosecutor named Rachel Mitchell. Everyone, not just the senators, would be listening for any weaknesses, inconsistencies, or awkward moments on Ford's part.

Ford wasn't fazed. To her it would have been like practicing for a test to which she already knew the answers. She was confident of which data she did and did not know. No practice would change that.

She was only worried about one aspect: "I'm not sure I can do this in front of cameras," she told the team. She reiterated a question she had been asking for days: Why couldn't she just field questions from the Senate Judiciary Committee in a closed hearing?

Now Seidman stepped in. In a one-on-one conversation with Ford, she reiterated what Katz and Banks had been saying to her for days: The only way she could ensure that her account was communicated with accuracy and integrity was in a televised hearing. That's what Kavanaugh would be doing. "Okay," Ford replied.

Seidman was finally convinced that Ford would follow through. But Katz and Banks weren't so sure.

That afternoon, Jodi took a train to Washington, looked up the address of Katz and Banks's law firm, found a coffee bar a few steps from their office, and prepared to wait there for many hours. Katz had not invited her. She had never met Banks and still had never exchanged a word with Ford. At this point, she and Megan knew only bits and pieces about what going on behind the scenes. When Jodi had told Katz she was buying a train ticket, the attorney had said she couldn't make any promises in terms of what Jodi would be able to see. But she and Megan had agreed that one of them had to be in Washington for what was about to happen, to witness it from the closest possible vantage point, as they sought to figure out what these events would mean.

Later that evening, Jodi was sitting in the same coffee bar when Katz and Banks showed up to retrieve her and take her upstairs to witness the tail end of their preparations. Upstairs the lawyers were in great spirits. Their office had been transformed into a command center, filled with reminders of the disparate reactions to the client's story. Because of the threats the lawyers had received, security guards stood at the door. But the space was also cluttered

with tokens of encouragement, like flower arrangements for Ford, sent by strangers, grouped haphaz-
ardly on Katz's desk. So many cookies had arrived
that they stood in stacks atop the file cabinets.

Only a small team of mostly female lawyers and
strategists who were volunteering to help Ford was
left in the office. Their mood was energized, optimistic, and defiant.

On her way to the elevator, Katz grabbed a print
copy of the **Times** off a desk and gestured triumphantly at the headline: "Bill Cosby, Once a Model
of Fatherhood, Is an Inmate." The day before, Bill
Cosby had been sentenced to three to ten years in
prison, a moment of accountability that many had
thought would never arrive. Commentators were
saying it was the first major verdict of the #MeToo
era. Katz felt like history was on her side.

But at the same moment, Trump was on television,
blasting the accusations against Kavanaugh as part
of one big Democratic "con job," among the developments that Megan was tracking back in New York.
The president was using the Kavanaugh case to reas-
sert his own innocence and position himself as a victim. "I've been a famous person for a long time, but
I've had a lot of false charges made against me, really
false charges," Trump said. "So when I see it, I view
it differently than somebody sitting home watching
television where they say, 'Oh, Judge Kavanaugh this
or that.' It's happened to me many times."

Trump once again took direct aim at Megan and

Barbaro's coverage of his treatment of women, calling it "false reporting" and "fake news." Trump also described "four or five women who got paid a lot of money to make up stories about me." There was no evidence to support Trump's claim. But Lisa Bloom's efforts to line up donations to potential Trump accusers from prominent Democrats had been documented by journalists, arming him with a talking point that, once altered and exaggerated, helped him make his case.

Ford went to bed at 10:00 p.m., hoping to get a solid night's sleep. Two hours later, she was up. She took a shower and watched television until dawn. "I was waiting and ready to go do it and be done," she said later.

The morning was a haze of preparation. A stylist showed up to do her hair, and when she glanced in the mirror, she didn't really look like herself, because the ends were curled. Some of her advisers had suspected, correctly, that the California academic didn't have the type of clothes normally worn to Congressional hearings, so they had ordered eleven different suits that were delivered to her hotel the day before. To Ford, the suits had looked so dark and expensive—so East Coast. She chose the one non-black option, in midnight blue, one that she would be able to wear teaching, and a tailor had materialized to adjust it.

Two colleagues from Stanford, one who had flown on the private jet, another who happened to be in town, joined her for breakfast in her hotel room. As they discussed the scientific papers each of them had been working on, Ford felt herself transitioning into the professional mode she intended to adopt in the hearing.

A Chevy Suburban SUV was waiting. She rode in the SUV to Capitol Hill with Katz, Banks, Bromwich, Robbins, and two of her security guards. The car pulled into an underground carpark, and then she was escorted through the bowels of Congress, down a hallway and up a stairwell into a wide corridor lined with office doors. People were peeking out, trying to catch a glimpse of her. Soon she and her team were in their own space, a room that looked like an office several doors down from the hearing chamber, where they would be able to rest and regroup during breaks. Ford was still editing the opening statement she carried in a binder, obsessing over each word choice. Ford said she crossed out a "screamed" and changed it to "yelled."

When Grassley stopped by her room, Ford smiled and exchanged pleasantries with him. She was still determined to be as congenial as possible every step of the way.

Ford's advisers had pushed the Judiciary Committee to hold the hearing in one of its smaller rooms, which they thought would help minimize Ford's jitters. None of them had explicitly told

Ford the extent to which the testimony would be broadcast: another move that glossed over how massive, how consequential, this dispute over one encounter in high school had grown. Katz and Banks were worried that if she knew she would freeze with fear.

As the proceedings came to order, Ford began to read her statement without much sense of the impression she was making. She had been telling this same story all summer. She had been up all night. At her first moment at the microphone, she had asked for caffeine. The room felt strange, with senators elevated above her. The lights were overwhelmingly bright, as if they were all in an operating theater.

Her voice was scratchy with emotion, but she did not break down. The words and images she had chosen so carefully were especially evocative. She spoke of Kavanaugh fumbling to get past the one-piece bathing suit she had worn under her clothes, and the sound of the boys "pinballing off the walls" on the way downstairs as she hid in a bathroom.

"I have had to relive this trauma in front of the world, and have seen my life picked apart by people on television, on Twitter, other social media, other media, and in this body, who have never met me or spoken with me," she said. "I am an independent person and I am no one's pawn. My motivation in coming forward was to be helpful and to provide facts about how Mr. Kavanaugh's actions have damaged my life, so that you could take into serious consideration as you make your decision about how to proceed."

Ford was used to question-and-answer exchanges from the many hours she had spent in scientific conferences, and now she drew on that experience, trying to speak clearly and precisely. She didn't mind her back-and-forths with Rachel Mitchell, the prosecutor to whom the Republicans had ceded their questioning. Unlike the senators, the prosecutor was seated at floor level, which helped make it feel like they were having a human-to-human interaction, she said. And her first rounds of questions felt respectful.

But as the session went on, Ford grew alarmed. The focus of Mitchell's inquiries was changing. How had Ford traveled to Washington? What were the circumstances of her polygraph test? This all seemed tangential and confusing to her, she said. By the final break, Ford was worn down. She did not want to go back in.

When her turn at the microphone was finally finished, Mitchell approached her.

"I'll be praying for your safety," the prosecutor said. That terrified Ford. Did she know about something specific that Ford should fear?

Back in their private room, Ford's advisers were smiling and commending her. She appreciated the feedback but still saw it in academic terms. "When you give a science talk, you just say what you know," she explained. "It's not 'great job!'" But in terms of transmitting her account, she felt like she had done well—left it all on the field, she said later, using one of her beloved sports analogies. When Republican senator Jeff Flake of Arizona, seen as a potential toss-up vote, stopped by to say hello, she greeted him warmly. She still had little sense of the power or resonance her voice had carried out across the land.

Jodi, who had borrowed a pass for the packed hearing room and slipped in near the end of Ford's turn, was absorbing her first impressions of Ford in person. She faced the senators, seated at a huge wooden table, flanked by Katz and Bromwich. With only the back of her head visible to Jodi, what had come through most strongly was her voice. It was unexpectedly girlish, but she had authority, in part because she was so precise. In her testimony, she seemed devoted to getting every answer right. Unlike in the Weinstein case, when the voices of victims had been mediated by journalists, the world had watched and heard unfiltered narration from the woman herself.

Many viewers thought she was such a compelling witness that the nomination was virtually dead. On C-SPAN, sexual assault survivors were calling in to share their stories. "I have not brought this up for years until I heard this testimony and it is just breaking my heart," said a seventy-six-year-old woman. Trump said he found Ford "very compelling" and "a very credible witness." At the **Times,** editors and reporters were poised to cover a Kavanaugh withdrawal if necessary.

Like many other viewers, Jodi and Megan weren't sure what to expect when it came time for Kavanaugh to speak at the hearing. Would the distinguished federal judge present himself as above it all, to remind the world how much respect he had accumulated over his career? Perhaps he would say that he sincerely could not remember any such incident but that he should be judged by his adult conduct. That tactic had helped other figures dismiss damaging reports from their youth. During the 2000 presidential race, George W. Bush had brushed away stories of excess drinking, by saying, "When I was young and irresponsible, I was young and irresponsible." It was one of the most effective lines of autobiographical spin ever, making the former party boy sound self-deprecating and sympathetic—no one wanted to be judged by their younger self's worst moments.

But it quickly became clear that that was not Kavanaugh's intention. As he took his turn at the polished wood table, he regained ground, giving a sweeping, forceful denial of Ford's accusation under oath. "I categorically and unequivocally deny the allegation against me by Dr. Ford. I never had any sexual or physical encounter of any kind with Dr. Ford. I never attended a gathering like the one Dr. Ford describes in her allegation. I've never sexually assaulted Dr. Ford or anyone," he said.

Jodi couldn't see his face either, just a brush of

brown-gray hair atop square shoulders. But she could hear him, and his rush of anger, almost as if he was spitting his opening statement into the air. His demeanor was the opposite of Ford's. She had sounded measured, calm, polite, not particularly political, and eager to please, sprinkling her testimony with scientific terminology, as if to help validate what she was saying. He sounded loud, biting, and openly partisan. "This whole two-week effort has been a calculated and orchestrated political hit, fueled with apparent pent-up anger about President Trump and the 2016 election," he said.

Over the course of several minutes, he put the listener in his shoes, describing a life of hard work upended by an escalating and out-of-control series of complaints. Over the previous week, Avenatti's client, Julie Swetnick, had finally come forward; in a sworn statement to the committee and then in a TV interview, she contradicted herself and was widely seen as not credible.

"The Swetnick thing is a joke," he said. "That is a farce."

"I wanted a hearing the day after the allegation came up," he said, referring to Ford's account. "Instead, ten days passed where all this nonsense is coming out," he said, mentioning some of the vaguer rumors that had circulated: "I'm on boats in Rhode Island, I'm in Colorado, you know, I'm sighted all over the place. And these things are printed and run, breathlessly, by cable news," he said.

"My family and my name have been totally and permanently destroyed by vicious and false additional accusations," he said. That word—**additional**—was telling.

He was driving a larger argument, making himself a focal point for male grievance, saying that he was the victim, that his entire lifetime of dedication and care, down to the hours he spent coaching his daughters in basketball, was being destroyed by women making irresponsible claims.

"If every American who drinks beer or every American who drank beer in high school is suddenly presumed guilty of sexual assault, we'll be in an ugly new place in this country," he said.

The Republican senators used their own question time to amplify his message. They sidelined Rachel Mitchell, who had been pressing Kavanaugh on the particulars of the alleged incidents, abandoning their plan to let a woman serve as their public voice. Instead, the all-male group of Republicans took turns expressing outrage at what they called the victimization of an upstanding man.

"It just keeps getting worse," said Senator John Cornyn of Texas. "It's this story that not even the **New York Times** would report, the allegation of Ms. Ramirez. And then Stormy Daniels's lawyer comes up with this incredible story, accusing you of the most sordid and salacious conduct. It's outrageous, and you're right to be angry."

"A disgrace," said Senator Orrin Hatch of Utah.

"This has been sadly one of the most shameful chapters in the history of the United States Senate," echoed Senator Ted Cruz of Texas.

During the testimony, the judge made some improbable statements. He called "Devil's Triangle," a term in his yearbook that had received media attention, a drinking game, when most people knew it as high school slang for a three-way liaison between two men and a woman. He claimed that Ford's story had been "refuted by the very people she says were there, including by a longtime friend of hers." That was not true: the friend, Leland Keyser, whom Ford recalled being at the party, had told the Judiciary Committee in a letter written by her attorney that she didn't remember the gathering and didn't know Kavanaugh, but she also had told the **Washington Post** she believed Ford was telling the truth. When Senator Amy Klobuchar, a Democrat from Minnesota, asked Kavanaugh if he had ever partially or fully blacked out from drinking, he countered by asking if **she** ever had, sounding defensive.

In the hearing room, Jodi was struck by something that wasn't as palpable on television: the small size of the room, packed not just with Ford and Kavanaugh supporters, but leaders and critics of #MeToo. When Ford had finished her testimony, cries of "Thank you, Doctor Ford" had mingled with a shout of "Confirm Brett!" The seats for visitors ran only eight abreast, not that much bigger than airplane rows. Women in Kavanaugh T-shirts were right up against those who had come for Ford. Tarana Burke, the founder of the #MeToo movement, had come in sneakers, so she could walk to the protest events happening all over Capitol Hill. She was sitting not far from Ashley Kavanaugh, the judge's wife, who wore an expression of horror. All of them were crammed into an official-looking box, with wood paneling and brass seals, for a fight with improvised rules and no impartial referee.

The next morning, Jodi met Katz in the lobby of the Watergate Hotel. In the narrow conference room where Ford had huddled with her team, the preparation gear was still lying around, neat arrangements of highlighters and peanut M&M's. A second later, Ford walked in.

She seemed completely similar, and utterly different, from the day before. The first words out of her mouth were the exact same thing she had said at the start of the hearings: She requested caffeine. She was as eager to please as she had been in the hearing, asking Katz if she had been gracious enough when Senator Flake had said hello. ("You were lovely," Katz reassured her.) But the formal suit was gone, replaced with a turquoise hoodie and blue rubber Birkenstock sandals, reminders that this person came with an identity and life that was only partially represented in her few hours on the public stage. She looked like a Californian again, her hair still mussed from sleep.

Around her wrist, she wore a thin silver bracelet that said "Courageous."

Since she had left Capitol Hill the day before, she finally allowed herself to collapse somewhat. She had not watched Kavanaugh's testimony. The previous night, her friends and family had congregated in a room at the Watergate for a little thank-goodness-it's-over gathering, her Palo Alto guests meeting her high school friends. One was going on television to be interviewed about Ford, and she thanked her for doing that. Her parents were there too. As everyone else was chatting and drinking, Ford had laid down on the little upholstered bench, right there in the party room, and closed her eyes.

Ford's airplane was leaving soon, and she was eager to return West, to fly away from the Washington ordeal. As she talked about when she could move back into her house, she focused on slipping back into her old life and routine. That hardly seemed possible: Her story was now having a seismic national, cultural, and political effect.

A few hours later, as the Judiciary Committee geared up to vote on whether to send the nomination to the full Senate, Katz and Banks watched the minute-by-minute television coverage from the conference room of their office. Jodi sat with them, observing the attorneys as they waited to find out if their client's testimony would truly influence the outcome of the nomination.

Katz paced the length of the conference table, texting with Ford, who was airborne. The wait was agonizing, and the outcome the lawyers wanted— for Senator Jeff Flake or another Republican to vote no—was unlikely. So as the headlines and images flicked by, without any real news yet, Jodi asked the lawyers a broader question: How much had really changed in the past year, and what would the legacy of Ford's testimony be?

"If he's confirmed, I question whether we're any better off," said Banks, the pessimist of the pair.

Katz, still the believer in the possible, could not let that answer stand. She felt Ford had challenged outdated social norms and had only been able to do so because the #MeToo movement had given her a window, because standards had already shifted. "A year ago she would never have been given an opportunity to testify," she argued.

"Things **have** qualitatively changed," she continued. "The institutions have **not** changed. The Senate has **not** changed. The power of this country is aggregated in the White House and in the Senate. But that doesn't say that this movement is a failure." Katz added that many of Ford's adversaries had not directly called her a liar, but, instead, floated an eccentric theory that she had been mistaken about the identity of the perpetrator. That was an odd form of progress, she said, but it was progress nonetheless.

"I'm not saying the movement's a failure," Banks retorted. "I'm saying despite the power of the movement, the results seem to be the same."

In the end, the television didn't offer clear answers. After being dramatically confronted by two sexual assault survivors in a Capitol Hill elevator, Flake negotiated a pause in the process, asking for an FBI investigation of Ford's allegation, as well as Ramirez's, before the full Senate voted on Kavanaugh's nomination. This was exactly what Katz and Banks had tried and failed to obtain weeks before. Now the Republicans on the committee and the White House signed off, eager to do whatever necessary to solidify Flake's support for the judge.

Jodi returned to New York and Megan arrived to continue shadowing the lawyers. On television and online, some observers were heralding the postponement of the vote and the launch of the FBI investigation as a victory for Ford, but Katz and Banks were skeptical. "We still don't know how all this will play out," Katz told Megan.

A few hours later, back in California that Friday, September 28, Ford had an emotional reunion with her husband and her two sons. The boys jumped up and down, smothering her with hugs, she said.

For the first time in months, Ford felt almost serene. There had been some embarrassment, sitting in front of all those cameras, and some awkwardness with Rachel Mitchell. But no one had actually tried to destroy her family or academic career. She assumed Kavanaugh would be confirmed, as she always had. Her victory had been telling her story to the world with dignity, she said. Maybe that would make it easier for the next generation of victims to come forward. And maybe the people vetting candidates for the court would be more careful next time.

Finally, Ford thought, she could return to her life. She turned down every interview request, telling her team: "I don't want to be **that** person, I just want to go back to teaching."

Instead, she came under attack, as Republicans sought to push Kavanaugh's confirmation through.

On Sunday night, Rachel Mitchell sent a five-page memo to the Senate Republicans taking aim at her credibility. ("A 'he said, she said' case is incredibly difficult to prove. But this case is even weaker than that.") Three nights later, Trump mocked her gleefully at a campaign rally in Southaven, Mississippi, letting loose more than ever before. ("'How did you get home?' 'I don't remember.' 'How did you get there?' 'I don't remember.' 'Where is the place?' 'I don't remember.' 'How many years ago was it?' 'I don't know. I don't know. I don't know.' 'What neighborhood was it in?' 'I don't know.' 'Where's the house?' 'I don't know.' 'Upstairs, downstairs, where was it?' 'I don't know.'")

As Trump spoke, Republicans on the Senate Judiciary Committee released a sworn statement from a man Ford had dated in the early 1990s claiming that he had seen Ford use her understanding of psychology to coach a roommate as she prepared to take a polygraph test as part of a job interview with federal law enforcement, a claim that appeared designed to cast doubt on the polygraph test that Ford had passed. Ford was furious. It was one thing for critics to take shots at her. But this lie also hurt her friend, Monica McLean, the former FBI agent who was forced to publicly deny having ever let Ford or anyone else prepare her for a polygraph exam.

It felt like everyone in the country had a reaction to what Ford had done. A server at Dale's restaurant in Southaven, Mississippi, the same town where Trump had just spoken, was among those who were outraged. "Any woman can say anything," she said of the #MeToo movement. "You know as well as I do, they bring it on themselves, to get up the ladder, to destroy somebody they don't care for. I think it's something that should be kept personal. Sure there's a lot of bad guys in this world doing a lot of things they shouldn't have been." Her own daughter was a rape victim, she said. "I mean, I understand it big-time. You go to counseling, for a year, two, whatever you need to do, but PTSD? No, I can't see that. That's just too much. My daughter has gone on just fine in life. You forgive, you forget. You don't carry that with you your whole stupid life."

Others were celebrating Ford as a hero. Victims of sexual violence everywhere were still pouring their hearts out in response to her testimony. She was receiving tens of thousands of letters from supporters confiding their own personal stories of abuse, assault, and harassment. Celebrities like Ellen DeGeneres and Connie Chung were going public for the first time about violations they said they had suffered, citing Ford as their motivation. Protestors were swarming Capitol Hill with an intensity that made the initial Kavanaugh demonstrations look mild. **Time** magazine created a visual testament to Ford on its cover, an image of her face made with lines from her testimony.

In speaking with the **Washington Post,** in testifying before cameras, Ford had sought to retain control over her own story, but now it was being undermined, heralded, and otherwise appropriated. Desperate for a final say, Ford turned back to her team. Was there something else she could do or say? Her team counseled her against it. She could show a video of the attack, Katz and Banks told her, and critics would still dismiss her. And there was no way she could assume the weight of every survivor's trauma.

"You can't take on all the hopes and prayers and dreams of every person who wants women to be treated respectfully," Katz later recalled telling her in a phone call. "You can't carry that."

Ford couldn't let go. On Thursday night, October 4, Ford called Katz and Banks. The next day, the Senate would finally take its first vote on whether to advance Kavanaugh's nomination. In the end, the FBI investigation of Ford's allegation had been extremely narrow; after interviewing Mark Judge, P. J. Smyth, Leland Keyser, and an attorney for one of the witnesses, the FBI had found "no corroboration." They had not interviewed Ford—or Kavanaugh. The questions about what had really happened three decades earlier had not been settled. (The investigation also found no corroboration of Ramirez's allegation.)

But Ford wanted a final say. That evening, she finished composing a secret letter she had begun drafting two days earlier. It was addressed to Senator Jeff Flake, thanking him for the kindness he had shown her.

Late that night, Banks sent the letter to the senator's private email address. The next morning, before the vote, a courier whisked a hard copy to his office.

That afternoon, Friday, October 5, the Senate advanced the nomination. The final vote would likely take place the next day. It was the exact first anniversary of Jodi and Megan's first Weinstein story, and the second anniversary of the release of the **Access Hollywood** tape almost to the day.

Megan took a train to Washington and found Katz outside her office. The lawyer's cell phone was cradled in her neck and tears were in her eyes. The vote had played out as they expected. She was talking to Ford, both women processing what was happening. Ford had done far more than she had ever planned. The judge was still going to be on the Supreme Court.

"You did your part, stay strong," Katz said into the phone.

The next day, Katz, Banks, and a junior attorney in their office walked past hundreds of protesters and into the halls of the Senate building, trailed by Megan, for the final vote on Kavanaugh's nomination. In the Senate gallery, the lawyers pushed open the wood doors, walked down the white marble stairs, and slid into the blue chairs. They were there to represent Ford right up to the very end, even if it meant simply sitting in the gallery, they said.

The lawyers watched with grim faces as Republican senators rose to talk about how innocent men everywhere were at risk of being unfairly targeted. Most of them did not directly attack Ford; they called her a pawn of those trying to defeat Kavanaugh's nomination. Democrats were doing the opposite, criticizing Kavanaugh, and praising his accusers, sympathizing with sexual assault victims everywhere. When Senator Dick Durbin, a Democrat from Illinois, heralded Ford as the definition of civic duty, and apologized for the treatment she had received, Katz bent her head, overcome.

The mounting concern on both sides of the debate had turned into fury. On Capitol Hill, anti-Kavanaugh protestors displayed massive signs that said WE BELIEVE CHRISTINE BLASEY FORD and WE BELIEVE

ALL SURVIVORS and confronted Republican senators in person, and even arrived at McConnell's house with beer cans, in reference to Kavanaugh's teenage habits, yelling "Chug, chug, chug" and "What do we do with a drunken justice?" Now some worked their way into the gallery for the final vote. One by one, they rose to shout their complaints. As security dragged them out, their cries echoed down the hall: "I stand with survivors." "This process is corrupt." "This is a stain on American history."

Across the room, Don McGahn, Trump's White House counsel, sat watching the proceedings with a smile on his face. When the vote was over, Senator McConnell held a press conference. Megan noted that he too radiated delight: He had gotten a new Supreme Court majority and maybe an unexpected political bonus too. The "virtual mob that's assaulted all of us in the course of this process has turned our base on fire," he said.

Kavanaugh's confirmation was certainly not the final measure of the fate of the #MeToo movement. A few weeks before, McDonald's workers, including Kim Lawson, the woman Jodi had interviewed, had held a coast-to-coast walkout over the company's weak sexual harassment policies. Historians were calling it the country's first sexual harassment–related strike in a century. Leslie Moonves, the chairman of CBS, stepped down, becoming the first Fortune 500 CEO to lose his job in the reckoning.

The day before, the Nobel Peace Prize committee had announced that its 2018 award would go to Nadia Murad and Denis Mukwage, two activists who had worked to end sexual violence. At that moment, the **Times** was finishing a shocking story about Google and secret problems among some of its top male executives, including the so-called father of Android phones, who had been paid $90 million to leave the company after another employee had accused him of forced oral sex, an allegation he denied.

The debate over Ford's allegations was helping people reassess high school behavior, even if only in private. That's where a lot of the most profound change was happening, with the cacophonous public conversations, so frequently unsatisfying, sparking more contemplative private ones.

Ford herself continued to fluctuate in her feelings over what had happened. In her interviews with Megan over the following months, she was often sad or confused, occasionally emboldened and angry, almost always still very anxious. Should she have shared her story? Would it have been better kept to herself? One day Ford was tallying all the reasons not to come forward about an assault. The next day, she would claim to have no regrets. The ambivalence she had originally felt about going public seemed like it might last a very long time.

At the height of the Kavanaugh fracas in Washington, the **Times** had asked readers if they had ever behaved toward women or girls in ways they had regretted. Hundreds replied, confessing transgressions from groping to gang rapes.

"I think 'conquering' her sexually was something I expected I needed to do," wrote Tom Lynch of forcing his hand up a girl's skirt at a prom in 1980.

Terry Wheaton, now eighty-two years old, recounted forcibly kissing a classmate around 1952.

"I'm sorry, Diane," he said.

THE GATHERING

During the final months of 2018, we returned to an idea we had first considered during the Weinstein investigation. Back then, as we struggled to persuade women to break their silence, we wondered if it might help to bring some of them together to talk in person. At the time the idea had seemed impossible, a threat to the secrecy of our reporting.

But we found ourselves thinking about the possibility again, for new reasons. We realized it might help answer lingering questions, which applied far beyond the Weinstein case: What happened to women who spoke up, and what did they make of everything that had transpired?

On January 16, 2019, twelve women who had been part of our reporting convened in Los Angeles, at our request, to try to answer those questions.

The gathering had been challenging to arrange. The women lived in three countries, and we had made many calls and sent many messages to sort through schedules and explain our intention. No, this wouldn't be a group therapy session. We wanted to conduct a joint interview, for journalistic purposes. We had looked for a hotel conference room where everyone could meet, but none seemed private enough. So Gwyneth Paltrow, who was planning to attend, offered her home in Brentwood, with us paying for the meals so as to avoid accepting anything of substantial financial value from a source. For some participants, travel expenses were a barrier, so we covered a few air tickets and hotel rooms.

It was raining at 6:00 p.m. that evening when we arrived, along with our sources and subjects. Our cars pulled past an inconspicuous gray fence, and we found ourselves inside the same kind of sheltered environment as Paltrow's house in the Hamptons, the location of our first in-person interview with her all those months ago. Inside, we congregated in the den, which would be our main meeting room for the evening and part of the next day, accepting drinks and settling on wide sofas in front of a crackling fireplace.

Around the room was a history of our reporting, come to life. Rachel Crooks, who had told Megan her account of being forcibly kissed by the president at the Trump Tower elevator, had traveled from Ohio, where she was still dealing with the fallout of sharing her story, which had brought her more opportunities and problems than she had ever imagined. Seeing the tall Midwesterner in the California home was jolting to Megan—but perhaps no more than everything else that had happened since the two had first spoken.

Ashley Judd was wearing sweats, because she had come straight from her flight from Germany, where she was living. Since the Weinstein story had been published, she had been praised as a heroine, received awards, and accepted a teaching post at Harvard University's Kennedy School, her alma mater. She was to begin in the fall of 2019, with a simple title: "Leader." She was joining the board of Time's Up, the organization to promote safe and fair workplaces that had started in Hollywood in the wake of the Weinstein scandal and spread far beyond it, and had filed her own lawsuit against the producer for harassment, defamation, and loss of career opportunities. Strangers often approached her to convey their gratitude, once even lining up to wait for her as she disembarked from an airplane.

Jodi wanted to see her shake hands with Laura Madden, the former Weinstein assistant with the account of being harassed in Dublin decades ago, who had traveled from Wales. These women were the first two who had gone on the record about the producer. For all the resolve she had shown in October 2017, Madden remained soft-spoken, tucking her soft brown hair behind her ear, explaining that she was unaccustomed to this type of sharing with strangers.

Madden had flown in with her fellow former Miramax employee Zelda Perkins, who had become an activist. A few weeks after the Weinstein story broke, she had held her breath and become the first of several women to break publicly their settlement nondisclosure agreements, speaking to the press about everything except the specific experience and identity of Rowena Chiu, the colleague she had been trying to protect. In effect, Perkins had dared Weinstein to come after her legally, and he had not. In the media and British Parliament, she had mounted a public case against confidential settlements, questioning the whole notion of hush money to silence accusations of sexual abuse and other wrongdoing. Perkins was a critic by nature—that trait had helped drive her to confront Weinstein years ago, and now to challenge accepted legal practice—and she sized up the room with an air of skepticism.

Walking into Paltrow's house felt strange to her: They had last seen one another working on **Shakespeare in Love** and other films but had never shared with each other their accounts of how Weinstein had behaved. After **Shakespeare in Love** had been released, Paltrow won her Oscar a few months after Perkins had signed the settlement papers that would erase her story for the next twenty years. Now the two blondes were seated side by side on a rug in conversation. Paltrow, still wearing a dress and makeup from a talk show taping, was an easy host, sitting back and letting us run the proceedings.

Kim Lawson, the McDonald's worker whom Jodi had first spoken to almost a year before, had come from Kansas City. Since that conversation, she had become a leader of the campaign to make the fast food giant, the second-largest employer in the nation, address sexual harassment on the job. She was accompanied by Allynn Umel, an organizer of the labor campaign. But Lawson didn't appear to need any hand-holding: She was vivacious, and judging from the laughter coming from her corner of the room, she seemed to bond quickly with others.

Christine Blasey Ford sat on the couch, flanked by Debra Katz and Lisa Banks, the two lawyers who had encouraged her to testify. This was a rare excursion: Three months after the Kavanaugh hearing, Ford remained mostly hidden. She was in a much different position than the other women in the room. She was still receiving death threats. She hadn't even returned to local shopping for fear of being approached by strangers, let alone to the teaching job she loved. But she had told Megan that coming to Los Angeles reflected her new determination to venture out.

In addition to those participants, women whom we had written about by name before, was Rowena Chiu, who joined but stood apart in an important way. Since the Weinstein story had broken, she had remained invisible, communicating with Jodi through her lawyer. She had never been publicly identified or broken her silence and wasn't sure if she ever would. We had invited her to join anyway, not in spite of her silence but because of it: So many women had kept terrible stories to themselves. Maybe

Chiu would speak to the consequences of that decision. But she had come on the condition that the
group keep her name confidential, if she never decided to come forward, and that her lawyer, Nancy
Erika Smith, attend too.

Because Chiu had stayed hidden, we had imagined
her as shy or stricken, but she was warm and confident and had an impressive camera slung over her
shoulder. Her parents had moved from Hong Kong
to the United Kingdom before she was born, and she
spoke with a British accent. She had left her life in
film behind many years ago, getting a law degree,
becoming a management consultant, moving to the
United States, and now wrote research papers for
the World Bank while raising four children. She lived
right down the road from Ford, as it happened. To
Jodi's relief, Chiu and her husband were not angry
about the awkward moment in the driveway; they understood how confusing the situation had been. She
and Perkins had finally been in touch again, trying
to figure out who they were to one another after all
this time. But she wasn't sure she would speak at the
gathering, she warned us. She had still never shared
her story out loud with another group of people.

Beginning to mingle, the women were friendly
but tentative. Almost all were strangers to one another, and the thing they had in common was so unusual. Each had obsessed over the decision to share
her account of harassment or assault, in many cases
with either Jodi or Megan coaxing and encouraging

them on the other end of the phone. We had asked them to come to the gathering prepared to answer one central question: After the leap of faith, what had they found on the other side?

We intended the interview, which would begin that evening and stretch into the next day, to be as egalitarian as possible. What each woman had to say was equally important. But there was no avoiding disparities among the participants. At McDonald's, Lawson was now making $10 an hour. Six months before, she had been homeless. We didn't mention that to the others, but every last detail of Paltrow's house—a one-story series of soothing gray-and-white rooms, scattered with small luxuries like soft throws and gilded teacups, all connected by an expansive kitchen—was a tangible reminder of differences between the women.

We made a quick round of introductions, explaining the role that each person had played in our journalism, and soon everyone was settling in at a long table with plates of Japanese food—skewers, salads, rice. The women went around the table, each saying something about how she had decided to speak up, essentially retelling the stories of theirs we have written, and the conversation began to warm up. During Paltrow's turn, she raised a glass and toasted Judd for being the first actress to break the silence about Weinstein.

"Ashley, honestly, what you did—it's very, very hard to be first into the breach," she said, acknowledging that in speaking on the record in the first Weinstein story, Judd had gone where she had not. "You really were the one who paved the way for all of us to come forward in your wake," she said.

"I always worried about you," Judd said back to her—meaning, back in the '90s and whether she was safe from Weinstein.

As the conversation went around the table, some common experiences began to surface. Crooks explained that some of her own family members had continued to support Trump, not her. Perkins said that for all the public attention she had received for her battle against secret settlements, some relatives had never once acknowledged her efforts.

After Madden spoke, she turned to Ford, mentioning that she had been able to speak out about Weinstein in part because she was confident her encounters with him were part of a broader predatory pattern.

"To stand up on your own was quite something," Madden said.

"Yeah, I didn't know if there were other people," Ford replied.

The anticipation in the room rose a notch. The group only knew Ford—her now-famous face and her now-familiar high voice—from her public testimony. She began taking them behind the scenes, recounting her Santa Cruz beachside deliberations over the summer, including her initial idea that she might phone Kavanaugh before he was nominated and ask him to reconsider.

"I was like, 'Why don't we just call him and just be, like: **Hey, let's save our families this whole thing,**'" she said.

When we got to Chiu, Jodi gave her an out, asking if she wanted to pass.

"Sure, I will take a turn," she said: brief words, but for her, momentous ones. "I'm the only person at the table who has not yet gone public with my story, so I've had very little practice in telling it," Chiu said. Aside from her husband, her family still knew nothing, she said.

"There are very few, I feel, Asian voices that come forward with this kind of story," she continued. "It's not because this kind of thing does not happen to Asian people, but I think certainly within the U.S. we have a whole culture around a model minority that doesn't make a fuss, that doesn't speak up, that puts their head down and works really hard and doesn't cause waves."

For those reasons and others, Chiu said, she was now contemplating breaking her silence. "The whole idea of coming out and speaking about something that would undoubtedly shock my friends, and shift the whole of my life, is really terrifying," she said. "It's really helpful to be here tonight to hear each of your perspectives, especially about how you've come forward and what made you come forward."

With that, the agenda became more urgent and concrete. For us, this gathering was an interview to share with readers. For her, it was potential help in making a life-defining choice.

Chiu gestured to her camera and asked if she could take some shots that night and the next day. She had given herself a perfect job: She could hide behind the lens, remaining invisible if she preferred, observing everyone else.

The group reassembled the next morning, forming a loose circle on the same couches and chairs in the den. At the center, a huge gray-and-white ottoman held cups of coffee—and flowerpots containing microphones. This was still an interview, and we were recording, as everyone knew. The plan for the next few hours was simple: We asked the women to take turns sharing stories about what happened after they came forward and hoped the conversation would build from there. Outside, it was still raining, adding to a sense of refuge.

Laura Madden was still nervous about speaking. She was self-effacing, and she had gotten relatively little credit for her bravery, continuing to rinse dishes and supervise homework in Swansea. But in her lilting accent, she told the other women what had happened, simply in her own head, in the wake of the Weinstein story: She had rewritten the history of her adult life.

"I suppose the last year, hearing other people's stories, and also seeing a documentary that was made, and it was really about the employees in London, and seeing how young I was . . . ," she trailed off, trying to describe what it had been like to see her own experience depicted objectively on-screen. "I could reframe it and see that it wasn't actually anything that I did wrong," she said. "It was what he did wrong."

No one could restore the years Madden, now forty-eight, had spent feeling uneasy about her time at Miramax or hand her a fresh career or financial success. But "just being able to see it as **his** problem has helped get some sense of myself back," she said.

Paltrow, sitting cross-legged on the rug by the warmth of the fireplace, described a very different kind of change in understanding her personal history and career. After the story had broken of Weinstein's misconduct, she learned that the producer had used her—her name, her Oscar, her success—as a means of manipulating other vulnerable women. Starting in the fall of 2017, Paltrow had spent many hours on the phone with other women who told her that Weinstein, while harassing or assaulting them, would routinely cite her and her soaring career, falsely implying she had yielded to him. "He was pointing to my career and saying, 'Don't you want what she has?'"

Some of the women had gone public. Others had told Paltrow that because they succumbed to

Weinstein sexually, they felt they could never speak out. Weinstein denied he had ever made those claims about Paltrow, but it seemed this was why he had been so worried about the prospect of her speaking up: Once others knew her story, his scheme would fall apart.

"That has by far been the hardest part of this, to feel like a tool in coercion of rape," Paltrow said through tears. "It almost makes me feel culpable in some way, even though it's completely illogical." As she spoke, her home's luxury suddenly looked a little different: Weinstein had taken Paltrow's enviable life and deployed it against other women.

Umel, the labor organizer for the McDonald's workers, passed the star a box of tissues.

As each woman spoke, the others focused intently, with few phone checks and no interruptions. Each one was a messenger from an unfamiliar world: the battleground Midwest; show business; the thunder dome of Supreme Court confirmation hearings. Those differences, rather than splitting the group, generated curiosity and drew the women together.

Kim Lawson, the twenty-six-year-old fast food worker, her hair in a neat braid, lived more than four thousand miles away from Zelda Perkins. The producer was two decades her senior, spoke with a crisp British accent, and was wearing a sweater with David Bowie's name embroidered on it. But both had thrown themselves into activism, and as they spoke in succession, their words echoed.

Perkins described how she had felt delivering testimony about confidentiality agreements to members of Parliament: "The most extraordinary thing for me was walking into the Palace at Westminster and realizing that as an individual, that this was actually mine—the Palace at Westminster was mine, the politicians were mine."

Lawson told the group about filing a complaint against McDonald's with the Equal Employment Opportunity Commission, the government agency charged with upholding workers' rights against discrimination. "I never felt so much power in my life," she said. Few women in the room had ever walked a picket line, and so she described the September strike: loud chanting and yells of solidarity, new people to meet, a sense of energy and camaraderie, and lots of men who turned out in support, deliberately marching behind the women. Lawson had delivered a speech, given interviews, and pushed her daughter the length of the march in a stroller. "Everyone's with you," she said. "It's like, you're going to hear me today if you heard me no other day, you know?" she said.

Their stories involved a kind of poetic reversal. They had suffered from harassment but gained new authority and respect from fighting it. Even at her young age, Lawson had become a kind of team coach to other female McDonald's employees across the country involved in the union push, counseling them on a text chain. Customers looked at her differently: "Weren't you on TV about sexual harassment?" they asked her.

"Since I've spoken I've been able to come into the person that I was growing into at twenty-four," Perkins said, citing the age she had been when she left Miramax.

But neither Perkins nor Lawson could report complete triumphs. Settlement laws had not changed in the UK, and Perkins did not know if they would. McDonald's was beginning to strengthen its policies, introducing new training for managers and a hotline, and making plans for posters giving employees instructions on how to report. But Lawson hadn't yet seen any of those changes materialize in her own store, and it was not yet clear how much the company's thousands of workplaces would shift.

"There's a huge part of me that can't wait for it all to be over and then to just go back to my horses, and my sheep, and never ever have to speak to a journalist, or be on TV, or do any of those things ever again," Perkins said.

Some of the women nodded. Together, they had all been part of a genuine realignment, but it was so incomplete. How much more of themselves did each want to donate to the effort?

———

After Rachel Crooks came forward about Trump in 2016, she suffered from crippling anxiety and self-consciousness, she said as she sat facing the others with her long legs tucked beneath her. She was the only one present who lived in a rural, conservative area—"more of a #himtoo community," as she called it.

After she got through a few television appearances and a press conference about the accusation, she received an unexpected invitation. Local Democrats wanted her to run for a seat in the state legislature—a terrible idea, she thought. Critics had already accused her of telling her Trump story for political ends. "It's confirming what everyone thought, that I was doing this for some sort of agenda," she explained.

But she cared about education and health care. As for the incumbent, he was "a rubber stamp for the Republican party," she told the group. Maybe she could use her new profile in a positive way, she thought. "Right or wrong, I would have more fundraising potential because I now had this national voice," she said. So Crooks ran for public office, learning to lead rallies and make speeches, she said. She had joined an unprecedented wave of female candidates across the country, campaigning to seize more political power than women had ever held in United States history.

The night she lost her race, she said, she didn't even cry or feel self-pity: Democrats had, for the most part, lost across Ohio. But months later, she was struggling with the way the campaign had solidified the tendency of others to view her only through her Trump story. On television, she was sometimes just labeled "Trump Accuser" at the bottom of the screen, a phrase her mother hated. "This has become your identity," a male friend told her recently.

"It has opened doors and provided this new path, but it also ties me to this awful human being," she said.

The group silently considered her dilemma. Crooks was living out one of the most common fears about coming forward: It could label you forever. Ford listened particularly closely. Her current fears matched what Crooks described having faced two years before, right down to a specific detail about avoiding local stores. Sitting on the couch, with her red glasses pushed up on her head, she began quizzing Crooks, as if she held a map to what lay ahead.

"I was wondering how long that lasted before you just sort of normally jump into your car and go to a restaurant without people looking at you and wondering if that's really you," Ford said. She was also struggling online, including with fake social media profiles of herself saying, "I recant my whole story."

"I'm, like, 'That's not true!'" Ford said. "But I'm not brave enough to get into that with them. And there's just too many of them, so . . . the social media piece . . . I don't do well with that," she said.

"Sometimes I write the replies, and I just never post them," Crooks told her. "It's very cathartic."

The reaction wasn't all negative, Ford acknowledged. She had been offered prizes, invitations, book and movie contracts. The mail for her was still accumulating, including many private stories of violence—"175,000 letters in Palo Alto," Katz interjected. Those were only the paper letters. There were many more electronic missives. In those, and everywhere else, the reactions to what she had done were so extreme.

For hours, the others had mostly been nodding and asking polite follow-up questions. Now they spoke up with purpose. Paltrow offered a football analogy of her own. "They only tackle you when you've got the ball," she said, explaining that she had once heard the phrase from the country singer Tim McGraw.

She and Judd—longtime experts in fielding public scrutiny and criticism—began to coach everyone else in how to deal with other people's judgments. Judd was direct: Stop reading about yourself online, she instructed Ford.

"If an alcoholic can stay away from a drink one day at a time, I can stay away from the comment section one day at a time," Judd said. "I'm participating in my own self-harm when I expose myself to that material," she continued.

"Do you just not really go on the internet much?" Ford asked Judd, incredulous.

"I'm completely abstinent from all media about myself and have been for probably almost twenty years," Judd said. She posted pictures and links on social media but tried not to read anything written about herself: that was part of why she had disappeared to the woods after the first Weinstein article had been published.

As she spoke, she was curled in a pink upholstered chair facing the group. She had sat there all day, absorbing what others had to say, speaking relatively little. She seemed like the one participant who had not really been transformed. She had always wanted to be an activist, and when she went on the record about Weinstein, the world affirmed her instincts.

"I have to know the hill on which I'm willing to die," she told the group. "The equality of the sexes is that hill for me."

Throughout the discussion, Chiu sat listening, saying little, occasionally clicking her camera in the direction of the others. No one pressed her on the momentous decision of whether she would say publicly what had happened to her all those years ago.

But during the final hours of the gathering, as Ford spoke more, Chiu seemed to hang on every word. Ford had become, in Chiu's mind, a kind of proxy for what she might undergo if she went public. The fact that the two women were neighbors only heightened the connection she felt. Even as Chiu kept her story hidden, she watched as friends and neighbors had organized a candlelight vigil and meal deliveries for Ford.

For months, Chiu had pictured the controversy and criticism that engulfed Ford happening to her instead. The analogy was inexact—the Weinstein case was far more settled and less controversial—but for her, it was real. "I imagined it would all come crashing down," Chiu admitted to the rest of the group. "There'd be news vans outside my door. I was worried my children would be followed to school."

That mental exercise was having an unexpected effect. Watching Ford from nearby—and now meeting her up close—had strengthened Chiu's desire to go public. She told the group that she could feel herself getting closer to joining them, to putting her name to her story. "I can't say that being in this room with so many of you—I can't say that doesn't inspire me," she said.

"I think it's really going to change who I am," she added. That had turned out to be the strongest unifying thread after the hours of discussion: Almost every member of the group who had spoken publicly had been transformed by it, and was stunned by the impact that sharing her own intimate story had on others.

The women around the room leaped in with expressions of support. "If you decide to come forward, that's a big step and that's a step of growth," Lawson said. "No matter how long it took you to say anything about it."

"If you do it, we have your back," Paltrow said.

Ford cut in with a note of caution. "Can I just say something to you?" she asked. "When I was in your position, I had a lot of people kind of telling me, 'You should do this. It's going to be great'—kind of the same kind of thing that's happening right now." But the advice, and especially the upbeat projections about how well it would all work out, had been impossible to take in. "I just didn't even hear any of it, it was so overwhelming to me," she said.

No one could ever predict how speaking out would go. Forecasting was futile. Once a story was publicly told for the first time, there was no telling what might happen, who might read it, or what others might echo, add, or disagree with. There was no guarantee of affirmation or impact. The results could be wrenching, empowering, or both.

But this was what everyone in the room, and more people beyond it, now understood: If the story was not shared, nothing would change. Problems that are not seen cannot be addressed. In our world of journalism, the story was the end, the result, the final product. But in the world at large, the emergence of new information was just the beginning—of conversation, action, change.

"We're still here," Perkins said, to laughter, in one of the group's final exchanges. She wasn't speaking directly to Chiu but the message was clear. "We're still smiling. None of us died from stepping forward. We walked through the fire, but we all came out the other side."

"I think we're probably all proud of the scars that we received," she said.

In summing up how the reckoning might be remembered over time, Laura Madden took an even longer view. "We're not the first people who've spoken up," Madden said. "We're not the first **women** who've spoken up."

"There isn't ever going to be an end," she said. "The point is that people have to continue always speaking up and not being afraid."

A few weeks later, Chiu called: She was ready to go on the record, and for us to share her name publicly.

She understood that more than eighty women had already come forward about Weinstein. She wasn't sure that the public would still care about her account. But she wanted to speak anyway. During the initial Weinstein investigation, she hadn't been ready, but the other women, in Los Angeles and around the world, had eased the way. She feared the legal cases against him might not be successful. So she wanted to help write the history and continue pushing for change.

"I'm not just going to let it slide away," she said.

ACKNOWLEDGMENTS

If you've read these pages, you already have some sense of the debts we owe. Those are only the beginning.

To all of our sources: Thank you for participating in our journalism. Some of you spoke with us at great personal risk or confided stories you never thought you would share with a stranger—and then shared even more for this book. Many of you submitted to lengthy, repeated questioning or uncomfortable lines of inquiry. A special measure of gratitude to everyone who provided the illuminating emails, texts, and other documents interspersed throughout this narrative. A much larger cast, from experts to silent tipsters we can never name, provided essential guidance, including stories and ideas that ring in our heads still.

In addition to the colleagues portrayed in this book, we're grateful to the **Times** journalists who joined our efforts on the Weinstein story, including Rachel Abrams, Ellen Gabler, Susan Dominus, Steve Eder, Jim Rutenberg, William Rashbaum, Barry Meier, Al Baker, Jim McKinley, and the audio team at **The Daily.** At every turn, we received crucial support from Arthur

Sulzberger Jr., A. G. Sulzberger, Sam Dolnick, our colleagues on the business side of the newspaper, and from subscribers, who make this journalism possible. Dean Baquet, Matt Purdy, David McCraw, Sheryl Stolberg, Emily Steel, Carolyn Ryan, and Michael Barbaro generously provided feedback on the manuscript.

The editor who is invisible in this book yet present on every page is Ann Godoff, our galvanizing force. Ann endowed this project with her vision, clarity, and decisiveness, and notes so inspiring we hung them on our office walls. For all of that, we are forever grateful. William Heyward and Casey Denis, Sarah Hutson and Gail Brussel, Carolyn Foley and Juliann Barbato all poured many hours and years of experience into helping us tell and share this story. Thank you for your extraordinary dedication.

Rebecca Corbett, our editor at the **Times,** is our true north. She not only steered us through our investigation of Weinstein but also read and commented on several versions of these chapters, helping us capture and explain what we witnessed.

Alexis Kirschbaum, our editor and ally in London, provided essential insight, feedback, and friendship. Thank you as well to Emma Bal and Jasmine Horsey of Bloomsbury Publishing.

Elyse Cheney is our agent, matchmaker, and guide, and we are grateful for her tenacity, judgment, and hustle. We're also indebted to her colleagues Claire Gillespie, Alice Whitwham, Alex Jacobs, and Allison Devereux. Charlotte Perman and Kristen Sena of Greater Talent Network have handled our speaking engagements with grace—particularly the campus visits, with questions from students that helped us articulate what we wanted to say in these pages.

Kelsey Kudak fact-checked the manuscript with sensitivity and commitment, moving through hundreds of pages of complicated investigative work and taking direction from two different authors with equanimity. Astha Rajvanshi provided research assistance on topics large and small.

For other essential help, we'd also like to thank Joseph Abboud, Kendra Barkoff, Kassie Evashevski, Natasha Fairweather, Jonathan Furmanski, Molly Levinson, Eleanor Leonard, Priya Parker, Melissa Schwartz, Felicia Stewart, Nancy Erika Smith, and Josh Wilkinson. For our author photos, we were lucky enough to have a photographer who knows a thing or two about portraits in the extended **She Said** family; many thanks to Martin Schoeller and his team for these pictures.

Anyone who has parented young children can instantly fill in the scenes of diaper changing, bottle-feeding, and sleep training that took place in between (and occasionally during) our reporting. We were saved again and again by our babysitters, our children's teachers, and most of all, our families.

From Jodi: Not everything in life happens in the order you expect. During the period described in this book, I needed my parents, Wendy and Harry Kantor, more than I have at any time since childhood, because of the constancy of their love and the way they frequently swept in to care for, entertain, and guide my own children. Mom and Dad; Charlene Lieber, my second mother; calm, brave Fred Lieber; and the entire extended Kantor Lieber clan: Thank you for seeing us through these frantic years. Donna Mitchell, thank you for being a force of calm and goodness in the lives of our daughters, and for sharing the biggest and smallest moments with us.

Ron: Even as you unearthed stories of financial wrongdoing and reported on your own book on what to pay for college, you backed this work with full force, encouraging, feeding, and sustaining me. One of the best gifts you ever gave me was the Post-it you left on my desk, a few days before the publication of the original Weinstein story, that read "You can do this." Yes, but only with your love, help, and devotion.

Talia, you are a light, a lockbox, and an increasingly formidable discussion partner and debater. You overheard things that no tween should hear, faithfully kept secrets, helped with your little sister, and kept your cool even as I was often absorbed in broader dramas. Watching you articulate who you really are, and begin to build a life, is the thrill of mine.

Violet, you were only a year and a half old when we started, and your innocence made you my refuge. Parents are supposed to console their children, but I frequently found solace in your curls, songs, made-up words, discoveries, and above all, in the fierceness of your embrace.

From Megan: I'm indebted to my parents, John and Mary Jane Twohey, who have served as my moral compass for decades, reinforcing my values, nudging me along the pursuit of truth, and picking me up whenever I stumble. Ben and Maya Rutman, Helen and Felix Rutman-Schoeller and Martin Schoeller, I am thankful for your endless kindness and joyous laughter. Jenny

Rattan-John, you are our rock, our teacher, and a cherished member of our family.

Jim: We had been married for less than a year and were brand-new parents when the Weinstein investigation began. Not once did you teeter in your support of the project and later this book, even when it meant canceled vacations, long stretches of single parenting, and fielding the intense emotions that came with this work. Your warm hugs, sharp listening skills, and encouraging texts propelled me forward, and your own expertise and judgment as a literary agent were delivered up at just the right moments.

Mira: you learned how to walk and talk during the course of this reporting, and the feistiness with which you tackled each stage of development served as a major source of inspiration. I am increasingly impressed by and grateful for your grit, cunning, and passion.

To our daughters, and to yours: May you know respect and dignity always, in the workplace and beyond.

NOTES

This book is based on three years of our reporting, stretching from the spring of 2016 through the spring of 2019, on President Donald J. Trump's treatment of women, Harvey Weinstein's decades of alleged sexual harassment and abuse, and Christine Blasey Ford's path to publicly accusing Brett Kavanaugh of sexual assault. These notes are intended to provide readers with a road map of which information in this book came from which sources.

We conducted hundreds of interviews, speaking with almost everyone depicted in this book, including Trump, Weinstein, and Ford, who detailed her experience to Megan over dozens of hours. Ford's legal team, Bob Weinstein, David Boies, Lance Maerov, Irwin Reiter, and most of the alleged victims portrayed granted us multiple interviews. Some of what we share was originally off the record, such as Jodi's early conversations with Reiter, and Weinstein's October 4, 2017, surprise visit to the **Times,** but through additional reporting, including returning to the parties involved, we were able to include the material. Over the past two years, we have sought comment from Weinstein on our findings multiple times, most recently in spring 2019. Kelsey Kudak spent five months fact-checking the book, often adding new information.

We reviewed thousands of pages of documents, cited below, including lawsuits filed against Trump, internal records from The Weinstein Company, and correspondence between Ford and her lawyers. Some text messages, emails, and other primary records are reproduced in the book so that readers can examine them directly.

We also drew on the reporting of other journalists, including Ronan Farrow, Emily Steel, and Michael Schmidt.

CHAPTER ONE: THE FIRST PHONE CALL

9 **"Here's the thing, I have been treated"**: Rose McGowan, email message to Jodi Kantor, May 11, 2017.

9 **"Because it's been an open secret"**: Rose McGowan (@rosemcgowan), "because it's been an open secret in Hollywood/ Media & they shamed me while adulating my rapist. #WhyWomenDontReport," Twitter, October 13, 2016, https://twitter.com/ rosemcgowan/status/786723360550035460.

10 **writing a memoir**: Rose McGowan, **Brave** (New York: HarperCollins, 2018).

10 **"tank that shows off cleavage (push up bras encouraged)":** Rose McGowan (@rosemcgowan), "casting note that came w/script I got today. For real. name of male star rhymes with Madam Panhandler hahahaha I die," Twitter, June 17, 2015, https://twitter.com/rosemcgowan/status/611378426344288256.

10 **"It is okay to be angry":** Rose McGowan (@rosemcgowan), "It is okay to be angry. Don't be afraid of it. Lean in. Like a storm cloud it passes, but it must be recognized. #readthis," Twitter, April 3, 2017, https://twitter.com/rosemcgowan/status/849083550448193536; "dismantle the system," Twitter, May 4, 2017, https://twitter.com/rosemcgowan/status/860322650962264064.

11 **"At some pt":** Jennifer Senior (@JenSeniorNY), "At some pt, all the women who've been afraid to speak out abt Harvey Weinstein are gonna have to hold hands and jump," Twitter, March 30, 2015, https://twitter.com/jenseniorny/status/582657086737289216.

12 **He had even participated:** Jodi Kantor (@jodikantor), "Harvey Weinstein at the January 2017 Women's March in Park City, Utah," Twitter, October 5, 2017, https://twitter.com/jodikantor/status/916103297097961472.

18   **described what it called a horrific group sexual assault:** Sabrina Rubin Erdely, "A Rape on Campus," **Rolling Stone,** November 4, 2014. Rolling Stone retracted the story on April 5, 2015, and commissioned a study by the **Columbia Journalism Review,** which was published by the magazine. Sheila Coronel, Steve Coll, and Derek Kravitz, "Rolling Stone and UVA: The Columbia University Graduate School of Journalism Report," **Rolling Stone,** April 5, 2015, https://www.rollingstone.com/culture/culture-news/rolling-stone-and-uva-the-columbia-university-graduate-school-of-journalism-report-44930; Ravi Somaiya, "Rolling Stone Article on Rape at University of Virginia Failed All Basics, Report Says," **New York Times,** April 5, 2015, https://www.nytimes.com/2015/04/06/business/media/rolling-stone-retracts-article-on-rape-at-university-of-virginia.html.

18   **a series of lawsuits:** Ben Sisario, Hawes Spencer, and Sydney Ember, "Rolling Stone Loses Defamation Case Over Rape Story," **New York Times,** November 4, 2016, https://www.nytimes.com/2016/11/05/business/media/rolling-stone-rape-story-case-guilty.html; Hawes Spencer and Ben Sisario, "In Rolling Stone Defamation Case, Magazine and Reporter Ordered to Pay $3 Million," **New York Times,** November 7, 2016, https://www.nytimes.com/2016/11/08/business/media/

in-rolling-stone-defamation-case-magazine-and-reporter-ordered-to-pay-3-million.html; Matthew Haag, "Rolling Stone Settles Lawsuit Over Debunked Campus Rape Article," **New York Times,** April 11, 2017, https://www .nytimes.com/2017/04/11/business/media/rolling-stone-university-virginia-rape-story -settlement.html; Sydney Ember, "Rolling Stone to Pay $1.65 Million to Fraternity Over Discredited Rape Story," **New York Times,** June 13, 2017, https://www.nytimes.com/2017/06/13/business/media/rape-uva-rolling-stone -frat.html.

18   **police had called the story "a complete crock":** Erik Wemple, "Charlottesville Police Make Clear That Rolling Stone Story Is a Complete Crock," **Washington Post,** March 23, 2015, https://www.washingtonpost.com/blogs/erik-wemple/wp/2015/03/23/charlottesville -police-make-clear-that-rolling-stone-story-is -a-complete-crock; Bill Grueskin, "More Is Not Always Better," **Columbia Journalism Review,** April 5, 2015, https://www.cjr.org/analysis/rolling_stone_journalism.php; Craig Silverman, "The Year in Media Errors and Corrections 2014," **Poynter Institute,** December 18, 2014, https://www.poynter.org/newsletters/2014/the -year-in-media-errors-and-corrections-2014.

20   **were shelving rape kits, robbing victims of the chance for justice:** Megan Twohey,

"Dozens of Rape Kits Not Submitted for Testing by Chicago Suburban Police Departments," **Chicago Tribune,** June 14, 2009, https:// www.chicagotribune.com/news/chi-rape-kits -14-jun14-story.html; Megan Twohey, "Illinois to Test Every Rape Kit," **Chicago Tribune,** July 6, 2009, https://www.chicagotribune.com/ news/ct-met-rape-kit-law-20100706-story.html; Megan Twohey, "Doctors Continue to Operate Unchecked," **Chicago Tribune,** August 23, 2010, https://www.chicagotribune.com/lifestyles/ health/chi-doctor-sex-charges-gallery-storygallery .html; Megan Twohey, "The Child Exchange," **Reuters,** September 9, 2013, https://www.reuters .com/investigates/adoption/#article/part1.

21 **"That must be a pretty picture, you dropping to your knees": Celebrity Apprentice: All- Stars,** Season 6, episode 1, aired March 3, 2013, on NBC; Mark Graham, "Did Donald Trump Just Utter the Most Blatantly Sexist Statement in the History of Broadcast Television?" VH1, March 5, 2013, http://www .vh1.com/news/84410/donald-trump-brande -roderick-on-her-knees.

21 **Most of Trump's former employees:** Associated Press, "For Many Trump Employees, Keeping Quiet Is Legally Required," **Fortune,** June 21, 2016, http://fortune.com/2016/06/ 21/donald-trump-nda; John Dawsey and Ashley Parker, "'Everyone Signed One': Trump

Is Aggressive in His Use of Nondisclosure Agreements, Even in Government," **Washington Post,** August 13, 2018, https://www.washingtonpost.com/politics/everyone-signed-one-trump-is-aggressive-in-his-use-of-nondisclosure-agreements-even-in-government/2018/08/13/9d0315ba-9f15-11e8-93e3-24d1703d2a7a_story.html.

22 **pieced together multiple allegations:** Michael Barbaro and Megan Twohey, "Crossing the Line: How Donald Trump Behaved with Women in Private," **New York Times,** May 14, 2016, https://www.nytimes.com/2016/05/15/us/politics/donald-trump-women.html.

22 **"kissed, fondled, and restrained" her from leaving:** Ibid.

23 **conducted a lengthy interview of the candidate:** Donald Trump, interview by Megan Twohey and Michael Barbaro, May 10, 2016.

23 **"went on Fox and Friends to dispute your story":** Fox and Friends, "Donald Trump's Ex-girlfriend Says She Was Misquoted in the **Times,"** Fox News, May 16, 2016, https://video.foxnews.com/v/4895612039001/#sp=show-clips.

24 **"The @nytimes is so dishonest":** Donald J. Trump (@realdonaldtrump), "The @nytimes

is so dishonest. Their hit piece cover story on me yesterday was just blown up by Rowanne Brewer, who said it was a lie!" Twitter, May 16, 2016, https://twitter.com/realdonaldtrump/status/732196260636151808; Donald J. Trump (@realdonaldtrump), "With the coming forward today of the woman central to the failing @nytimes hit piece on me, we have exposed the article as a fraud!" Twitter, May 16, 2016, https://twitter.com/realdonaldtrump/status/732230384071680001.

25   **His argument was absurd:** Erik Wemple, "Bill O'Reilly Follows Donald Trump into the Racist Hellhole," **Washington Post,** June 7, 2016, https://www.washingtonpost.com/blogs/erik-wemple/wp/2016/06/07/bill-oreilly-follows-donald-trump-into-racist-hellhole.

25   **audiotape from the gossip show <u>Access Hollywood</u> from 2005:** David A. Farenthold, "Trump Recorded Having Extremely Lewd Conversation about Women in 2005," **Washington Post** (updated), October 8, 2016, https://www.washingtonpost.com/politics/trump-recorded-having-extremely-lewd-conversation-about-women-in-2005/2016/10/07/3b9ce776-8cb4-11e6-bf8a-3d26847eeed4_story.html.

26   **Trump apologized for his words:** Video, "Trump Responds in 2016 to Outrage over

Comments," **New York Times,** October 8, 2016, https://www.nytimes.com/video/us/politics/100000004698416/trump-responds-to-outrage-over-lewd-remarks.html; Maggie Haberman, "Donald Trump's Apology That Wasn't," **New York Times,** October 8, 2016, https://www.nytimes.com/2016/10/08/us/politics/donald-trump-apology.html.

26 **"No, I have not":** "Transcript of the Second Debate," **New York Times,** October 10, 2016, https://www.nytimes.com/2016/10/10/us/politics/transcript-second-debate.html.

26 **two other women:** Megan Twohey and Michael Barbaro, "Two Women Say Donald Trump Touched Them Inappropriately," **New York Times,** October 12, 2016, https://www.nytimes.com/2016/10/13/us/politics/donald-trump-women.html.

27 <u>**The Apprentice**</u> **had gone on the air:** Rachel Crooks, interviews by Megan Twohey, October 2016 through spring 2019.

27 **Before that, the only man who had ever kissed her:** Eli Saslow, "Is Anyone Listening?" **Washington Post,** February 19, 2018, https://www.washingtonpost.com/news/national/wp/2018/02/19/feature/trump-accuser-keeps-telling-her-story-hoping-someone-will-finally-listen.

29   **"You are disgusting!" Trump shouted:**
Donald Trump, interview by Megan Twohey,
October 11, 2016.

29   **Minutes later, Trump stepped onstage:**
Video, "Presidential Candidate Donald Trump
Rally in Panama City, Florida," C-SPAN,
October 11, 2016, https://www.c-span.org/
video/?416754-1/donald-trump-campaigns
-panama-city-florida.

30   **Some Republicans were saying he should
drop out:** Jessica Taylor, "'You Can Do
Anything': In 2005 Tape, Trump Brags about
Groping, Kissing Women," National Public
Radio, October 7, 2017, https://www.npr.org/
2016/10/07/497087141/donald-trump-caught
-on-tape-making-vulgar-remarks-about-women;
Alan Rappeport, "John McCain Withdraws
Support for Donald Trump after Disclosure
of Recording," **New York Times,** October 10,
2018, https://www.nytimes.com/2016/10/08/
us/politics/presidential-election.html; Jonathan
Martin, Maggie Haberman, and Alexander
Burns, "Lewd Donald Trump Tape Is a
Breaking Point for Many in the G.O.P.," **New
York Times,** October 8, 2016, https://www
.nytimes.com/2016/10/09/us/politics/donald
-trump-campaign.html.

30   **An explosive civil lawsuit alleged:** Josh
Gerstein, "Woman Suing Trump over Alleged

Teen Rape Drops Suit, Again," **Politico,** November 4, 2016, https://www.politico.com/ story/2016/11/donald-trump-rape-lawsuit -dropped-230770; Jane Coaston and Anna North, "Jeffrey Epstein, the Convicted Sex Offender Who Is Friends with Donald Trump and Bill Clinton, Explained," **Vox,** February 22, 2019. https://www.vox.com/2018/12/3/ 18116351/jeffrey-epstein-trump-clinton-labor -secretary-acosta.

31 **as a woman tearfully recounted:** abc.com Staff, "Woman Accuses Trump of Inappropriate Sexual Conduct at 1998 US Open," ABC, October 20, 2016, https://abc7.com/politics/ woman-accuses-trump-of-inappropriate-sexual -conduct-at-1998-us-open/1565005.

31 **a link to a post from a conservative news site:** Katie Mettler, "She Accused Trump of Sexual Assault, Lou Dobbs Tweeted Her Phone Number," **Washington Post,** October 14, 2016, https://www.washingtonpost.com/news/ morning-mix/wp/2016/10/14/shc-accused -trump-of-sexual-assault-lou-dobbs-tweeted-her -phone-number.

33 **"Failure to do so will leave my client":** Marc Kasowitz, "re: Demand for Retraction," letter from Marc Kasowitz to David McCraw, October 12, 2016, https://assets.donaldjtrump .com/DemandForRetraction.PDF.

33 **"It would have been a disservice":** David McCraw, "re: Demand for Retraction," letter from David McCraw to Marc Kasowitz, October 13, 2016, https://www.nytimes.com/ interactive/2016/10/13/us/politics/david-mccraw -trump-letter.html.

35 **had covered up repeated allegations:** Emily Steel and Michael S. Schmidt, "Bill O'Reilly Thrives at Fox News, Even as Harassment Settlements Add Up," **New York Times,** April 1, 2017, https://www.nytimes.com/ 2017/04/01/business/media/bill-oreilly-sexual -harassment-fox-news.html.

36 **advertisers like Mercedes-Benz:** Karl Russel, "Bill O'Reilly's Show Lost More Than Half Its Advertisers in a Week," **New York Times,** April 11, 2017, https://www.nytimes .com/interactive/2017/04/11/business/oreilly -advertisers.html.

36 **other women at Fox started:** Emily Steel and Michael S. Schmidt, "Bill O'Reilly is Forced Out at Fox News," **New York Times,** April 19, 2017, https://www.nytimes.com/2017/04/19/ business/media/bill-oreilly-fox-news-allegations .html.

36 **Roger Ailes, the Republican power broker:** John Koblin and Jim Rutenberg, "Accused of Sexual Harassment, Roger Ailes Is Negotiating

Exit from Fox," **New York Times,** July 19, 2016, https://www.nytimes.com/2016/07/20/business/media/roger-ailes-fox-news-murdoch.html.

37 **Shaunna Thomas, a feminist activist:** Shaunna Thomas, interview by Jodi Kantor, April 2017.

CHAPTER TWO: HOLLYWOOD SECRETS

39 **red carpet photos:** "2017 Cannes Film Festival Red Carpet Looks," photos, **New York Times,** May 20, 2017, https://www.nytimes.com/2017/05/20/fashion/2017-cannes-film-festival-red-carpet-looks.html.

40 **given an interview to <u>Variety</u> in 2015:** Ramin Setoodeh, "Ashley Judd Reveals Harassment by Studio Mogul" **Variety,** October 6, 2015, https://variety.com/2015/film/news/ashley-judd-sexual-harassment-studio-mogul-shower-1201610666.

40 **"I am so sorry, my lawyer":** Judith Godrèche, email message to Jodi Kantor, June 13, 2017.

42 **wasn't a Weinstein victim:** Marissa Tomei, interviews by Jodi Kantor, 2017–18.

43 **"You have to ask for money":** Elizabeth Rubin, "Spy, Mother, Comeback Kid: All Eyes

Are on Claire Danes," **Vogue,** July 14, 2013, https://www.vogue.com/article/all-eyes-on -claire-homeland-claire-danes-and-damian-lewis.

45   **a gushing tweet a few months before:** Lisa Bloom (@LisaBloom), "BIG ANNOUNCEMENT: My book SUSPICION NATION is being made into a miniseries, produced by Harvey Weinstein and Jay Z!," Twitter, April 7, 2017, https://twitter.com/ lisabloom/status/850402622116855809.

45   **made getting in touch with Ashley Judd simple:** Ashley Judd and Maryanne Vollers, **All That Is Bitter and Sweet** (New York: Ballantine, 2015).

46   **she had a personal story to tell:** Ashley Judd, interviews by Jodi Kantor and Megan Twohey, June 2017–January 2019.

49   **She yearned for playmates and company:** Many of the details of Judd's upbringing are chronicled in her 2015 autobiography, Judd and Vollers, **All That Is Bitter and Sweet.**

51   **a law school professor named Diane Rosenfeld:** Diane Rosenfeld, interview by Jodi Kantor, May 11, 2018.

52   **"I propose a model":** Ashley Judd, "Gender Violence: Law and Social Justice" (master's

thesis, Harvard's Kennedy School of
Government, 2015), 2010.

54 **"I'm not as nasty":** "#NastyWoman,"
YouTube video, 00:06:43, Live at State of the
Word, posted by Nina Mariah, December 11,
2016, https://www.youtube.com/watch?v=
dvN0On85sNQ.

54 **Judd was fired:** Ashley Judd, interview by Jodi
Kantor, 2017; Copper Fit executives, interview
by Jodi Kantor, 2019.

54 **The call ended with a plan:** Jill Kargman,
interview by Jodi Kantor, June 2017.

54 **Kargman urged Jodi:** Jenni Konner, interviews
by Jodi Kantor, 2017; Lena Dunham, interviews by
Jodi Kantor, 2017.

55 **told Jodi she had delivered a similar warning:**
Tina Brown, interview by Jodi Kantor,
September 26, 2017.

56 **Paltrow shared the unknown side of the
story:** Gwyneth Paltrow, interviews by Jodi
Kantor and Megan Twohey, 2017–19.

59 **the producer's mother:** Anita Gates, "Miriam
Weinstein, Mother and Backbone of Original
Miramax, Dies at 90," **New York Times,**
November 4, 2016, https://www.nytimes.com/

2016/11/04/movies/miriam-weinstein-died
-miramax.html.

60   **a sixty-six-dollar:** "Jade Egg," Goop, https://
shop.goop.com/shop/products/jade-egg?country
=USA: Bill Bostock, "Gwyneth Paltrow's
Goop settles $145,000 lawsuit over baseless
vaginal eggs health claims," **Business Insider,**
September 5, 2018, https://www.businessinsider
.com/gwyneth-paltrows-goop-lawsuit-vaginal
-egg-claims-2018-9.

60   **"Organically sourced, fair trade urine pH
sticks":** Jen Gunter, "Dear Gwyneth Paltrow,
I'm a Gynecologist and Your Vaginal Jade Eggs
Are a Bad Idea," **Dr. Jen Gunter,** January 17,
2017, https://drjengunter.com/2017/01/17/dear
-gwyneth-paltrow-im-a-gyn-and-your-vaginal
-jade-eggs-are-a-bad-idea.

64   **She did not reply:** Uma Thurman, interviews
and emails with Jodi Kantor, 2017–19.

64   **While reporting on DNA evidence:** Linda
Fairstein, interview by Megan Twohey,
conducted in 2009 while reporting at the
Chicago Tribune.

69   **liked to boast of his coziness with media:**
Ryan Tate, "Why Harvey Weinstein Thinks
He Owns New York Media," **Gawker,** April 2,
2008, http://gawker.com/5004915/why

-harvey-weinstein-thinks-he-owns-new-york
-media.

69   **based in part on Corbett:** David Simon,
interview and email with Jodi Kantor, 2018–19.

69   **when two <u>Times</u> reporters discovered:** James
Risen and Eric Lichtblau, "Bush Lets U.S. Spy
on Callers without Courts," **New York Times,**
December 16, 2005, https://www.nytimes.com/
2005/12/16/politics/bush-lets-us-spy-on-callers
-without-courts.html.

CHAPTER THREE: HOW TO SILENCE A VICTIM

73   **the corresponding state agencies:** The New
York Division of Human Rights, https://dhr
.ny.gov, and the California Department of Fair
Employment and Housing, https://www.dfeh.ca
.gov.

73   **obtained a report:** Generated in 2017 by the
California Department of Fair Employment
and Housing.

75   **On the afternoon of July 14:** Meeting
notes and documents from Katie Benner and
Jodi Kantor.

75   **Two weeks before, Katie Benner:** Katie
Benner, "Women in Tech Speak Frankly on
Culture of Harassment," **New York Times,**

June 30, 2017, https://www.nytimes.com/2017/
06/30/technology/women-entrepreneurs-speak
-out-sexual-harassment.html.

76   **a blog post describing the harassment
and retaliation:** Susan Fowler, "Reflecting
on One Very, Very Strange Year at Uber,"
Susan Fowler, February 19, 2017, https://
www.susanjfowler.com/blog/2017/2/19/
reflecting-on-one-very-strange-year-at-uber.

76   **One of the men and one of the firms:** Katie
Benner, "A Backlash Builds against Sexual
Harassment in Silicon Valley," **New York
Times,** July 3, 2017, https://www.nytimes.com/
2017/07/03/technology/silicon-valley-sexual
-harassment.html.

76   **Steel was hearing alarming accounts:** Emily
Steel, "At **Vice,** Cutting-Edge Media and
Allegations of Old-School Sexual Harassment,"
New York Times, December 23, 2017, https://
www.nytimes.com/2017/12/23/business/media/
vice-sexual-harassment.html.

76   **conversations with restaurant, retail, hotel,
and construction workers:** Catrin Einhorn,
"Harassment and Tipping in Restaurants: Your
Stories," **New York Times,** March 18, 2018,
https://www.nytimes.com/2018/03/18/
business Einhorn and Rachel Abrams, "The
Tipping Equation," **New York Times,**

March 12, 2018, https://www.nytimes.com/
interactive/2018/03/11/business/tipping-sexual
-harassment.html.

76 **male blue-collar workplaces:** Susan Chira and
Catrin Einhorn, "How Tough Is It to Change a
Culture of Harassment? Ask Women at Ford,"
New York Times, December 19, 2017, https://
www.nytimes.com/interactive/2017/12/19/us/
ford-chicago-sexual-harassment.html; Susan
Chira and Catrin Einhorn, "The #MeToo
Moment: Blue-collar Women Ask, 'What
About Us?'" **New York Times,** December 20,
2017, https://www.nytimes.com/2017/12/20/
us/the-metoo-moment-blue-collar-women-ask
-what-about-us.html; Susan Chira, "We Asked
Women in Blue-collar Workplaces about Sexual
Harassment: Here Are Their Stories," **New
York Times,** December 29, 2017, https://www
.nytimes.com/2017/12/29/us/blue-collar-women
-harassment.html; Susan Chira, "The 'Manly'
Jobs Problem," **New York Times,** February 8,
2018, https://www.nytimes.com/2018/02/08/
sunday-review/sexual-harassment-masculine-jobs
.html.

78 **If they received subpoenas compelling
them to talk:** Emily Steel, "How Bill O'Reilly
Silenced His Accusers," **New York Times,**
April 4, 2018, https://www.nytimes.com/2018/
04/04/business/media/how-bill-oreilly-silenced
-his-accusers.html.

80   **Even the EEOC:** Chai Feldblum, interview by
Jodi Kantor, May 11, 2017.

82   **relinquished control of Miramax, their first
movie company:** After selling Miramax to
Disney for $80 million in 1993, the Weinsteins
separated themselves from Disney in 2005. Laura
M. Holson, "How the Tumultuous Marriage
of Miramax and Disney Failed," **New York
Times,** March 6, 2005, https://www.nytimes
.com/2005/03/06/movies/how-the-tumultuous
-marriage-of-miramax-and-disney-failed.html.

88   **to the home of John Schmidt:** John Schmidt,
interviews by Megan Twohey, September 2017
through spring 2019.

89   **One Friday evening:** Amy Israel, interviews by
Jodi Kantor, 2017–19.

92   **Three weeks later:** Zelda Perkins, interviews
by Jodi Kantor, 2017–19.

95   **Much later, Chiu told Jodi:** Rowena Chiu,
interviews by Jodi Kantor, May–June 2019.

97   **with a more senior figure:** Donna Gigliotti,
emails to Jodi Kantor and Kelsey Kudak,
November 2017–June 2019.

97   **she questioned whether Gigliotti could:**
Megan Twohey, Jodi Kantor, Susan Dominus,

Jim Rutenberg, and Steve Eder, "Weinstein's Complicity Machine," **New York Times,** December 5, 2017, www.nytimes.com/interactive/2017/12/05/us/harvey-weinstein-complicity.html.

103 **driven up to Chiu's house:** Andrew Cheung, interview by Jodi Kantor, July 2017.

106 **Amy Israel had recommended:** Laura Madden, interviews by Jodi Kantor, July 2017 through January 2019.

114 **Allred's autobiography:** Gloria Allred, **Fight Back and Win** (New York: HarperCollins, 2006); Gloria Allred, interviews by Megan Twohey, October 2016 through spring 2019.

115 **In 2011, she and a partner:** Emily Steel, "How Bill O'Reilly Silenced His Accusers," **New York Times,** April 4, 2018, https://www.nytimes.com/2018/04/04/business/media/how-bill-oreilly-silenced-his-accusers.html.

115 **Allred was working on a settlement:** Rebecca Davis O'Brien, "USA Gymnastics, McKayla Maroney Had Confidentiality Agreement to Resolve Abuse Claims," **Wall Street Journal,** December 20, 2017, https://www.wsj.com/articles/usa-gymnastics-reached-settlement-over-abuse-claims-with-gold-medalist-mckayla-maroney-1513791179; Will Hobson, "McKayla

Maroney Sues USA Gymnastics, Saying It Tried to Buy Her Silence on Abuse," **Washington Post,** December, 20, 2017, https://www .washingtonpost.com/sports/mckayla-maroney -sues-usa-gymnastics-saying-it-tried-to-buy-her -silence-on-abuse/2017/12/20/1e54b482-e5c8 -11e7-a65d-1ac0fd7f097e_story.html.

115 **in 2004, Allred's firm had also negotiated a settlement:** Ashley Matthau, interviews by Megan Twohey, October 2017 through spring 2019.

117 **a group of consumer lawyers in California:** Consumer Attorneys of California, https://www .caoc.org.

118 **On a tense phone call with lobbyists:** Various participants on the call, interview by Megan Twohey, 2018.

CHAPTER FOUR: "POSITIVE REPUTATION MANAGEMENT"

119 **his parents' Creole restaurant:** Brett Anderson, "A History of the Baquets, New Orleans Restaurant Family: From the T-P Archives," NOLA, originally published July 20, 2004, republished May 15, 2014, https:// www.nola.com/dining/2014/05/from_the_t-p _archives_a_short.html; Brett Anderson, "The Importance of Eddie's: The Late-great Baquet

Family Restaurant, Remembered," NOLA, May 16, 2014, https://www.nola.com/dining/2014/05/the_importance_of_eddies_the_l.html.

120   **but Baquet was contacted by David Boies:** Information taken from Megan Twohey interviews, from 2017 through spring 2019, of Boies and those familiar with his representation of Harvey Weinstein, and emails and other records that included comments made by Boies from 2015 through 2017, as well as the following articles about him: Daniel Okrent, "Get Me Boies!" **Time,** December 25, 2000, http://content.time.com/time/world/article/0,8599,2047286,00.html; Andrew Rice, "The Bad, Good Lawyer: Was David Boies Just Doing Right by Harvey Weinstein? Or Did He Cross an Ethical Line?" **New York** magazine, September 30, 2018, http://nymag.com/intelligencer/2018/09/david-boies-harvey-weinstein-lawyer.html.

120   **"I'm not calling as Harvey's lawyer":** Dean Baquet, interviews by Megan Twohey and Jodi Kantor, 2018.

124   **On August 3:** Lanny Davis, interview by Megan Twohey and Jodi Kantor, August 3, 2017.

133   **In 2002, the <u>New Yorker</u> writer:** Auletta heard about the settlements while working on a profile

of Harvey Weinstein. Ken Auletta, "Beauty and the Beast," **New Yorker,** December 8, 2002, https://www.newyorker.com/magazine/2002/12/16/beauty-and-the-beast-2.

134 **Auletta, David Remnick, the magazine's editor:** Ken Auletta, Bob Weinstein, David Boies, interviews by Megan Twohey, 2019.

138 **The producer had long relied on private detectives:** Megan Twohey, Jodi Kantor, Susan Dominus, Jim Rutenberg, and Steve Eder, "Weinstein's Complicity Machine," **New York Times,** December 5, 2017, www.nytimes.com/interactive/2017/12/05/us/harvey-weinstein-complicity.html.

139 **Under the terms of a contract:** Alana Goodman, "Harvey Weinstein's ORIGINAL contract with ex-Mossad agents ordered them to prove he was the victim of a 'negative campaign' in what was dubbed 'Operation Parachute'—spying on actresses, close friend designer Kenneth Cole and amfAR," **Daily Mail,** November 8, 2017, https://www.dailymail.co.uk/news/article-5062195/Harvey-Weinstein-agreed-pay-1-3m-ex-Mossad-agents.html.

139 **Seth Freedman, a British freelance journalist:** Twohey and Kantor interviews of McGowan, Kendall, and others who were contacted by Seth

Freedman in 2016 and 2017, and emails sent by Freedman.

139   **Black Cube went to work on Benjamin Wallace:** Benjamin Wallace, interview by Megan Twohey, 2018, and 2016 emails between Wallace and Seth Freedman.

140   **By May 2017:** Ronan Farrow, "Harvey Weinstein's Army of Spies," **New Yorker,** November 6, 2017, www.newyorker.com/news/news-desk/harvey-weinsteins-army-of-spies.

140   **Under the contract that Boies helped revise:** "Read: The Contract Between a Private Security Firm and One of Harvey Weinstein's Lawyers," **New Yorker,** November 6, 2017, https://www.newyorker.com/sections/news/read-the-contract-between-a-private-security-firm-and-one-of-harvey-weinsteins-lawyers.

141   **Jodi received a series:** "Diana Filip," email to Jodi Kantor, August 8, 2017. The associated website, Reuben Capital Partners, has been stripped; screenshots of the website were published. Alana Goodman, "EXCLUSIVE: The SPY Who Duped Rose McGowan UNMASKED! This is the blonde Israeli military veteran who worked undercover for disgraced mogul Harvey Weinstein and tricked the actress into sharing her memoirs," **Daily Mail,** November 8, 2017, https://www.dailymail

.co.uk/news/article-5064027/Israeli-military-vet
-duped-Rose-McGowan-revealed.html.

144 **profile of Gloria Allred and Lisa Bloom:**
Alexandra Pechman, "Gloria Allred and Lisa
Bloom Are the Defenders of Women in 2017,"
W, July 21, 2017, https://www.wmagazine.com/
story/gloria-allred-lisa-bloom-donald-trump-blac
-chyna-lawyer.

146 **Megan had never spoken to Bloom:** Megan
Twohey, email to Lisa Bloom, November 1, 2016.

146 **Bloom convened a press conference:** Stephen
Feller, "Trump Rape Accuser Cancels Press
Conference after Death Threats," **United Press
International,** November 3, 2016, https://www
.upi.com/Top_News/US/2016/11/03/Trump
-rape-accuser-cancels-press-conference-after
-death-threats/2381478150421.

147 **Bloom acknowledged that she solicited
money:** Kenneth P. Vogel, "Partisans, Wielding
Money, Begin Seeking to Exploit Harassment
Claim," **New York Times,** December 31, 2017,
https://www.nytimes.com/2017/12/31/us/
politics/sexual-harassment-politics-partisanship
.html.

147 **spent months vetting Jane Doe:** Lisa Bloom,
interview by Kantor and Twohey, 2019; Lisa
Bloom email to Megan Twohey, June 2019.

147   **Steel had quietly begun interviewing:** Tamara
      Holder, interviews by Megan Twohey, summer
      2018 through spring 2019; emails between
      Tamara Holder and Lisa Bloom; Lloyd Grove,
      "Clients Turn on 'Champion for Women' Lisa
      Bloom after Her Scorched-earth Crusade for
      Harvey Weinstein," **Daily Beast,** October 26,
      2017, https://www.thedailybeast.com/lisa-bloom
      -has-files-on-rose-mcgowans-history-inside-her
      -scorched-earth-crusade-for-harvey-weinstein;
      Emily Steel, "Fox Is Said to Settle With Former
      Contributor Over Sexual Assault Claims,"
      New York Times, March 8, 2017, https://www
      .nytimes.com/2017/03/08/business/fox-news
      -roger-ailes-sexual-assault-settlement.html.

149   **As the show struggled to get off the ground:**
      Twohey's amfAR reporting included interviews
      of amfAR board members, including its then
      chairman Kenneth Cole, Harvey Weinstein,
      David Boies, Charles Prince, and others with
      knowledge of the $600,000 raised at an
      amfAR charity auction that flowed to **Finding
      Neverland** investors. It also included emails
      and other documents from 2015 to 2017 that
      outlined the financial transaction, concern
      about the transaction among certain members
      of amfAR's staff and board, and how Weinstein
      responded to attempts to investigate it; Megan
      Twohey, "Tumult after AIDS Fund-Raiser
      Supports Harvey Weinstein Production," **New
      York Times,** September 23, 2017, https://www

.nytimes.com/2017/09/23/nyregion/harvey
-weinstein-charity.html.

149 **Megan was meeting Tom Ajamie:** Tom
Ajamie, interviews by Megan Twohey, summer
2017 through spring 2019.

151 **Bloom had already been working with the
producer:** December 2016 billing records from
Lisa Bloom's law firm, The Bloom Firm.

157 **"Based on social media activity and
comments":** Sara Ness, Draft Report submitted
to Harvey Weinstein, July 2017.

CHAPTER FIVE: A COMPANY'S COMPLICITY

163 **To keep the dialogue over email going:** Irwin
Reiter emails to Jodi Kantor, September 2017.

164 **On Monday night, September 18:** Irwin
Reiter, interviews by Jodi Kantor and Megan
Twohey, September 2017 through May 2019.

167 **Cosby's TV projects and tour dates evaporated:**
Frank Pallotta and Molly Shiels, "NBC Says It's
Not Moving Forward with Bill Cosby Project,"
CNN, November 19, 2014, https://money.cnn
.com/2014/11/19/media/cosby-nbc-sitcom/
index.html; Goeff Edgers, "Bill Cosby's 'Far
from Finished' Tour Pushes On: But Will It Be
His Last?" **Washington Post,** March 24, 2015,

https://www.washingtonpost.com/entertainment/
bill-cosbys-far-from-finished-tour-pushes-on-will
-it-be-his-last/2015/03/24/d665bee4-cf1f-11e4
-8a46-b1dc9be5a8ff_story.html; Todd Leopold,
"Cancellations Have Dogged Cosby's Tour,"
CNN, February 21, 2015, https://www.cnn
.com/2015/02/20/entertainment/feat-cosby-tour
-cancellations/index.html.

168   **By her second day of work:** From emails and
other internal Weinstein Company records from
2014 and 2015.

169   **"She said he was very persistent":** Ibid.

170   **Shari pressed forward:** Shari Reiter, interview
by Jodi Kantor, October 25, 2018.

170   **Rehal was Weinstein's personal assistant:**
Sandeep Rehal, interviews by Jodi Kantor,
November 2018.

171   **$2.5 million in 2015:** Harvey Weinstein's
contract with The Weinstein Company.

172   **Reiter wrote to Tom Prince:** Email exchanges
between Tom Prince and Irwin Reiter, February
2015.

173   **was having eerily similar conversations:**
Michelle Franklin, interviews by Jodi Kantor,
2017–19.

174   **On the afternoon of September 19:** Harvey
      Weinstein, Jason Lilien, Lanny Davis, Charlie
      Prince, Roberta Kaplan, and Karen Duffy,
      interview by Megan Twohey and Rebecca
      Corbett, September 19, 2017.

181   **"I'm worse":** Harvey Weinstein interview by
      Jodi Kantor, September 19, 2017.

182   **eager to see him charged:** Megan Twohey,
      James C. McKinley Jr., Al Baker, and
      William K. Rashbaum, "For Weinstein, a Brush
      With the Police, Then No Charges," **New York
      Times,** October 15, 2017, https://www.nytimes
      .com/2017/10/15/nyregion/harvey-weinstein
      -new-york-sex-assault-investigation.html.

183   **Boies and Abramowitz shared the
      documents:** Ken Auletta, David Boies,
      interviews by Megan Twohey, 2019.

184   **Weinstein paid Gutierrez:** Twohey interviews
      of people familiar with the settlement and
      internal Weinstein Company records from
      2015.

184   **copy of the audio recording:** Ronan Farrow,
      "Harvey Weinstein's Secret Settlements,"
      New Yorker, November 21, 2017, https://
      www.newyorker.com/news/news-desk/harvey
      -weinsteins-secret-settlements.

185   **No one had more incentive to hold Weinstein accountable:** Based on Megan Twohey interviews in 2018 and 2019 of Bob Weinstein, Megan Twohey and Jodi Kantor interviews of those who worked with him, as well as emails and other internal Weinstein Company records.

187   **When Harvey Weinstein needed money:** Megan Twohey interview of Bob Weinstein; Ronan Farrow, "Harvey Weinstein's Secret Settlements," **New Yorker,** November 21, 2017, https://www.newyorker.com/news/news-desk/harvey-weinsteins-secret-settlements.

187   **One day in 2010 or 2011:** Bob Weinstein, interview by Megan Twohey, 2018; and Irwin Reiter, interviews by Jodi Kantor, 2017-19.

189   **Bob sent David Boies an email:** Bob Weinstein, email to David Boies, August 16, 2015.

196   **But Lance Maerov, who had been appointed:** Lance Maerov interviews by Megan Twohey, September 2016 through spring 2019; interviews of those who worked with Maerov; emails and other internal Weinstein Company records.

199   **Rodgin Cohen, one of the most prominent corporate lawyers:** H. Rodgin Cohen, email to

Philip Richter, an attorney for The Weinstein Company board, September 4, 2015.

202   **The New York Attorney General's office:** Megan Twohey and William K. Rashbaum, "Transactions Tied to Weinstein and AIDS Charity Are Under Investigation," **New York Times,** November 2, 2017. https://www.nytimes .com/2017/11/02/nyregion/harvey-weinstein -amfar.html.

204   **a long, detailed complaint:** Internal Weinstein Company records from 2015 and 2016.

CHAPTER SIX: "WHO ELSE IS ON THE RECORD?"

229   **At the start of his newspaper career:** Dean Baquet, interviews by Jodi Kantor and Megan Twohey, 2018.

234   **When the call itself began:** Harvey Weinstein, Charles Harder, Lisa Bloom, and Lanny Davis, interview by Jodi Kantor, Megan Twohey, and Rebecca Corbett, October 3, 2017.

234   **Harder had made a name:** Eriq Gardner, "Ailes Media Litigator Charles Harder on His Improbable Rise with Clients Melania Trump and Hulk Hogan," **Hollywood Reporter,** September 22, 2016, https://www .hollywoodreporter.com/thr-esq/ailes-media -litigator-charles-harder-930963.

234   **shut down the gossip website Gawker:** Sydney
      Ember, "Gawker and Hulk Hogan Reach
      $31 Million Settlement," **New York Times,**
      November 2, 2016, https://www.nytimes.com/
      2016/11/03/business/media/gawker-hulk-hogan
      -settlement.html.

235   **He had represented Roger Ailes:** Brian
      Stelter, "Roger Ailes Enlists Lawyer behind
      Hulk Hogan and Melania Trump Suits," **CNN
      Money,** September 5, 2016, https://money.cnn
      .com/2016/09/05/media/roger-ailes-charles
      -harder/index.html.

235   **After he negotiated a $2.9 million settlement:**
      Tom Hamburger, "Melania Trump Missed
      Out on 'Once-in-a-Lifetime Opportunity' to
      Make Millions, Lawsuit Says," **Washington
      Post,** February 7, 2017, https://www
      .washingtonpost.com/politics/melania-trump
      -missed-out-on-once-in-a-lifetime-opportunity
      -to-make-millions-lawsuit-says/2017/02/06/
      3654f070-ecd0-11e6-9973-c5efb7ccfb0d_story.
      html?utm_term=.1f8e8f635b8c&tid=a
      _inl_manual; Emily Hell, "When They Go
      Low, Melania Trump Calls Her Lawyers,"
      Washington Post, January 30, 2019,
      https://www.washingtonpost.com/lifestyle/
      style/when-they-go-low-melania-trump
      -calls-her-lawyers/2019/01/30/d3892a1e
      -240a-11e9-ad53-824486280311_story.
      html?utm_term=.09e90f097c14; Glenn

Feishman, "Trump Hires Harder, Hulk Hogan's Gawker-Toppling Lawyer in Dispute Against Omarosa," **Fortune,** August 14, 2018, http://fortune.com/2018/08/14/trump-charles-harder -gawker-lawyer-hulk-hogan-omarosa.

235 **"the very notion of a free press":** Jason Zengerle, "Charles Harder, the Lawyer Who Killed Gawker, Isn't Done Yet," **GQ,** November 17, 2016, https://www.gq.com/story/charles-harder-gawker-lawyer.

240 **"it's going to be bad":** Lance Maerov, David Boies, and David Glasser, interviews by Megan Twohey, 2018 and 2019.

240 **"We can nip at it around the edges":** Lisa Bloom, email to Harvey Weinstein, Lanny Davis, Charles Harder, and David Boies, October 4, 2017.

CHAPTER SEVEN: "THERE WILL BE A MOVEMENT"

244 **Megan called David Glasser:** David Glasser, interviews by Megan Twohey, October 2017 and spring 2019.

245 **At 1:43 p.m., Team Weinstein's answer landed:** Charles Harder, email to Diane Brayton, Arthur Sulzberger Jr., Dean Baquet, Jodi Kantor, and Megan Twohey, October 4, 2017.

250 **At 3:33 p.m., McCraw forwarded the reporters:** David McCraw, email to Charles Harder, October 4, 2017.

255 **Jodi and Megan sat down to read about themselves:** Brent Lang, Gene Maddaus, and Ramin Setoodeh, "Harvey Weinstein Lawyers Up for Bombshell **New York Times, New Yorker** Stories," **Variety,** October 4, 2017, https://variety.com/2017/film/news/harvey -weinstein-sexual-new-york-times-1202580605; Kim Masters, Chris Gardner, "Harvey Weinstein Lawyers Battling **N.Y. Times, New Yorker** Over Potentially Explosive Stories," **Hollywood Reporter,** October 4, 2017, https:// www.hollywoodreporter.com/news/harvey -weinstein-lawyers-battling-ny-times-new-yorker -potentially-explosive-stories-1045724.

258 **"My mom is just my mom":** Gracie Allen, interview by Jodi Kantor, 2018.

261 **Suddenly, Weinstein himself was on the phone:** Weinstein and Bloom, interview by Jodi Kantor and Megan Twohey, October 5, 2017.

268 **Tolan pushed the button:** Jodi Kantor and Megan Twohey, "Harvey Weinstein Paid Off Sexual Harassment Accusers for Decades," **New York Times,** October 5, 2017, https://www .nytimes.com/2017/10/05/us/harvey-weinstein -harassment-allegations.html.

269   **most of the directors would resign:** Bruce
Haring, "Fifth Weinstein Company Board
Member Resigns, Leaving Three Remaining,"
Deadline, October 14, 2017, https://deadline
.com/2017/10/fifth-weinstein-company
-board-member-resigns-leaving-three-left
-1202188563.

271   **Katherine Kendall said:** The stories of Tomi
-Ann Roberts, as well as Katherine Kendall,
Dawn Dunning, and Judith Godrèche, were
all depicted in the **New York Times** in the
following weeks. Jodi Kantor and Rachel
Abrams, "Gwyneth Paltrow, Angelina Jolie
and Others Say Weinstein Harassed Them,"
New York Times, October 10, 2017, https://
www.nytimes.com/2017/10/10/us/gwyneth
-paltrow-angelina-jolie-harvey-weinstein.html;
the stories of Hope d'Amore and Cynthia Burr
were depicted thereafter. Ellen Gabler, Megan
Twohey, and Jodi Kantor, "New Accusers
Expand Harvey Weinstein Sexual Assault
Claims Back to '70s," **New York Times,**
October 30, 2017, https://www.nytimes.com/
2017/10/30/us/harvey-weinstein-sexual-assault
-allegations.html.

272   **Ronan Farrow was finishing:** Ronan Farrow,
"From Aggressive Overtures to Sexual Assault:
Harvey Weinstein's Accusers Tell Their Stories,"
New Yorker, October 10, 2017, https://
www.newyorker.com/news/news-desk/from

-aggressive-overtures-to-sexual-assault-harvey
-weinsteins-accusers-tell-their-stories.html.

272   **Lauren Sivan, a television journalist:**
Yashar Ali, "TV Journalist Says Harvey
Weinstein Masturbated in Front of Her,"
Huffington Post, October 6, 2017,
https://www.huffingtonpost.com/entry/
weinstein-sexual-harassment-allegation_us
_59d7ea3de4b046f5ad984211.

273   **when Megan later revealed in the paper:**
Nicole Pelletiere, "Harvey Weinstein's
Adviser, Lisa Bloom, Speaks Out: 'There
was misconduct,'" ABC, October 6, 2017,
https://abcnews.go.com/Entertainment/
harvey-weinsteins-adviser-lisa-bloom-speaks
-misconduct/story?id=50321561; Megan Twohey
and Johanna Barr, "Lisa Bloom, Lawyer Advising
Harvey Weinstein, Resigns Amid Criticism From
Board Members," **New York Times,** October 7,
2017, https://www.nytimes.com/2017/10/07/
business/lisa-bloom-weinstein-attorney.html.

CHAPTER EIGHT: THE BEACHSIDE DILEMMA

276   **When Jodi got a tip:** Melena Ryzik, Cara
Buckley, and Jodi Kantor, "Louis C. K. Is
Accused by 5 Women of Sexual Misconduct,"
New York Times, November 9, 2017, https://
www.nytimes.com/2017/11/09/arts/television/
louis-ck-sexual-misconduct.html.

278   in search of a woman named Stormy Daniels:
Michael Rothfeld and Joe Palazzolo, "Trump
Lawyer Arranged $130,000 Payment for Adult-
Film Star's Silence," **Wall Street Journal,**
January 12, 2018, https://www.wsj.com/
articles/trump-lawyer-arranged-130-000
-payment-for-adult-film-stars-silence
-1515787678; Megan Twohey and Jim
Rutenberg, "Porn Star Was Reportedly Paid to
Stay Quiet about Trump," **New York Times,**
January 12, 2018, https://www.nytimes.com/
2018/01/12/us/trump-stephanie-clifford-stormy
-daniels.html.

278   in 2016, American Media Inc.: Joe Palazzolo,
Michael Rothfeld, and Lukas I. Alpert,
"**National Enquirer** Shielded Donald Trump
from Playboy Model's Affair Allegation," **Wall
Street Journal,** November 4, 2016, https://
www.wsj.com/articles/national-enquirer
-shielded-donald-trump-from-playboy-models
-affair-allegation-1478309380; Ronan Farrow,
"Trump, a Playboy Model, and a System
for Concealing Infidelity," **New Yorker,**
February 16, 2018, https://www.newyorker
.com/news/news-desk/donald-trump-a-playboy
-model-and-a-system-for-concealing-infidelity
-national-enquirer-karen-mcdougal; Jim
Rutenberg, Megan Twohey, Rebecca R. Ruiz,
Mike McIntire, and Maggie Haberman, "Tools
of Trump's Fixer: Payouts, Intimidation and
the Tabloids," **New York Times,** February 18,

2018, https://www.nytimes.com/2018/02/18/
us/politics/michael-cohen-trump.html; Ronan
Farrow, "Harvey Weinstein's Army of Spies,"
New Yorker, November 6, 2017, https://
www.newyorker.com/news/news-desk/harvey
-weinsteins-army-of-spies; Mike McIntire,
Charlie Savage, and Jim Rutenberg, "Tabloid
Publisher's Deal in Hush-Money Inquiry
Adds to Trump's Danger," **New York Times,**
December 12, 2018, https://www.nytimes.com/
2018/12/12/nyregion/trump-american-media
-michael-cohen.html.

280   **"He's now experiencing all the things
he's put everybody else through":** Melena
Ryzik, "Weinstein in Handcuffs Is a 'Start to
Justice' for His Accusers," **New York Times,**
October 25, 2018, https://www.nytimes.com/
2018/05/25/nyregion/metoo-accusers-harvey
-weinstein.html.

282   **Democrats were split:** Laura McGann, "The
Still Raging Controversy Over Al Franken's
Resignation, Explained," **Vox,** May 21, 2018,
https://www.vox.com/2018/5/21/17352230/
al-franken-accusations-resignation-democrats
-leann-tweeden-kirsten-gillibrand.

283   **Brafman gave a radio interview:** "Defending
'Brilliant' Harvey Weinstein," BBC, June 15,
2018, https://www.bbc.co.uk/sounds/play/
p0664pjp.

284   **Kim Lawson, a twenty-five-year-old:** Kim
Lawson, interviews by Jodi Kantor, 2018–19.

286   **The attorney Debra Katz, who specialized in
sexual harassment:** Debra Katz, interviews by
Jodi Kantor and Megan Twohey, 2018–19.

290   **Her name was Christine Blasey Ford:**
Christine Blasey Ford, interviews by Megan
Twohey, December 2017 through May 2019,
and written communication between Ford and
her friends, members of the Senate Judiciary
Committee, and one of her lawyers. The
paper in question can be found at https://
www.researchgate.net/publication/327287729
_Attenuation_of_Antidepressant_Effects_of
_Ketamine_by_Opioid_Receptor_Antagonism.

292   **"She said she was eventually able to escape":**
"Declaration of Russell Ford," Senate Judiciary
Committee Investigation of Numerous
Allegations Against Justice Brett Kavanaugh
During the Senate Confirmation Proceedings,
November 2, 2018, https://www.judiciary
.senate.gov/imo/media/doc/2018-11-02%20
Kavanaugh%20Report.pdf, 55-56.

293   **In the spring of 2016, she and a friend:** Keith
Koegler, interview by Megan Twohey, 2019;
Christine Blasey Ford, interviews by Megan
Twohey, 2018–19.

295 **Their second date had taken place:** Jessica Contrera, Ian Shapira, Emma Brown, and Steve Hendrix, "Kavanaugh Accuser Christine Blasey Ford Moved 3,000 Miles to Reinvent Her Life: It Wasn't Far Enough," **Washington Post,** September 22, 2018, https://www .washingtonpost.com/local/christine-blasey-ford -wanted-to-flee-the-us-to-avoid-brett-kavanaugh -now-she-may-testify-against-him/2018/09/22/ db942340-bdb1-11e8-8792-78719177250f_story .html.

298 **The next morning, July 10, Ford returned:** WhatsApp messages from Christine Blasey Ford to **Washington Post** Tip Line, Senate Judiciary Committee Investigation of Numerous Allegations Against Justice Brett Kavanaugh During the Senate Confirmation Proceedings, November 2, 2018, https://www.judiciary .senate.gov/imo/media/doc/2018-11-02%20 Kavanaugh%20Report.pdf, 46.

298 **a mother who raved:** Julie O'Brien, "I Don't Know Kavanaugh the Judge, but Kavanaugh the Carpool Dad Is One Great Guy," **Washington Post,** July 20, 2018, https://www.washingtonpost.com/opinions/ i-dont-know-kavanaugh-the-judge-but -kavanaugh-the-carpool-dad-is-one-great -guy/2018/07/10/a1866a2c-8446-11e8-9e80 -403a221946a7_story.html.

299 On July 18, she met with Karen Chapman:
Christine Blasey Ford, interviews by Megan
Twohey, 2018–19; Mathew McMurray, email to
Kelsey Kodak, June 17, 2019.

304 "Got it!" the aide wrote back: Email from
Dianne Feinstein's office to Christine Blasey
Ford, July 2018.

**305 "She did not try to minimize the gaps in her
memory":** Lawrence Robbins, interview by
Megan Twohey, January 2019.

307 Her law partner, Lisa Banks: Depiction of
Debra Katz based on Megan Twohey and Jodi
Kantor interviews of Katz from August 2017
through spring 2019; Lisa Banks, interviews by
Megan Twohey and Jodi Kantor, October 2017
through spring 2019; written communications
to and from the lawyers.

310 took on another adviser: Barry Coburn,
interview by Megan Twohey, February
2019.

313 In August, Ronan Farrow: Ronan Farrow,
"Les Moonves and CBS Face Allegations of
Sexual Misconduct," **New Yorker,** August 6,
2018, https://www.newyorker.com/magazine/
2018/08/06/les-moonves-and-cbs-face
-allegations-of-sexual-misconduct.

313 **Louis C.K. made his first appearance:** Melena Ryzik, "Louis C.K. Performs First Stand-up Set at Club Since Admitting to #MeToo Cases," **New York Times,** August 27, 2018, https://www.nytimes.com/2018/08/27/arts/television/louis-ck-performs-comedy.html.

313 **was about to release his latest book:** Hillel Italie, "Next O'Reilly Book Coming in September," Associated Press, April 23, 2018, https://www.apnews.com/f00002d9107742b991fecb982312243b.

CHAPTER NINE: "I CAN'T GUARANTEE I'LL GO TO DC"

319 **Five days later, on Tuesday:** Christine Blasey Ford, interview by Megan Twohey, 2018–19.

319 **a reference to Margaret Atwood's dystopian feminist novel:** Sheryl Gay Stolberg, Adam Liptak, and Charlie Savage, "Takeaways from Day 1 of Brett Kavanaugh's Confirmation Hearings," **New York Times,** September 4, 2018, https://www.nytimes.com/2018/09/04/us/politics/kavanaugh-confirmation-hearing-updates.html.

319 **Republicans, unified behind Trump's pick, were lashing back:** Ibid.

321   **On Wednesday, September 12, an article
appeared:** Ryan Grim, "Dianne Feinstein
Withholding Brett Kavanaugh Document
from Fellow Judiciary Committee Democrats,"
The Intercept, September 12, 2018, https://
theintercept.com/2018/09/12/brett-kavanaugh
-confirmation-dianne-feinstein.

321   **the senator announced by press release:**
Dianne Feinstein, "Feinstein Statement
on Kavanaugh," United States Senator for
California, Dianne Feinstein, September 13,
2018, https://www.feinstein.senate.gov/public/
index.cfm/press-releases?ID=FB52FCD4-29C8
-4856-A679-B5C6CC553DC4.

324   **people were absorbing the article:** Emma
Brown, "California Professor, Writer of
Confidential Brett Kavanaugh Letter, Speaks
Out about Her Allegation of Sexual Assault,"
Washington Post, September 16, 2018, https://
www.washingtonpost.com/investigations/
california-professor-writer-of-confidential
-brett-kavanaugh-letter-speaks-out-about
-her-allegation-of-sexual-assault/2018/09/16/
46982194-b846-11e8-94eb-3bd52dfe917b_story
.html.

325   **Kavanaugh's denial, issued the Friday before:**
Seung Min Kim, "Kavanaugh Denies Decades-
old Allegation of Potential Sexual Misconduct,"
Washington Post, September 14, 2018,

https://www.washingtonpost.com/politics/
kavanaugh-denies-decades-old-allegation-of
-potential-sexual-misconduct/2018/09/14/
60ee3ae8-b831-11e8-94eb-3bd52dfe917b_story
.html?utm_term=.7d6c36ca93cf.

326 **"You've got to deny, deny, deny":** Bob
Woodward, **Fear: Trump in the White House**
(New York: Simon & Schuster, 2018), 175.

326 **the president had mocked:** Aaron Blake, "'I
Don't Believe Them': Trump Doubts Sexual
Abuse Accusers and Sides with an Ally—Again,"
Washington Post, July 6, 2018, https://www
.washingtonpost.com/news/the-fix/wp/2018/
07/06/i-dont-believe-them-trump-doubts-sexual
-abuse-accusers-and-sides-with-an-ally-again.

327 **"I oppose Kavanaugh's nomination":** Rosa
Brooks (@brooks_rosa),"Tweet 1 of a bunch: I
oppose Kavanaugh's nomination, think senators
should vote no based on his judicial record,
but am uncomfortable with asserting that
his behavior as a teen tells us anything about
his "character" now," Twitter, September 16,
2018, https://twitter.com/brooks_rosa/status/
1041482381625122816.

328 **Katz was on morning news shows:** "Lawyer:
Kavanaugh Accuser Willing to Testify," CNN,
September 17, 2018, https://www.cnn.com/
videos/politics/2018/09/17/kavanaugh-accuser

-christine-ford-attorney-debra-katz-newday-sot
.cnn.

329   **Senate, Judiciary Committee chairman
Chuck Grassley:** Descriptions of the
negotiations between Ford's team and the
Republican staff of the US Senate Judiciary
Committee based on Twohey and Kantor
interviews of Katz and Banks; Twohey interview
of Mike Davis; written communication included
in Senate Judiciary Committee Investigation
of Numerous Allegations Against Justice Brett
Kavanaugh During the Senate Confirmation
Proceedings, November 2, 2018, https://
www.judiciary.senate.gov/imo/media/doc/
2018-11-02%20Kavanaugh%20Report.pdf;
additional emails provided by Katz.

329   **That summer, the Senate Judiciary
Committee:** Lydia Weaver, "Senate Judiciary
Urges Response to Sexual Harassment in Federal
Courts," **The Hill,** June 13, 2018, https:/
/thehill.com/regulation/392075-senate
-judiciary-wants-response-to-sexual-harassment
-in-federal-courts.

330   **"She should not be ignored":** "Kellyanne
Conway Says Kavanaugh Accuser 'Should
Not Be Ignored,'" NBC, September 17, 2018,
https://www.nbcnews.com/video/kellyanne
-conway-says-kavanaugh-accuser-should
-not-be-ignored-1322246211718.

332   **Anita Hill worried aloud:** Anita Hill, "How to Get the Kavanaugh Hearings Right," **New York Times,** September 18, 2018, https://www.nytimes.com/2018/09/18/opinion/anita-hill-brett-kavanaugh-clarence-thomas.html.

333   **Judge had written two memoirs:** Dwight Garner, "What a Book Critic Finds in Mark Judge's 'Wasted' 21 Years Later," **New York Times,** October 2, 2018, https://www.nytimes.com/2018/10/02/books/wasted-mark-judge-memoir.html.

333   **Instead, his staff accepted a written statement from Judge:** Senate Judiciary Committee Investigation of Numerous Allegations Against Justice Brett Kavanaugh During the Senate Confirmation Proceedings, November 2, 2018, https://www.judiciary.senate.gov/imo/media/doc/2018-11-02%20Kavanaugh%20Report.pdf, 79.

334   **The staff also accepted a similar written statement from P. J. Smyth:** Senate Judiciary Committee Investigation of Numerous Allegations Against Justice Brett Kavanaugh During the Senate Confirmation Proceedings, November 2, 2018, https://www.judiciary.senate.gov/imo/media/doc/2018-11-02%20Kavanaugh%20Report.pdf, 90–91.

335   **part of a coordinated strategy:** Mike Davis, interview by Megan Twohey, June 2019.

337   **"You lying fucking cunt!":** Barry Coburn and
      Christine Blasey Ford, interviews by Megan
      Twohey, 2019.

338   **CNN was flashing a confidential list of
      demands:** Transcript, "Trump's Star Gets
      Bars; Kavanaugh Accuser Open to Testifying;
      Conway's Interview Reviewed," CNN,
      September 21, 2018, http://transcripts.cnn.com/
      TRANSCRIPTS/1809/21/nday.06.html.

338   **Trump was now directly casting doubt
      on Ford's allegation:** Donald J. Trump (@
      realdonaldtrump), "I have no doubt that, if
      the attack on Dr. Ford was as bad as she says,
      charges would have been immediately filed with
      local Law Enforcement Authorities by either
      her or her loving parents. I ask that she bring
      those filings forward so that we can learn date,
      time, and place!" Twitter, September 21, 2018,
      https://twitter.com/realdonaldtrump/status/
      1043126336473055235.

338   **At a gathering of Evangelical activists:**
      "'We're going to plow right through it,'
      McConnell says on Kavanaugh nomination,"
      Washington Post, September 21, 2018, https://
      www.washingtonpost.com/video/politics/were
      -going-to-plow-right-through-it-mcconnell
      -says-on-kavanaugh-nomination/2018/09/21/
      39beef50-bdac-11e8-8243-f3ae9c99658a_video
      .html?utm_term=.56cd2476da50.

338   **the entire committee would vote:** "Judiciary Committee Continues Effort to Accommodate Testimony from Dr. Ford Next Week," Senate Judiciary Committee, September 21, 2018, https://www.judiciary.senate.gov/press/rep/ releases/judiciary-committee-continues-effort -to-accommodate-testimony-from-dr-ford-next -week.

339   **Grassley tweeted out word of his concession:** The time stamp on Grassley's tweet has defaulted to Pacific Coast time, which is why the tweet reads 8:42 p.m. Pacific time, but Grassley actually published this tweet at 11:42 p.m. Eastern time. Chuck Grassley (@ChuckGrassley), "Judge Kavanaugh I just granted another extension to Dr Ford to decide if she wants to proceed w the statement she made last week to testify to the senate She shld decide so we can move on I want to hear her. I hope u understand. It's not my normal approach to b indecisive," Twitter, September 21, 2018, https://twitter.com/ChuckGrassley/status/ 1043344767684366336.

341   **the account of Deborah Ramirez:** Ronan Farrow and Jane Mayer, "Senate Democrats Investigate a New Allegation of Sexual Misconduct, from Brett Kavanaugh's College Years," **New Yorker,** September 23, 2018, https://www.newyorker .com/news/news-desk/senate-democrats

-investigate-a-new-allegation-of-sexual
-misconduct-from-the-supreme-court-nominee
-brett-kavanaughs-college-years-deborah-ramirez.

342 **At practically the same moment, Michael
Avenatti:** Lisa Ryan, "What 'Credible
Information' Does Michael Avenatti Have on
Kavanaugh?" **The Cut,** September 24, 2018,
https://www.thecut.com/2018/09/michael
-avenatti-kavanaugh-judge-client-tweets.html.

345 **"I'll sleep with you":** Rebecca Corbett,
interviews by Megan Twohey and Jodi Kantor,
2018–19.

345 **that evening's article about the politics of
Ford's upcoming testimony:** Sheryl Gay
Stolberg and Nicholas Fandos, "Christine Blasey
Ford Reaches Deal to Testify at Kavanaugh
Hearing," **New York Times,** September 23,
2018, https://www.nytimes.com/2018/09/23/
us/politics/brett-kavanaugh-christine-blasey-ford
-testify.html.

346 **Now, in an appearance on CBS This
Morning:** Emily Tillett, "Kellyanne Conway
says Brett Kavanaugh allegations feel like
'a vast left-wing conspiracy,'" **CBS This
Morning,** September 24, 2018, https://www
.cbsnews.com/news/kellyanne-conway-says
-brett-kavanaugh-accusers-allegations-feel
-like-a-vast-left-wing-conspiracy-2018-09-24.

346   **"shameful smear campaign":** "McConnell slams 'shameful smear campaign' against Kavanaugh," **Washington Post,** September 24, 2018, https://www.washingtonpost.com/video/ politics/mcconnell-slams-shameful-smear -campaign-against-kavanaugh/2018/09/24/ f739f09a-c02f-11e8-9f4f-a1b7af255aa5_video .html?utm_term=.6d2f69646c81.

346   **Kavanaugh released a letter:** "Brett Kavanaugh defends himself in letter to Senate Judiciary Committee," CNN, September 24, 2018, https://www.cnn.com/2018/09/24/ politics/read-brett-kavanaugh-letter-senate -judiciary-committee/index.html.

346   **"He jumped into this thing":** Mike Davis, interview by Megan Twohey, June 2019.

351   **"Bill Cosby, Once a Model of Fatherhood":** Graham Bowley and Joe Coscarelli, "Bill Cosby, Once a Model of Fatherhood, Sentenced to Prison," **New York Times,** September 25, 2018, https://www.nytimes.com/ 2018/09/25/arts/television/bill-cosby-sentencing .html.

351   **Trump was on television:** Press Conference by President Trump," The White House, September 27, 2018, https://www.whitehouse .gov/briefings-statements/press-conference -president-trump-2.

354   **As the proceedings came to order, Ford began to read her statement:** Christine Blasey Ford, Opening Statement, Kavanaugh Hearing, September 27, 2018, https://www.c-span.org/video/?c4760434/christine-blasey-ford-opening-statement.

356   **sexual assault survivors were calling in:** "Brenda from Missouri calls into C-SPAN," C-SPAN, September 27, 2018, https://www.c-span.org/video/?c4751718/brenda-missouri-calls-span.

356   **Ford "very compelling":** "Trump's Evolving Statements on Christine Blasey Ford," Associated Press, October 3, 2018, https://apnews.com/04e24ef006f4487282e2f9be3faf0a01.

357   **George W. Bush had brushed away stories:** Jim Yardley, "Bush, Irked at Being Asked, Brushes Off Drug Question," **New York Times,** August 19, 1999, https://www.nytimes.com/1999/08/19/us/bush-irked-at-being-asked-brushes-off-drug-question.html.

358   **"This whole two-week effort has been a calculated and orchestrated political hit":** "Kavanaugh Hearing: Transcript," **Washington Post,** September 27, 2018, https://www.washingtonpost.com/news/national/wp/2018/09/27/kavanaugh-hearing-transcript.

358   **widely seen as not credible:** David Bauder,
        "NBC Faces Scrutiny for Interview with
        Kavanaugh Accuser," Associated Press,
        October , 2018, https://www.apnews.com/
        42674fffa6dd4c108ccd908bee7c856e.

360   **That was not true:** Senate Judiciary Committee
        Investigation of Numerous Allegations Against
        Justice Brett Kavanaugh During the Senate
        Confirmation Proceedings, November 2, 2018,
        https://www.judiciary.senate.gov/imo/media/
        doc/2018-11-02%20Kavanaugh%20Report
        .pdf, 93; Seung Min Kim, Sean Sullivan, and
        Emma Brown, "Christine Blasey Ford Moves
        Closer to Deal with Senate Republicans to
        Testify against Kavanaugh," **Washington
        Post,** September 23, 2018, https://www
        .washingtonpost.com/politics/lawyers-for
        -christine-blasey-ford-say-she-has-accepted
        -senate-judiciary-committees-request-to
        -testify-against-kavanaugh/2018/09/22/
        e8199c6a-be8f-11e8-8792-78719177250f_story
        .html?utm_term=.296382a233b1.

365   **a five-page memo:** Rachel Mitchell,
        "Memorandum, Analysis of Dr. Christine Ford's
        Allegations," September 30, 2018, https://
        www.jimhopper.com/pdf/mitchell_memo
        _highlighted.pdf.

365   **Three nights later, Trump mocked her
        gleefully:** Allie Malloy, Kate Sullivan, and Jeff

Zeleny, "Trump mocks Christine Blasey Ford's testimony, tells people to 'think of your son,'" CNN, October 4, 2018, https://www.cnn.com/2018/10/02/politics/trump-mocks-christine-blasey-ford-kavanaugh-supreme-court/index.html.

366 **Monica McLean, the former FBI agent who was forced to publicly deny:** Gregg Re and John Roberts, "Christine Blasey Ford Ex-boyfriend Says She Helped Friend Prep for Potential Polygraph; Grassley Sounds Alarm," Fox News, October 2, 2018 https://www.foxnews.com/politics/christine-blasey-ford-ex-boyfriend-says-she-helped-friend-prep-for-potential-polygraph-grassley-sounds-alarm; Peter Baker, "Christine Blasey Ford's Credibility Under New Attack by Senate Republicans," **New York Times,** October 4, 2018, https://www.nytimes.com/2018/10/03/us/politics/blasey-ford-republicans-kavanaugh.html.

366 **A server at Dale's restaurant in Southaven:** Susan Chira and Ellen Ann Fentress, "In a Mississippi Restaurant, Two Americas Coexist Side by Side," **New York Times,** October 8, 2018, https://www.nytimes.com/2018/10/08/us/politics/trump-kavanaugh-mississippi-.html.

366 **"You don't carry that":** "Who Is Believed and Who Is Blamed?," **The Daily,** October 10,

2016, https://www.nytimes.com/2018/10/10/
podcasts/the-daily/kavanaugh-assault-metoo
-women-girls-respond.html.

367 **Celebrities like Ellen DeGeneres and
Connie Chung:** Savannah Guthrie, "Ellen
DeGeneres Opens up about Being a Victim of
Sexual Abuse," **Today Show,** October 4, 2018,
https://www.today.com/video/ellen-degeneres
-opens-up-about-being-a-victim-of-sexual
-abuse-1336566851633; Connie Chung, "Dear
Christine Blasey Ford: I, Too, Was Sexually
Assaulted—and It's Seared into My Memory
Forever," **Washington Post,** October 3, 2018,
https://www.washingtonpost.com/opinions/
dear-christine-blasey-ford-i-too-was-sexually
-assaulted—and-its-seared-into-my-memory
-forever/2018/10/03/2449ed3c-c68a-11e8-9b1c
-a90f1daae309_story.html.

368 **"no corroboration":** Senate.gov, "Supplemental
FBI Investigation Executive Summary,"
October 5, 2018, https://www.grassley.senate
.gov/news/news-releases/supplemental-fbi
-investigation-executive-summary.

370 **arrived at McConnell's house with beer
cans:** Jenna Amatulli, "Brett Kavanaugh
Protesters Bring Beer, Chant 'Chug' Outside
Mitch McConnell's House," **Huffington Post,**
October 5, 2018, https://www.huffpost.com/
entry/brett-kavanaugh-protesters-bring-beer

-chant-chug-outside-mitch-mcconnells-house_n
_5bb75543e4b028e1fe3cdc5a.

370 **A few weeks before, McDonald's workers:**
Rachel Abrams, "McDonald's Workers across
the U.S. Stage #Metoo Protests," **New York
Times,** September 18, 2018, https://www
.nytimes.com/2018/09/18/business/mcdonalds
-strike-metoo.html.

370 **the chairman of CBS, stepped down:**
Edmund Lee, "CBS Chief Executive Les
Moonves Steps Down after Sexual Harassment
Claims," **New York Times,** September 9, 2018,
https://www.nytimes.com/2018/09/business/les
-moonves-longtime-cbs-chief-may-be-gone-by
-monday.html.

371 **Google and secret problems:** Daisuke
Wakabayashi and Katie Benner, "How
Google Protected Andy Rubin, 'Father of
Android,'" **New York Times,** October 25,
2018, https://www.nytimes.com/2018/10/25/
technology/google-sexual-harassment-andy
-rubin.html.

371 **At the height of the Kavanaugh fracas in
Washington:** Alicia P. Q. Wittmeyer, "Eight
Stories of Men's Regret," **New York Times,**
October 18, 2018, https://www.nytimes.com/
interactive/2018/10/18/opinion/men-metoo
-high-school.html.

EPILOGUE: THE GATHERING

373 **twelve women:** This chapter is based on audio recordings of the group interview that took place over two days.

376 **the first of several women:** Matthew Garrahan, "Harvey Weinstein: How Lawyers Kept a Lid on Sexual Harassment Claims," **Financial Times,** October 23, 2017, https://www.ft.com/content/1dc8a8ae-b7e0-11e7-8c12-5661783e5589.

376 **a public case against confidential settlements:** Holly Watt, "Harvey Weinstein Aide Tells of 'Morally Lacking' Non-disclosure Deal," **The Guardian,** March 28, 2018, https://www.theguardian.com/film/2018/mar/28/harvey-weinstein-assistant-zelda-perkins-i-was-trapped-in-a-vortex-of-fear; House of Commons Women and Equalities Committee, "Sexual Harassment in the Workplace, Fifth Report of Session 2017–2019," **House of Commons,** July 18, 2018, https://publications.parliament.uk/pa/cm201719/cmselect/cmwomeq/725/725.pdf.

387 **Crooks ran for public office:** Matthew Haag, "Rachel Crooks, Who Accused Trump of Sexual Assault, Wins Legislative Primary," **New York Times,** May 9, 2018, https://www.nytimes.com/2018/05/09/us/politics/rachel-crooks-ohio.html.

387   **an unprecedented wave of female candidates:**
Karen Zraick, "Night of Firsts: Diverse
Candidates Make History in Midterm
Elections," **New York Times,** November 11,
2017, https://www.nytimes.com/2018/11/07/us/
politics/election-history-firsts-blackburn-pressley
.html.

393   **more than eighty women had already come
forward:** Sara M. Moniuszko and Cara Kelly,
"Harvey Weinstein Scandal: A Complete List of
the 87 Accusers," **USA Today,** October 27, 2017,
https://www.usatoday.com/story/life/people/
2017/10/27/weinstein-scandal-complete-list
-accusers/804663001.Index

INDEX

ABOUT THE AUTHORS

JODI KANTOR and **MEGAN TWOHEY** are investigative reporters at the **New York Times.** Kantor has focused on the workplace in her reporting, and particularly the treatment of women, covered two presidential campaigns, and is the author of **The Obamas.** Twohey has focused much of her attention on the treatment of women and children, and, in 2014, as a reporter with Reuters News, was a finalist for the Pulitzer Prize for Investigative Reporting. Kantor and Twohey shared numerous honors for breaking the Harvey Weinstein story, including a George Polk Award and, along with colleagues, the Pulitzer Prize for Public Service.

shesaidthebook.com